Essentials for Today's Nursing Assistant

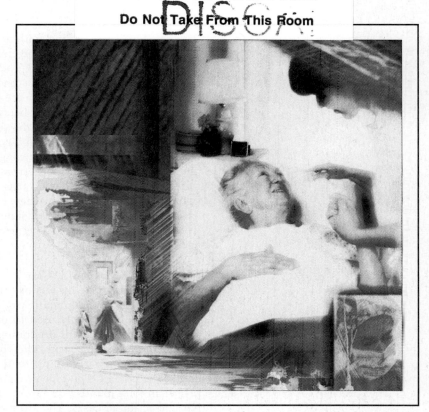

Peggy A. Grubbs, RN, BSN

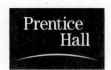

Prentice
Hall

Upper Saddle River, New Jersey 07458

Library of Congress Cataloging-in-Publication Data

Grubbs, Peggy A.
    Essentials for today's nursing assistant/Peggy A. Grubbs.
— Special ed.
        p. ; cm.
    Includes index.
    ISBN 0-13-099087-6 (alk. paper)
        1. Nurses' aides—Handbooks, manuals, etc. 2. Clinical
competence. I. Title.
    [DNLM: 1. Nurses' Aides—Handbooks. 2. Clinical
    Competence—Handbooks 3. Nursing Care—Handbooks.
    WY 49 G885e 2003]
    RT84.G78 2003
    610.73'06'98—dc21   2003021010

Publisher: Julie Levin Alexander
Assistant to Publisher: Regina Bruno
Executive Editor: Maura Connor
Aquisitions Editor: Barbara Krawiec
Editorial Assistant: Sheba Jalaluddin
Director of Manufacturing and Production: Bruce
    Johnson
Managing Production Editor: Patrick Walsh
Production Liason: Mary C. Treacy
Production Editor: Linda Begley, Rainbow Graphics
Manufacturing Manager: Ilene Sanford
Manufacturing Buyer: Pat Brown
Design Director: Cheryl Asherman
Senior Design Coordinator: Maria Guglielmo Walsh
Senior Marketing Manager: Nicole Benson
Product Information Manager: Rachele Strober
Marketing Coordinator: Janet Ryerson
Composition: Rainbow Graphics
Cover Printer: Phoenix Color
Printer/Binder: Banta Harrisonburg

Pearson Education LTD.
Pearson Education Australia PTY, Limited
Pearson Education Singapore, Pte. Ltd
Pearson Education North Asia Ltd
Pearson Education, Canada, Ltd
Pearson Educación de Mexico, S.A. de C.V.
Pearson Education–Japan
Pearson Education Malaysia, Pte. Ltd
Pearson Education, Upper Saddle River

*I would like to dedicate
this book to my grandchildren who are
the light of my life*

NOTICE

The procedures described in this textbook are based on consultation with nursing assistant authorities. The author and publisher have taken care to make certain that these procedures reflect currently accepted clinical practice; however, they cannot be considered absolute recommendations.

The material in this textbook contains the most current information available at the time of publication. However, federal, state, and local guidelines concerning clinical practices, including, without limitation, those governing infection control and universal precautions, change rapidly. The reader should note, therefore, that new regulations may require changes in some procedures.

It is the responsibility of the reader to familiarize himself or herself with the policies set by federal, state, and local agencies, as well as the supplements written to accompany it, disclaim any liability, loss, or risk resulting directly or indirectly from the suggested procedures and theory, from any undetected errors, or from the reader's misunderstanding of the text. It is the reader's responsibility to stay informed of any new changes or recommendations made by any federal, state, and local agency as well as by his or her employing health care institution or agency.

NOTE ON GENDER USAGE

The English language has historically given preference to the male gender. Among many words, the pronouns, "he" and "his" are commonly used to describe both genders. The male pronouns still predominate our speech, however, in this text "he" and "she" have been used interchangeably when referring to the Nursing Assistant and/or the patient. The repeated use of "he or she" is not proper in long manuscript, and the use of "he or she" is not correct in all cases. The authors have made great effort to treat the two genders equally. Throughout the text, solely for the purpose of brevity, male pronouns and female pronouns are often used to describe both males and females. This is not intended to offend any reader of the female or male gender.

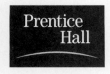

10 9 8 7 6 5 4 3 2 1
ISBN 0-13-099087-6

Brief Contents

CONTENTS

List of Procedures

- Handwashing
- Removing Gloves
- Putting on a Gown
- Removing a Gown
- Putting on a Mask
- Removing a Mask
- Applying a Soft Belt Restraint
- Applying a Vest Restraint
- The Heimlich Maneuver
- Care of the Unconscious Person with an Airway Obstruction
- One-Rescuer CPR
- Stripping a Bed
- Making a Closed Bed
- Making an Open Bed
- Making an Occupied Bed
- Making a Surgical Bed
- Admitting a Patient
- Transferring a Patient
- Discharging a Patient
- Assisting the Patient to Move Up in Bed
- Moving the Patient Up in Bed with a Lift Sheet
- Moving the Patient to the Side of the Bed
- Assisting the Patient to Turn Away from You
- Assisting the Patient to Turn Toward You
- Logrolling the Patient
- Assisting the Patient to a Sitting Position
- Assisting the Patient to Sit on the Side of the Bed (Dangle)
- Assisting the Patient to Transfer from the Bed to a Chair or Wheelchair
- Using a Gait/Transfer Belt to Assist the Patient in Transferring from the Bed to a Chair or Wheelchair
- Using a Mechanical Lift
- Moving the Patient from the Bed to a Stretcher
- Using a Gait/Transfer Belt to Assist the Patient to Ambulate
- Performing Range-of-Motion Exercises
- Assisting the Patient to Brush the Teeth
- Giving Oral Care to the Comatose Patient
- Care of Dentures
- Giving a Backrub

- Giving a Complete Bed Bath
- Assisting a Self-Care Patient with a Partial Bath
- Assisting the Patient to Shower
- Assisting the Patient with a Tub Bath
- Perineal Care
- Giving a Bed Shampoo
- Shaving the Male Patient
- Assisting the Patient to Dress
- Taking an Oral Temperature Using a Glass Thermometer
- Taking an Oral Temperature Using an Electronic Thermometer
- Taking a Rectal Temperature Using a Glass Thermometer
- Taking an Axillary Temperature Using an Electronic Thermometer
- Taking a Rectal Temperature Using an Electronic Thermometer
- Taking an Axillary Temperature Using a Glass Thermometer
- Taking a Tympanic, or Aural (Ear), Temperature
- Taking a Radial Pulse
- Measuring an Apical Pulse
- Counting Respirations
- Measuring the Blood Pressure
- Intake and Output
- Assisting the Patient with a Bedpan
- Providing Catheter Care
- Giving a Cleansing Enema
- Giving a Commercially Prepared Enema
- Inserting a Rectal Tube
- Using a Standing Balance Scale
- Collecting a Routine Urine Specimen
- Collecting a Clean-Catch Urine Specimen
- Collecting a Urine Specimen from an Infant
- Collecting a Stool Specimen
- Providing Postmortem Care
- Shaving the Operative Area (Skin or Surgical Prep)
- Deep Breathing and Coughing Exercises
- Foot and Leg Exercises
- Bottle-Feeding the Infant
- Diapering the Infant
- Giving an Infant a Sponge Bath

List of Guidelines

- Health
- Personal Hygiene and Appearance
- Managing Stress
- Developing Professionalism
- Medical Asepsis
- Standard Precautions
- Accident Prevention
- Correct Body Mechanics
- Using a Restraint
- Applying a Soft Limb Restraint
- Oxygen Safety
- Assisting Victims of Domestic Violence
- Fainting
- Seizures
- Emergency Care for a Stroke
- Effective Communication
- Communicating with the Elderly
- Communicating with Children
- Communicating with People from Diverse Cultures
- Communicating with the Vision-Impaired Patient
- Communicating with the Hearing-Impaired Patient
- Hearing Aid Care
- Communicating with the Speech-Impaired Patient
- Communicating with the Confused Patient
- Communicating with the Developmentally Disabled
- Communicating with Visitors
- Using the Telephone
- Recording Patient Information
- Prevention of Pressure Ulcers
- Care of the Patient with Arthritis
- Care of the Patient with Respiratory Problems
- Care of the Patient with Circulatory Problems
- Care of the Patient with Digestive Problems
- Care of the Patient with Urinary Problems
- Care of the Patient Who Has Had a Stroke
- Care of the Patient with Diabetes Mellitus
- Care of the Patient with Reproductive Problems
- Care of the Patient with Cancer
- Dealing with Cultural Diversity
- Assisting Patients with Psychosocial Needs
- Assisting Patients to Meet Spiritual Needs

- Assisting Patients with Sexual Needs
- Restorative Care
- Cleaning Equipment
- Maintaining the Patient's Unit
- Handling Clean Linen
- Handling Dirty Linen
- Bedmaking
- Repositioning the Patient in a Wheelchair
- Protecting the Falling Patient
- Using Assistive Ambulation Devices
- Assisting with a Specialty Bath
- Nail Care
- Foot Care
- Combing and Brushing the Patient's Hair
- Reading a Glass Thermometer
- Using a Stethoscope
- Using the Food Guide Pyramid
- Serving Food Trays
- Feeding a Patient
- Assisting Patients with Dysphagia
- Care of the Patient with a Feeding Tube
- Care of the Patient with an IV
- Providing Patients with Drinking Water
- Assisting a Patient with a Bedside Commode
- Using a Urinal
- Care of a Urinary Drainage System
- Applying an External Catheter
- Emptying a Urinary Drainage Bag
- Restorative Bladder Retraining
- Restorative Bowel Retraining
- Inserting a Suppository
- Performing Ostomy Care
- Assisting the Patient Who Is Receiving Oxygen
- Care of the Patient in Traction
- Cast Care
- Collecting a Fresh-Fractional Urine Specimen
- Collecting a 24-Hour Urine Specimen
- Straining Urine
- Collecting a Sputum Specimen
- Administering a Vaginal Irrigation
- Applying Elastic Support Hose
- Applying Elastic Bandages
- Safe Application of Heat and Cold
- Meeting the Needs of the Geriatric Patient
- Care of Patients with Alzheimer's Disease

List of Guidelines *(cont.)*

- Care of the Confused Patient
- Care of the Aggressive/Combative Patient
- Care of the Depressed Patient
- Care of Children with HIV Infection
- Assisting Family and Friends of HIV-Infected Patients
- Infant Safety
- Assisting with Breast-Feeding
- Cord Care
- Care of the Toddler
- Care of the Preschool Child
- Care of the School-Age Child
- Care of the Ventilator Patient
- Care of the Patient with a Tracheostomy
- Care of the Patient with an Infusion Therapy Pump
- Changing the Clothes of a Patient with an IV
- Care of the Patient with an Enteral Nutrition Pump

- Care of Patient with a Gastrointestinal Suction Pump
- Caring for a Patient on Dialysis
- Assisting the Homebound Patient with Medication
- Safety in the Home
- Infection Control in the Home
- Disposing of Regulated Medical Waste
- Using Cleaning Products
- Laundry and Care of Clothing
- Grocery Shopping
- Preparing Foods
- Using a Microwave Oven
- Conducting a Job Search
- Interviewing for a Job
- Surviving the Probationary Period
- Resigning from a Job
- Following Standards of Care
- Participating in a Successful Survey

Preface

Much has been written about the high cost of health care today. In fact, many of the changes we have seen in the delivery of health care are in response to this problem. There has also been an increase in the cost of health care education. In the last few years, the cost of textbooks has been spiraling upward until today, textbooks are often the most expensive component in an educational program. We have talked to students and educators from all across the country who are struggling with a sluggish economy and overextended school systems. You told us that there was a desperate need for a comprehensive, affordable nursing assistant textbook. You have asked for relief, and we have heard you.

The author and a dedicated team at Prentice Hall Publishing have designed a textbook that both meets your needs scholastically and is cost-effective. In forging this new design we were determined not to sacrifice quality or content. The standards we set were rigorous. The book had to be well written, readable, and understandable. It had to be comprehensive and complete so that it could stand alone without the need for a student workbook. Knowing that "a picture is worth a thousand words," we decided to continue using the large number of photographs and illustrations that made the first edition so popular.

Essentials for Today's Nursing Assistant, Special Edition, focuses on health care as it is being practiced today. It incorporates recent changes in procedures and philosophies in diverse areas of the health care delivery system. Although this textbook presents new procedures using new equipment such as the tympanic thermometer, it includes tried-and-true practices that have not changed over the years. Our goal was to include procedures and practices that are used in the majority of health care facilities in the United States.

This edition of *Essentials for Today's Nursing Assistant* continues with the holistic, humanistic approach and restorative focus that was the unifying element of the first edition. The concern with meeting the needs of the whole person, physically and psychosocially, coincides with a national trend to provide this kind of care. In the multicultural world of today, respect for the individual has become a necessity. Restorative, holistic care has proven to be an effective tool in reducing health care costs and enhancing quality of life. The sooner we can return patients to independence and as nearly normal function as possible, the sooner they can get on with their lives.

Essentials for Today's Nursing Assistant, Special Edition, emphasizes the role of the nursing assistant in the delivery of quality health care. It stresses the importance of taking care of oneself and developing a professional attitude. It addresses the need for continuing education and identifies new directions nursing assistants can take to accomplish their own career goals.

Special Edition Highlights

- Continued emphasis on the restorative, holistic approach to quality health care
- Increased emphasis on cultural awareness
- Discussion of interpersonal relationships with specific communication guidelines
- Simple language and a clear writing style for all levels of learning skills and styles
- Concise, measurable objectives and a glossary of key vocabulary terms with definitions that open each chapter
- Boxed procedures for easy identification with simple directions and beginning and ending steps separated from the body of the procedure
- Boxed guidelines for easy identification
- Comprehensive glossary and cross-referenced index for student convenience
- An anatomy and physiology insert for students and instructors who want more detailed information

Special Edition Changes and Additions

- Clean, crisp, uncluttered design that allows students to concentrate on content
- Chapters 2 and 3 combined and reorganized for a more-in-depth chapter on "The Role of the Nursing Assistant"
- Chapters 11 and 12 combined and reorganized into "Communicating with Co-workers"
- Rehabilitation and restorative care moved to a more appropriate location in Unit Four
- "Employability Skills" added to give students the information they need to get a job and keep it
- A new chapter, "Surveys and Accreditation," which provides guidelines to help students understand how the survey process helps to ensure quality patient care
- End-of-life issues incorporated into the text
- Workplace violence addressed when appropriate

- Infection control, communicable diseases, and emergency care all updated, with the latest recommendations by the American Heart Association included
- Expanded computer information
- Increased emphasis on nursing assistant education and training based on OBRA guidelines
- New procedures added
- New guidelines to help nursing assistants meet patient needs
- Exciting expansion of the end-of-chapter exercises to facilitate student learning. The "four R's" used in the first edition now cover fill-in-the-blank questions (Review), key points to remember (Remember), case studies (Reflect), and multiple choice questions (Respond).

This textbook is a complete learning package in itself. The end-of-chapter material offers a variety of interactive exercises to stimulate critical thinking. The fact that no student workbook is required makes *Essentials for Today's Nursing Assistant, Special Edition,* an excellent and affordable choice. An Instructor's Guide containing teaching strategies, quizzes, quiz answer keys, and answer keys to end-of-chapter exercises is available for the convenience of instructors.

To the Student

You, the student, are the reason that authors write textbooks. You are the focus of our concern, the basis for our industry, and the light that guides our way. As an author, I have consistently tried to keep you at the center of this project. I have tried to write a book that will enable you to read and learn easily. My goal is to provide you with a textbook that will help you become a competent, compassionate nursing assistant. I sincerely hope this book meets that goal.

This edition of *Essentials for Today's Nursing Assistant* continues the tradition set by the first edition. It emphasizes the importance of the role of the nursing assistant in providing quality patient health care. It includes the latest information on safety issues such as infection control and emergency care. It contains procedures and guidelines that are used in the majority of health care facilities. Some of these procedures may not be used in your area, and some you may not be allowed to do. Your instructor will identify the procedures and guidelines that you will be required to learn.

As you begin your study, keep in mind these guides to finding materials in the text:

- The table of contents tells you where specific information is located and in what order it is presented. All headings, procedures, and guidelines are listed with the appropriate page number for convenience.
- The list of procedures contains all the procedures in the text for easy reference. Procedures are boxed for easy identification and illustrations are provided to demonstrate some of the steps.
- Use the list of guidelines to locate a specific guideline. This list contains all of the guidelines presented in the text. Guidelines are also boxed and illustrated.
- Read the objectives listed at the beginning of each chapter. Objectives are the goals you will

be expected to reach. You will often find the objectives identified in the headings and subheadings. After completing the chapter, review the objectives and be sure that you have met all of them. If you have met the objectives, you should have a clear understanding of the material presented in the chapter.

- Study the glossary at the beginning of each chapter. The glossary is a list of the key vocabulary words or terms introduced in the chapter. The terms are printed in italics in the text to make them easier to identify. The definition is provided in the same sentence. Knowledge of the vocabulary words or terms will help you to answer quiz questions correctly.
- Read headings and subheadings to get a clear idea of the material provided in the chapter. Headings and subheadings are printed in large, boldfaced type that stands out from the rest of the text. Use the headings and subheadings to locate information needed to answer questions and meet objectives.
- Study the illustrations and photographs to help you understand what the author is trying to say. Line drawings are used when they demonstrate procedural steps more clearly. Charts and tables are helpful to reinforce information.
- Do the end-of-chapter exercises. The Review section uses thought-provoking fill-in-the-blank type questions. They are designed to help you review the glossary or vocabulary terms. The Remember section contains a list of the important points of the chapter. Read and study this list to help you remember the key issues. The Reflect section includes a case study and related questions that help you reflect on the issues and use the information you have learned. The Respond section contains multiple-choice questions that will help you learn the material and develop test-taking skills.

Acknowledgments

For me, writing a textbook is a labor of love. It is the fulfilment of a dream to help raise the quality of health care through education and training. I would like to express my gratitude to the many people who helped me achieve my dream.

I want to thank my family and friends for their unwavering support and understanding. They exulted in my success and suffered with me through revisions and deadlines. I am especially grateful to my friends and neighbors on Little Gasparilla Island, who aided and abetted me every step of the way.

Special thanks to all those health care professionals who willingly shared their knowledge and expertise: Sandra L. Wolever, RN, my daughter and colleague, who has been my lifeline to modern trends and technology; Barbara A. Blasband, RN, BA, my friend and coauthor of *The Long-Term Care Nursing Assistant*, a book that I frequently use as a reference; and Leeann Matthews, RN, for helping me understand the special needs of her students.

The team I worked with at Prentice Hall is one of the best in the business, and I want to thank them. Special thanks to Julie Alexander, Publisher, for assembling this great team; Barbara Krawiec, Aquisitions Editor, for her vision and creativity; Michael Sirinides, Editorial Assistant, for his dedication and efforts to keep me on track and on time; and Michal Heron for stunning, detailed photographs that always deliver the message.

Finally, I want to thank all the students who assisted in this project. Their dedication and hard work inspired me to do my very best to provide you with a textbook that would help you care for the most important people in the world—our patients.

No textbook would be worth its salt without dedicated, informed reviewers. For the countless hours they spent critiquing this book for content, accuracy, and readability, I thank them.

Reviewers

Marie Baker, RN, MS
Nursing Instructor
Rock Valley College
Rockford, IL

Salley Flesh, Ph.D, RN
Professor Allied Health Department
Black Hawk College
Moline, IL

Teri King, MA, NREMT-P, LP
Science/HST Instructor
McNeil High School
Austin, TX

Julie Postai, RN, MSN, ARNP
Allied Health Coordinator
Fort Scott Community College
Ft. Scott, KS

Juanita Wells, RN, BSN
Nursing Instructor
Mott Community College
Flint, MI

Katherine Williford
Director of NEWH Nursing Consortium
NEWH Nursing Consortium
Rocky Mount, NC

Chapter One

Introduction *to* Health Care

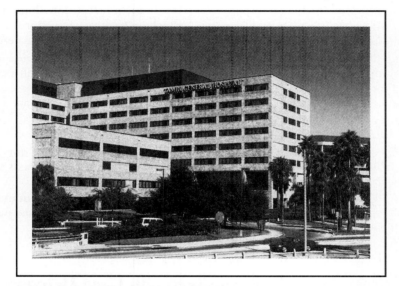

OBJECTIVES

After studying this chapter, you will be able to

1. Briefly describe the history of health care in the United States.

2. Explain what is meant by holistic health care.

3. Identify three recent changes in the health care delivery system.

4. Explain the relationship between cross-training and unlicensed assistive personnel (UAP).

5. Identify the purpose of government regulations.

6. Describe four types of health care facilities.

7. Explain the importance of the chain of command.

8. Identify three members of the health care team.

9. Define the roles of three members of the nursing department.

10. Describe the educational requirements for nursing assistants under the Omnibus Budget Reconciliation Act (OBRA).

chain of command   The order of authority within a facility.

competency   The knowledge and skill required to perform tasks correctly.

cross-training   An approach to health care education that involves training a staff member to perform basic skills that have traditionally been considered the responsibility of another member of the health care team.

holistic health care   An approach to health care in which the whole person is treated, both physically and emotionally. It involves treatment of both the physical illness and the person's emotional response to the illness.

humanistic health care   An approach to health care in which each person is treated as an individual. A person's culture and beliefs are considered as well as their illness or disease.

licensed practical nurse (LPN)   Health care team member who is educated and licensed to assist the registered nurse in planning and providing nursing care.

Medicaid   State-funded program designed to help meet the medical needs of low-income families.

Medicare   Federal program that helps provide medical and hospital care to persons who are 65 years or older or are permanently disabled.

nursing assistant (NA)   Health care team member who provides care for the patients under the supervision of a nurse.

Omnibus Budget Reconciliation Act (OBRA)   Federal act whose purpose is to improve the quality of health care. This act addresses the safety, happiness, and well-being of patients.

registered nurse (RN)   Health care team member who is educated and licensed to assess, plan, provide, coordinate, and evaluate nursing care.

rehabilitation   The process of restoring the patient to as nearly normal function as possible.

restorative care   A type of nursing care that assists patients in meeting their needs as independently as possible.

unlicensed assistive personnel (UAP)   Unlicensed health care workers who assist nurses in providing patient care.

You have chosen a wonderful time to enter the health care field. Today, nursing offers more opportunities than ever before. As a nursing assistant, you will be an important member of a team dedicated to caring for the sick and the afflicted. You will work with and care for people from many different cultural backgrounds. Your role will be both challenging and rewarding.

The health care system in which you will be working has changed dramatically in recent years and is still changing. To understand the vital role that you will play as a nursing assistant, it will help to know a little about its history.

The History of Health Care

Health care began many centuries ago in the home. The care and healing of the sick was the responsibility of the family and the community. Certain individuals within a town or village were often designated as caregivers or healers. These early caregivers went into the patient's home to administer health care. (See Figure 1–1.)

The first hospitals were located in monasteries and other church buildings where members of religious groups provided care for the sick. Individuals who wanted to become caregivers often came to the hospital to live and work. These early caregivers received no pay, and patients were not usually charged for their medical care. Over the years, responsibility for caring for the sick shifted from religious groups to the public or government.

Health Care Delivery in the United States

Hospitals in the early years of the United States' history were crude by today's standards. There were no safety- or disease-control policies in place and few government regulations. Many of the people who practiced medicine and cared for the sick were untrained. Although some health care facilities pro-

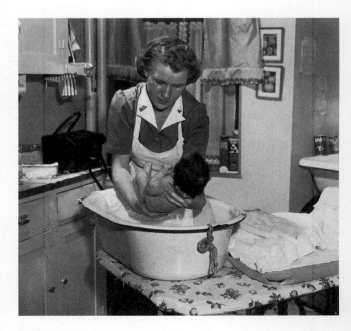

FIGURE 1–1

In the 1930s, health care was often delivered in the patient's home.

vided training, there was no legal requirement to do so. Eventually, laws were passed to regulate health care facilities and to protect the public from untrained workers.

In 1945, by the end of World War II, the delivery of health care in hospitals had improved. Most facilities had well-trained personnel and equipment to handle complex medical situations. Safety and disease control became important considerations. New medications such as penicillin were being used to treat diseases. Equipment was available that could artificially perform the function of a kidney and artificially maintain breathing. Because of this increased technology, health care delivery shifted away from the home and into institutions such as hospitals and long-term care facilities.

By 1980, hospital care had become very expensive. For many types of illnesses, it became easier and less expensive to provide quality health care in the patient's own home. Hospitals were reserved for patients requiring the special type of care that only the hospital could provide. Thus, we have seen the delivery of health care go full circle, beginning and ending in the home. (See Figure 1–2.)

From Family Physicians to Specialists

For many years, the leader of the health care team was the family physician. The physician treated patients in his office, visited them in their homes, and admitted them to a hospital, if necessary. He was a family friend as well as a physician. He listened to their problems and knew their histories. He delivered their babies and closed their eyes at death.

Toward the middle of the twentieth century, health care became more specialized and fragmented. The family doctor was replaced by various specialists. Dealing with several health care providers rather than one familiar doctor frequently caused the patient confusion and misunderstanding. This kind of health care was very expensive, and the individual patient seemed to get lost in the system. Concerns began to arise that the health care delivery system in this country had developed a serious problem. One of the solutions to that problem has been holistic health care.

Holistic and Humanistic Health Care

Holistic Health Care

Holistic health care means treating the whole person, both physically and emotionally. It involves not only treating the patient's illness, but also exploring how he or she thinks and feels about the illness. It is concerned with how the disease affects the person's quality of life. For example, a woman who has had a breast removed because of cancer may be considered "cured" according to medical standards. However, if she is depressed about her appearance, feels unloved by her husband, or is afraid to socialize, then she is not really healthy. Holistic care focuses on the psychological and social aspects of the patient's recovery as well as on the medical progress. (See Figure 1–3.)

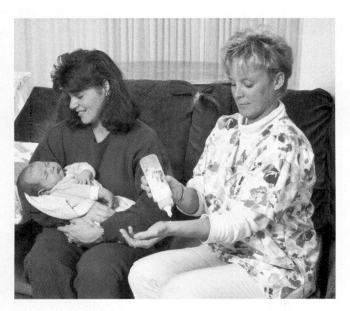

FIGURE 1–2
Today, there is a return to caring for patients at home.

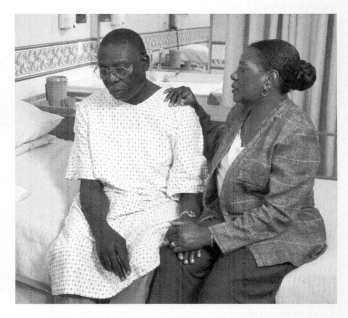

FIGURE 1–3
It is important to consider how the patient feels about his or her illness.

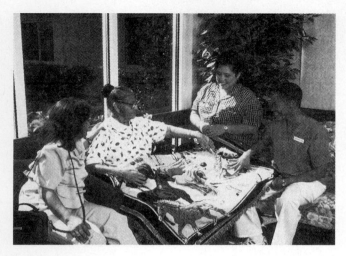

FIGURE 1–4
We all have a right to enjoy our differences.

Humanistic Health Care

By the late 1980s the word "humanistic" was added when talking about health care delivery. *Humanistic health care* means treating each person as an individual. It emphasizes respecting all cultures and beliefs and acknowledges that people cannot be classified by groups or diseases. Each and every one of us reacts differently to an illness, just as we react differently to other situations. We have a right to have those differences recognized and respected. (See Figure 1–4.)

Holistic health care has been embraced by more and more health care workers. As a nursing assistant, you have the opportunity to provide holistic care. You spend more time with the patient than any other health care provider. You have the opportunity to listen as you perform necessary, and sometimes lengthy, procedures. A personal commitment to the holistic approach can help you provide quality patient care. Although the delivery of quality health care is the responsibility of the facility, it is provided one person at a time. Remember, you can make an enormous difference in a patient's quality of life.

Changes and Trends in the Health Care System

Major advances in health care in the United States include new medications, new methods of treatment, improved maternal and infant care, improved hygiene and sanitation, and the control of many communicable diseases. While these changes have contributed to an increased life expectancy, they have also influenced where health care takes place

and how much that health care costs. The United States spends more money on health care than any other country in the world, and the costs continue to increase. This rise in costs has prompted many changes in the health care delivery system.

Diagnostic Related Groups

Under the diagnostic related group (DRG) system, an average cost and length of stay was established for each disease having a related diagnosis. Reimbursement to health care facilities was based on "average stays." Hospitals were not provided additional payment for patients who remained beyond the established length of stay. Under this system, many patients were discharged "quicker and sicker," meaning they were sent home after the designated stay, though they were still very sick. "Average stays" do not take into consideration the needs of individual patients. For example, while a 25-year-old patient may be well enough to go home on the second day after surgery, an 85-year-old may have only begun the recovery process.

Health Maintenance Organizations

Health maintenance organizations (HMOs) were developed by insurance companies and other groups to offer complete heath care coverage through their own providers. In an HMO, a group of health care professionals, called a network, join together to care for participating members. The price of services to members is reduced as long as they use health care providers within the network. Many companies also offer other types of insurance coverage, which allows the patient a larger choice of providers.

Managed Care

Managed care or case management involves the coordination of health care services to meet an individual patient's needs in a cost-effective manner. A case manager is assigned to each patient and is responsible for assessing the patient, planning the care, and coordinating the services that the patient may receive from a variety of providers. Providers are encouraged to move the patient through all phases of recovery in a "timely" manner. While case management helps to improve the coordination of patient care and to reduce costs, it also limits the patient's choice of where to go for health care. See Figure 1–5 for a comparison of the methods to reduce health care costs.

Cross-Training

In an effort to cut costs, the responsibilities of many health care workers has begun to change and ex-

Methods to Reduce Health Care Costs

Diagnostic Related Groups (DRGs)

Determines average length of stay for each disease or illness having a related diagnosis. A facility is not provided additional payment for patients who remain beyond the established time. Patients go home "quicker and sicker."

Health Maintenance Organization (HMO)

A group of professionals joined together in a network to care for members. The price of services is reduced as long as patients stay within the network. Limits the patient's choice of providers.

Managed Care/Case Management

Services are coordinated to meet the patient's individual needs in a cost-effective manner. A case manager assesses the patient, plans and coordinates services, and evaluates the results. The goal is to reduce costs and improve the quality of care. Limits the patient's right to make decisions.

FIGURE 1–5 Examples of three methods to reduce health care costs.

pand. Nurses now perform procedures that once were done only by physicians, and nursing assistants have assumed some tasks once reserved for licensed nurses. These changes require advanced training in order to assure safe and effective performance.

Cross-training involves training a staff member to perform a skill that has traditionally been considered the responsibility of another member of the health care team. For example, the nursing assistant may be trained to draw the patient's blood (phlebotomy) for testing. This procedure is traditionally done by doctors, nurses, or phlebotomists. Nursing assistants may also be trained to perform basic physical therapy tasks. Cross-training produces a multiskilled health care worker ready to adapt to the changing world of health care. It is a relatively new trend that may not be practiced in all areas or facilities. You might want to ask if cross-training is available when you apply for a job.

Unlicensed Assistive Personnel

Unlicensed assistive personnel (UAP) is a broad term used to describe unlicensed health care workers who assist nurses in providing patient care. They may also be called patient care assistant (PCA), patient care

technician (PCT), or nursing care technician (NCT). While UAPs provide basic patient care such as bathing and grooming, they also may perform more advanced procedures. They may be taught to draw blood, obtain electrocardiograms (ECGs), or insert urinary catheters. Training and experience vary widely.

Many hospitals hire state-tested nursing assistants for UAP positions. This cost-effective measure works well for everyone. The patient receives quality care, the employer gets a worker who is already trained in the basics, and the employee gets additional training and education at no expense. Once you have successfully completed your nursing assistant training program, you might want to consider becoming a UAP. The cross-training you receive will increase your chance of advancement in the workplace.

The Expansion of Home Health Care and Outpatient Units

Early discharge of very sick patients due to cost-saving measures led to another development—the rapid expansion of home health care. Many patients arrived home still needing skilled nursing care. Home health agencies could deliver that care less expensively than hospitals. Other cost-saving changes included the establishment of outpatient clinics and outpatient surgery units. These facilities provided a less expensive environment for many emergency and surgical procedures.

Subacute Care Units

The subacute care unit was designed to care for groups of patients who share specific needs. For example, a subacute care unit may specialize in rehabilitation, respiratory care, or chronic illness. Patients in subacute care units are not necessarily "less sick," and in fact may require more health care services than other patients. However, many of their problems are similar, and they often require the same types of services. Concentrating resources, equipment, and trained personnel in one setting is more efficient and more cost-effective. Subacute care is discussed in more detail in Chapter 31.

Rehabilitation and Restorative Care

One of the most important changes in health care involved rehabilitation and restorative care. The emphasis on restorative care started in rehabilitation departments and spread into all types of health care facilities. *Rehabilitation* is the process of restoring the

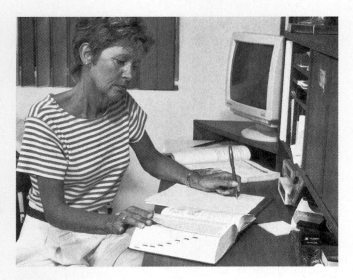

FIGURE 1–6
A new and expanded role requires education and training.

patient to as nearly normal function as possible. *Restorative care* is the nursing care that assists patients in meeting their needs as independently as possible. The approach is holistic, caring, and positive. For years this type of care has been practiced with certain types of patients, such as those with spinal cord injuries. Today, however, it is believed that all patients can benefit from restorative nursing care. Restorative care techniques are emphasized throughout the text. Rehabilitation and restorative care are described in more detail in Chapter 14.

Future Trends in the Health Care Delivery System

Most of the future trends expected in health care are continuations of recent changes. Continued growth in home health care, outpatient units, and subacute care units is expected. The most important factor is the aging of the American population. The large number of "baby boomers" born between 1945 and 1964 will soon be reaching 65. The fastest-growing age group continues to be over 85. Older people have more chronic diseases and require more health care services.

Other types of facilities are being developed to meet the needs of individuals who require assistance with daily living in order to maintain independence. One of the options currently available is an **ALF** (assisted living facility) that provides help with activities such as bathing, dressing, and toileting. Some facilities also function as group homes that provide meals, laundry, supervision, and house-keeping services to people who are unable to live alone. Most of these types of facilities do not provide nursing services.

When you complete your nursing assistant training, you will have only just begun your entry into the health care delivery system. You will need to be continually updating information and skills. The facility in which you work will provide many educational opportunities for you. However, the responsibility for being a well-educated, well-trained health care worker is yours. (See Figure 1–6.)

Government Regulations and Programs

The Purpose of Government Regulations

Health care facilities are regulated by the federal, state, and local governments. The purpose of these regulations is to protect patients and promote quality patient care in all health care settings. Government survey teams make regular inspections to make sure that each facility follows the regulations. A facility that does not meet the standards may be warned, fined, or even closed. It is the responsibility of each employee in every department to follow the regulations. As a nursing assistant, you need to be aware of these regulations and do your part to uphold them.

Omnibus Budget Reconciliation Act

The *Omnibus Budget Reconciliation Act* (*OBRA*) is a federal act passed in 1987 to improve the quality of health care. It is concerned with the safety, happiness, and well-being of patients. Patient rights such as confidentiality and freedom of choice are specifically addressed. Educational requirements and standards of care for nursing assistant training are a part of this federal legislation.

OBRA also addresses the provision of licensed nurses and social workers. It recognizes that patient assessment and evaluation require the services of an adequate number of professional personnel. OBRA requires the development of quality assurance programs to determine and follow up on problems that affect quality patient care.

Other areas of concern include safety, infection control, and nutrition. Specific rules were established regarding rehabilitation and the use of restraints. Although OBRA focuses on long-term care facilities, the law is designed to improve the quality of patient care in all health care settings.

Occupational Safety and Health Administration

The Occupational Safety and Health Administration (OSHA) is a government agency that is concerned with the safety and health of workers in industry. In health care, these concerns include disease control practices, chemical safety, accident prevention, and other safety issues.

Medicare and Medicaid

Two government programs that have had a tremendous impact on the health care system are Medicare and Medicaid. *Medicare* is a federal program that helps provide medical and hospital care to persons who are 65 years or older or are permanently disabled. It is funded by Social Security, and eligibility is based on age rather than income. A person who is 65 years old is eligible for Medicare, regardless of how much money he or she makes. Medicare also provides health care to the disabled under certain circumstances. *Medicaid* is a program funded by each state that is designed to help meet the medical needs of low-income families. For example, a single parent making minimum wage might be eligible for Medicaid benefits. Guidelines to qualify for Medicaid vary from state to state. Some individuals may qualify for both Medicare and Medicaid. The 75-year-old person receiving Medicare benefits and trying to live on a fixed income might also qualify for Medicaid. The primary difference between the two programs is that Medicare is based on age, while Medicaid is based on income.

Health Care Facilities

There are several types of facilities that provide health care services in the United States. Some provide a variety of services, while others, such as long-term care facilities and mental hospitals, are designed to meet specialized needs. Functions of most health care facilities include the prevention, diagnosis, and treatment of injury or disease and the delivery of rehabilitation and restorative care. Types of health care facilities are shown in Figure 1–7.

- **General Hospitals** provide treatment for a variety of problems, including acute illness and surgery. Maternity care may also be provided.
- **Specialty Hospitals** treat patients of a certain age group or those who have a specific health problem. Examples of this type of facility include children's, women's, cancer, and mental hospitals.
- **Long-Term Care Facilities** (also called nursing homes, extended care facilities, skilled nursing homes, or convalescent centers) treat patients who are unable to care for themselves at home, but do not need to be in a hospital.
- **Home Health Agencies** provide health care to patients with varying diseases in their own homes. Some home health agencies may be associated with hospitals, are privately owned, or are operated by a government agency.
- **Hospice** treats patients who are terminally ill and offers support services to their families. Hospice may care for patients at home, in a section of the hospital, or in its own building.
- **Assisted Living Facilities (ALFs)** provide patients help with activities such as bathing, dressing, and toileting. Meals, laundry, and housekeeping are available. An ALF may be in a private home or a part of an existing health care facility.

FIGURE 1–7
Types of health care facilities.

Health Care Facility Organization

Although there is little change in the way health care facilities are organized today, there have been changes in titles of individuals and departments. Traditionally, an administrator was responsible for the entire facility. He or she was trained in business administration and reported to the board of trustees. Today, the administrator may be called the president, the director, or some other title that indicates top management.

Each facility has an organizational chart that includes every employee classification. This chart indicates the order of authority in each department and in the entire facility. The organizational chart provides information on the relationship between different departments. It identifies to whom each employee is responsible and indicates how each employee fits into the organization of the facility.

The Chain of Command

The *chain of command* is the order of authority within a facility. Authority begins at the top and moves downward through each department. The goal is to keep communication flowing smoothly and to avoid misunderstandings. Employees should take problems, questions, and reports to the person directly above them in the chain. If the problem is not resolved there, it should be taken to the next level on the chain. Problems are handled within a department whenever possible. For example, if a nursing assistant has a problem with a dietary aide, the nursing assistant should go to the nurse. The nurse will discuss the problem with the dietary aide's supervisor. Skipping links in the chain by going around the appropriate person or interfering in another department can cause problems and confusion and is not acceptable.

In Figure 1–8, the first level above the nursing assistant is the staff nurse (sometimes called the charge nurse). This is the person you should go to if you have a problem or an observation to report. This nurse is aware of your assignment and the condition of the patients with whom you will be working.

Always take problems, questions, or information about a patient to the nurse in charge. If she or he cannot help you, you can go to the supervisor, proceeding up the chain as necessary.

The Health Care Team

The health care team includes all of the people who provide care and services for the patient. At the center of the team are the patient and the patient's family. (See Figure 1–9.) The team works together, with each team member playing an important role. Doctors, nurses, social workers, and physical therapists are examples of team members who provide direct care for patients. Members of the housekeeping department, dietary department, and business office provide services that are necessary for the health and well-being of patients. As a nursing assistant, you are an important member of the health care team because you provide personal care for the patient on a daily basis.

The Nursing Team

Structure of the Nursing Department

The largest department in most health care facilities is the nursing department. Members of this department provide most of the direct patient care. The person responsible for the entire nursing department is a registered nurse who may be called a director of nurses (DON), vice president, or nurse manager. Most facilities have an assistant director of nurses (ADON) who assists the DON. Nursing supervisors, also registered nurses, are responsible for a particular shift or an area. Each team or nursing station is the responsibility of a nurse who may be called a charge nurse, team leader, or head nurse. This nurse may be either a registered nurse or a licensed practical nurse, depending on facility policy. Nursing assistants work under the direct supervision of nurses.

The Nursing Staff   .

The nursing staff is composed of registered nurses, licensed practical nurses, and nursing assistants. There may also be other unlicensed personnel performing specific duties in the department. Individual responsibility depends on education, training, and facility policy.

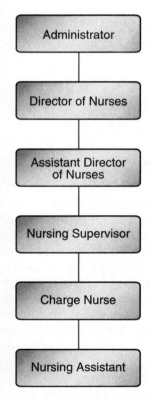

FIGURE 1–8
An example of a nursing department chain of command.

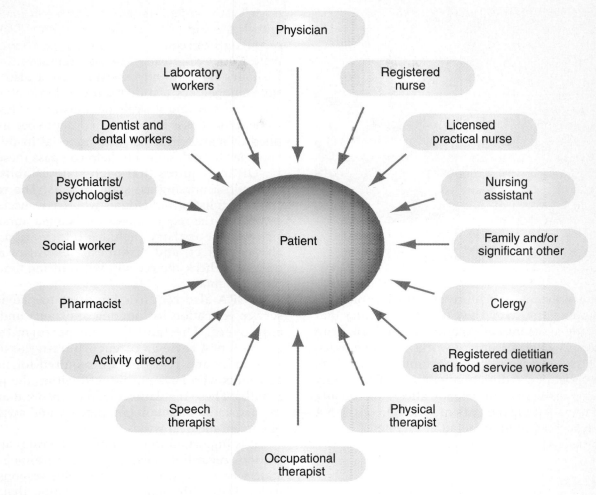

FIGURE 1–9
The patient and the family are at the center of the health care team.

Registered Nurse

The *registered nurse* (*RN*) is a person who is educated and licensed to assess, plan, provide, coordinate, and evaluate nursing care. Registered nurses supervise the work of licensed practical nurses, nursing assistants, and other unlicensed personnel. They provide education in health promotion and disease prevention for coworkers, patients, families, and the community. To become a registered nurse, the student must complete a two-year, three-year, or four-year nursing program and pass a state Board of Nursing examination. Two-year nursing programs are offered at colleges and universities. A graduate of a two-year program receives an associate degree in nursing (ADN). Three-year nursing programs are offered by hospitals. Students who complete a three-year program are usually called diploma graduate nurses. Four-year nursing programs are offered by universities and focus on administration, research, and teaching. A graduate of a four-year program receives a bachelor of science degree in nursing (BSN). A reg-

istered nurse may also earn a master's degree or a doctoral degree in nursing.

Licensed Practical Nurse/Licensed Vocational Nurse

The *licensed practical nurse* (*LPN*) is educated and licensed to assist the registered nurse in planning and providing nursing care. In some states this nurse is called a licensed vocational nurse (LVN). LPNs practice under the supervision of registered nurses. To become an LPN, the student must complete a 12- to 18-month nursing program and pass a state Board of Nursing examination. LPN nursing programs may be offered by a hospital, a local school district, or a community college.

Nursing Assistant

The *nursing assistant* (*NA*) provides patient care under the supervision of a nurse. (See Figure 1–10.) A nursing assistant may be called a nurse aide, pa-

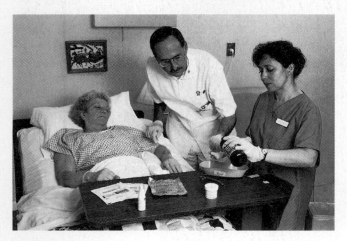

FIGURE 1–10
Nursing assistants help the nurses with patient care.

tient care assistant, patient care technician, or a certified nursing assistant. The title CNA indicates that the nursing assistant has received a certificate from the state in which he or she works. Nursing assistant competency is very important because NAs provide most of the direct patient care. The quality of nursing assistant competency affects the quality of care provided for the patient. The role of the NA will be discussed in more detail in Chapter 2.

Nursing Assistant Training

OBRA legislation sets up minimum requirements for nursing assistant training. States may enlarge the program in content or number of hours required. The goal is to ensure that all nursing assis-

tants, nationwide, can demonstrate *competency* (the knowledge and skill required to perform tasks correctly). OBRA requires that nursing assistants complete a state-approved training program of at least 75 hours. The nursing assistant must also take a state competency test that is divided into two parts: a written test and a skills demonstration test. The student must pass both tests in order to become certified or state approved. The material in this textbook has been designed to help you pass these tests.

OBRA requires that each state establish and maintain a nursing assistant registry. The registry contains a list of individuals who have successfully completed the requirements for being a nursing assistant. The registry includes information about abuse, neglect, and dishonesty. Facilities are required to check the registry when hiring new nursing assistants.

OBRA also requires facilities to provide inservice education for nursing assistants and other employees. The facility must perform regular competency reviews of each nursing assistant. Retraining and retesting are required for nursing assistants who have not worked within the past 24 months. These regulations help to ensure that nursing assistants maintain competency and awareness of current medical issues.

It is important that you know the rules and regulations regarding nursing assistant training in the state where you will work. It is your responsibility to keep up with changes in legislation that affect your employment. Remember, if you stop working as a paid nursing assistant for 24 consecutive months, your certificate will no longer be valid, and you will have to repeat your training.

 ## Review

Read each sentence and fill in the blank with the vocabulary term that best completes the sentence.

1. The nursing care that assists patients in meeting their needs as independently as possible is called _____.

2. _____ is the knowledge and skill required to perform tasks correctly.

3. _____ is the program that helps low-income families meet their medical needs.

4. A _____ is a type of health care facility that specializes in caring for patients who are terminally ill.

5. A nurse who assists registered nurses in planning and providing care is a/an _____.

 ## Remember

1. Learning about the history of health care will help you understand the role you play in providing health care.

2. Holistic health care means treating the whole person, physically and emotionally.

3. Humanistic health care emphasizes respect for the culture and beliefs of the individual.

4. Many of the recent changes and trends in health care are a result of efforts to cut costs.

5. Cross-training produces a multiskilled worker ready to adapt to the changing world of health care.
6. Restorative care assists and encourages patients in meeting their needs as independently as possible.
7. The purpose of federal and state regulations is to protect patients and ensure quality care.
8. Medicare provides health care to the elderly, and Medicaid provides health care to low-income families.
9. It is important that employees follow the chain of command in the facility.
10. The health care team includes all the people who provide care and services to the patient.
11. Members of the nursing department provide most of the direct patient care in a health care facility.

 Reflect

Read the following case study and answer the questions.

Case Study
Melody worked as a nursing assistant in a local hospital. She entered a patient's room just as the housekeeping aide was leaving. Noticing a banana peel under the bed, she called the housekeeping aide back into the room and scolded her for not doing a better job. Melody threatened to tell the director of nurses. The housekeeping aide burst into tears and ran out of the room. The patient in the room asked Melody what was going on. Melody replied, "I was just trying to protect you."

1. Should Melody have corrected the housekeeping aide? Why or why not?
2. Did Melody follow the chain of command?
3. What would have been the appropriate way to handle the problem?
4. How could Melody's behavior affect the patient?

 Respond

Choose the best answer for each question.

1. The first hospitals were usually located in
   A. Churches and monasteries
   B. Big cities
   C. Governmental buildings
   D. Small towns

2. Holistic and humanistic health care focuses on
   A. The sickest patient
   B. The most religious patient
   C. The individual patient
   D. The nicest patient

3. Many of the current changes and trends in health care are a result of
   A. Better insurance plans
   B. Efforts to control infection
   C. A shortage of doctors
   D. Efforts to cut costs

4. What is the advantage of hiring nursing assistants to become UAPs?
   A. Patients receive quality care.
   B. Employers get workers trained in the basics.
   C. Employees get additional training and education.
   D. All of the above.

5. The primary purpose of OBRA legislation is to
   A. Provide less expensive health care
   B. Improve the quality of health care
   C. Protect health care facilities from lawsuits
   D. Raise federal taxes

6. Which of the following programs is designed to help meet the medical needs of low-income families?
   A. Medicaid
   B. Medicare
   C. OBRA
   D. OSHA

7. The nursing assistant reports observations and problems first to the
   A. Physician
   B. Charge nurse

   C. Supervisor

   D. Administrator

8. The director of nurses must be

   A. An RN

   B. An LPN

   C. A nursing assistant

   D. A physician

9. The minimum number of hours for nursing assistant training required by OBRA is

   A. 50

   B. 75

   C. 100

   D. 125

10. Which of the following statements about the nursing assistant competency test is FALSE?

   A. The nursing assistant must first complete a state-approved training program.

   B. The competency test is divided into two parts.

   C. The nursing assistant is required to pass only one part of the test.

   D. One part of the test involves demonstrating skills.

Chapter Two

The Role
of the Nursing Assistant

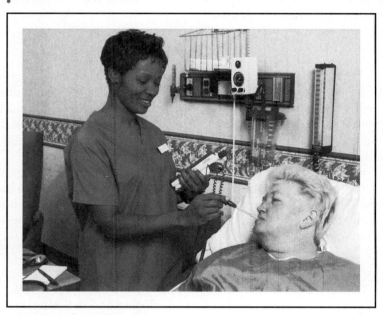

OBJECTIVES

After studying this chapter, you will be able to _____

1. Identify six responsibilities of the nursing assistant.

2. List six desirable personal qualities of the nursing assistant.

3. List four guidelines for proper personal hygiene and appearance.

4. Describe six guidelines for stress management.

5. Identify three professional qualities and skills that will improve job performance.

6. Explain the six steps of the problem-solving process.

7. Identify four guidelines a nursing assistant may use in developing professionalism.

8. Describe three expanded roles of the nursing assistant.

9. List two ways to continue your education.

activities of daily living (ADLs)   Personal care activities that individuals usually perform every day.

empathy   The ability to share another person's point of view and understand his or her feelings.

flexibility   The ability to adjust to change.

hygiene   The observance of rules for health and cleanliness.

job description   A list of tasks and responsibilities to be performed in a certain job.

mobility   One's ability to move about.

organize   To arrange information, tasks, or things in an orderly manner.

priority, prioritize   To arrange information or tasks in their order of importance.

stress   Mental and physical tension or strain.

Although the role of the nursing assistant has changed in recent years, it is still based on caring. It involves showing kind, compassionate concern for the needs of others. It means being respectful of the culture and individuality of each patient. As a nursing assistant, you will assist patients in meeting their physical and emotional needs and will play an important role in the delivery of quality health care. This chapter will give you a clearer idea of the tasks that nursing assistants perform and the basic skills and qualities possessed by good nursing assistants. (See Figure 2–1.)

Responsibilities of the Nursing Assistant

Nursing assistants are responsible for performing many tasks and procedures. This textbook is con-

cerned with instructing you in the proper way to assist patients in performing these tasks as independently as possible. Sometimes you will help the nurse and other times you may work alone, but as a nursing assistant you must always work under the supervision of a nurse.

One of the most important responsibilities of the nursing assistant is to assist patients with activities of daily living. *Activities of daily living (ADLs)* are personal care activities that individuals usually perform every day. ADLs include:

- Bathing and hygiene
- Grooming and dressing
- Eating and drinking
- Toileting
- Exercising and moving about

Your employer will provide you with a *job description* (a list of your tasks and responsibilities in that facility). (See Figure 2–2.) The job description varies from facility to facility. You are responsible for knowing which tasks that you may or may not do in the facility in which you work or train.

The job description of the nursing assistant may include the following:

- Assist patients with ADLs.
- Make beds and keep units neat.
- Measure patients' temperature, pulse, respirations, and blood pressure.
- Measure fluid intake and output.
- Measure height and weight.
- Assist in admitting, transferring, and discharging patients.
- Communicate effectively with patients, visitors, and co-workers.
- Observe, report, and record information.
- Assist patients with restorative care.
- Protect patient privacy.
- Follow safety rules.
- Follow facility policies.

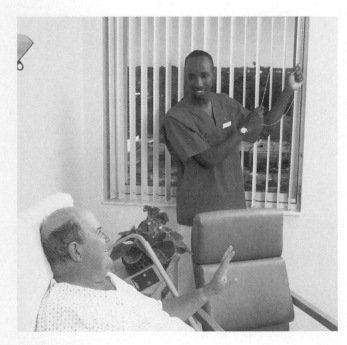

FIGURE 2–1
Providing for the patient's comfort helps meet physical needs.

CITY MEMORIAL HOSPITAL
CRITERIA-BASED
JOB DESCRIPTION

Title: Nursing Assistant
Department: Nursing
Dept. Number: Various   Status: Nursing Assistant
Job Code: 123   Grade: Step:
Reports to:

Educational & Experience Requirements
High School graduate. Nurse Aide Certification. Medical terminology.

Primary Function
The Nursing Assistant is directly responsible to the staff nurse and assists in the care of the patient by performing simple procedures.

Duties and Responsibilities
1. Effectively communicates mission of City Memorial Hospital.
   A. Communicates mission statement through daily activities

2. Responsible for actively demonstrating City Memorial Hospital's philosophy of Customer Relations, individual respect, teamwork, and productivity.

3. Provides direct patient care under the supervision of a staff nurse.
   A. Gives complete AM or PM care to assigned patients, including complete or partial bath, back rub, care of hair, oral hygiene, and bedmaking.
   B. Assists the staff nurse in the care of critical patients or patients in isolation.
   C. Assists patients with their meals and feeds patients where indicated. Provides between-meal nourishment and liquids.
   D. Records intake and output when ordered.
   E. Measures and records Foley catheter drainage on output sheet.
   F. Assists in transportation of patients to other departments or for discharge as requested.
   G. Assists in the admission, discharge, and transfer of patients.
   H. Notes patient's condition changes and reports to the staff nurse responsible for the patient.
   I. Assists in the provision of postmortem care.
   J. Applies restraints under the direction of a staff nurse.
   K. Empties drain receptacle. Measures and records draining output.

4. Performs procedures outlined in procedure manual under the supervision of a staff nurse.
   A. Applies ice caps/bags.
   B. Applies nonsterile dressings.
   C. Gives routine cleansing enemas.
   D. Takes and records vital signs.
   E. Performs skin preps not involving sterile procedures.
   F. Collects urine (nonsterile), sputum, and stool specimens.
   G. Collects voided specimens for Ketodiastix testing.

FIGURE 2–2
A sample job description.

There are some tasks that nursing assistants are not allowed to do. These vary according to state and local laws. However, there are two basic rules that always apply:

1. Never do anything that you have not been trained to do, regardless of who asks.
2. Never do anything that is not included in your job description or is against facility policy. The fact that you know how to perform a task does not mean that you will be allowed to do it.

Individual responsibilities of a nursing assistant are determined by education, training, governmental guidelines, and facility policy. There may be procedures outlined in this text that you will not be taught because nursing assistants in your area are not allowed to perform those tasks. You may also learn procedures in your training program that your employer will not allow you to do. Your employer may provide you with special training to do procedures that are not included in a basic training program, or you may be cross-trained to do tasks that are normally performed by other health care workers.

Providing Quality Patient Care

All the responsibilities of the nursing assistant revolve around the delivery of quality patient care. The holistic approach, which emphasizes individuality and culture, helps ensure that tasks are performed in a way that meets each patient's needs. Nursing care delivered in a restorative manner is essential to providing quality care and promoting patient independence. Although it may be quicker and easier to do a

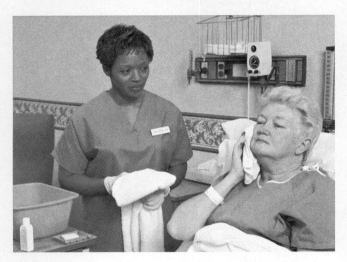

FIGURE 2–3
Encourage the patient to be as independent as possible.

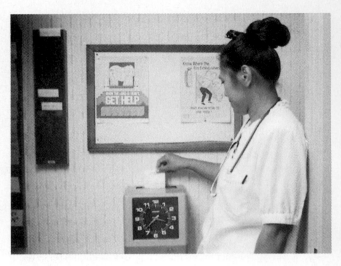

FIGURE 2–4
Coming to work on time demonstrates dependability.

task yourself, the patient will benefit more if allowed to help. For example, it may be hard to watch the patient who is slowly, and with much difficulty, washing her face. You may want to take the washcloth and do it for her, but an effective nursing assistant will encourage patients to do as much as they are able to do—independently. (See Figure 2–3.)

Personal Qualities of the Nursing Assistant

There are many desirable qualities and characteristics that are necessary in order to be an effective nursing assistant. Some of these qualities you may already have and others you will need to develop. An effective nursing assistant will be:

Caring: Liking people and being willing to care for them is essential to providing quality health care.

Respectful: Every patient has the right to be treated with respect and dignity regardless of physical or mental limitations. Be respectful of all cultures and religions. Treat family members, visitors, and co-workers with respect as well.

Dependable: A dependable person comes to work when scheduled and arrives on time. Assignments are carried out in a timely manner. (See Figure 2–4.)

Honest and trustworthy: The patient, your employer, and your coworkers should be able to trust you to do your job correctly and completely.

Empathetic: *Empathy* is the ability to share another person's point of view and understand

his or her feelings. It involves thinking how you would feel if you were in the same situation.

Considerate: Be concerned for other people's feelings. Think about how they might be affected by what you do or say.

Culturally aware: Be knowledgeable about different cultures in your area. Identify issues that are important to the patient or are different from the ordinary routine. Help patients meet their individual cultural needs.

Patient: Accept the fact that some patients may be slow or have difficulty following directions. Allow time for them to perform activities as independently as possible.

Supportive: Encourage patients to do as much as possible for themselves. Maintain a positive attitude and praise all efforts no matter how slight.

Enthusiastic: Come to work ready and willing to do your job. Be cheerful and show people that you like what you do.

Proud: Be proud that you are a nursing assistant, an important member of the health care team.

Taking Care of Yourself

If you want to become a successful nursing assistant, you must first learn to take care of yourself. Caregivers are givers—they give of their time, their energy, and their affection. They are often so involved in caring for others that they forget about their own needs. Although that may sound very generous, in reality it is not wise. If you do not take care of yourself, you will not be able to care effectively for others.

Guidelines for Health

- Eat a well-balanced diet including a variety of foods.
- Start the day with a good breakfast.
- Try to maintain a healthy weight.
- Get sufficient rest and sleep.
- Exercise regularly.
- Avoid using alcohol or drugs.
- See your doctor for a regular checkup. (See Figure 2–5).

Health Maintenance

One of your responsibilities as a nursing assistant is to protect your own health. The work of a nursing assistant is challenging and sometimes exhausting. You will need to be able to move and think fast. The job requires physical energy, emotional stability, and good health.

Do not bring alcohol or drugs to work, and do not come to work under the influence of alcohol or drugs. The use of these substances will endanger the patients and will risk your losing your job. Be aware that you may be required to undergo routine drug testing where you work.

Personal Hygiene and Appearance

Hygiene involves cleanliness and health maintenance, so personal hygiene refers to keeping yourself clean and healthy. Cleanliness promotes health

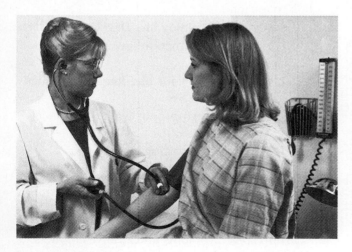

FIGURE 2–5
See your doctor for a regular checkup.

and helps prevent the spread of disease. It is important that you look clean and well groomed on the job. A nursing assistant who looks professional helps build confidence in others. The patient will be more likely to listen to you and to trust you. How can you convince the patient of the importance of personal hygiene and appearance if you do not follow these practices yourself?

Emotional Needs

Your emotional needs are determined by your inner feelings. One of the most important of the emotional needs is one's opinion of oneself, called self-esteem. Self-esteem helps you feel good about yourself and to believe in your own abilities. Although other people influence your self-esteem, it is your own opinion that matters most. Think well of yourself and remind yourself how special you really are.

Human beings are social animals—we live in families, groups, and communities. We all need interaction with other people to be socially healthy. Social needs are met through friendships, families, churches, clubs, and other organizations. Best friends, casual acquaintances, and co-workers are all part of your social circle. (See Figure 2–6.)

Try to make new friendships and work hard to maintain existing friendships. Join a club or take part in community affairs. Reach out beyond your immediate circle to extend your social network. It is

Guidelines for Personal Hygiene and Appearance

- Take a daily bath or shower.
- Brush your teeth after every meal.
- Use deodorant or antiperspirant.
- Shampoo your hair at least once a week.
- Clean and trim your fingernails as needed.
- Male nursing assistants should shave daily and keep beards and mustaches trimmed neatly.
- Wear a clean uniform every day.
- Clean and polish your shoes daily.
- Keep your shoes and clothing in good repair.
- Apply cosmetics lightly and avoid perfumes.
- Avoid using fingernail polish or artificial nails.
- Wear your hair in a style that is off your face and collar.
- Avoid wearing jewelry.
- Avoid smoking while in uniform.
- Use correct posture.

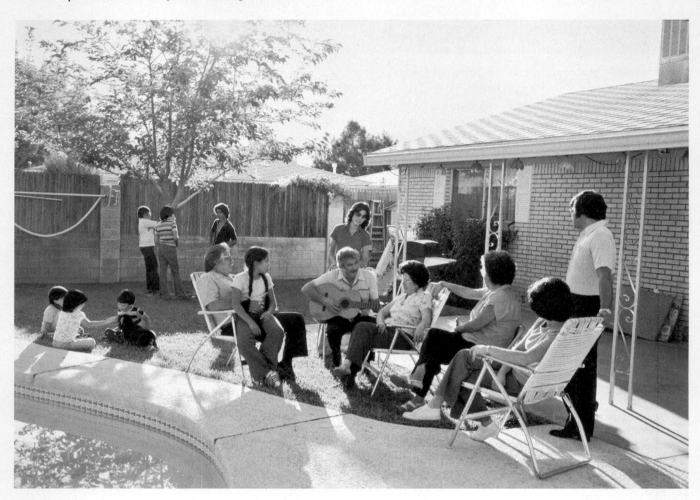

FIGURE 2–6
We need interactions with others to be socially happy.

also important to maintain close family relationships, because family members are often more supportive than anyone else.

Stress Management

Stress is mental and physical tension or strain. When you are stressed, your body goes into overdrive. Heart rate increases, body temperature rises, muscles tense, and respiration increases. For a short time, you will become physically stronger and faster. Mentally and emotionally, stress narrows your focus, and this is helpful in an emergency. When stress occurs and is not soon relieved, it is hard to see the whole picture. If this situation continues, you will soon be exhausted physically and mentally.

Your job as a nursing assistant in a health care facility can be very stressful. You care for sick people on a daily basis. Their health and well-being are affected by how well you do your job. If you make a mistake, someone may suffer needlessly. You may

Guidelines for Managing Stress

- Share your feelings with others. It helps to talk to a friend.
- Learn to relax and enjoy life. Develop a hobby.
- Treat yourself like someone special. Give yourself a reward.
- Add some humor to your life. Read the comics or watch a funny movie.
- Exercise. A relaxing outdoor walk helps relieve stress.
- Get a library card. Reading is relaxing.
- Be assertive and stand up for what you believe is right.
- Let go and realize that there are some things you cannot control.
- Learn to solve problems and resolve conflicts. This can sometimes prevent stress.

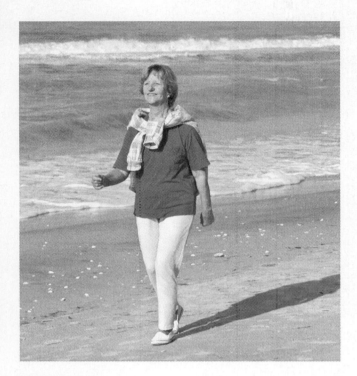

FIGURE 2–7
A relaxing outdoor walk helps to relieve stress.

also be worrying about problems of your own. You know that you should not bring personal problems to work, but sometimes it is hard to put them out of your mind. Eliminating stress is not always possible. The key is to learn how to manage the stress in your life. (See Figure 2–7.)

Job Skills and Performance

In addition to the personal qualities just described, there are special skills and professional qualities one must develop to be an effective nursing assistant. You will want to make certain that your job performance will satisfy your supervisors. Job performance includes your work habits, how you interact with people, and your competency (the knowledge and skill required to perform tasks correctly). One of the first steps is to become familiar with the policies and guidelines of the facility and to follow them consistently.

How well you do your job is very important to your own success. Your job performance is constantly being observed and evaluated. A formal evaluation and discussion will be done at least once a year. Your salary and opportunities for advancement are affected by your evaluation, so it is in your best interest to improve your job performance. You can improve your evaluation by developing the qualities and characteristics listed earlier in this chapter. Three skills that improve job performance include being a team player, being flexible, and organizing your work.

Being a Team Player

The ability to get along with other people is a necessary skill for any health care worker. In order to be an effective team player, you will need to be respectful, considerate, and cooperative. Cooperation benefits both the patient and the staff members. Many procedures are easier when employees work together. For example, two people can get a weak patient out of bed easier than one person can. It is also safer because there is less chance of accident or injury to either the patient or the health care worker. The presence of two people helps the patient feel safer, and a patient who feels secure is more likely to move independently. (See Figure 2–8.)

Assist your co-workers whenever possible and ask for help if you need it. However, you are responsible for completing your assignment, so do not expect others to do your work for you. If you complete your assignment early, help your co-workers finish theirs.

A good team player is able to follow directions, so listen carefully when the nurse is giving orders or instructions. If there is anything that you do not understand, ask the nurse to explain more clearly. If you have a problem or a concern, talk to the nurse. State the facts clearly and simply in a respectful manner.

You will probably be working with health care employees whose cultural backgrounds are not the same as your own. They may speak a different language. Respect their beliefs and customs. Make sure that you understand clearly when communicating. Be patient and help them to understand as well.

Being Flexible

Flexibility (the ability to adjust to change) is necessary because your schedule and your assignment may not always be the same. Care of the patients is

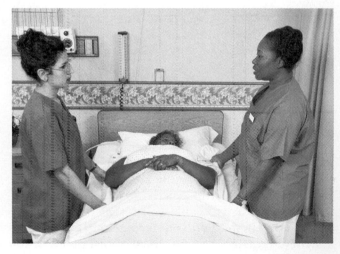

FIGURE 2–8
The patient feels more secure when two people are assisting.

divided among the nursing staff members who are on duty. Although the goal is consistency of care by assigning the same staff members to the same patients each day, this is not always possible. If some of the people who are scheduled to work do not come to work, an area may be short-staffed. When that happens, you may have to leave your regular unit and work in a different area. Complete your assignment to the best of your ability. Speak to the nurse if you are unable to carry out all the duties you are assigned.

Organizing Your Work

The word *organize* means to arrange information, tasks, or things in an orderly manner. In order to be organized you will need to arrange your tasks in a way that allows you to perform them quickly and safely. Organization improves your job performance and makes you more efficient. It reduces stress by helping you figure out how to complete your assignment. Being organized will improve your evaluation and add to your sense of satisfaction. Organization involves planning, collecting supplies and equipment, setting priorities, and managing your time. It also includes organizing the way you perform each task.

Planning

As soon as you get a report from the nurse, make rounds and check on all of your assigned patients. Take care of their immediate needs and reassure them that you will be back later. Make a list of the procedures that are identified on your assignment sheet. Include tasks that are done at scheduled intervals, such as "turn the patient every two hours." List appointments the patients need to keep, such as a doctor's visit or an occupational therapy treatment. Check the calendar for activities the patients might enjoy, such as a movie or a birthday party. Include on your list staff meetings or classes that you are required to attend. (See Figure 2–9.)

Collecting Supplies and Equipment

In addition to being organized about the tasks or procedures you are assigned to do, it is also important to approach each task in an organized manner. Before you begin any procedure, determine what supplies you will need in order to complete the task, and take the necessary supplies to the area in which you will be working. This will improve your performance of the task as well as enable you to get it done more quickly. If you find that you need help in completing a procedure, have the equipment and supplies available before your co-worker arrives. Being prepared shows courtesy and saves time for both of you.

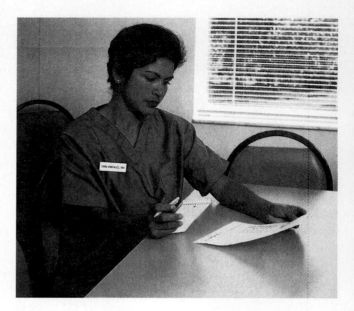

FIGURE 2–9
Take time to plan your workday at the beginning of the shift.

Setting Priorities

When the list is completed, rate each task according to *priority* (order of importance). Place procedures and events that are scheduled at specific times high on your priority list. The sickest patients are usually cared for first. Long, involved procedures, such as a complete bed bath, are best done early in the shift. Your list may need to be adjusted several times during the shift. For example, a new admission or a sudden change in the condition of one of the patients can change the order of your priorities. Regardless of the changes, setting priorities helps you get the most important tasks done on time.

Guidelines for Managing Time

■ Keep small talk to a minimum during working hours. Chatting with a co-worker about subjects that are not related to work can be a real time-waster.

■ Be aware that while planning takes time, it saves time in the long run.

■ Anticipate and handle problems before they get out of hand. They can be resolved more quickly if you catch them early.

■ Know the correct sequence of steps for procedures. Avoid needless actions and repetition.

■ Group tasks together when possible. In one trip down the hallway you might dispose of dirty linens, pick up an extra pillow for a patient, and make arrangements for a co-worker to help you move a heavy patient.

Managing Time

You can't really manage time—you can manage only your own actions and how you use your time. The preceding guidelines will help you to use your time more effectively.

Developing Professionalism

The term "professionalism" means to be worthy of the standards of a profession. Professionals follow the legal and ethical principles of their profession. They continuously seek to increase their knowledge and improve their skills. You, as a nursing assistant, need to develop professionalism.

All the things you learn in this course will help you to become more professional. One of the most important steps is to develop pride in your work. You are a nursing assistant, a job that not just anyone can do. So hold your head high and be proud that you are a part of a caring profession.

Problem Solving and Conflict Resolution

Problem Solving

The ability to solve problems is one of the major differences between successful and unsuccessful people. Problem solving is a skill that is easily learned and well worth developing. The problem-solving process involves six steps: identifying the problem,

collecting information, listing possible solutions, planning and taking action, and evaluating the outcome. (See Figure 2–10.) It does not matter if the problem is large or small, the same process can be used.

Identifying the Problem

You cannot solve a problem until you identify and define it. Sometimes that is easy. For example, you can't pay the rent today, because you went out last night and spent all your money. It is not difficult to identify the problem in that situation, is it? However, most problems are not that simple. To identify and define a problem, you have to break it down into its parts and determine the main issue. If it is a complex problem, you may have to treat each part as a separate problem and solve it one part at a time.

Collecting Information

Gather information and get the facts together by using reliable sources and making sure that all the information relates to the problem. Are there legal or ethical issues involved? What will happen if the problem is not resolved? These questions help you decide how important the problem really is.

Listing Possible Solutions

Make a list and write down every idea. Do not limit your ideas—the more you have, the more likely you will be able to come up with the right one. Consider all suggestions, no matter how unlikely they sound. This is a trial-and-error method, so do not get discouraged.

Making a Decision

Look at all the possible solutions and start narrowing them down until only two or three remain. Eliminate ideas that are unethical or compromise your own values. Think about the consequences or

---

Guidelines for Developing Professionalism

- Behave in a legal and ethical manner.
- Maintain a neat, clean appearance and dress appropriately.
- Develop skills in problem solving and conflict resolution.
- Be flexible and adaptable to change.
- Develop job performance skills.
- Respect all cultures and religions. Think about how your actions might affect others.
- Continue your education. Be a lifetime learner.
- Have pride in your job.

The Six Steps of Problem Solving

1. Identify the problem.
2. Collect information.
3. List possible solutions.
4. Make a decision.
5. Plan and take action.
6. Evaluate the outcome.

FIGURE 2–10
The problem-solving process.

results of a certain action and what will happen if you choose it. The idea that best suits the situation and has the least impact on others is usually a wise decision.

Planning and Taking Action

It doesn't matter how many decisions you make, if you do not put them into action you will not be able to solve the problem. Develop a plan of action and get started. List the steps to be taken and set up a time frame for completion. Collect any materials that may be required and anticipate barriers you may have to overcome.

Evaluating the Outcome

Evaluating involves judging whether or not the chosen solution has worked and if the outcome is acceptable. If the original problem is resolved, you can feel proud of yourself. The next time a similar problem arises, you will know how to handle it. Do not get discouraged if the solution did not work. Return to your list of possible solutions and try something different. If none of your ideas seem appropriate, you may need to start back at the beginning and reevaluate the situation. Did you correctly identify the problem? Do you need to collect more information? Some problems take more time to solve than others, so do not rush the process.

Conflict Resolution

Conflict involves a disagreement of ideas. Resolution is the solving of a problem—a solution. So conflict resolution means finding a solution to a disagreement. Conflict occurs anywhere there are people whose needs, values, and cultures differ. You may find conflict at work, in a community gathering, in your family, or within yourself. (See Figure 2–11.)

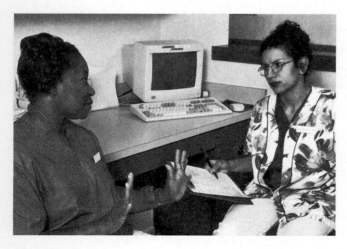

FIGURE 2–11
Conflict involves a disagreement of ideas.

What causes conflict? It occurs when people have opposing beliefs and each one feels that he or she is right. Conflict might involve two individuals or large groups of people. The issue of abortion is an example of conflict. The people who are against abortion firmly believe they are right, while those who are for free choice are equally committed to their choice. The result is a major conflict of worldwide proportions.

As a nursing assistant, you may experience conflict with a patient, a co-worker, or your supervisor. Conflict is not always bad because it can increase creativity, identify problems, draw out the facts and clear the air. The problem with conflict is that while it lasts, efficiency and morale decline. The key to conflict resolution is to learn different methods to resolve different situations. The following responses can help you resolve conflicts more effectively:

- **Agreement:** Be cooperative, but not assertive. "Okay, if that's what you want to do, I'll try it."
- **Avoidance:** Be unassertive and uncooperative. "Do whatever you want to. It doesn't matter to me."
- **Combination:** Combine your beliefs and be fully assertive and cooperative. "Let's work on this together and combine our ideas."
- **Competition:** Be assertive and uncooperative. "We're going to do it my way whether you like it or not."
- **Compromise:** Be moderately assertive and cooperative. "We'll do it your way first, and then try it my way."

Since one response will not work for all problems, you will have to decide which method to use. Do not assume that someone must win and someone must lose. In fact, the best conflict resolution is when everybody wins. Consider the following example:

> You have a conflict with a patient. The nurse tells you to help Mr. Diaz get bathed and dressed for a 10 o'clock appointment, but Mr. Diaz does not want to get out of bed. Here's a way that you might resolve the conflict. You say to the patient, "Mr. Diaz, I need to help you and Mr. Brown with your baths. Would you like to take your bath now, or do you want me to help Mr. Brown first?" Mr. Diaz responds, "I want to be first," and eagerly goes off to the bathroom with you. Who won and who lost? Both of you won and nobody lost. You got to assist him with his bath, and he got to make a choice.

The next time you find yourself involved in a conflict, try using one of the methods you have learned. If one does not work, try another. Remember, there is more than one way to handle a difficult situation.

New and Expanded Roles of the Nursing Assistant

In the past, most nursing assistants were employed in hospitals; today, the majority of NAs work in home health or long-term care facilities. There are jobs available for nursing assistants in assisted care facilities, rehabilitation centers, clinics, and many other health care settings.

Changes in the health care system have produced some new and expanded roles for nursing assistants, such as the restorative nursing assistant, subacute care aide, patient care technician, hospice aide, psychiatric aide, and activity aide. These roles are usually available to nursing assistants who have work experience and an interest in a specific type of health care. Additional training and education are necessary for most of these new and expanded roles.

The Restorative Nursing Assistant

Restorative nursing assistants (RNAs) work with members of the rehabilitation team to help patients maintain and regain independence. The primary focus is on *mobility* (the ability to move about) and activities of daily living (ADLs). These aides may also work with patients who have eating and swallowing problems. They may work with other restorative programs provided by the facility. Restorative aides may work in a specific department, such as physical therapy, or the job may require knowledge of several rehabilitation areas.

The Subacute Aide

The subacute unit in a hospital or long-term care facility provides specialized care to patients. Some units specialize in rehabilitation, while others provide care for patients who have complex medical problems. Nursing assistants who are hired to work in these units are usually experienced, competent, and efficient. Because the focus of subacute units varies, so do nursing assistant responsibilities. The subacute unit presents a challenging experience for the nursing assistant. Nursing assistants who are experienced in subacute care will be very much in demand in the future.

The Hospice Aide

Hospice provides care for terminally ill patients and their families. Most hospices hire nursing assistants who have also completed home health aide training. They usually prefer individuals who have at least one year of experience in a health care facility. Hospice provides its own special training program

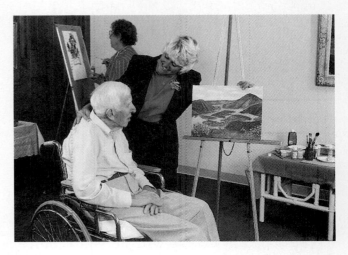

FIGURE 2–12
The activity aide helps patients meet their social needs.

to help employees learn more about the dying process and caring for the dying patient and the patient's family. Caring for the dying can be stressful, but it is also very satisfying.

The Psychiatric Aide

Psychiatric units or hospitals care for people who have psychological or mental problems. The nursing assistant may be employed in a psychiatric unit assisting patients with ADLs. Special training is necessary to learn how to deal with the physical and emotional problems of these patients. While some facilities expect the person to complete a training course before employment, others provide the training themselves.

The Activity Aide

The activity aide helps patients to meet social needs through planned activities. They provide recreation, arts and crafts, and parties to help patients to celebrate holidays. Nursing assistants who have an interest in this type of work may be hired and trained to help the activity director in planning programs, preparing materials, and helping patients participate. The activity department is very helpful in long-term care facilities where patients often stay for long periods of time. (See Figure 2–12.)

Continuing Your Education

One reason for continuing your education is to move up to a higher level of nursing. That is certainly a worthwhile idea, if that is your goal. But suppose your goal was to become a nursing assistant and you are satisfied with having achieved that goal. Is it wrong to feel that way? Absolutely not! Dedicated nursing assistants are always needed, and that job is very important.

However, the fact that you have reached your goal of becoming a nursing assistant does not mean that you are through learning. You will need to keep up with the many changes in health care. You may be required to learn new skills or techniques. For example, as new equipment arrives, you will need to learn how to use it.

Health care facilities usually provide continuing education classes, called in-services, for their employees. You will be required to attend some of these, while others will be your choice. Remember that regular attendance at in-services helps to improve your evaluation and your job performance.

There are many opportunities in the community for continuing education. Convenient classes are often available through the public school system or at community colleges. Courses may also be offered on public television or on the Internet. If you make continuing education a part of your life plan, you will become more professional and increase your chances of success.

Moving Up or Across the Career Ladder

A career is often compared to a ladder. You can either go up the ladder or across it. The nursing assistant is on the first rung of the nursing career ladder. The next step up the ladder is the licensed practical nurse (LPN), and above that is the registered nurse (RN). At the RN level there are several more rungs, ranging from an associate degree to a doctoral degree.

There is another method of movement called cross-laddering (moving sideways on the career ladder). Suppose you have worked as a nursing assistant but you do not want to become a nurse. However, you do want to transport the skills and knowledge you have acquired into a new job. The basic nursing assistant skills you have learned will be useful in many other positions.

Cross-training, as described in Chapter 1, is another way to gain additional skills and knowledge. You will be exposed to a different job without leaving the security of the one you already have. This provides an opportunity for you to decide

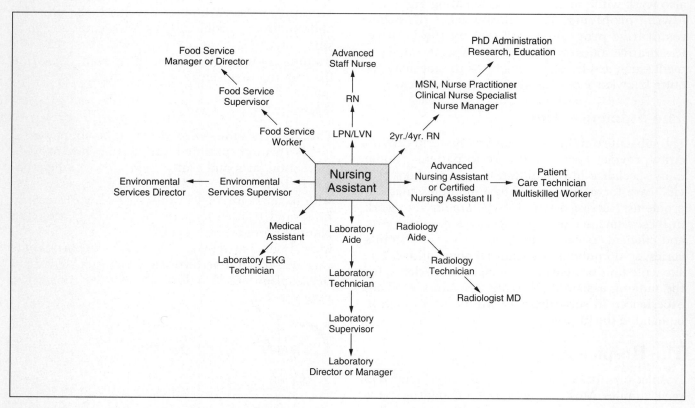

FIGURE 2–13
You can transport your nursing assistant skills into other jobs in the health care field.

whether you would like to move into that branch of health care. For example, if you have been cross-trained to draw blood, you might decide to become a full-time phlebotomist.

Scholarships and financial assistance are available for deserving students who might not otherwise be able to continue their education. Many facilities have financial assistance available for the continuing education of their employees. You might ask about this type of benefit when you apply for a job.

Health care is one of the fastest-growing industries today. You are entering the field as a nursing assistant, an entry-level position. You can take the knowledge and the skills you will learn and transport them into any other job in the health care field. The decision as to where and how far to go is in your hands. (See Figure 2–13.)

Review

Read each sentence and fill in the blank with the vocabulary term that best completes the sentence.

1. A list of your tasks and responsibilities is included with a _____.
2. _____ is the observance of rules for health and cleanliness.
3. The word _____ means to arrange things in an orderly manner.
4. It helps to rate each task according to _____ or order of importance.
5. _____ is mental and physical tension or strain.

Remember

1. The nursing assistant always works under the supervision of a nurse.
2. You are responsible for knowing which tasks you may or may not perform in the facility in which you work or train.
3. The holistic, humanistic approach is the key to providing quality patient care.
4. One of the most important qualities of a nursing assistant is dependability.
5. If you do not take care of yourself, you will not be able to care effectively for others.
6. Never use alcohol or drugs while working, and never bring alcohol or drugs to the workplace.
7. Your personal hygiene and appearance affect your professionalism.
8. Three skills that improve job performance include being a team player, being flexible, and organizing your work.
9. Planning, prioritizing, and managing time are important organizational skills.
10. The first step in problem solving is to identify and define the problem.
11. Conflict occurs when people have opposing strong beliefs and each believes he or she is right.
12. The majority of nursing assistants work in home health or long-term care facilities.
13. Most of the expanding roles of the nursing assistant require additional training and education.
14. Make continuing education a part of your life plan.
15. You can transport your skills as a nursing assistant up or across the health care career ladder.

Reflect

Read the following case study and answer the questions.

Case Study
Joel works as a nursing assistant in a nursing home. Because they are short of help one morning, he has been assigned more patients than usual. He takes time to plan his schedule and make rounds. Knowing he must work fast in order to get everything done, Joel politely refuses to help another nursing assistant move a heavy patient. Joel tells one of the residents, Mr. Evans, to hurry up and finish his bath. This upsets Mr. Evans, who puts down the washcloth and starts to cry. Joel says, "Don't cry Mr. Evans, that won't help anything. I'll bathe you

and get you dressed." Joel quickly finishes bathing and dressing all the residents that he has been assigned to care for that morning.

1. List Joel's actions that indicate good nursing care.

2. What should Joel have done about his co-worker's request for help?
3. What would have been a more restorative way to handle Mr. Evans?
4. Was Joel's verbal response to Mr. Evans appropriate? Why or why not?

 Respond

Choose the best answer for each question.

1. Which of the following statements about nursing assistants is TRUE?
   A. Never bathe a patient who has heart disease.
   B. Never do anything you have not been trained to do.
   C. Nursing assistants may give medicines.
   D. Nursing assistants may take verbal orders from a doctor.

2. A patient tells you that in her culture people do not bathe daily. What is your best response?
   A. "Well, that's not the way we do things here."
   B. "You'll feel better if you bathe daily."
   C. "I'll let the nurse know and we can add it to your care plan."
   D. "You people always want to be different."

3. The ability to share another person's point of view and understand their feelings is called
   A. Dependability
   B. Enthusiasm
   C. Empathy
   D. Honesty

4. Which of the following is a guideline for health?
   A. Eat a well-balanced diet.
   B. Get sufficient sleep.
   C. Exercise regularly.
   D. All of the above.

5. You will look more professional if your fingernails are
   A. Polished bright red
   B. Applied artificially
   C. Short and clean
   D. Long and pointed

6. Which of the following is the healthiest way to relieve stress?

A. Talk to a friend.
B. Have a good cry.
C. Go on a shopping spree.
D. Have a few drinks.

7. You observe that a co-worker is having difficulty moving a heavy patient up in bed. What is your best response?
   A. Get busy and finish your own work.
   B. Volunteer to help her.
   C. Ask one of the male nursing assistants to help her.
   D. Tell the charge nurse.

8. The FIRST step in problem solving is to
   A. Collect information
   B. Make a decision
   C. Take action
   D. Identify the problem

9. If you work as a hospice aide, your duties will focus on
   A. Caring for terminally ill patients
   B. Planning activities for nursing home residents
   C. Working in a subacute unit
   D. All of the above

10. Which statement about continuing education is FALSE?
    A. You will be required to attend some in-services where you work.
    B. There are educational opportunities in the community.
    C. You can move up or sideways on the career ladder.
    D. Your education ends when you graduate the nursing assistant program.

Chapter Three

Ethical *and*
Legal Considerations

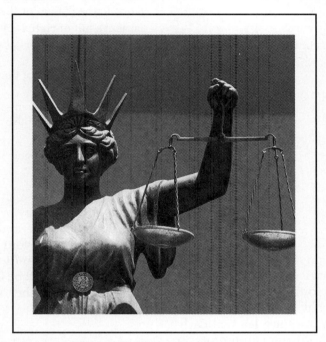

1. Identify four ethics that the nursing assistant might follow.

2. Describe three central themes of end-of-life issues.

3. Briefly explain the purpose of advance directives.

4. Describe four rights of the patient in a health care facility.

5. Describe four legal issues that may affect the nursing assistant.

After studying this chapter, you will be able to

6. Describe two residents' rights in long-term care.

7. Identify three types of abuse.

8. Explain two ways the nursing assistant can help to prevent abuse.

abandonment Being left without care or support.

accountability   To accept responsibility for your own actions.

advance directive   A document giving instructions regarding a person's desires about health care treatment in the event that he or she is no longer able to voice such desires.

assault   Any threat to do bodily harm.

autonomy   The ability to be in control of one's own life.

battery   The act of touching another person's body without permission.

confidentiality   The act of keeping information about patients private and disclosing it only to appropriate health care team members.

ethics   Guidelines for right and wrong behavior.

false imprisonment   The act of restricting or restraining a person's movements without proper consent.

invasion of privacy   Failure to protect a person's body from exposure or failure to keep personal information confidential.

negligence   Failure to give proper care, which results in harm to the patient or the patient's property.

patient's bill of rights   A list of the basic rights to which all patients are entitled. Such lists exist for different health care settings.

restraint   Any device that restricts movement or normal access to one's body.

slander To injure the name and reputation of another person by making a false statement.

Ethics

Today's health care workers are faced with many issues that present a challenge both ethically and legally. *Ethics* are guidelines for right and wrong behavior. The decision as to what is right and what is wrong is based on values. Values are learned early in life from family, friends, and the community in which one lives. From those values you develop a set of rules to guide you through life.

You will learn about professional ethics that apply to members of your profession. Doctors, nurses, and other health care workers have developed standards for their profession called medical ethics. The goal of medical ethics is to do as much good for the patient as possible and to do no harm. This principle is basic to all health care.

Nursing assistants must also behave in an ethical manner. A set of ethics for nursing assistants may include the following:

- Respect each patient's culture and religion.
- Respect each patient as an individual.
- Protect the patient from harm.
- Protect the patient's privacy.
- Be honest and trustworthy.
- Avoid spreading gossip.
- Be aware of the limits of your role.
- Perform your job to the best of your ability.

Gifts and Tips

It is considered unethical and against the policy of most health care facilities to accept tips. Never ac-

cept a gift or money from a patient or family member. Politely refuse and explain that caring for the patient is part of your job. Sometimes people will send flowers or candy to show their appreciation. These items should be taken to the nurse's station to be shared with other members of the health care team.

End-of-Life Issues

The issue of what to do in the last days of life has become an important topic in recent years. New technology and medications allow health care providers to extend life even after body organs fail. We are now starting to seriously compare quantity of life with quality of life. In other words, are the extra months or years gained worthwhile? Do we want to let death come naturally or do we want everything possible done to delay death? Those are decisions that each individual must eventually make and discuss with his or her loved ones. (See Figure 3–1.)

End-of-life issues are greatly influenced by culture and religion. For example, some religious groups do not allow medical treatment that interferes with the natural process. Others believe that life must be preserved at all costs. It is important for most individuals to be able to live up to cultural expectations. As health care workers, we can help patients by being respectful of their beliefs and customs.

End-of-life issues revolve around three central themes—being in control, making choices, and being comfortable and pain free.

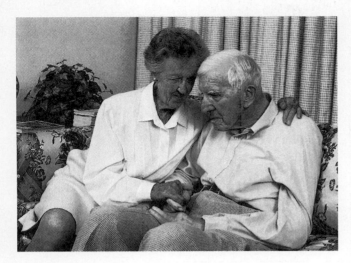

FIGURE 3–1
Discuss end-of-life issues with your loved ones.

Control

Patients in all health care settings frequently complain about losing control. This loss can cause depression, frustration, or anger. Most people want to be in control of their own lives. They want to make decisions about their own health care and direct the course of treatment. All patients do not want the same thing. Some people want to die at home in as natural a way as possible and without the support of machinery or artificial means. Others want to be in a hospital and have everything done that is possible to prolong life. Health care workers need to be advisors and supporters, not controllers.

Choice

Individuals have the right to make informed choices about their health care. These choices might include:

- How much or how little treatment is given
- Who is to deliver these treatments
- Where they will be during their final days
- What information is to be given out to others
- Whether or not live-saving measures are to be taken
- Who is to make decisions when they cannot

You, as a nursing assistant, can help by allowing patients to make choices whenever possible and by being supportive of their choices.

Comfort and Pain Control

No one wants to suffer needlessly or die in pain. Caretakers must be knowledgeable about comfort measures and pain control. Comfort measures may include repositioning, bathing, and massage as well as pain medications. Providing a clean, dry bed and giving a relaxing back rub are comfort measures the nursing assistant can give. You will also need to be aware of signs of discomfort and report your observations to the nurse.

The hospice movement has long advocated returning health care control to the patients who are involved. This organization focuses on the care of terminally ill patients and their families. They provide trained workers and support services that allow patients to be at home or in a home-like setting, cared for by their loved ones. Hospice is discussed in more detail in Chapter 26.

As a nursing assistant, your role is to do all that you can to make the last days of patients as comfortable as possible. Be nonjudgmental and supportive of the patient's end-of-life decisions. Sometimes their decisions will go against your own feelings and beliefs. You will wonder if their choices are ethical. Just remember, it is their decision and their ethics involved. The use of advance directives gives legal support to patients and caregivers regarding these end-of-life issues.

Advance Directives

Adults have the right to control their own health care. They can accept or refuse any medical or surgical treatment. It is easy to exercise that right when they are well and can tell others what they want. However, the most difficult health decisions often occur during a severe illness when patients may not be able to speak for themselves. This is when the need for advance directives arrives. An *advanced directive* is a document that gives instructions as to the patient's desires about health care treatment. The directive becomes effective only if the patient is unable to make decisions or state his or her wishes.

Patient Self-Determination Act

In 1990, Congress passed the Patient Self-Determination Act, which included two rights:

1. The right to make decisions about one's own medical care, including the right to refuse medical or surgical treatment
2. The right to prepare legally binding advance directives

Health care facilities are required to give information regarding advance directives during the patient's admission. While the aim of the law is to encourage people to prepare advance directives, it does not require them to do so.

Living Wills

A living will is a document that contains instructions about whether or not a person wants his life prolonged by artificial means if he becomes terminally ill. It provides a legal method to state one's wishes about treatment and to make sure those wishes are expressed to family members, doctors, and health care facilities. A living will should also

cover the issue of food and fluids. If that is not specifically included, food and fluids may be given, even if other means of life support are not used. (See Figure 3–2.)

Power of Attorney for Health Care

The Patient Self-Determination Act also recommended that a person appoint a power of attorney for health care, sometimes referred to as a health

---

LIVING WILL

Declaration made this_____ day of _____ , 20____.

I,_____ willfully and voluntarily make known my desire that my dying not be artificially prolonged under the circumstances set forth below, and I do hereby declare:

If at any time I have a terminal condition and if my attending or treating physician and another consulting physician have determined that there is no medical probability of my recovery from such condition, I direct that life-prolonging procedures be withheld or withdrawn when the application of such procedures would serve only to prolong artificially the process of dying, and that I be permitted to die naturally with only the administration of medication or the performance of any medical procedure deemed necessary to provide me with comfort care or to alleviate pain.

It is my intention that this declaration be honored by my family and physician as the final expression of my legal right to refuse medical or surgical treatment and to accept the consequences for such refusal.

In the event that I have been determined to be unable to provide express and informed consent regarding the withholding, withdrawal, or continuation of life-prolonging procedures, I wish to designate, as my surrogate to carry out the provisions of this declaration:

Name:_____ Phone:_____

Address: _____
      (City)   (State)   (Zip)

I understand the full import of this declaration, and I am emotionally and mentally competent to make this declaration.

Additional instructions (optional):

☐   I do not desire that the artificial administration of nutrition and hydration be withheld or withdrawn even when the application of such procedures would serve only to prolong artificially the process of dying.

☐   Other (specify):_____

_____

_____

Signed: _____

Witness: _____

Address:_____

                                    Zip Code

Phone: (____)_____

Witness: _____

Address: _____

                                    Zip Code

Phone: (____)_____

FIGURE 3–2
Example of a living will.

care surrogate. This gives a person selected by the patient the legal right to make decisions regarding medical treatment if the patient is not able.

The legality of a living will, power of attorney for health care, or health care surrogate varies from state to state. The right to discontinue food and fluids also differs. However, an advance directive expresses the patient's personal wishes and provides guidelines for family members and health care providers.

Legal Issues and Laws

There are specific legal issues and laws that concern health care workers. Laws are a set of rules that are enforced by the courts, and breaking the law can cause you serious problems. Legal issues that affect the nursing assistant are discussed in this section.

Assault

A threat to do bodily harm is called *assault*. Assault and battery are often considered together, but in assault there is no physical contact. Threats of punishment or shaking a fist at someone are forms of assault. (See Figure 3–3.)

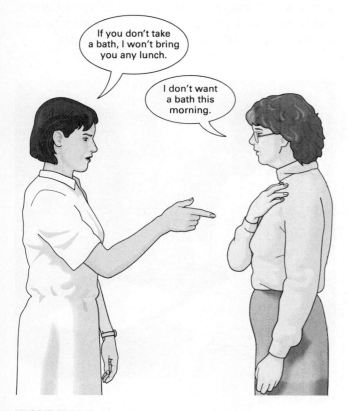

FIGURE 3–3
Any threat may be considered assault.

Battery

Touching another person's body without permission is called *battery*. This might involve hitting, pinching, or pushing a patient. Treating a patient roughly or forcing him or her to do something is also considered battery. Patients have the right to refuse any treatment or procedure.

False Imprisonment

Restricting or restraining a person's movements without proper consent is called *false imprisonment*. False imprisonment can be compared to placing a person in prison when that person has not committed a crime. False imprisonment frequently involves the use of restraints. A *restraint* is any device that restricts movement or normal access to one's body. Locking a patient in a room or tying a patient to a chair to prevent wandering are examples of false imprisonment.

Invasion of Privacy

Failing to protect the privacy of the patient's body or the privacy of personal information is *invasion of privacy*. Unnecessary exposure of the patient's body by failing to close the patient's door or not pulling the curtains are examples of invasion of privacy. Entering the patient's room without knocking is also an invasion of privacy.

Personal and medical information about the patient must be kept confidential. *Confidentiality* means keeping information that you have learned about the patient to yourself. Do not discuss patients at break time, during lunch, or after work. Be careful with the patient's medical records, and do your charting in the proper area. Questions from family or friends concerning medical treatment should be referred to the nurse.

Negligence

Failure to give proper care, which results in harm to the patient or the patient's property, is called *negligence*. You can be negligent when you fail to perform a task or you perform a task in a careless manner. You are also negligent if you harm the patient by doing something you are not allowed to do. Examples of negligence include:

- The wheels on the patient's bed were not locked. The bed rolled as the patient attempted to lie down. The patient fell and broke a leg.
- A patient fell and broke his arm while trying to get to the call signal, which had not been left within reach. (See Figure 3–4.)

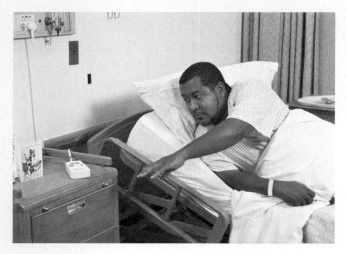

FIGURE 3–4
Failure to place the call signal within the patient's reach can result in negligence.

■ A patient complained of chest pain. The nursing assistant did not report this to the nurse, and the patient had a heart attack.

Slander and Libel

Injuring the name and reputation of another person by making a false statement is called *slander*. Slander that is put in writing is called libel. To avoid these legal problems, do not talk or write about a patient's actions or lifestyle. Avoid listening to or repeating gossip about another person.

Abandonment

Leaving or deserting a patient whose care you are responsible for is called *abandonment*. You have a duty to each patient to whom you are assigned, and it is unlawful to fail to meet that duty. Walking off the job without permission is an example of abandonment. Notify the nurse and get permission if you need to leave the job for any reason. There must be someone equally qualified to take your place in caring for the patient. This is especially important in home health when you may be the only health care worker in the home.

Legal Accountability

Accountability is taking responsibility for your own actions. Legal accountability means that you are legally responsible for your actions. If you are guilty of assault, battery, false imprisonment, invasion of privacy, negligence, slander, or anything else that harms a patient, a legal action can be brought against you.

It is your responsibility to know what tasks a nursing assistant is allowed to do in your facility.

You will be held legally accountable if you perform a task that a nursing assistant is not allowed to do and the patient is harmed. If the nurse or anyone else asks you to do one of these forbidden tasks, you must politely refuse. Do not be rude or defensive. The following example may help you understand this principle.

> The nurse puts the patient's medication in a dish of ice cream and asks you to feed it to him. You must refuse this request because nursing assistants are not allowed to give medications. You might say something such as "I'm sorry, but I am not allowed to give medications."

Although the nursing assistant always works under the supervision of a nurse, there may be times when you will need more information before you can carry out the nurse's order. If you do not understand what the nurse wants you to do, you must ask him or her to explain the order more clearly. Do not proceed until you are sure of the instructions. (See Figure 3–5.)

Wills

A patient or a family member may ask you to witness or help prepare a will. You should politely refuse and direct the person to the nurse. Getting involved in other people's legal transactions is seldom a wise thing to do. Always let the nurse know if a patient talks about making a will. It may be that the patient is really concerned about dying.

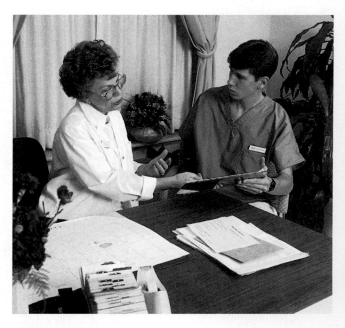

FIGURE 3–5
Discuss your concerns with the nurse if you are not sure what action to take.

The Patient's Bill of Rights

A *patient's bill of rights* is a list of the basic rights to which all patients are entitled. "A Patient's Bill of Rights" for hospital patients was issued in 1973 by the American Hospital Association (AHA). It was soon followed by the Resident's Bill of Rights for long-term care residents. The basic rights of individuals are included in both, but the Resident's Bill of Rights contains additional rights that apply only to the long-term care setting. Home health agencies have adopted a similar bill.

A more recent goal of patients' rights has been to improve patient autonomy and independence. *Autonomy* means being in control of one's own life. In order for individuals to share responsibility for their own health, they need to be informed. A detailed list of patients' rights is provided in Figure 3–6.

Patient's Bill of Rights
A health care facility must protect and promote the rights of each patient, including the following:
1. The right to considerate and respectful care
2. The right to be informed of his/her medical condition and treatment and to take part in planning the care
3. The right to know the name and classification of assigned personnel
4. The right to be informed of responsibility for charges and services
5. The right to refuse medication and treatment
6. The right to have an advance directive (living will, durable power of attorney, health care surrogate)
7. The right to personal privacy and confidentiality of information
8. The right to inspect his/her records
9. The right to receive adequate and appropriate health care
10. The right to informed consent
11. The right to continuity of care
12. The right to be free from unnecessary physical restraints and drugs
13. The right to be free from verbal, mental, sexual, or physical abuse
14. The right to equal policies and practices regardless of source of payment
15. The right to be treated without discrimination

FIGURE 3–6 A patient's bill of rights.

Some of the patients' rights are described in the following paragraphs.

The Right to Be Treated with Consideration and Respect

Every patient has the right to be different and a right to be accepted as such. Respect must be shown for patients of all cultures and nationalities, regardless of their physical or mental condition. When you are considerate and respectful, you help the patient maintain dignity and self-esteem.

The Right to Full Disclosure

The patient has the right to obtain current information about his or her health status or treatment. The patient has the right to know the names and titles of physicians, nurses, nursing assistants, and anyone else who provides care. Students, interns, and other trainees must be identified as such. However, it is not the responsibility of the nursing assistant to supply this information. These types of questions should be referred to the nurse.

The Right to Make Decisions

The patient has the right to make decisions regarding his or her plan of care. The patient has the right to have an advance directive, if desired. You can help by encouraging and assisting the patient in planning his or her own care. Allowing the patient to make decisions helps him or her maintain independence.

The Right to Privacy and Confidentiality

The patient has the right to personal privacy. This involves privacy of the patient's body, of personal belongings, and of information. OBRA specifically addresses confidentiality of patient information and patient health care records. A violation of this right is an invasion of privacy. You must keep patient information confidential and protect the patient's privacy while providing care.

The Right to Appropriate Care

The patient has the right to receive appropriate care, services, and reasonable continuity of care. This means that the patient's care plan must be followed by all who provide patient care. It also means that the same health care providers should care for the patient whenever possible. You protect this right by carrying out all the procedures and tasks that you are assigned to do. Check the patient's care plan frequently to be sure that you are giving appropriate care.

The Right to Refuse

A patient has the right to refuse medication and treatment. Be very careful while providing personal care that you do not violate this right. You cannot force a procedure on a patient, even if you think it will be beneficial. For example, you cannot make a patient take a bath if the patient refuses to do so.

The Right to Informed Consent

Patients have the right to be informed, in terms they can understand, about any tests or treatments that are being considered. They must also be informed and give permission before being involved in human experimentation or research.

The Right to Be Treated Without Discrimination

Every person has the right to be treated in a way that is not discriminatory. Health care workers need to be sensitive to culture, religion, race, language, age, gender, and other patient differences.

*R*esident's Rights

The patient's bill of rights, when applied to residents of long-term care facilities, is called the resident's bill of rights. Additional rights have been added to cover the special situations found in long-term care. Although the resident's bill of rights has been in existence for years, it has been emphasized and strengthened by OBRA. The resident's bill of rights is discussed in this section.

The Right to Be Free from Harm or Abuse

Abuse in any form is illegal. Many patients in long-term care facilities are sick and helpless, and it is the responsibility of the health care facility to protect them. As a member of the health care team, you share in that responsibility.

The Right to Be Free from Physical or Chemical Restraints

Restraints require a physician's order and can be used only to protect the patient from harm. A violation of this right is considered false imprisonment and abuse, so check with the nurse before applying a restraint. Restraints are discussed in more detail in Chapter 6.

The Right to Personal Choice

The resident has the right to choose activities in which he or she wishes to participate. The resident's personal preferences and culture must be considered regarding clothing, diet, and schedules. You can help protect this right by encouraging the resident to make choices. (See Figure 3–7.)

The Right to Participate in Group Activities

The resident has the right to participate in resident and family group activities. Some groups may meet to express residents' concerns and grievances. Some groups help plan resident activities, and others provide support and reassurance. Other groups meet cultural and spiritual needs. Participation in group activities helps meet the patient's social needs. It builds self-esteem and helps protect the patient's independence. Let the nurse know if the resident has expressed a desire to participate in a group.

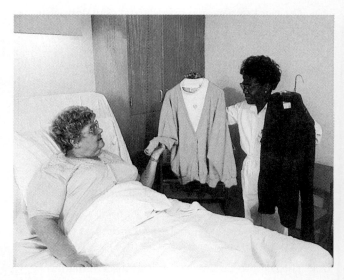

FIGURE 3–7
Encourage the patient to make choices.

The Right to Personal Belongings

The resident has the right to retain and use personal possessions and clothing as space permits. Residents and their families are encouraged to bring photographs and mementos from home. A resident may also bring items of furniture, such as a rocking chair or a sewing table. Always handle all the resident's belongings carefully.

The Right to Privacy for Married Couples

A married couple has the right to privacy during visitation. They are also permitted to share a room when both are residents of the same facility. Allow the residents to close the door for privacy, and knock before entering.

If you violate one of the patient's or resident's rights, you may also be breaking the law. Knowledge of the rights to which patients and residents are entitled will help to protect patients, residents, and yourself.

Patient Abuse

Persons who are abused are usually not physically or mentally able to defend themselves. Children and the elderly are most at risk. Abuse may be physical, emotional, sexual, material, or a combination.

Physical abuse can include hitting or handling a patient roughly. Neglecting a patient by failing to change a wet bed or not providing adequate fluids is also considered physical abuse.

Emotional abuse involves verbal statements that frighten or threaten the patient. Belittling or mocking a patient or failing to be respectful is also emotional abuse.

Sexual abuse can involve actual physical contact or threats of physical contact. Most sexual abuse is a combination of both physical and emotional abuse.

Material abuse involves misuse of the patient's personal possessions. Stealing the patient's money or eating the patient's food are examples of material abuse.

Protecting the Patient from Abuse

One of the most important responsibilities of the nursing assistant is to protect patients from abuse. Remember, abuse can take place in a hospital, a nursing home, a private home, or any other health care setting. Abusers may be health care workers, family members, or other patients. Those being abused may not be able to protect themselves because of physical or mental impairment. They may be afraid to report the abuse because they are dependent on the abuser for care or financial support.

One of the best ways to protect the patient from abuse is by being observant. Be aware of the signs and symptoms of abuse that might include the following:

- Bruises or skin tears
- Anxiety and nervousness
- Fear and avoidance to touch
- Withdrawal or depression
- Frequent crying
- Changes in personality

Be observant for changes in the patient's personality and report any unusual patient behavior to the nurse. Encourage the patient to talk about fears and anxieties. While giving care, observe the patient's skin for bruises or skin tears that might be the result of rough handling. Report any suspicious observations to the nurse immediately. State the facts and do not offer your opinion or make unfounded accusations. It is your moral, ethical, and legal duty to report patient abuse.

You may call the abuse hotline or the Ombudsmen Committee to report abuse. The Ombudsmen Committee is made up of concerned citizens who investigate complaints of patient abuse. In most areas the members are appointed by the governor of the state. (See Figure 3–8.)

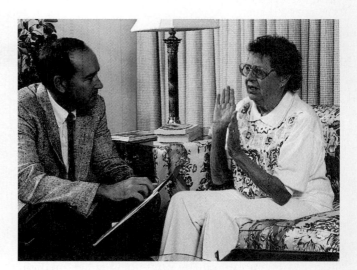

FIGURE 3–8
Ombudsmen Committee members investigate complaints of patient abuse.

Review

Read each sentence and fill in the blank with the vocabulary term that best completes the sentence.

1. Leaving a patient without care or support is called _____.
2. A _____ is a device that restricts movement or normal access to one's body.
3. A threat to do bodily harm is _____.
4. _____ is failure to give proper care that results in harm to the patient or the patient's property.
5. The act of touching another person's body without permission is called _____.

Remember

1. The goal of medical ethics is to do as much good for the patient as possible and to do no harm.
2. Never accept a gift or money from a patient or family member.
3. End-of-life issues include being in control, making choices, and being comfortable and pain free.
4. Advance directives give patients control of their own health care when they are not able to express their wishes.
5. Personal and medical information must be kept confidential.
6. Negligence is failure to give proper care that results in harm to the patient or his property.
7. You are legally accountable for your own actions.
8. Patients have the right to refuse medication or treatment.
9. Residents of long-term care facilities have the right to retain and use personal belongings as space permits.
10. A change in the patient's personality or behavior might indicate abuse.
11. It is your moral, ethical, and legal responsibility to report patient abuse.

Reflect

Read the following case study and answer the questions.

Case Study

Mrs. Jannus is a diabetic patient who has been admitted to the hospital after an insulin reaction. She is on multiple medications for various complications of diabetes. She is confused at times. Jerry is a nursing assistant who has been assigned to care for Mrs. Jannus. Jerry suspects that she has been hiding extra food in her closet. While she is sleeping, he searches her closet and removes two candy bars from her purse. When the nurse brings her medication, Mrs. Jannus refuses to take a pill so the nurse hides it in her applesauce. The nurse tells Jerry to feed the applesauce to Mrs. Jannus. Mrs. Jannus doesn't want the applesauce, but Jerry feeds it to her anyway. At lunchtime he tells everyone about that "crazy Mrs. Jannus" and how difficult she has been.

1. List the patient's rights that Jerry violated.
2. Did he do anything illegal?
3. What should Jerry have done about the candy bars?
4. What should Jerry have done when the nurse asked him to feed Mrs. Jannus the applesauce that contained medication?

Respond

Choose the best answer for each question.

1. Which statement about ethics is TRUE?
   A. It is alright to accept a tip if you have given a patient really good care.
   B. Talking about patients makes break time more relaxing.
   C. Show respect for the patient's culture and religion.
   D. There are no ethical standards for nursing assistants.

2. Loss of control can cause patients to be
   A. Angry
   B. Depressed
   C. Frustrated
   D. All of the above

3. The Patient Self-Determination Act focused on
   A. The right to make decisions about one's own health care
   B. The right to be free from restraints
   C. The right to privacy and confidentiality
   D. The right to use one's own personal belongings in the health care facility

4. A Power of Attorney for Health Care gives a designated person
   A. The right to manage the patient's money
   B. The right to sell the patient's house
   C. The right to make health care decisions for the patient
   D. The right to make all decisions for the patient

5. The ability to be in control of one's own life is called
   A. Autonomy
   B. Assault
   C. Ethics
   D. Negligence

6. Shaking your fist at a patient is an example of
   A. Assault
   B. Battery
   C. Negligence
   D. Slander

7. Forcing a resident to take a bath after he refused is an example of
   A. Assault
   B. Battery
   C. Negligence
   D. Libel

8. You get mad at your supervisor and walk off the floor. This is an example of
   A. Assault
   B. Battery
   C. Slander
   D. Abandonment

9. Which of the following is NOT included in the Patient's Bill of Rights?
   A. The right to refuse
   B. The right to free medical care
   C. The right to appropriate medical care
   D. The right to privacy

10. Laughing at or making fun of a patient is an example of
    A. Physical abuse
    B. Emotional abuse
    C. Sexual abuse
    D. Material abuse

Chapter Four

Infection Control

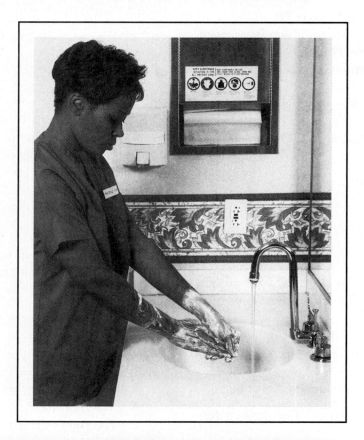

OBJECTIVES

After studying this chapter, you will be able to

1. Explain the importance of infection control.

2. Briefly describe the infection process.

3. Describe three signs and symptoms of infection.

4. Explain two ways the body defends itself against infection.

5. Describe the purpose and goals of the infection control professional (ICP).

6. List four guidelines for medical asepsis.

7. Explain why frequent handwashing is important for health care workers.

8. List six guidelines for standard precautions.

9. Identify the three categories of isolation included in transmission-based precautions.

10. Describe the holistic approach to isolation.

11. List three requirements of the OSHA Bloodborne Pathogens Standard.

12. Perform the procedures described in this chapter.

asepsis   A condition free from pathogens.

biohazardous waste   Material that has been contaminated with blood or body fluids.

bloodborne pathogens   Disease-causing microorganisms that are found in blood, human blood components, any body fluid that contains blood cells, and products made from human blood tissue.

contamination   The condition of items or areas that have been exposed to disease-causing microorganisms.

disinfection   The process of destroying pathogens on objects and surfaces.

HIV (human immunodeficiency virus) infection   A disease that destroys the immune system and leaves the body unable to fight infection.

infection   The invasion and growth of disease-causing microorganisms in the body.

isolation   The practice of separating the infected patient from others to prevent the spread of infection.

microorganism   General term for any small plant or animal that cannot be seen without the aid of a microscope.

nonpathogens   Microorganisms that are not harmful and do not cause infection.

normal flora   Microorganisms that live and grow in certain locations of the body.

pathogens   Harmful microorganisms that can cause infection upon entering a person's body.

standard precautions   Procedures to be used with all patients to protect the health care worker against exposure to blood, body fluids, and body substances.

sterile   The condition of being free from all microorganisms.

susceptible   One who is likely to develop an infection or disease when exposed to pathogens.

transmission-based precautions   Procedures used when a patient is known to be infected or suspected of being infected with certain contagious diseases or conditions.

The Importance of Infection Control

Infection control includes the practices used to prevent the spread of infection. *Infection* is the invasion and growth of disease-causing microorganisms in the body. In health care facilities, where there are so many sick people, microorganisms are abundant. As a health care worker, you will be exposed to infection frequently. Although every exposure to infection does not result in disease, preventing exposure is the best way to prevent infection. (See Figure 4–1.)

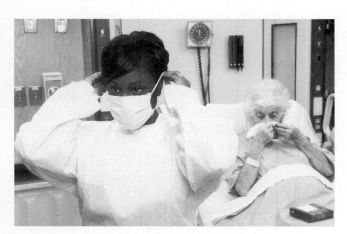

FIGURE 4–1
Health care workers are frequently exposed to infection.

Individuals who are sick enough to enter a health care facility are often not able to care for themselves. It then becomes the responsibility of health care workers to provide for their care and protection. A patient who is weak and frail is likely to get a nosocomial infection (an infection that the patient acquires after entering a health care facility). All it takes to cause a nosocomial infection is one careless act.

The health of the patient, as well as your own health, depends on the infection control precautions and procedures described in this chapter. The safest way to provide quality patient care is by following the infection control policies where you work. As you study this textbook, pay close attention to infection control issues in each chapter.

Microorganisms

Microorganism is the general term for any small plant or animal that cannot be seen without the aid of a microscope. Microbe is another name for a microorganism. Microorganisms are everywhere in our environment. They are on our bodies, in the food we eat, and in the air we breathe. Some harmful microorganisms (commonly called germs) can enter the body, multiply, and cause infection. However, all microorganisms are not harmful.

Types of Microorganisms

The three basic types of microorganisms are non-pathogens, pathogens, and normal flora. *Pathogens* are harmful microorganisms that can cause infection when they enter the body. *Nonpathogens* are microorganisms that are not harmful and do not cause infection. *Normal flora* are microorganisms that live and grow in certain locations of the body. As long as they remain in their normal locations, they act as nonpathogens and help keep the body healthy, but they can cause infection if they enter another part of the body.

Environmental Factors that Affect Microorganisms

Because microorganisms are living beings, they require food and water to grow and reproduce. While most need oxygen, some microorganisms can live without it. Although they can live almost anywhere, microorganisms thrive in a warm, moist, dark environment. Areas of the body that provide excellent conditions for the growth of microorganisms include the mouth, underarms, and genitals. In the home or health care facility, bathrooms, kitchens, and dining rooms provide a favorable environment for microorganisms.

The growth and reproduction of microorganisms are slowed at very cold temperatures, while very hot temperatures usually destroy them. For example, if you place a package of fresh meat in the freezer, the cold temperature will not kill the microorganisms—it will only slow their growth. However, boiling the meat for a period of time will destroy the microorganisms.

Infections and How They Occur

When harmful microorganisms invade the body, an infection can occur. Most of this chapter is concerned with teaching you techniques to prevent the transmission of infection. First, however, let's look at how infection occurs, how it affects the body, and how the body fights infection.

The Infection Process

Infection follows a chain of events that can be broken at any point. (See Figure 4–2.)

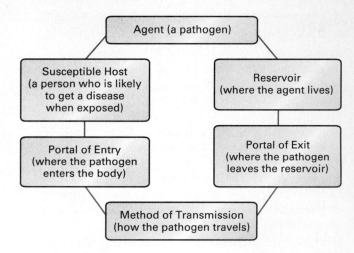

FIGURE 4–2
The chain of infection.

- **Agent**—a pathogen, a microorganism that can cause disease.
- **Reservoir**—a place where microorganisms can live and grow. Humans, animals, birds, insects, food, and water are all reservoirs for pathogens.
- **Portal of entry and exit**—natural body openings, such as the mouth, nose, and rectum or a break in the skin, where microorganisms may enter or exit from the body.
- **Method of transmission**—food, water, air, insects, animals, rodents, body fluids, and body substances. Pathogens can also be transmitted by handling contaminated dishes, utensils, medical equipment, and personal care items. Infections are frequently transmitted on the hands of health care workers.
- **Susceptible host**—a person who is *susceptible* (likely to catch an infection or disease when exposed). Patients in health care facilities are more susceptible to infection because they are already ill.

Contamination

Contamination refers to items or areas that have been exposed to disease-causing microorganisms. The terms "clean" and "dirty" or "soiled" are used in health care to indicate whether an item or area has been used or contaminated. "Clean" items have not been used and are placed in a "clean" area. "Dirty" items have been used and are placed in a "dirty" area. The facility will have a clean utility room for items that are clean, and a dirty utility room for items that are contaminated. It is important not to take contaminated items such as dirty bedpans into the clean utility room.

Signs and Symptoms of Infection

An infection may be located in one part of the body (a local infection), or it may affect the whole body (a systemic infection). Signs and symptoms of a local infection may include:

- Redness
- Swelling
- Heat
- Pain
- Drainage

In addition to local signs and symptoms, the patient with a systemic infection might also suffer from headache, fever, chills, nausea, vomiting, or diarrhea. Observing for signs and symptoms of infection is an important responsibility of the nursing assistant. Infections identified early may be minor and easily treated. Any signs or symptoms of infection should be reported immediately to the charge nurse. You play a key role in protecting the patient from infection.

The Body's Defense Against Infection

A healthy individual has many defenses against infection. For example, unbroken skin is a barrier to harmful microorganisms. Hairs in the nose can filter out pathogens and also provide a barrier. The immune system has special cells called lymphocytes that are produced in the spleen, thymus, and bone marrow to help fight infection. Their function is to attack and destroy invading microorganisms. This action is called the immune response.

A healthy immune system can successfully fight off many infections. When the immune system is weakened, pathogens may enter the body, multiply, and cause disease. The immune system can be weakened by poor nutrition, chronic illness, and stress. Some medications can also weaken the system.

Preventing the Spread of Infection

Infection Control Professional

Modern infection control has gone global. Infectious diseases such as HIV infection are worldwide problems. *HIV (human immunodeficiency*

virus) infection is a disease that destroys the immune system and leaves the body unable to fight other infections. Today, there are programs concerned with the health and welfare of the general public at an international level. These programs are supervised by infection control professionals (ICPs). The ICP may be a doctor, nurse, or medical technologist.

All health care facilities use ICPs to prevent infection, follow up on outbreaks, and provide education. They keep up with new medications and procedures in the ever-changing world of infection control. Their goal is to decrease disease transmission to other patients and to health care workers. This, in turn, prevents infections from spreading into the community.

The ICP works closely with other staff members. As a nursing assistant, you can help by using good infection control practices at all times. Attend facility in-services and ask questions when you don't understand. Know how to recognize signs and symptoms of infection and report your observations to the nurse or ICP immediately.

Every facility has written policies and procedures to help prevent the spread of infection. These policies reflect federal, state, and local regulations, as well as the needs of the individual facility. They are also influenced by guidelines and recommendations from the Centers for Disease Control and Prevention (CDC) and from the Occupational Safety and Health Administration (OSHA). Although all facilities do not have the same policies and procedures, the principles are similar. Most facilities will have policies and procedures that include the following:

- **Medical asepsis**—all the techniques used to prevent the spread of infection. *Asepsis* means absence of pathogens.
- **Disinfection**—the process of destroying pathogens on objects and surfaces. (See Figure 4–3.)
- **Sterilization**—method used to kill all microorganisms. An item that is *sterile* is free from all microorganisms.
- **Isolation**—separating the infected patient from others to prevent the spread of infection.
- **Barrier practices**—using barriers such as gloves, gowns, and masks to prevent the spread of microorganisms.
- **Blood and body fluid precautions**—practices used to prevent the spread of microorganisms from blood and body fluids.
- **Sharps precautions**—practices used in handling and disposing of needles and syringes and other sharp objects.

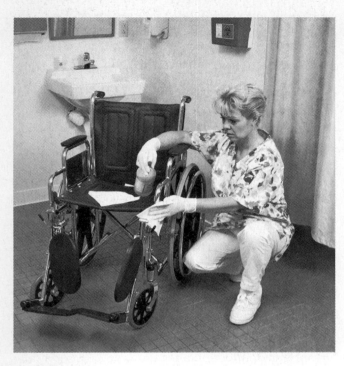

FIGURE 4–3
Disinfectants are used to destroy pathogens on objects and surfaces.

Guidelines for Medical Asepsis

- Cover your mouth and nose when sneezing. Wash your hands immediately afterward.
- Hold all items away from your clothing.
- Discourage sharing personal items such as combs and brushes.
- Do not take equipment and supplies from one patient's room to another.
- Empty urinals and bedpans immediately: Clean and cover them after use.
- Take all dirty or contaminated items to the dirty utility room.
- Keep the overbed table clean. Do not place bedpans, urinals, dirty linen, or other soiled items on it.
- Do not put dirty linen on the floor. (See Figure 4–4.)
- Report any signs or symptoms of infection immediately.

- **Waste disposal**—proper disposal of *biohazardous waste* (material that has been contaminated with blood or body fluids).

Preventing the spread of infection and lowering its risk to patients, visitors, and employees is an important responsibility of all health care workers. You also need to be concerned with protecting yourself and your family. The first concept you must learn is asepsis, the basis of all infection control.

Medical Asepsis

The goal of medical asepsis is to prevent the spread of pathogens. Medical asepsis is also known as "clean technique." It involves keeping everything (including oneself) as clean as possible. Aseptic technique should be practiced by everyone, everywhere, all the time. You can use these techniques in your own home to help you and your family stay healthy.

The Importance of Handwashing

Handwashing is the easiest and the most effective way to prevent the spread of infection. Your hands

come in contact with microorganisms as you go about your daily routine, and they provide an ideal environment for the growth of pathogens. The hands are the most common carriers of disease. If you do not wash them frequently, pathogens can be transmitted from your hands to the patient or from the patient to you. Using the correct procedure for handwashing will protect the patients, visitors, and staff members. It also helps protect you and your family from disease. You should wash your hands

- Before and after caring for each patient
- Before and after using gloves

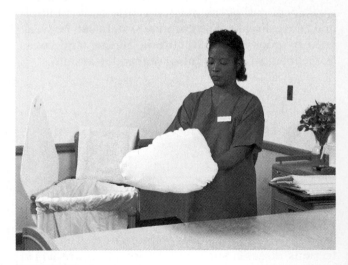

FIGURE 4–4
Never put dirty linens on the floor.

Procedure for Handwashing

1. Remove your watch or push it up out of the way.

2. Stand far enough away from the sink so that your uniform does not touch the sink and become contaminated.

3. Use a paper towel to turn the water on. (In some facilities this step is not considered necessary. Both the water faucet and your hands are "dirty.")

4. Adjust the water to a warm temperature. Discard the paper towel in the wastebasket.

5. Wet the hands and wrists thoroughly by holding them under running water. Hold the hands, fingertips down, lower than the elbows so that water runs off the finger tips.

6. Apply soap to the hands and work up a lather.

7. Wash the hands and wrists vigorously for at least 15 seconds. Apply friction to all surfaces of the hands as follows:

    a. Wash the palms and backs of the hands. Do not forget the outside surface of the thumb. (See Figure 4–5A.)

    b. Interlace the fingers and thumbs. Move the hands back and forth. (See Figure 4–5B.)

    c. Wash the wrists and lower arms 3 or 4 inches above the wrists using rotating movements.

8. Clean under each fingernail separately with an orange stick, as needed.

9. Rinse well, starting above the wrist and ending with the fingertips, keeping your hands lower than the elbows and the fingertips down. (See Figure 4–5C.)

10. Dry your hands thoroughly, using a separate paper towel for each hand. Discard the towels in the wastebasket.

11. Use dry paper towels to turn the water off and open the door. (See Figure 4–5D.) Discard the paper towels in the wastebasket.

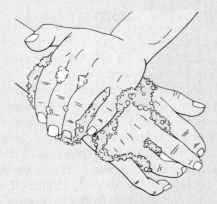

A. Wash the palms and backs of the hands.

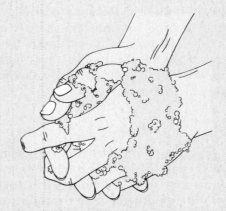

B. Interlace the fingers and thumbs and move the hands back and forth.

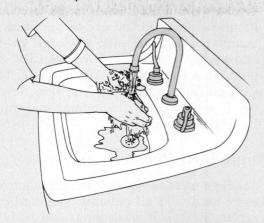

C. Keep your hands lower than your elbows with the fingertips down.

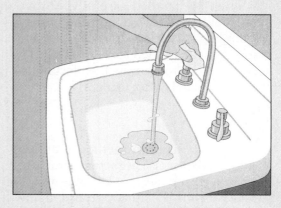

D. Use a dry paper towel to turn off the water faucet.

FIGURE 4–5
Handwashing procedure.

- Before and after eating
- After coughing, sneezing, or blowing your nose
- After combing your hair
- After using the toilet
- Before handling "clean" items
- After handling "dirty" items
- Before and after smoking
- Before handling contact lenses, using lip balm, or applying makeup

Proper handwashing requires the use of an antimicrobial soap. This type of soap helps destroy microorganisms. Most facilities provide liquid antimicrobial soap in dispensers. Bar soap is not recommended because pathogens can live on the surface of the bar. Use a lot of friction (rubbing your hands together), and be sure to wash between the fingers, the thumb area, and three or four inches above the wrist. Rinse your hands under running water that is not too hot because hot water irritates the skin.

There is much confusion today concerning the amount of time that hands should be washed. For many years it was believed that the hands should be washed for one full minute. Recent studies have shown that with vigorous friction and the use of antimicrobial soap, 15 seconds is sufficient. The CDC recommends washing the hands for at least 15 seconds. Your instructor will teach you the accepted time frame in your area.

Disinfection

Disinfection is the process of destroying pathogens on nondisposable items that have become contaminated. These items are usually cleaned with soap and water before disinfecting. Some examples of chemical disinfectants are hydrogen peroxide, alcohol, bleach, and Lysol. Disinfectants are strong chemicals and must be handled carefully. Always wear gloves and avoid inhaling any fumes that may be present. Do not wipe dry; allow the surface to air dry. Disinfectants must be labeled and stored in a secure place. It is important to return a disinfectant to its proper place immediately after using it.

Sterilization

The most common sterilization method requires bringing the object to a very high temperature, under pressure, for a period of time. The objective is to kill all microorganisms. For this purpose, many facilities use an autoclave, which produces steam under pressure, much like a pressure cooker. (See Figure 4–6.) Sterile items are placed in a sealed package. If the seal is broken, the item is no longer sterile. Special training is necessary to learn to per-

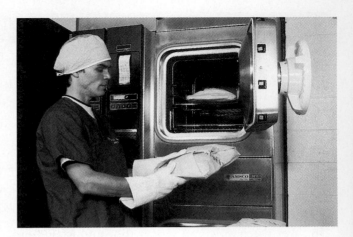

FIGURE 4–6
An autoclave is used to sterilize objects.

form sterile procedures correctly. Inserting urinary catheters and changing surgical wound dressings are examples of sterile procedures. In most facilities, nursing assistants are not allowed to perform sterile procedures.

Isolation Precautions

Isolation (separating a person from others) has been used as a method of infection control for many years. In the beginning, all persons infected with certain diseases were placed in separate hospitals to isolate them from uninfected persons. Later, infected persons were isolated according to their disease. Today, we treat **all** patients as potentially infectious, but we do not isolate all of them.

For several years the CDC recommended the use of universal precautions, a method of infection control that assumed that all human blood and body fluids were potentially infectious. Universal precautions included basic aseptic practices such as handwashing and the use of personal protective equipment barriers, such as gloves, gowns, masks, and eye protectors. In 1996 the CDC issued new guidelines for isolation precautions. The revised CDC guidelines consist of two tiers (levels) of precautions—standard precautions and transmission-based precautions.

Standard Precautions

Standard precautions are infection control practices to be used with **all** patients. Standard precautions replace universal precautions and body substance isolation. It stresses the importance of all body fluids, secretions, and excretions in the transmission of infection. Standard precautions are used when there is a possibility of contact with any of the following:

Guidelines for Standard Precautions

- Use standard precautions when caring for **all** patients.
- Wash hands after contact with blood, body fluids, secretions, excretions, or contaminated items.
- Wash hands after removing gloves and between patient contacts.
- Wear gloves when touching blood, body fluids, secretions, excretions, and contaminated items.
- Remove gloves promptly after use and before touching or going to another patient.
- Wear gowns when performing procedures where your clothing might come into contact with blood, body fluids, secretions, excretions, or contaminated items.
- Remove the used gown as soon as possible and wash your hands.
- Wear masks, face shields, and protective eyewear when contact with droplets or splashes of blood, body fluids, secretions, or excretions is possible.
- Remove masks, face shields, and protective eyewear as soon as possible and wash your hands.
- Handle soiled equipment in a manner that prevents contact with skin, mucous membranes, or clothing. Clean and disinfect soiled equipment according to facility policy.
- Treat all soiled linen as potentially infectious.
- Carefully dispose of sharp objects in the proper container.

- Blood
- All body fluids, secretions, and excretions
- Nonintact skin (sores, skin tears, and other injuries)
- Mucous membranes (thin sheets of tissue that line body openings)

Transmission-Based Precautions

The second tier of precautions is called *transmission-based precautions* and are to be used when the patient is known to be infected or suspected of being infected with certain contagious diseases or conditions. Transmission-based precautions are to be used in addition to standard precautions. Transmission-based precautions condense all types of isolation into three categories: contact precautions, droplet precautions, and airborne precautions.

Contact Precautions

In addition to standard precautions, contact precautions are used to prevent the spread of infection by direct contact (touching the infected area) or indirect contact (touching an object that has been in contact with the infected area). Examples of diseases that are spread by contact include skin or wound infections, infected pressure ulcers, pediculosis (lice), scabies ("the itch"), diphtheria, enteric (intestinal) infections, impetigo, conjunctivitis ("pink eye"), hepatitis A, herpes zoster (shingles), and *Escherichia coli* (*E. coli*) infections. The chart in Figure 4–7 provides instructions for following contact precautions.

Contact Precautions

Visitors report to nursing station before entering room.

- *Patient Placement*: Private room (if not available, place patient with another patient with similar microorganism, but with no other infection).
- *Gloves*: Wear gloves when entering the room and for all contact of patient and patient items, equipment, and body fluids.
- *Gown*: Wear a gown when entering the room if it is anticipated that your clothing will have substantial contact with the patient, environmental surfaces, or items in the patient's room.
- *Masks and Eyewear*: Indicated if potential for exposure to infectious body material exists.

Always use Standard Precautions.

- *Handwashing*: After glove removal, while ensuring that hands do not touch potentially contaminated environmental surfaces or items in the patient's room.
- *Transport*: Limit the movement and transport of the patient.
- *Patient Care Equipment*: When possible, dedicate the use of noncritical patient care equipment to a single patient.
- *Place Contact Precautions* sign on the door of the patient's room.

FIGURE 4–7
Contact precautions.

Droplet Precautions

Visitors report to nursing station before entering room.

- *Patient Placement*: Private room (if not available, place patient with a patient who has active infection with the same microorganism).

- *Gloves*: Must be worn when in contact with blood and body fluids.

- *Gowns*: Must be worn during procedures or situations where there will be exposure to body fluids, blood, draining wounds, or mucous membranes.

- *Masks and Eyewear*: In addition to *Standard Precautions*, **wear mask when working within three feet of patient** (or when entering patient's room).

Always use Standard Precautions.

- *Handwashing*: Hands must be washed before gloving and after gloves are removed.

- *Transport*: Limit the movement and transport of the patient from the room to essential purposes only. If necessary to move the patient, minimize patient dispersal of droplets by masking the patient if possible.

- *Patient Care Equipment*: When using common equipment or items, they must be adequately cleaned and disinfected.

- *Place Droplet Precautions* sign on the door of the patient's room.

FIGURE 4–8
Droplet precautions.

Droplet Precautions

In addition to standard precautions, droplet precautions are used to reduce the risk of spreading pathogens that are carried by large droplets that are produced either when the patient infected with a mouth or respiratory infection coughs, sneezes, or talks or by procedures that cause the patient to cough. Examples of diseases spread by droplets include pneumonia, influenza, meningitis, diphtheria, pertussis (whooping cough), rubella (measles), mumps, and streptococcal throat infections. The chart in Figure 4–8 provides instructions for following droplet precautions.

Airborne Precautions

In addition to standard precautions, airborne precautions are used to reduce the risk of spreading infections that are carried by small droplets that can

Airborne Precautions

Visitors report to nursing station before entering room.

- *Patient Placement*: Private room. Negative air pressure in relation to the surrounding areas. Keep doors closed at all times.

- *Gloves*: Same as *Standard Precautions*.

- *Gown or Apron*: Same as *Standard Precautions*.

- *Masks and Eyewear*: For known or suspected pulmonary tuberculosis: Mask: N-95 (respirator) must be worn by all individuals prior to entering room. For known or suspected airborne viral disease (for example, chickenpox or measles) standard mask should be worn by any person entering the room unless the person is not susceptible to the disease. When possible, persons who are susceptible should not enter the room.

Always use Standard Precautions.

- *Handwashing*: Hands must be washed before and after gloves are removed. Skin surfaces must be washed immediately and thoroughly when contaminated with body fluids or blood.

- *Patient Transport*: Limit the transport of the patient to essential purposes only. If transport is necessary, place a mask on the patient if possible.

- *Patient Care Equipment*: When using equipment or items (stethoscope, thermometer), they must be adequately cleaned and disinfected before use by another patient.

- *Place an Airborne Precautions* sign on the door of the patient's room.

FIGURE 4–9
Airborne precautions.

remain suspended in the air and be inhaled by an uninfected person. Examples of airborne diseases include measles, varicella (chickenpox), herpes zoster, and tuberculosis. The chart in Figure 4–9 provides instructions for following airborne precautions.

Isolation Practices

In recent years, isolation practices and procedures have changed dramatically. Many of these changes came about as a result of the concept of treating all patients as potentially infectious. For example, the dishes and eating utensils of patients in isolation are treated no differently than those of other patients because all used dishes and utensils are considered infectious. Therefore, double bagging of trays and dishes from isolation rooms is no longer necessary. The use of disposable dishes and utensils is rarely used for the same reason. Each facility has policies and procedures regarding contaminated dishes and eating utensils.

All used linen is considered infectious and should be handled carefully. Double bagging of linen and the use of meltaway bags have been discontinued in most facilities. Each facility has policies and procedures for handling contaminated linen.

Another change involves protective, or reverse, isolation. In this type of isolation the patient was isolated to help prevent him or her from being infected by others. Studies have shown that this procedure was not very effective in protecting the patient. However, some facilities may use special precautions to protect patients with weakened immune systems, such as those with AIDS or severe burns.

The best way to protect the patient, yourself, and others is to know and follow the policies and procedures of the facility in which you work. If you work in a facility that still practices procedures such as double bagging or protective isolation, your employer will provide the necessary training.

Protective Procedures

Protective procedures are those procedures necessary to protect you from, and prevent the spread of, infection. Health care facilities are required to provide whatever personal protection equipment is necessary at no charge to the employee. They must also provide training in the use of available equipment. This textbook gives instructions in the use of the most commonly used equipment: gloves, gowns, and masks.

Using Gloves

Gloves should be worn anytime there is a possibility that you will come into contact with blood, body fluids, secretions, excretions, or contaminated items. Put on gloves before touching mucous membranes or nonintact skin. Before putting on gloves, check them carefully for holes or other defects. Wash your hands, take a clean pair of gloves from the box, and put one on each hand. Avoid contaminating the gloves by touching an unclean surface. A clean pair of gloves must be worn for each patient and for each task performed. Gloves should be removed before leaving the patient's room. Never wear gloves out into the hallway.

When you are ready to remove the gloves, keep in mind that the outside surfaces are considered "dirty," and the inside surfaces of the gloves are considered "clean." Therefore, the outside of the gloves should not touch your skin or any clean area. After removing gloves, wash your hands and dispose of the gloves appropriately. (See Figure 4–10.) The procedure for removing gloves is located on page 48.

Using a Disposable Gown

A gown should be worn anytime there is a possibility that your clothing might come into contact with blood, body fluids, secretions, excretions, nonintact skin, or mucous membranes. The gown must be large enough to cover the entire uniform in order to protect it from contamination. Some gowns have ties at the waist and neck to secure the gown, and others are used as a "pullover." Adhesive strips may be used instead of ties. Most gowns are disposable and are discarded after one use. Remove soiled gowns as promptly as possible and wash your hands. Gowns are usually fluid resistant, but if the gown becomes damp it must be changed immediately. The following procedure is for a disposable gown with ties. Keep in mind that the ties at the neck are considered clean and are untied last when removing the gown. When gloves are worn, they should come up over the cuffs of the sleeves of the gown. See Figure 4–11 on page 49 for putting on a gown. See Figure 4–12 on page 50 for removing a gown.

Using a Mask

A mask is needed when there is a danger of infection by inhaling airborne organisms and to prevent blood, body fluids, secretions, or excretions from getting into your mouth or nose. Protective eyewear,

Procedure for Removing Gloves

1. Remove the first glove using the following steps:
   a. Grasp the glove at the palm of the hand, with the gloved fingers of the other hand (Figure 4–10A).
   b. Pull the glove over your hand, while turning the glove inside out (Figure 4–10B).
2. Continue holding the removed glove with the gloved hand.

3. Place the ungloved index and middle fingers under the cuff of the remaining glove (Figure 4–10C).
4. Carefully turn the cuff downward, pulling it inside out over your hand and over the other glove (Figure 4–10D).
5. Discard the gloves according to facility policy.
6. Wash your hands.

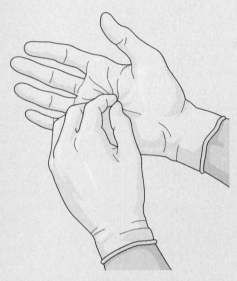

A. Grasp the glove at the palm of the hand with the gloved fingers of the other hand.

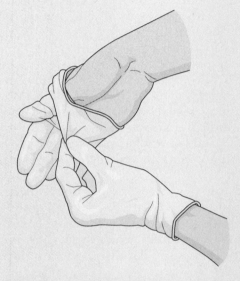

B. Pull the glove over your hand while turning the glove inside out.

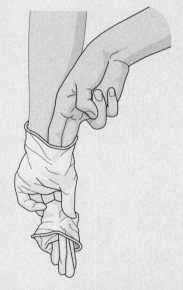

C. Place the ungloved index and middle fingers under the cuff of the remaining glove.

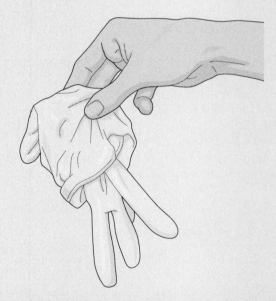

D. Turn the cuff downward, pulling it inside out over your hand and over the other glove.

FIGURE 4–10
Removing gloves.

Procedure for Putting on a Gown

1. Wash your hands.
2. Unfold the clean gown so the opening is in the back. Do not shake the gown or allow it to touch an unclean surface.
3. Slide your hands and arms through the sleeves of the gown.
4. Make sure the gown is snug at the neck and covers your uniform.
5. Tie the ties at the neck of the gown.
6. Overlap the back of the gown to cover your entire uniform.
7. Fasten the ties at the waist of the gown.
8. Gloves should be pulled up over the cuffs of the gown. (See Figure 4–11.)

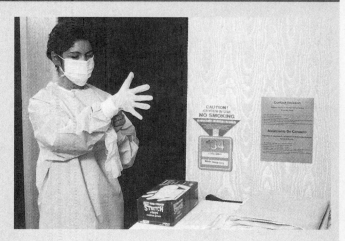

FIGURE 4–11
Pull the gloves up over the cuffs of the gown.

such as goggles or a face mask, may also be necessary in this situation. If the mask becomes damp before you are finished with your task, the mask must be changed immediately. Do not drape the mask around your neck where it can contaminate your uniform. Do not wear it out of the patient unit. Discard the mask as soon as you remove it. There are several types of masks available. (See Figure 4–13.) The procedures on page 51 are for the type with string ties at the bottom and top.

Patient Care Equipment

Disposable patient care equipment should be discarded in the proper container as soon as possible. Reusable equipment soiled with blood, body fluids, secretions, or excretions must be handled carefully. Avoid contact with skin, mucous membranes, or clothing. Clean and disinfect used equipment before using it to care for another patient. Use cleaning procedures according to facility policy.

Linen

Consider all used linen as potentially infectious. Linen that has been soiled by blood, body fluids, secretions, or excretions should be handled and transmitted in a manner that prevents skin contact, clothing contamination, and transfer of microorganisms. Double bagging is not required.

Handling Needles and Other Sharp Objects

Sharps injuries involving needle sticks are a common source of work-related infections in health care workers. Infection control policies and procedures have targeted the problem for years. According to the CDC, most needle-stick injuries can be avoided by using safer needle-stick devices. Some examples include needleless devices, shielded needles, and blunt needles. Advances in technology have made it possible to eliminate sharps for many uses. Placing sharps containers within easy reach in every patient's room also reduces the risk. Recent legislation requires the use of safer devices to prevent sharps injuries.

As a nursing assistant you will not use needles and syringes as often as nurses or lab technicians. However, with cross-training and multitasking the risk will increase. Remember that razors are also considered sharps, so be careful when handling them. The rules apply to everyone and are there to protect you and other health care workers.

Needles and syringes should be disposed of promptly and should never be bent, broken, or recapped. Wear gloves and handle sharp items, such as razor blades, carefully. All sharp objects should be disposed of immediately after use in a puncture-proof container. Do not force an item into the container, and notify the nurse when the container is full.

Procedure for Removing a Gown

1. Untie the ties at the waist of the gown.
2. If you are wearing gloves, remove them.
3. Wash your hands.
4. Untie the ties at the neck without touching your neck or the outside of the gown.
5. Pull each sleeve off by grasping each shoulder on the inside of the gown, at the neck line (see Figure 4–12A).
   a. Do not contaminate your hands by touching the outside of the gown.
   b. Turn the sleeves and gown inside out as you slide your arms up through them (see Figure 4–12B).

6. Holding the gown away from your body by the inside of the shoulder seams, fold it inside out, bringing the shoulders together (see Figure 4–12C).
7. Roll the gown up with the soiled side inside, and do not let it touch your uniform. Discard it in the appropriate container (see Figure 4–12D).
8. Wash your hands (see Figure 4–12E).

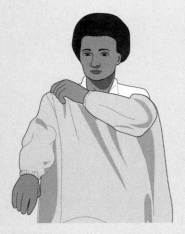

A. Pull each sleeve off by grasping each shoulder on the inside of the gown at the neckline.

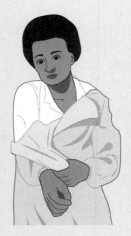

B. Turn the sleeves and gown inside out as you slide your arms up through the sleeves.

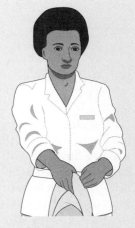

C. Holding the gown away from your body, fold it inside out, bringing the shoulders together.

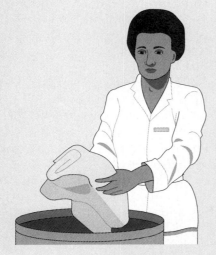

D. Roll the gown up with the soiled side inside and discard it in the appropriate container.

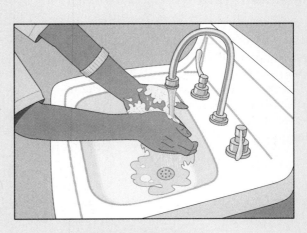

E. Wash your hands after you remove the gown.

FIGURE 4–12
Removing a gown.

Procedure for Putting on a Mask

1. Wash your hands.
2. Place the upper edge of the mask over the bridge of your nose. Be careful not to touch the part of the mask that will cover your face.
3. Tie the upper ties over your ears.
4. Adjust the lower edge of the mask under your chin.

5. Tie the lower ties at the nape of your neck.
6. If the mask has a metal strip in the upper edge, form it to your nose for a close fit. If you are wearing glasses or goggles, the mask should be under the bottom of the glasses or goggles.

Procedure for Removing a Mask

1. Wash your hands.
2. Untie the ties.

3. Discard the mask by touching only the strings. Dispose of the mask in the proper container.
4. Wash your hands.

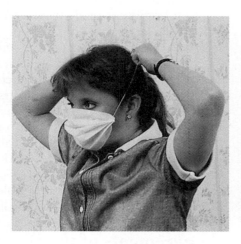

A. Fasten the mask to fit snugly over the nose and mouth.

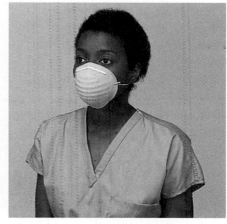

B. The rigid mask snaps easily into place.

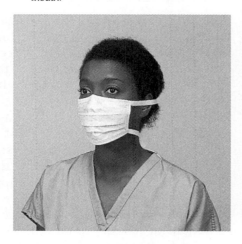

C. This type of mask provides extra filtration.

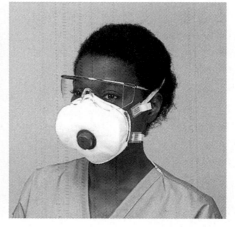

D. Goggles or eyeglasses may be worn with the mask.

FIGURE 4–13
Types of isolation masks.

A Holistic Approach to Isolation

Patients may be isolated at bedside in their unit or in a separate room. Isolation can have a negative impact on the patient's well-being. To be separated from others, to be alone, somehow suggests that the isolated patient is "bad" or has done something wrong. In many cultures isolation is a form of punishment, and the isolated patient may feel "dirty" or ashamed. Feelings of unworthiness can damage self-esteem.

Isolation affects the patient physically, emotionally, and socially. These needs must be addressed for quality care to be delivered. Be sensitive to each patient's needs. Use empathy—try to think how you would feel if you had to be isolated. Being alone might be a pleasant relief for a while, but what if it went on for hours or days? How would you feel?

Staff members often become the major support system of the isolated patient. To be truly supportive, you will need to examine your attitude toward isolation and infection. If you are afraid, these feelings will interfere with your ability to help the patient. Knowledge and experience can help you to overcome your fears. Talk with the nurse about your feelings and ask questions that concern you. The more times you perform isolation procedures, the more confident you will become.

Encourage communication while you are in the isolation room. Listen to the patient's fears, concerns, and complaints and solve any problems that you can. Show the patient that you care by offering an additional touch, such as a backrub, a touch on the hand, or a hug if it seems appropriate. Touch can be a powerful communicator.

Bring the isolated patient disposable reading materials, such as newspapers or magazines. If there is a telephone in the room, encourage the patient to talk to friends and family members. Assist visitors with protective equipment as necessary and help to make their visits as pleasant as possible. You can make a difference in the quality of life of the isolated patient. (See Figure 4–14.)

Bloodborne Pathogens Standard

As mentioned previously, OSHA is a governmental agency that is concerned with the health and safety of workers. The Bloodborne Pathogens Standard was written by OSHA to help protect health care workers who come into contact with blood or other infectious materials.

Bloodborne pathogens are disease-causing microorganisms that are found in blood, human blood components, any body fluid that contains blood cells, and products made from human blood tissue. They are transmitted by direct or indirect contact with blood or body fluids and by needle sticks and injuries from sharp objects that are contaminated. The bloodborne diseases of most concern in health care today are hepatitis B, hepatitis C, and HIV infection. These diseases are discussed in Chapter 5.

Recent OSHA amendments to the Bloodborne Pathogens Standard require all health care facilities to use safer devices to protect workers from sharps injuries. These actions are designed to reduce health care workers' exposure to blood and prevent occupational transmission of bloodborne diseases.

Requirements of the Bloodborne Pathogens Standard

Employers must establish an exposure control plan that identifies workers at risk for occupational exposure to blood and other infectious material. The plan must include methods to protect and train employees. Bloodborne pathogens training must be provided annually at no cost to the worker. Personal protective equipment, such as gowns, gloves, and masks, must be provided at no cost to the health care worker. Puncture-resistant boxes must be available for needles and other disposable sharp objects. Needles must not be recapped, broken, or bent.

Employers are required to offer hepatitis B vaccinations at no cost to all employees who have a high risk of occupational exposure to the disease. The vaccine is given in three doses. It is up to the employee to choose whether or not to take the vaccine.

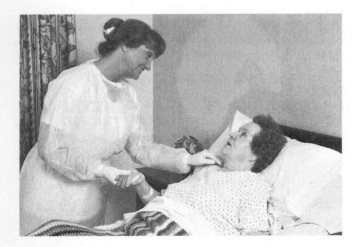

FIGURE 4–14
You can make a difference in the quality of life of the isolated patient.

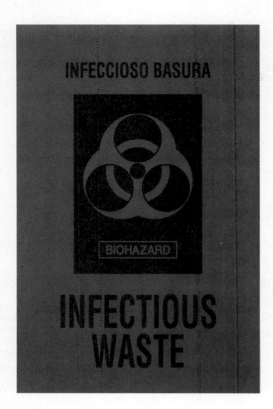

FIGURE 4–15
A biohazard label indicates that the contents are infectious.

Infectious Waste

There are requirements for the housekeeping and maintenance departments regarding decontamination and disposal of biohazardous waste (items contaminated by blood, body fluids, or body substances that can cause infection). All bags, boxes, and other containers of biohazardous waste must be clearly identified with a biohazardous label. (See Figure 4–15.) They cannot be disposed of in the regular trash.

Exposure Incidents

OSHA requires that all exposures to bloodborne pathogens such as needle sticks and blood splashes be recorded and reviewed regularly. Exposure incidents are to be reported immediately. Medical follow-up is offered free to employees. Free testing is available at the time of the incident or at a later date if the employee requests it. If you are involved in an exposure incident, report it to your supervisor at once.

Health care workers are still responsible for protecting themselves, by attending training programs and by consistently following infection control practices such as handwashing. All the laws in the world will not help if health care workers do not practice infection control or follow standard precautions.

Review

Read each sentence and fill in the blank with the vocabulary term that best completes the sentence.

1. _____ is the term for any small plant or animal that cannot be seen without a microscope.
2. A microorganism that is harmful and can cause disease is called a _____.
3. _____ refers to items or areas that have been exposed to disease-causing microorganisms.
4. A person who is likely to develop an infection or disease when exposed to pathogens is said to be _____.
5. Microorganisms that live and grow in certain locations of the body are called _____.

Remember

1. Always follow the infection control policies where you work or train.
2. Pathogens are microorganisms that cause infection; nonpathogens do not cause infection.
3. Microorganisms thrive in a warm, dark, moist environment.
4. Infection follows a chain of events that can be broken at any time.
5. It is important to recognize the signs of infection and report them immediately.
6. The infection control professional (ICP) works to prevent infection, follows up on outbreaks, and provides education.
7. Infection control is the responsibility of all health care workers.
8. Handwashing is the most effective method of preventing the spread of infection.
9. Standard precautions should be followed while caring for **all** patients.

10. In addition to standard precautions, transmission-based precautions should be used when the patient is known to be infected or suspected of being infected with certain communicable diseases.

11. Needles and syringes should be disposed of promptly and carefully in a special sharps container.

12. Your attitude toward infection and isolation will affect your response to the isolated patient.

13. The Bloodborne Pathogens Standard is designed to reduce health care workers' exposure to blood and prevent occupational transmission of bloodborne pathogens.

14. Containers of biohazardous waste must be clearly identified with a biohazardous label.

 Reflect

Read the following case study and answer the questions.

Case Study

Tiffany Moore is a 10-year-old patient who is in the hospital with a broken leg. She has impetigo on her other leg and has been placed on contact isolation. James, her nursing assistant for the day, wears gloves while bathing her. When he is through, he goes out of the room to the dirty utility room to remove his gloves and wash his hands. He washes his hands for 15 seconds with antimicrobial soap. He holds his hands with the fingertips pointed upward while drying them. He uses a separate paper towel for each hand.

1. What protective equipment will James need to wear while bathing Tiffany?

2. Since she is on contact precautions, will standard precautions be necessary?

3. What steps of the handwashing procedure did James do correctly? What steps were incorrect?

4. What should James have done about removing his gloves after bathing Tiffany?

 Respond

Choose the best answer for each question.

1. An infection that a patient acquires after entering a health care facility is called
   A. An enteric infection
   B. A nosocomial infection
   C. A social infection
   D. An aerobic infection

2. Which of the following statements about microorganisms is TRUE?
   A. Microorganisms thrive in a warm, dark, moist environment.
   B. Pathogens are microorganisms that do not cause disease.
   C. All microorganisms are harmful.
   D. Microorganisms are killed by cold temperatures.

3. A place where microorganisms live and grow is called a/an
   A. Portal of entry
   B. Susceptible host
   C. Agent
   D. Reservoir

4. The initials ICP stand for
   A. Infection control policy
   B. Infection control professional
   C. Infection control place
   D. Infection control procedure

5. Which of the following is a guideline for medical asepsis?
   A. Take all contaminated items to the clean utility room.
   B. It is alright to place soiled linen on the floor.
   C. Wash your hands after sneezing.
   D. Place the bedpan on the overbed table.

6. When rinsing your hands, hold your fingertips
   A. Pointed upward
   B. Pointed downward
   C. Against the side of the sink
   D. Over the waste basket

7. You can be certain an item is sterile if
   A. The seal is unbroken
   B. It is labeled "sterile"
   C. It is in the clean utility room
   D. It is wrapped in sterile paper

8. Which type of isolation would be used for tuberculosis?
   A. Contact
   B. Enteric
   C. Bloodborne
   D. Airborne

9. When would it be necessary to wear gloves?
   A. When feeding a patient
   B. When performing routine care
   C. When touching nonintact skin
   D. When combing the patient's hair

10. Which of the following statements about bloodborne pathogens is FALSE?
    A. HIV infection is caused by a bloodborne pathogen.
    B. The Bloodborne Pathogen Standard is enforced by OSHA.
    C. Biohazardous waste must all be labeled.
    D. Your employer can charge you for the hepatitis B vaccine.

Chapter Five

Communicable Diseases

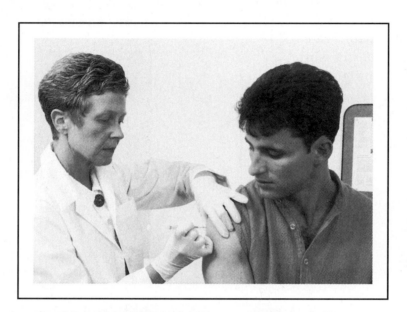

OBJECTIVES

*A*fter
studying
this chapter,
you will
be able to
_____

1. Explain how most childhood communicable diseases can be prevented.

2. List three methods of transmission of HIV.

3. Identify two ways to prevent the spread of HIV infection.

4. Explain how hepatitis A, hepatitis B, and hepatitis C are transmitted.

5. Briefly describe the process for controlling sexually transmitted diseases in the United States.

6. List four risk groups for tuberculosis.

7. Identify three methods to prevent and control the spread of tuberculosis.

8. Describe the TB skin test that is mandatory for most health care workers.

9. Identify three emerging infectious diseases.

A *communicable disease* is a disease that spreads easily from one person to another. In the past, most communicable diseases were uncontrollable. Some were deadly killers. However, many of these diseases have been eliminated or brought under control in the United States. Diseases like yellow fever, cholera, smallpox, diphtheria, and typhoid fever are rarely seen in America today. Many unimmunized children, though, still get diseases such as measles and chickenpox. Other diseases, like tuberculosis, hepatitis B, and HIV, are on the increase.

Communicable diseases are caused by pathogens, and preventing transmission of the disease depends on how the pathogen is spread. Frequent handwashing and following standard precautions is especially important because patients are usually *infectious* (capable of spreading infection) before symptoms appear. (Standard precautions were explained in Chapter 4. A review may be helpful.)

Childhood Communicable Diseases

Even though they can be prevented by *immunization* (a procedure to make a person more resistant to a specific disease), the most common communicable diseases that infect children today are chickenpox, whooping cough, mumps, and measles. A substance that is given to increase immunity against specific pathogens is called a vaccine. Antibodies, a substance that is produced by the immune system when a foreign body (a virus, for example) invades the body, are produced when a vaccine is given. These antibodies protect the person from getting the disease.

Current immunization schedules recommend that more immunizations be given at a single visit and that children be immunized fully by the age of two. Recommended immunizations include DTP (diphtheria, tetanus, and pertussis), MMR (measles, mumps, and rubella), chickenpox, oral polio vaccine, influenza, and hepatitis B. In the United States, immunizations are required for all children to be able to attend school. Most childhood diseases could be prevented by proper immunizations. (See Figure 5–1.)

Due to public misunderstanding and mistrust, many children do not receive immunizations. Poor access to services and crowded clinics contribute to the problem in some areas.

However, cultural and religious bias is the major cause of misunderstanding. Some religious groups discourage or forbid the use of vaccines. While most Americans are familiar with immunization programs, people from other parts of the world may be distrustful. The concept of giving medicine to healthy children may be entirely foreign to them. Explanations must be given and often repeated in a language they can understand. Your support and encouragement will be helpful.

Chickenpox (Varicella)

Chickenpox is caused by a virus that enters the body through the respiratory system. It is transmitted by direct or indirect contact with droplets from the respiratory tract of an infected child. Symptoms of chickenpox include fever, fatigue, and a rash that may appear all over the body. Complications can include pneumonia, encephalitis, and meningitis. The time period between exposure to a disease and the appearance of symptoms is called the incubation period. The incubation period for chickenpox is two to three weeks. It is most *contagious* (easily transmitted) one to two days be-

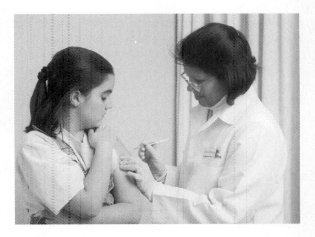

FIGURE 5–1
Many childhood diseases can be prevented by immunization.

fore the rash appears and remains contagious until crusts form on the rash. One attack usually provides lifelong immunity, and second attacks are rare. A vaccine is available.

Whooping Cough (Pertussis)

Whooping cough is caused by a virus that infects the respiratory system and is transmitted by contact with droplets from the respiratory tract of an infected child. Whooping cough usually affects children under the age of seven who have not been immunized. Symptoms of whooping cough include spasms of hard coughing that end in a high-pitched whooping sound. Nausea and vomiting commonly occur. Complications can include pneumonia, ear infection, and bleeding of lung tissue. The incubation period for whooping cough is 7 to 21 days. It is highly contagious before symptoms actually appear and continues to be so for about three weeks. Having the disease provides lifelong immunity. A vaccine is available.

Mumps (Parotitis)

Mumps is caused by a virus that is transmitted by saliva or droplets from an infected person. Symptoms include localized *edema* (swelling of a body part due to fluid in the tissues) of one or more of the salivary glands in the neck. It may occasionally spread to other glands, including the testes in males. The incubation period for mumps is two to three weeks. It is contagious from six days before symptoms appear through nine days after they appear. An attack provides lifelong immunity. A vaccine is available to prevent mumps.

Measles

There are two types of measles—rubeola and rubella. Measles may also occur in adults. Vaccines are available for both types.

Rubeola (Red or Hard Measles)

Rubeola is the more common measles and is caused by a virus that invades the respiratory system. It is transmitted directly or indirectly through respirations from an infected person. Symptoms vary from mild to severe and include fever, bronchitis, and a red, blotchy rash that starts on the face and spreads over the entire body. The rash usually lasts four to seven days. Complications can include ear infection, eye infection, pneumonia, and encephalitis. The incubation period for rubeola is one to two weeks. It is contagious from two to four days before the rash appears until two to five days after it appears. There is permanent immunity after an attack.

Rubella (German Measles)

German measles, also known as "three-day measles" is caused by a virus and is transmitted by contact with secretions from the nose or throat of an infected person. In pregnant women, infection in the first trimester (three months) can cause birth defects or death of the unborn baby. Symptoms of rubella include fever, fatigue, headache, swollen glands, and a rash. Complications are rare. The incubation period is 14 to 21 days, and it is most contagious from seven days before the rash appears through four days after it appears. One attack provides lifelong immunity.

Communicable Diseases			
Name	Incubation	Symptoms	Transmission
Chickenpox (Varicella)*	14–21 days	Rash, fever, fatigue	Virus; respiratory droplets
Whooping cough (Pertussis)*	7–21 days	Hard coughing spasms, nausea, vomiting	Virus; respiratory droplets
Mumps (Parotitis)*	13–21 days	Edema of salivary glands	Virus; respiratory droplets
Measles (Rubeola)*	7–14 days	Rash, fever, cough	Virus; direct or indirect contact; droplets
Measles (Rubella)*	14–21 days	Rash, fever, fatigue, swollen glands	Virus; direct or indirect contact; droplets

*Immunization available

FIGURE 5–2
Common communicable diseases of children.

Most of the childhood communicable diseases spread quickly because they are highly contagious before symptoms appear. A school-age child infected with chickenpox can expose an entire class before a rash ever appears. (See Figure 5–2.)

Scabies and Lice

Scabies and lice generally begin in environments in which hygiene is poor, but because they are highly contagious they can spread to anyone. Scabies and lice infect adults as well as children.

Scabies

Scabies, commonly called "the itch," is caused by mites that burrow into the skin. A rash and skin sores develop around the fingers, wrists, underarms, and genitals. Folds of skin under the breasts and around the abdomen and buttocks may be affected. Intense itching results and is usually more severe at night, so rest and sleep may be disturbed. Scabies is transmitted by direct contact with infected individuals. Hot baths with thorough cleansing of the involved areas is recommended. Starch or medicated baths may be ordered. Clean underclothing and bed linens are necessary. The physician will order ointments to relieve itching and medications to destroy the mites.

Lice (Pediculosis)

Lice may infect the skin or the hair. The presence of head lice is determined by close visual inspection of the scalp for nits (eggs of the lice). The nits mature in 3 to 14 days and produce more lice. Itching is severe, and scratching may result in an infection of the scalp. Transmission occurs through personal contact or contact with contaminated objects, such as combs and hats. A medicated shampoo or cream is available that usually destroys the lice and the nits. Treatment must be repeated in a week to kill newly hatched lice. Combs, brushes, bed linens, mattresses, and pillows must also be thoroughly cleansed.

Body lice may be found on the skin and clothing of infected persons. Treatment focuses on destroying the lice with insecticides. Thorough cleansing of the body, clothing, bed linens, mattresses, pillows, and upholstery is necessary.

The Common Cold

The common cold is caused by assorted viruses that are often called "rhino viruses" (*rhino* means "nose"). The nose frequently runs, stops up, gets red, and becomes sore. It usually involves an acute infection of the upper respiratory system. Although

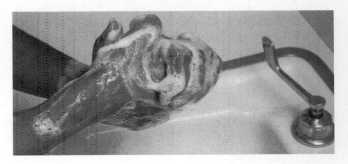

FIGURE 5–3
Handwashing helps to prevent transmission of the common cold.

the pathogens that cause the common cold are airborne, transmission generally occurs through direct or indirect contact with droplets or secretions on the hands. Touching the eyes, nose, or mouth with contaminated hands can carry the virus into the body. Symptoms include sore throat, sneezing, headache, fatigue, body aches and pains, and fever. Taste and smell may be affected, and a cough may develop. Complications can include ear infection or laryngitis. Symptoms usually last 4 to 10 days, regardless of treatment.

Although handwashing helps to prevent transmission of the common cold, there is no method of prevention, and no vaccine available. Treatment is aimed at symptom control. Antibiotics are not indicated unless a secondary infection occurs.

Patients who have colds or any other type of respiratory infection can help to prevent spreading the infection to others. Remind them to cover the mouth or nose when coughing or sneezing. Disposable tissues are safer than handkerchiefs. When possible, tissues should be discarded by the patient into a plastic bag. (See Figure 5–3.)

Influenza

Influenza (commonly called the flu) is caused by several types of viruses. New ones appear each year. The disease can range from a few isolated cases to an epidemic. The term *epidemic* means that a large number of people in a certain area are infected with the same disease. The onset of respiratory influenza is sudden, with chills, fever, aches, and pains. Headache, sore throat, cough, and fatigue usually follow. Symptoms fade as the fever decreases, but weakness may continue for days. Complications can include secondary bacterial infections. Influenza can be fatal to infants and to the frail elderly. The incubation period for influenza is one to three days. Influenza vaccine is available each year that may prevent or lessen the severity of the attack of certain types of influenza. The Centers for Disease Control and Prevention (CDC) recommends that health care workers get the vaccine yearly. Annual flu immunizations are also recommended for persons who are elderly or who have a chronic illness or a weakened immune system.

HIV Infection

HIV (human immunodeficiency virus) infection is a disease that destroys the immune system and leaves the body unable to fight infection. Originally, the disease was called **AIDS** (acquired immune deficiency syndrome), and the term is still frequently used. However, the correct term is HIV infection, or HIV disease, while the term AIDS refers to the acute stage of the disease. Although the rates of HIV infection and AIDS-related deaths in the United States appear to be leveling off, a worldwide epidemic continues. AIDS is the leading cause of death in some countries.

Cause

HIV infection is caused by a virus called HIV (human immunodeficiency virus). The virus enters the bloodstream and lives in the cells of the immune system (the body's defense system). The virus attacks and destroys certain white blood cells of the immune system called T4 cells. The death of these cells results in the person becoming immune deficient. (See Figure 5–4.) The term "immune deficient" means that the immune system does not have enough cells to defend the body against invading diseases. Once a person is infected with HIV, he or she is infectious and can transmit the disease to someone else. HIV-2 is also a virus that causes AIDS. Most of the people infected with HIV-2 are from West Africa or are the sexual partners of people from that part of the world.

Risk Groups

A risk group consists of people who share similar characteristics that make them likely to be exposed to a certain disease. Individuals who are at high risk of getting HIV are:

■ Men who have sex with men
■ Injectable drug users
■ Sexual partners of persons infected with HIV
■ Babies born to HIV-infected mothers
■ Individuals who receive blood transfusions contaminated by HIV
■ Hemophiliacs

Hemophilia is a disease in which the factor that causes blood to clot is missing. The hemophiliac

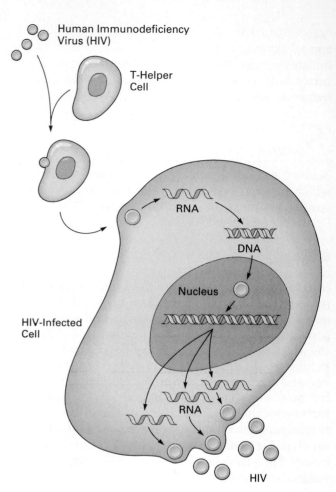

FIGURE 5–4
HIV enters the bloodstream and destroys the defense cells of the immune system.

can bleed to death from a minor cut or other injury. Treatment for hemophilia is frequent transfusion of blood or blood products. Frequent exposure to blood, blood products, or transfusions places the hemophiliac at increased risk of HIV infection.

Transmission

The most common methods of transmission of HIV are:

■ Sexual contact with an infected person
■ Sharing HIV-contaminated needles and syringes
■ HIV-infected mother to baby
■ Transfusion of blood contaminated by HIV

HIV infection is primarily a *sexually transmitted disease (STD)*, a disease in which the major route of transmission is sexual. Since the CDC first began tracking HIV, the highest risk group in the United States has been homosexual males. However, in recent years, the percentage of persons infected through the use of illegal injectable drugs has increased rapidly. Worldwide, the most frequent transmission of HIV is heterosexual contact with an infected person. Sexual behavior that involves exposure to blood is likely to increase the risk of HIV transmission.

Today, all blood collected for transfusions in the United States is tested for evidence of the virus. This practice has reduced the risk to hemophiliacs and others who receive blood transfusions or blood products. However, some people were already infected by contaminated blood before 1985, when testing the blood supply for HIV began.

HIV is not highly communicable because the virus is not airborne, and it can live only in certain body fluids. The concentration of HIV is greatest in blood, semen, vaginal secretions, and body fluids containing visible blood. There is no evidence that HIV is spread by casual contact, toilet seats, mosquitos, coughing or sneezing, or working and eating with an HIV-positive person.

Prevention

Since HIV is transmitted primarily by sexual contact, behavioral changes must be made in order to stop the rapid spread of disease. People must be aware of the danger of casual sex and of having multiple sex partners. Using condoms also helps to prevent the spread of HIV. The safest behavior is to have a mutually trusting relationship with only one sexual partner who is not HIV infected. Sharing contaminated needles and syringes can transmit the virus. Realizing that injectable drug users usually do not quit in spite of the risk of HIV, some states are providing clean needles and syringes to persons who use injectable drugs. Pregnancy is not recommended for women who are HIV positive. However, medication is available that can be given to the pregnant woman to reduce the risk of infecting the baby. It is also recommended that an HIV-positive mother not breastfeed her infant.

Most of the efforts for prevention of pediatric HIV is focused on counseling parents. In the beginning of the AIDS epidemic, most HIV infections in children were caused by contaminated blood and blood products. That problem was brought under control by effective screening of donors and the blood supply. Today, the primary route of HIV transmission in children is from an infected mother to her baby.

Occupational Exposure

The risk of getting HIV infection on the job is very slight if infection control practices are followed. Only a small number of occupational transmissions of HIV have been documented. Most of those involved instances where nurses or laboratory workers accidentally injected a large dose of HIV-infected blood into themselves.

Needles and sharp objects were involved in the majority of occupational exposures. A razor is an example of a sharp object that nursing assistants use. Handle razors carefully and avoid nicking the patient or yourself. As soon as you are through using any sharp object, dispose of it in a puncture-proof biohazardous container. (See Figure 5–5.)

Regular infection-control practices, especially handwashing, are very important in preventing the transmission of HIV infection in the workplace. Use standard precautions when caring for all patients, because you probably will not know which patients are infected. HIV is a fragile virus that is easily destroyed by chemicals that are commonly found in health care facilities, such as alcohol, Lysol, peroxide, and any other approved germicide. A mixture of one part bleach and nine parts water, prepared fresh every 24 hours, will also kill the virus.

If you think you have been exposed to blood or body fluids, report the incident to the nurse immediately. Health care workers who have had a documented exposure to HIV may be included in a postexposure program (PEP). This program offers testing, counseling, and drug regimes.

Education

Education helps to prevent the spread of HIV. Health care facilities are required to provide in-service education about HIV infection. New information about the disease appears regularly in newspapers, in magazines, and on television. The infection control nurse in your facility will have the most up-to-date information. It is your responsibility to stay informed with current, correct information about HIV infection.

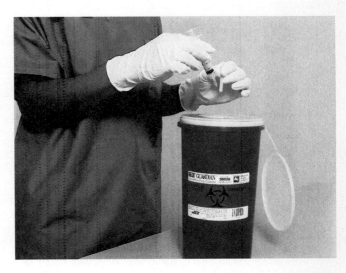

FIGURE 5–5
Dispose of sharp objects in a biohazardous container immediately after use.

Education has been concentrated on young, sexually active adults within the highest-risk groups. School programs are usually determined by state regulation, with the focus on teenagers. Little attention has been given to people over the age of 50. In recent years there has been a dramatic increase in STDs, including HIV infection, in the elderly. Educators are now targeting that group of people.

Signs and Symptoms

An individual who is infected with HIV may have no symptoms at all and may not even feel sick. The person may not even realize that he or she is infected. When symptoms appear, they may include fatigue, diarrhea, weight loss, fever, night sweats, and loss of appetite. Wasting syndrome, with significant weight loss, lack of appetite, and diarrhea, leaves the patient even more susceptible to other infections. The emotional devastation is as great as the physical problems. Anger, fear, guilt, and depression are all possible. An opportunistic disease may develop.

Opportunistic Diseases

An opportunistic disease is a disease that takes advantage of the body's loss of immunity and infects the body. Pneumonia, cancer, tuberculosis, thrush, fungal infections, and shingles are examples of opportunistic diseases that may occur in patients with HIV infection. The infection may lead to AIDS dementia with symptoms such as confusion, seizures, mood changes, or blindness. Most AIDS patients die of either pneumocystis carinii pneumonia (PCP), a rare form of pneumonia, or Kaposi's sarcoma (KS), a rare form of cancer.

Testing

The antibody to the HIV virus has been identified, and tests are available for screening purposes. Tests are available to determine if a person has developed antibodies to the virus. However, it takes several weeks after infection for the body to develop antibodies. During that time, a person who was infected might test negative but would already be infectious and able to transmit the disease. If no antibodies develop within five or six months after an exposure to HIV, the exposed person probably has not been infected. Every exposure to HIV does **not** result in infection.

Treatment of HIV Infection

At the present time, there is no vaccine available to prevent HIV infection, and there is no cure for AIDS. However, many drugs are now available for treatment. Azidothymidine (AZT), Didanosine (ddI), and pentamidine have been effectively used for several years. Protease inhibitors, which prevent replication (making more viruses), are now available. Treatment usually includes a combination of drugs. All of these drugs can have serious side effects. They are not effective in all cases and are very expensive. With early, aggressive treatment, AIDS patients are living longer and more comfortable lives. Unfortunately, because of expense and the lack of health care delivery systems, drug treatment is not available to people in some parts of the world.

Legal Issues

Federal and state laws have been passed concerning HIV reporting, education, testing, confidentiality, and discrimination. Laws are constantly changing in an effort to protect the rights of both HIV-infected patients and the public. Although your facility will provide regular HIV education, it is your responsibility to keep up with current legal issues in your area.

Nursing Care

As a nursing assistant, you may be caring for patients with HIV disease and AIDS. You will need to develop a supportive, nonjudgmental attitude in order to provide quality care. Care of the patient with HIV infection is discussed in Chapter 28.

Hepatitis

Hepatitis is a disease that affects the liver and causes the skin to look yellow (jaundice). Symptoms other than jaundice include fatigue, abdominal pain, loss of appetite, nausea, and vomiting. There are several types of hepatitis but the three most common are hepatitis A, hepatitis B, and hepatitis C. While all three are contagious, they are not transmitted in the same way. (See Figure 5–6.) There is no cure for hepatitis.

Hepatitis A

Hepatitis A is usually transmitted through contaminated food and water. Although it is not a major threat in the United States, it is still a problem in many underdeveloped countries where proper hygiene and sanitation practices are not in use. An attack of hepatitis A provides lifelong immunity. There is no carrier state and complications are rare. A vaccine is available, but in the United States it is recommended only for children between the ages of 2 and 18. Prevention involves using good hygiene and sanitation procedures.

Hepatitis			
	Hepatitis A	Hepatitis B	Hepatitis C
Transmission	Oral–fecal, poor sanitation, contaminated food and water	Bloodborne: sexual activity, drug abuse, contaminated needles, perinatal	Bloodborne: sexual activity, drug abuse, perinatal
Complications	Rare	Chronic liver disease, liver cancer	Chronic infections, chronic liver disease, liver failure
Carrier State	None	10% become chronic carriers	High number become chronic carriers
Risk to Health Care Workers	Poor handwashing increases risk	High risk for contact with infected blood or contaminated sharps	High risk for contact with infected blood or contaminated sharps
Vaccine	Approved for ages 2–18	HBV vaccine very effective, recommended for all health care workers, infants, and others at risk	None
Prevention	Handwashing, proper hygiene, and sanitation practices	Handwashing, standard precautions, avoiding illegal drugs	Handwashing, standard precautions, counseling to reduce high-risk practices

FIGURE 5–6
Comparison between hepatitis A, hepatitis B, and hepatitis C.

Hepatitis B

Hepatitis B is caused by a bloodborne pathogen. It is spread in the same way that HIV is transmitted—through sexual contact, blood, and certain body fluids. Unlike the fragile HIV virus, the hepatitis B virus (HBV) is more difficult to kill and is able to live longer outside the body. An estimated 10 percent of persons who are infected with HBV become chronic carriers (persons who are infected and can infect others, but may show no symptoms of disease). Hepatitis B is a threat to health care workers because you may care for patients who are carriers. You, in turn, can become infected and you may not even be aware of it.

Prevention of hepatitis B includes the practice of safer sex, avoidance of illegal drugs, handwashing, and standard precautions. A vaccine is available to prevent hepatitis B infection. The HBV vaccine is very effective and has few side effects. Health care facilities are required to offer the vaccine at no charge to their employees. You would be wise to take advantage of this opportunity if you have not already had the vaccine.

Hepatitis C

Although hepatitis C is not a new disease, its seriousness was not recognized until the late 1980s. It is now the most common disease caused by a blood-borne pathogen. The CDC estimates that nearly 4 million people in the United States are infected with the hepatitis C virus (HCV), and most of these have chronic infections. Hepatitis C is closely linked to cirrhosis, a deadly liver disease, and to liver cancer. HCV infection is the leading cause of liver transplants in the United States.

Blood transfusions used to account for most HCV infections but today, the majority are linked to injectable drug use. It may also be spread sexually. The disease progresses slowly and severe liver damage may occur before symptoms appear. A high number of chronically infected people will develop serious complications. There is no vaccine available for hepatitis C.

Prevention includes using good handwashing and standard precautions. Counseling is aimed at reducing high-risk behaviors such as illegal drug abuse.

Sexually Transmitted Disease (STD)

A disease in which the primary method of transmission is sexual is called an STD. This type of disease has been documented far back in history. Syphilis, one of the most common STDs, has been known to exist for thousands of years. An STD can lead to chronic illness, sterility, and death. Since the discovery of antibiotic medications, many STDs can be treated and cured, if diagnosed early. A person with an STD can infect others through sexual contact. Many STDs can also be passed on to the unborn child of an infected mother. Three of the most common STDs are gonorrhea, syphilis, and herpes. HIV infection and hepatitis B are also considered STDs.

Much progress has recently been made in the United States in controlling the spread of STDs. Doctors are required to report all STDs to the local health department. Sexual contacts named by the infected person are notified and asked to come in for testing and treatment. Confidentiality is extremely important to the success of this method.

Tuberculosis

Tuberculosis (TB) is caused by bacteria that enters through the respiratory system and causes infection. The lungs are the most common site of infection, but it may occur in other organs. It is transmitted primarily by airborne droplets from a person with active tuberculosis. (Persons who have inactive TB are not infectious.) Coughing, sneezing, talking, or singing can send the droplets into the air. Normal air currents can keep the droplets airborne for long periods of time and spread them throughout the room or building. Infection occurs when a susceptible person inhales droplets containing the TB pathogen. If the pathogen reaches the lungs, it can spread throughout the body.

A person may be exposed to tuberculosis and not get infected, and only about 10 percent of those who are infected develop active disease. A person who has been successfully treated for active tuberculosis is said to have inactive or latent tuberculosis. Active tuberculosis is infectious whereas inactive or latent tuberculosis is **not** infectious. Once a person is infected, he or she will always test positive for TB.

TB was a leading cause of death until the 1940s, when medications were developed for treatment. In 1986, the number of cases in America started to rise again. Many persons infected with HIV also became infected with TB. At risk for tuberculosis are individuals who are:

- In close contact with persons who have active TB
- In crowded, poor, unsanitary living conditions
- From countries where TB is a problem
- Suffering from a chronic illness
- HIV infected
- Alcoholics and drug addicts
- Homeless

- In prisons
- In schools
- In health care facilities

Wherever a large number of people share one area, the risk of tuberculosis transmission increases. This is known as the "shared air concept."

Symptoms

Symptoms of tuberculosis include a chronic cough, fever, chills, night sweats, fatigue, weight loss, and loss of appetite. As the disease advances, the person may start coughing up blood. Diagnosis is made by history, chest x-ray, microscopic examination of *sputum* (mucus from the lungs) specimens, and lung washings or biopsies.

Treatment

Treatment of tuberculosis involves taking multiple drugs over an extended period of time. It is a complicated program that requires close monitoring. The infected person must complete the drug therapy in order for it to be effective.

Multidrug-Resistant Tuberculosis

Multidrug-resistant tuberculosis (MDRTB) is a strain of TB that is resistant to current drugs and is frequently fatal. It develops when TB patients do not follow the drug program and the pathogens that remain become resistant to treatment. Patients who have MDRTB can remain infectious for a long time. This increases the risk of transmitting the disease to other patients and to health care workers.

Prevention and Control

Prevention and control of tuberculosis is accomplished in the following ways:

- Screening—Identify persons at risk.
- Testing—Tuberculosis skin test is mandatory in many schools and in most health care facilities.
- Isolation—Transmission-based precautions must be used for persons with suspected or diagnosed tuberculosis. Special isolation rooms that have an air filtration system must be used.
- Medical treatment and monitoring—An individualized plan is developed for each patient.
- Personal protection equipment—Specific isolation techniques are used, including respirator type masks and any other necessary equipment.
- Patient responsibility—Patients are instructed to cover coughs and sneezes with tissues to contain droplets.

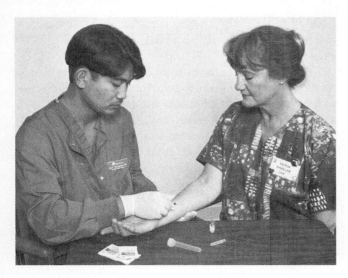

FIGURE 5–7
TB skin testing helps to control the spread of tuberculosis.

■ Education—Education of health care workers, appropriate to the job category, is mandated.

TB Testing

Routine screening and testing is the major method used to control the spread of TB. Annual TB skin testing is required for all health care workers.

Upon employment you will probably be given a two-step Mantoux skin test. A substance, purified protein derivative (PPD), is injected under the skin of your forearm. A thickened, hard area at the site of the test after 48 hours indicates that you have been infected with the TB bacteria. This is called a positive TB test. It **does not** mean that you have active tuberculosis. It means that at some point in your life, you were exposed to active TB and the bacteria entered your system. (Inactive or latent TB will also cause a positive skin test.) If you have a positive TB skin test, you will be sent for a chest x-ray. Sputum specimens may be necessary to determine if you have active tuberculosis. (See Figure 5–7.)

*E*merging Infectious Diseases

The CDC defines emerging infectious diseases as diseases that have increased or threatened to increase in the past two decades. Included are HIV, hepatitis C, and tuberculosis, which we have already discussed. Other emerging infectious diseases are MRSA, *E. coli*, Lyme disease, and mad cow disease. There are many reasons for the increase in incidence of these diseases, but overuse of antibiotics has contributed to the problem. This leads to the develop-

ment and growth of pathogens that are resistant to many of the drug treatments that are now available.

Methicillin-Resistant *Staphylococcus aureus*

Methicillin-resistant *Staphylococcus aureus* (MRSA) is a disease caused by a pathogen that is resistant to many antibiotics. It is usually found in warm, moist areas of the body like the nose and mouth. It primarily affects people whose resistance is low, such as the elderly or those with chronic diseases. MRSA occurs frequently in hospitals and nursing homes. It is highly contagious and difficult to contain.

Signs and symptoms of MRSA include redness, fever, and drainage. Transmission occurs by direct or indirect contact with the pathogens. In health care facilities, MRSA is usually spread by employees who have not properly washed their hands. The infected health care worker can then infect others. The best prevention method involves using infection control practices and standard precautions with the emphasis on handwashing.

Escherichia coli

Escherichia coli (*E. coli*) is a bacteria that is normal flora in the intestinal system of humans and animals. If it enters another part of the body, such as the urinary tract, it becomes a pathogen and causes infection. *E. coli* urinary infections are often a result of improper hygiene. *E. coli* can also be spread by contaminated food. A few years ago, outbreaks of *E. coli* infection were linked to undercooked hamburgers in a fast-food restaurant chain.

E. coli prevention involves a two-pronged attack. The first line of defense is practicing good infection control regarding handwashing and personal hygiene. The second prevention tactic is for the food service industry to reinforce standards of adequate cooking times and temperatures.

Lyme Disease

Lyme disease is caused by bacteria transmitted through the bite of an infected tick. These types of ticks are concentrated in the northern part of the United States. This disease is not transmitted person to person. It is a multisystem disorder with flu-like symptoms, which can include fever, chills, fatigue, and sore throat. Serious complications such as joint disease, cardiac problems, or neurological disorders may occur.

Prevention of Lyme disease focuses on avoiding tick-infested areas when possible, wearing protective clothing, and using insect repellents. The tick must be removed carefully. A preventative vaccine is available but is not completely effective. Early diagnosis and treatment helps to prevent complications.

Mad Cow Disease

Mad cow disease is a fatal brain disease of cattle that can be transmitted to humans through meat or by-products from infected cows. The disease was first recognized in England before it spread to other European countries. Infected cows exhibited un-usual behavior, which resulted in the name "mad cow disease." In humans, it causes a fatal nervous system disorder with progressive dementia and vi-sion problems.

Prevention centers on stopping the contamina-tion of cattle feed and by destruction of infected ani-mals. Whole herds of cattle have been destroyed in an effort to prevent mad cow disease. Many coun-tries, including the United States, banned the sale and shipment of English beef. These control mea-sures have resulted in a decrease in the incidence of mad cow disease.

 *R*eview

Read each sentence and fill in the blank with the vo-cabulary term that best completes the sentence.

1. A _____ is a disease that spreads easily from one person to another.
2. _____ is a procedure to make a person more resistant to a specific disease.
3. Swelling of a body part due to fluid in the tissue is called _____.
4. Patients who are _____ are capable of spread-ing disease.
5. _____ is mucus from the lungs.

 *R*emember

1. A communicable disease spreads easily from one person to another.
2. Proper immunization could prevent most child-hood communicable diseases.
3. Most of the childhood communicable diseases are highly contagious before symptoms appear.
4. There is no method of prevention, and no vac-cine available, for the common cold.
5. There are several types of influenza viruses, and new ones appear each year.
6. HIV infection is a disease that destroys the im-mune system and leaves the body unable to fight infection.
7. Every exposure to HIV does not result in infec-tion.
8. The risk of HIV infection or hepatitis in the workplace is very low if standard precautions are practiced.
9. The hepatitis B virus is more difficult to kill than the virus that causes HIV infection.
10. Hepatitis C infection is the leading cause of liver transplants in the United States.
11. Many sexually transmitted diseases can be treated and cured if diagnosed early.
12. Pulmonary tuberculosis is transmitted primar-ily by airborne droplets from a person with ac-tive TB.
13. Annual TB testing is required for all health care workers.
14. MRSA, *E. coli*, Lyme disease, and mad cow dis-ease are examples of infectious diseases that have increased in the past 20 years.

 *R*eflect

Read the following case study and answer the ques-tions.

Case Study
Magda Olavitch is a 5-year-old patient in the hospi-tal where you work as a nursing assistant. She has pneumonia that developed as a complication of chickenpox. Some of her rash remains but it is dry and crusts have formed. It no longer itches or both-ers Magda. However, she has a productive cough and sneezes often. Magda has had none of the childhood immunizations because her mother is afraid the shots will make her sick. The doctor and the nurses have been explaining to Mrs. Olavitch

how important it is for Magda to be fully immunized.

1. Will you need to wear gloves, gown, or mask when caring for Magda? Explain your answer.
2. What steps can you take to protect yourself from infection while caring for Magda?

Respond

Choose the best answer for each question.

1. Which of these communicable diseases has been brought under control in the United States?
   A. HIV disease
   B. Hepatitis B
   C. Typhoid fever
   D. Lyme disease

2. There is NOT a vaccine available to prevent the occurrence of
   A. Chickenpox
   B. Whooping cough
   C. Hepatitis B
   D. Hepatitis C

3. The common cold is most often transmitted by
   A. Contact with droplets or secretions on the hands.
   B. Eating contaminated food
   C. Contaminated needles and syringes
   D. Sexual contact with an infected person

4. The primary route of transmission of HIV in children is from
   A. An infected mother to her baby
   B. Contaminated needles and syringes
   C. Contaminated blood transfusions
   D. Living in a home with an infected person

5. Which of the following statements about HIV is TRUE?
   A. HIV is transmitted by casual contact.
   B. A vaccine is available to prevent HIV transmission.
   C. HIV is transmitted by mosquitos.
   D. Increased numbers of elderly people are infected with HIV.

3. Will you need to be concerned about contracting chickenpox from Magda? Explain your answer.
4. What might you say to Mrs. Olavitch to support what the doctor and nurses have told you about immunizations?

6. Hepatitis A is most commonly transmitted through
   A. Contaminated needles and sharps
   B. Contaminated blood transfusions
   C. Contaminated food and water
   D. Contaminated bed linens

7. Which of the following diseases is NOT caused by a bloodborne pathogen?
   A. Hepatitis B
   B. Hepatitis C
   C. HIV disease
   D. Lyme disease

8. The leading cause of liver transplants in the United States is
   A. Hepatitis C infection
   B. Hepatitis A infection
   C. HIV disease
   D. Lyme disease

9. The pathogen that causes tuberculosis is primarily spread by
   A. Airborne transmission
   B. Direct contact transmission
   C. Indirect contact transmission
   D. Bloodborne transmission

10. Which of the following diseases is caused by a pathogen that is resistant to many antibiotics?
    A. Lyme disease
    B. *E. coli*
    C. MRSA
    D. Mad cow disease

Chapter Six

Safety *and* Accident Prevention

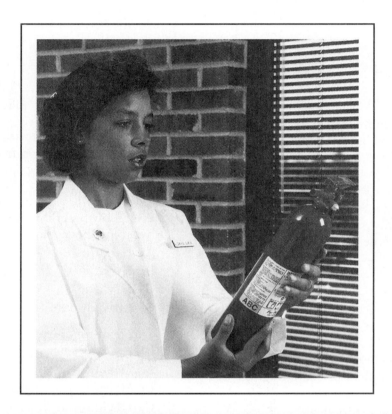

OBJECTIVES

After studying this chapter, you will be able to

1. Describe two risk factors that contribute to patient accidents.

2. Identify four guidelines for accident prevention.

3. List six guidelines for correct body mechanics.

4. Describe the OSHA Hazard Communication Standard.

5. Identify four alternatives to restraints.

6. List four guidelines to be followed when using restraints.

7. Explain the purpose of emergency management planning.

8. Describe the four steps of the RACE system for fire safety.

9. List five guidelines for assisting victims of domestic violence.

10. Describe three ways to protect yourself from workplace violence.

11. Perform the procedures described in this chapter.

body mechanics   The process of using the body safely and efficiently.
comatose   A condition in which a person is unconscious.
incontinence   The inability to control urine or bowel movement.

paralysis   The inability to move a body part.
suffocation   A condition in which breathing stops due to lack of oxygen.
toxic   Capable of causing poisonous reactions.

One of the most important responsibilities of health care workers is to protect patient safety. Patients have the right to an environment in which they can feel safe and secure from harm. As a nursing assistant, you have many opportunities to observe safety problems and hazards. You may be the first one to notice that a patient is weaker and more likely to fall. You may also be the one to discover faulty equipment, such as a broken footrest on a wheelchair.

One of your primary safety concerns is the prevention of accidents. Accidents are one of the leading causes of death in the United States. The cost of accidents, both financially and in human suffering, are staggering. This chapter focuses on accident prevention and other safety issues. Basic safety principles are emphasized throughout the text.

*R*isk Factors

Patients in health care facilities are more at risk of accidents than the general public. Several factors that contribute to patient accidents include disease, confusion, medications, lack of mental awareness, and age.

Disease or Injury

Either disease or injury can interfere with a patient's ability to protect him- or herself. For example, diseases like muscular dystrophy affect balance and mobility. An injury that causes *paralysis* (inability to move a body part) makes it harder to avoid danger. A stroke may leave the patient mentally or physically impaired.

Medications

Certain medications may cause weakness, dizziness, or confusion. Vision or hearing may be temporarily disturbed. Even desired reactions to medication can contribute to accidents. For example, medications given to remove excess body fluid cause frequent urination. A patient may have an accident while hurrying to the bathroom.

Decreased Mental Awareness

Confused patients often place themselves in danger because their judgment is impaired. They may be unable to distinguish safe from unsafe. Confused patients may walk out in front of a moving wheelchair or food cart. They may unknowingly burn themselves or drink harmful substances. *Comatose* (unconscious) patients are totally helpless and dependent on others for safety. Special precautions are necessary when caring for comatose patients. For example, this type of patient should have the side rails raised when care is completed.

Age

The two age groups that have the most accidents are children and the elderly. If another factor such as weakness or confusion is present, the risk is even greater. Close observation is necessary if you are working with either of these age groups. Remember, however, to focus on individual behavior rather than the patient's age. For example, a proud, elderly patient may take risks in an effort to maintain independence.

Staff Negligence

Most negligence is not intentional but is a result of carelessness or haste. Remember that you are legally responsible for accidents that occur because of your negligence whether it is intentional or not. Some examples of negligence include incorrect lifting techniques, improper use of restraints, or failure to clean up a spill. (See Figure 6–1.)

*T*ypes of Accidents

The most common accidents in health care are falls, burns, poisoning, and *suffocation* (a condition in which breathing stops due to lack of oxygen).

Falls

The most frequent accident in a health care facility is a fall, and the most common cause of a fall is wet,

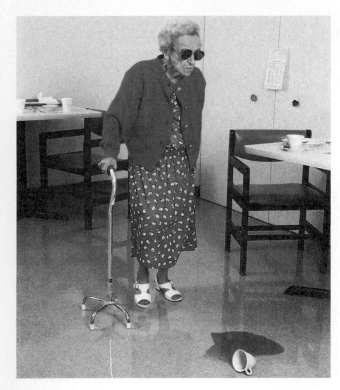

FIGURE 6–1
Failure to clean up a spill on the floor could cause a patient to fall.

slippery floors. Falls may also be caused by equipment that is damaged or improperly used. Environmental hazards, such as poor lighting or cluttered halls, can contribute to falls.

Accident Prevention

Safety should be uppermost in your mind at all times. Always check the safety of each of your patients as soon as you receive your assignment.

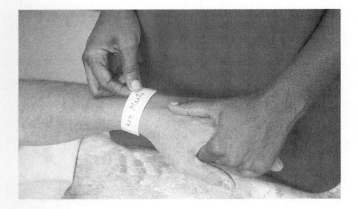

FIGURE 6–2
The safest way to identify the patient is by checking the identification bracelet.

Guidelines for Accident Prevention

- Identify the patient by checking the ID bracelet. Correctly identify each patient before you give care. (See Figure 6–2.)
- Place the call signal within the patient's reach regardless of the patient's physical or mental condition.
- Answer call signals promptly so patients who need assistance do not try to get up alone.
- Clean up water or other spills immediately. Observe "Wet Floor" signs and remind patients and visitors to avoid these areas.
- Follow facility policy regarding side rails. It is your responsibility to know which patients need side rails raised.
- Lock the wheels on wheelchairs, beds, stretchers, and other equipment when transferring patients.
- Keep frequently used articles, such as the telephone or television control, within easy reach of the patient.
- Return the bed to its lowest position when you leave the patient's room.
- Report building hazards, such as loose handrails or plumbing leaks, immediately.
- Report broken or faulty equipment immediately. Follow correct procedures when using equipment.
- Make sure the patient is wearing well-fitting footwear that has a closed heel and toe and nonskid soles. Wear this same type of shoe yourself when you are working.
- Get help when it is needed. Do not take chances with the safety of the patient or yourself.
- Check the water temperature before placing a patient in the tub or shower and make sure that food and fluids are not too hot.
- Keep cleaning products and other *toxic* (poisonous) substances in their original containers and store them in a safe area.
- Follow fire safety rules and be familiar with the emergency management plan in your facility.
- Follow standard precautions.
- Practice correct body mechanics at all times.

Body Mechanics

Body mechanics refers to using the body safely and efficiently. Using correct body mechanics makes your

Guidelines for Correct Body Mechanics

- Keep your back straight and use proper posture.
- Stand with your feet apart and your weight evenly balanced.
- Face the patient or the object that you are moving.
- Move close to the patient or hold the object close to your body.
- Use the large muscles of your legs to lift and the muscles of your arms to support.
- Shift the position of your feet when turning. Do not twist your body.
- Bend from the knees, not the waist.
- Push or pull an object whenever possible, rather than lift it.
- Use groups of muscles when it is possible. Two hands work better than one.
- Use smooth, coordinated motions.
- Let the patient know what you are going to do.
- Encourage the patient to help as much as possible.

work go more smoothly and helps you avoid injury or fatigue. Correct body mechanics begins with proper posture. Stand with your feet parallel and separated. Tighten the stomach muscles, flatten the abdomen, and straighten the spine. Raise your chest, spread your shoulders, and keep your head erect. Now, you are ready to move or lift efficiently. (See Figure 6–3.)

OSHA Regulations

The Occupational Safety and Health Administration (OSHA) issues many regulations and standards that concern the safety of health care workers. You learned about the regulations that relate to infection control in Chapter 4. OSHA conducts regular inspections to ensure that health care facilities follow the rules and regulations. It is your responsibility to know and use the safety practices and equipment provided by your facility.

Hazard Communication Standard

The Hazard Communication Standard states that health care workers have the right to know what hazards or dangers they are exposed to in the workplace. All hazardous chemicals and other dangerous mater-

ial must be labeled. Your employer is required to provide training to help you understand the labels and the safety procedures you must follow when using hazardous material. The health care facility is also required to provide Material Safety Data Sheets (MSDS) for all chemicals used. These forms address safety, health risks, and first aid procedures that might be needed.

Ergonomics Standard

In 2001 the OSHA Ergonomics Standard was passed and then repealed. The purpose of the standard was to reduce the number and severity of musculoskeletal (muscle and bone) disorders caused by risk factors on the job. Ergonomics is the study of human performance in the workplace. It involves designing equipment and practices that allow workers to perform their jobs safely.

Even though the standard was repealed, many facilities are following its recommendations that control measures be developed to eliminate or reduce known hazards. An example of these measures might be a policy requiring two persons for procedures that involve lifting. Some facilities provide back support belts to help prevent injuries. (See Figure 6–4.) In Chapter 18 you will learn about special procedures and equipment to use when moving and lifting patients.

Reporting Accidents and Errors

Accidents and errors are reported on a special form called an incident report. This form provides written documentation of an incident that may involve a patient, visitor, or employee. An incident report must be written whether or not a person is injured. A report must also be written if an error is made that could result in injury. Missing equipment, medications, or patient belongings also require an incident report. Defective or broken equipment may be included as well.

An incident report must be written any time you are involved in an accident, witness an incident, or make an error that could result in an injury. Information necessary to fill out the report includes the names of the persons involved; the date, time, and location of the incident; witnesses; and possible injuries. The report should be accurate and specific. When possible, use quotes to describe what someone tells you. Get the names and addresses of anyone who witnessed the incident.

An incident report must be written regardless of whether or not there are injuries. This is because

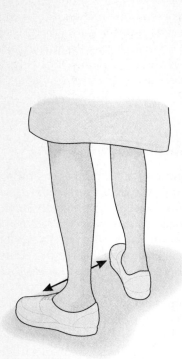

Feet 8–12 inches apart

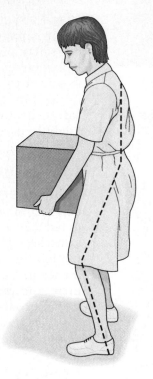

Knees bent, back straight

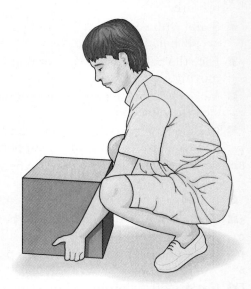

Use large muscles of thighs to lift

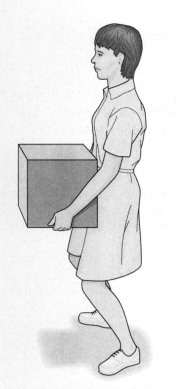

Hold object close to body

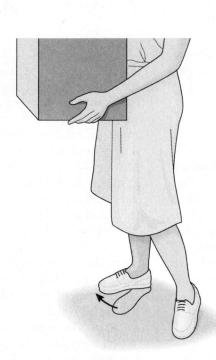

Turn whole body; don't twist

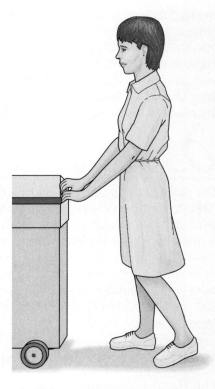

Push or pull rather than twist

FIGURE 6–3
Correct body mechanics.

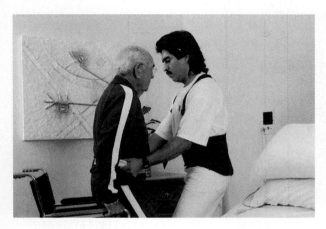

FIGURE 6–4
Back support belts may be worn to help prevent back injuries.

some injuries are not immediately apparent. Incident reports protect the patients, visitors, and employees. Incident reports are also used to identify safety problems. Facilities routinely study incident reports to find out why an incident occurred and how it can be prevented from happening again.

Restraints

A restraint is any device that restricts movement or normal access to one's body. Federal and state laws restrict the use of restraints in health care facilities. OBRA (Omnibus Budget Reconciliation Act) specifically addresses the use of restraints in long-term care facilities. The rules regarding restraints are not the same in every type of facility. It is your responsibility to know the policies concerning the use of restraints in your facility.

The use of a restraint always requires a physician's order. A restraint may only be used to ensure the safety of the patient or other patients. A restraint may **not** be used for discipline or staff convenience. Only commercially designed devices may be used as restraints, so do not use a sheet or other type of linen for this purpose. Never restrain a patient to the toilet or bedside commode. Stay with a weak or confused patient during toileting to prevent a fall or other accident.

Harmful Effects of Restraints

Restraints produce many harmful effects. Physical effects can include muscle weakness, loss of mobility, *incontinence* (inability to control urine or bowel movement), and skin breakdown. Restraints limit opportunities for activity and exercise. Many of the physical effects of restraints are the result of this decrease in activity. The restrained patient is dependent on others to meet toileting needs.

If these needs are not met promptly, the patient may lose the ability to control urine or bowel elimination. The desire for food and fluids may be affected.

Emotional responses to restraints include anger, fear, humiliation, resignation, and denial. There is a decrease in communication and social interaction with others. The loss of independence leads to a decrease in dignity and self-esteem. If the patient is angry or combative, a restraint will only increase the anger. Patients who are restrained tend to give up and lose interest in life.

Alternatives to Restraints

Action must be taken if a patient is in danger of injuring himself or herself. However, restraints are not the only solution. Many times, other more acceptable ways to protect the patient may be used. Some of the following alternatives may be used as a substitute for restraints:

- Find and treat the cause of behavior that might lead to the need for restraints.
- Provide diversional activities, such as television, music, or games.
- Allow wandering in a safe area.
- Provide a consistent, soothing environment.
- Observe, listen, and be attentive to patients.
- Encourage participation in planned activities.
- Provide opportunities for exercise.
- Encourage family participation.
- Use bed, door, and arm alarms to signal if a patient is in danger.

Guidelines for Using a Restraint

- Follow the nurse's directions about applying a restraint.
- Explain to the patient and the family, even if the patient is confused.
- Apply the restraint properly over the patient's clothing. Do not apply over bare skin.
- Pad bony areas to prevent injury.
- Tie a knot that can be easily released. Do not tie the restraint to the side rail or a part of the bed that would cause the restraint to tighten if the bed or rail were adjusted.
- Make sure that the patient is comfortable and that the call signal is within reach.
- Check the restraint frequently to guarantee safety.
- Remove the restraint and release the patient every two hours for at least 10 minutes. Provide toileting, exercise, fluids, and restorative care.

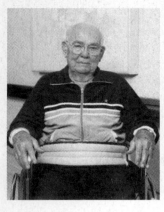

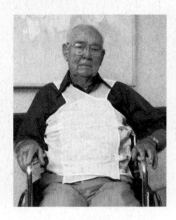

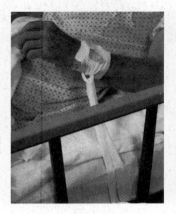

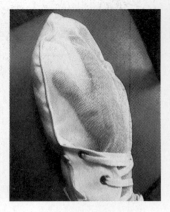

A. A SOFT BELT RESTRAINT   B. A SAFETY VEST RESTRAINT   C. A SOFT LIMB TIE RESTRAINT   D. A SOFT MITT RESTRAINT

FIGURE 6–5
Types of restraints.

Types of Restraints

The doctor's order specifies the type of restraint to be used, the reason for the restraint, and for how long it is to be applied. Some types of restraints in common use include the following:

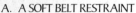 **A soft belt restraint** is applied around the waist to prevent falling from a chair or wheelchair (see Figure 6–5A). Some styles may have a front-opening or self-release buckle.

■ **A safety vest or jacket** is applied over the chest and back to prevent falling from a chair or wheelchair. It provides more support than a belt. If the vest is the criss-cross type, the straps must cross in the front (see Figure 6–5B).

■ **A soft limb tie** is a soft padded strap used to immobilize an arm or a leg to prevent the patient from pulling out tubes or interfering with treatment (see Figure 6–5C). This type of restraint must be checked frequently to prevent interruption of circulation.

■ **A soft mitten restraint** restricts use of the fingers but allows arm movement. It is less restrictive than a soft limb tie (Figure 6–5D).

■ **A roll belt restraint** is applied around the waist to prevent falling from the bed. The belt allows freedom for the patient to roll from side-to-side or sit up in bed.

■ **A pelvic support** is applied between the thighs to prevent a patient from sliding out of a chair.

Procedure for Applying a Soft Belt Restraint

Beginning Steps
■ Identify the patient and explain the procedure.
■ Collect necessary equipment and supplies.

■ Wash your hands and use standard precautions.
■ Protect the patient's privacy.
■ Use correct body mechanics.

1. Place the belt around the patient's waist and cross the strap through the loops in the back.
2. Adjust the belt to fit and make sure there are no wrinkles.
3. Secure the ties to the chair frame or the bed frame using a slip knot or half-bow that can be easily released. (See Figure 6–6.)
4. Make sure the restraint is not too tight. You should be able to insert four fingers under the restraint.

Ending Steps
■ Protect the patient's privacy.
■ Check to see that the patient is comfortable.
■ Lower the bed to the floor and raise the side rails if appropriate.
■ Place the call signal within the patient's reach.
■ Wash your hands.
■ Report and record your observations.

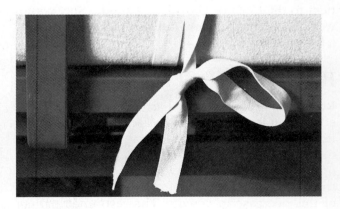

FIGURE 6–6
An example of a knot that can be easily released.

Procedure for Applying a Vest Restraint

Beginning Steps

- Identify the patient and explain the procedure.
- Collect necessary equipment and supplies.
- Wash your hands and use standard precautions.
- Protect the patient's privacy.
- Use correct body mechanics.

1. Slip the patient's arms through the armholes, with the vest crossing in front and the solid side in the back.
2. Bring the ties through the slots in the vest.
3. Adjust the vest to fit and make sure there are no wrinkles (Figure 6–7).
4. Secure the ties to the chair frame or a moveable part of the bedframe, using a slip knot or half-bow knot that can be released with one pull. Do not tie a restraint to the siderails.
5. Make sure the restraint is not too tight. You should be able to insert four fingers under the restraint.

Ending Steps

- Protect the patient's privacy.
- Check to see that the patient is comfortable.
- Lower the bed to the floor and raise the side rails if appropriate.
- Place the call signal within the patient's reach.
- Wash your hands.
- Report and record your observations.

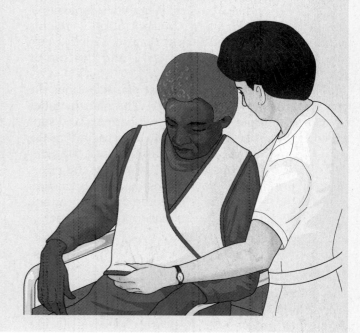

FIGURE 6–7
Adjust the vest to fit and make sure there are no wrinkles.

Guidelines for Use of a Soft Limb Restraint

- Check the restraint every 15 minutes to make sure it is not interfering with circulation in the extremity.
- You should be able to insert two fingers between the restraint and the patient's limb (see Figure 6–8).
- Check for swelling, cold skin temperature, or blue skin color in the restrained limb.
- Listen for patient complaints of pain, numbness, or tingling.
- If the restraint is too tight, loosen it and let the nurse know immediately.

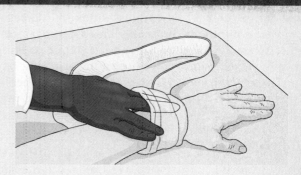

FIGURE 6–8
Insert two fingers under the wrist restraint to make sure it is not too tight.

Remember, when a patient is restrained, you are responsible for meeting all of his or her needs. The patient will not be able to get a drink of water or go to the bathroom without someone's assistance. Check frequently to see if the patient needs anything.

Emergency Management Planning

Emergency management planning outlines steps to be taken in the event of a fire or other disaster. The plan covers floods, hurricanes, tornados, and other severe weather disturbances. It includes explosions, bomb threats, and major transportation accidents (airplanes, trains, and buses). It also addresses an interruption in water, electricity, and heating or cooling systems.

The emergency management plan identifies the responsibility of each employee. The plan includes policies and procedures to protect patients and staff members. Instructions are given for evacuating the building and a safe shelter is designated. Disaster drills are held at regular intervals to test the effectiveness of the plan. Sometimes the facility coordinates with a community disaster drill to evaluate the entire community's response to an emergency.

Fire Safety

The threat of fire is always frightening, and this is especially true in health care facilities. Because patients may not be able to protect themselves, the health care facility staff is responsible for assuring their safety. Fire exits, closed stair wells, sprinkler systems, and automatic door closers are provided. Fire safety education classes are offered at regular intervals. Fire safety planning and education help to prevent fires and provide information about what to do if a fire occurs.

Causes of Fires

Fires can be caused by careless smoking, defective electrical equipment, improper trash disposal, or a lightning strike. Fires may also occur while cooking, using flammable substances, or administering oxygen. Because oxygen is frequently used in health care settings, it is important that you understand and follow the guidelines for oxygen safety.

Fire Emergency Plan

Every employee must be familiar with the fire emergency plan so they will know what to do in the event of a fire in the facility. The plan identifies the responsibilities of employees and the actions to be taken during a fire. Fire safety classes will be offered to provide this information and fire drills will be held to test the staff's response to a fire. It is too late to start planning once a fire breaks out. Everybody must know what to do and react appropriately. Knowing your responsibilities will help you to stay calm.

If a fire occurs, your first responsibility is to remove all patients who are in immediate danger. Reassure patients and visitors as you assist them to a safe area. Immediately close all doors and clear the halls of equipment. Many public facilities use the RACE system. (See Figure 6–9.) This system helps you remember what to do. In a health care facility, you would probably not get beyond step one or two before someone else began to help. But in a

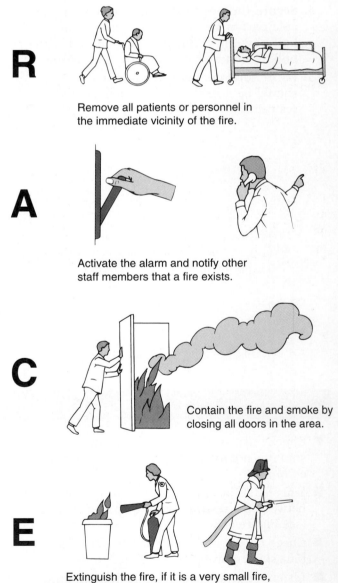

R Remove all patients or personnel in the immediate vicinity of the fire.

A Activate the alarm and notify other staff members that a fire exists.

C Contain the fire and smoke by closing all doors in the area.

E Extinguish the fire, if it is a very small fire, or allow the fire department to extinguish it.

FIGURE 6–9
The RACE system.

Guidelines for Oxygen Safety

- Remember that oxygen is combustible and will support fire.
- Post a "No Smoking" sign outside the patient's door and over the bed.
- Avoid using electrical equipment such as razors, hair dryers, and other small appliances that might provide a spark.
- Use cotton blankets instead of wool, nylon, or synthetic fabrics to prevent static.

home situation, you might be the one to carry out all four steps.

- **R—Remove** patients from the immediate area. Staff members, visitors, and others should also leave the area.
- **A—Activate** or sound the alarm and notify others that there is a fire.
- **C—Contain** or confine the fire to a small area by closing all the doors.
- **E—Extinguish** a small fire that has not begun to spread by using a fire extinguisher.

Fire Extinguishers

It is important that you know which fire extinguisher to use and how to operate it correctly. Fire extinguishers are usually labeled A, B, or C, according to the type of fires on which they should be used.

- **Type A** is used on paper, wood, or trash can fires.
- **Type B** is used on flaming liquids, such as oil or grease.
- **Type C** is used for electrical fires.
- **Type ABC** is used for all kinds of fires and is the most common type found in health care facilities.

The correct way to use a fire extinguisher is to remove the safety pin, point the nozzle toward the base of the fire, and push down on the handle. Use a sweeping motion over the base of the fire. Be certain the fire is completely extinguished before you leave the area. Your facility will provide in-service classes to show you how to use the types of extinguishers that are available.

*D*omestic *Violence*

In the past 20 years, domestic violence has become recognized as a serious problem in the United

States. Domestic violence may be defined as intimate partner or family member abuse. It may also be called spouse abuse or battering. Most domestic violence is committed by a spouse or boyfriend, either currently or formerly living in the same household. Domestic violence has no racial, ethnic, social, or financial barriers and occurs in all kinds of family settings.

Victims of Domestic Violence

The majority of victims of reported domestic violence are women, although the violence may be directed at anyone in the home. It is estimated that a woman is battered every 15 seconds in this country. Children who live in violent homes are at risk for abuse and for emotional damage as they grow older. Elderly people may become victims of domestic violence in the home. They may be abused by their spouses, partners, children, or caregivers. Patient abuse is discussed in Chapter 3 of this text. It would be helpful to review that material at this time.

Signs and Symptoms of Domestic Abuse

Victims of domestic violence may suffer emotional and physical abuse, which can result in disease, injury, or death. They make frequent visits to doctor's offices and emergency rooms, often with vague complaints. These are silent cries for help because many victims try to minimize real injuries and deny the abuse. They may have multiple injuries that ap-

Guidelines for Assisting Victims of Domestic Violence

- Know how to recognize injuries and behaviors associated with domestic violence.
- Report your observations and suspicions to your supervisor.
- Encourage the victim to talk about their problem.
- Avoid being judgmental.
- Encourage the victim to make plans to get out of the abusive situation.
- Remind the victim that domestic violence is a crime and that law enforcement officers can help.
- Provide resource information and telephone numbers.
- Protect the victim's confidentiality.
- Don't get personally involved in the situation.

pear to have occurred over a period of time. Injuries are usually on parts of the body that are normally covered by clothing.

Assisting Victims of Domestic Violence

Because of the number of individuals affected, it is likely that you will know and care for victims of domestic violence. The guidelines on page 77 will help you to assist the victims.

Workplace Violence

Workplace violence is on the increase, especially in health care. Several factors contribute to the problem, including the public's frustration with the health care delivery system. It may be the result of a person's inability to cope with sickness and death. Sometimes domestic violence spills over into the workplace. Violence can occur in a patient's room, in a common area, or in the parking lot. The bigger the facility, the more potential there is for violence because there are more dark, remote areas with fewer people around.

OSHA Guidelines

Health care facilities are required by OSHA to maintain a safe workplace. OSHA recommends that all facilities have written policies addressing violence and how to prevent it, safety and health training, and hazard prevention and control. Many facilities have developed violence response teams that may include health care professionals, security guards, and local law enforcement officers.

Protection Against Workplace Violence

The best protection against violence is to prevent the problem when possible. Be aware of your sur-

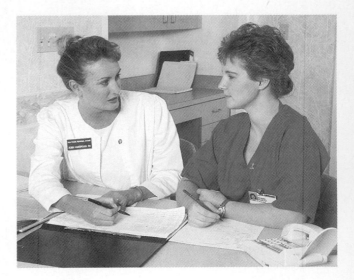

FIGURE 6–10
Notify your supervisor if you sense danger in the workplace.

roundings at all times and consider the potential for violence. Notify your supervisor or the security guard if you sense danger. (See Figure 6–10.) In home health it may be necessary to call the police as well as your supervisor. Report any threats, attempts, or actual violence immediately.

Be careful and use your common sense. Let the nurse know if you are going to leave your work unit to go to an isolated area such as the supply room or the basement. Try to leave the building when other people are in the parking lot. If you must go alone, ask a security guard to escort you. Be especially careful in a home health setting where there may be no one around to help you.

If a person near you becomes angry or hostile, be careful what you do or say. Do not argue or become defensive. Listen respectfully and try to remain calm. Watch for unspoken hostility such as muscle tension or pacing. In Chapter 27 you will find techniques for dealing with aggressive or combative persons. It would be helpful to review that material at this time. The safest solution is to calmly and politely turn the situation over to your supervisor.

Review

Read each sentence and fill in the blank with the vocabulary term that best completes the sentence.

1. _____ (the inability to move a body part) makes it harder to avoid injury.

2. A patient who is _____ (unconscious) is totally dependent on others for safety.

3. _____ occurs when breathing stops due to lack of oxygen.

4. It is important to store products that are _____ (poisonous) in a safe place.

5. _____ refers to using the body safely and efficiently.

Remember

1. Protecting patient safety is one of the most important responsibilities of health care workers.
2. The two age groups that have the most accidents are children and the elderly.
3. The most frequent accident in a health care facility is a fall.
4. Place the call signal within the patient's reach regardless of his or her physical or mental condition.
5. Identify the patient by checking the identification bracelet before you give care.
6. Use correct body mechanics and stand with your feet apart and your back straight.
7. OSHA conducts regular inspections to ensure that facilities follow safety rules and regulations.
8. A restraint may be used only to protect the safety of the patient or other patients.
9. Remove the restraint and release the patient every 2 hours for at least 10 minutes.
10. An emergency plan outlines actions to be taken should an accident occur.
11. The first step in the event of a fire is to remove patients who are in immediate danger.
12. Domestic violence has no racial, ethnic, social, or financial barrier and occurs in all kinds of family situations.
13. Be aware of your surroundings at all times and consider the potential for workplace violence.

Reflect

Read the following case study and answer the questions.

Case Study

Mrs. Wilson is a resident of the nursing home where Amy works as a nursing assistant. Mrs. Wilson had a stroke, which left her weak and slightly confused. She asks Amy to help her get out of bed and into a chair. Because Mrs. Wilson is not always able to cooperate, Amy tries to find a co-worker who will help her. No one is available and the mechanical lift is broken. Amy explains the situation to Mrs. Wilson, who starts crying. Amy responds, "Okay, I'll try to get you up, but if you get hurt, it's not my fault." First, she helps Mrs. Wilson to sit on the side of the bed. Then, with her knees locked and feet firmly to-gether, Amy lifts and moves Mrs. Wilson to a wheelchair. Although Mrs. Wilson is supposed to wear a soft belt restraint, Amy doesn't apply one because she is afraid it will upset Mrs. Wilson even more. Amy's back has started hurting and she immediately reports it to the nurse.

1. What should Amy have done when no one was available to help her get Mrs. Wilson out of bed?
2. Did Amy use correct body mechanics while getting Mrs. Wilson out of bed?
3. Did Amy make the proper decision regarding the restraint? Why or why not?
4. Was it really necessary for Amy to report her backache?

Respond

Choose the best answer for each question.

1. The most frequent accidents in health care facilities are
   A. Burns
   B. Falls
   C. Poisoning
   D. Suffocation

2. The safest way to identify a patient is to
   A. Call him by his name
   B. Check the room number
   C. Ask his roommate
   D. Check his identification bracelet

3. When a patient is comatose, the call signal should be placed
   A. On the wall above her bed
   B. Within her reach
   C. Within the nurse's reach
   D. Out of the way

4. Which of the following is an example of correct body mechanics when moving a patient?

A. Stand with your feet together.

B. Lock your knees as you lift.

C. Keep your back straight.

D. Bend from the waist.

5. It is not necessary to write an incident report if the accident causes no apparent injury.

A. True

B. False

6. The purpose of the OSHA Hazard Communication Standard is to

A. Reduce the risk of fire

B. Reduce the risk from hazardous materials

C. Reduce the risk of musculoskeletal injuries

D. Reduce the risk of chemical poisoning

7. How often must you check a patient with a wrist restraint?

A. Every 15 minutes

B. Every hour

C. Every 2 hours

D. Every shift

8. The FIRST step in the event of a fire is to

A. Remove patients from danger

B. Contain the fire

C. Call the fire department

D. Put out the fire

9. The majority of victims of domestic violence are

A. Children

B. The elderly

C. Women

D. Men

10. A hospital visitor has threatened to kill you. What should you do?

A. Ignore it. He is just upset.

B. Tell him that if he hits you, you will hit him back.

C. Report it to the nurse immediately.

D. Call the police immediately.

Chapter Seven

First Aid *and* Emergency Care

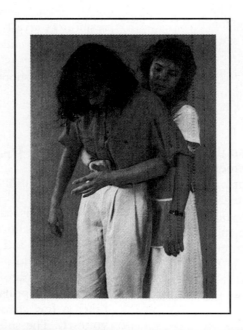

OBJECTIVES

After studying this chapter, you will be able to _____

1. Describe the use of standard precautions while providing emergency care.

2. List three rules for basic first aid.

3. Describe three life-threatening situations.

4. Identify the A,B,Cs of emergency care.

5. Describe the emergency care for airway obstructions, cardiac arrest, and respiratory arrest.

6. Describe the emergency care for hemorrhage, shock, and stroke.

7. List four guidelines each for fainting and seizures.

8. Demonstrate the procedures described in this chapter.

aspiration   Choking due to inhaling food or fluid into the airway.

assess   To examine or evaluate.

cardiac arrest   Condition in which the heart stops beating.

cardiopulmonary resuscitation (CPR)   Emergency procedure used to restore heart and lung function.

cyanosis   A bluish discoloration of the skin due to lack of oxygen.

first aid   The immediate care given for injury or sudden illness.

Heimlich maneuver   Procedure performed to dislodge a foreign body from the airway.

hemorrhage   Severe bleeding.

pulse   Heartbeat felt as blood pushes through arteries.

respiration   Breathing; the process of inspiration and expiration.

respiratory arrest   A condition in which breathing stops.

seizure   The sudden contraction of muscles caused by abnormal brain activity, also called a convulsion.

ventilate   To supply the lungs with air.

Knowledge of first aid can mean the difference between life and death in an emergency situation. Someone falls, chokes, or has a heart attack. A child swallows a poisonous cleaning fluid or falls in the swimming pool. Would you know what to do? This chapter deals with the more common emergencies that you might encounter. It provides guidelines and procedures for basic first aid and emergency care. It includes the most recent changes in basic life support recommended by the American Heart Association (AHA).

Basic First Aid

First aid is the immediate care that is given for injury or sudden illness. It is the "first" thing that you do to "aid" the victim. Proper care, given quickly, can prevent further injury and might save a life. As a health care worker, you will be expected to know basic first aid and emergency care. First aid courses are offered by the National Safety Council and the American Red Cross. Basic life support courses are offered by the National Safety Council, the American Red Cross, and the American Heart Association.

Legal Issues

In the health care facility, your responsibility is to stay with the patient, notify the nurse, and begin first aid. When the nurse arrives, you may be asked to assist. Outside your job, you are not legally required to render first aid. If you decide to help, you must perform correctly, within your training limits. You must also continue first aid until you are exhausted, someone else relieves you, or help is no longer needed. Many states have Good Samaritan laws that protect the legal rights of the person offering first aid. As long as you act within the guidelines of your training, you are usually safe from legal judgments.

Standard Precautions

While providing first aid, you will need to protect yourself against infection from unknown infected persons. This can be accomplished by following standard precautions. It is important to wear gloves during first aid to prevent contamination from blood, body fluids, secretions, excretions, non-intact skin, and mucous membranes (see Figure 7–1). First aid response must occur quickly, but it only takes a few seconds to put on gloves and protect yourself. The safest technique for rescue breathing is a pocket face mask with a one-way valve (see Figure 7–2).

Basic Rules of First Aid

There are certain basic rules of first aid that apply in all situations. Helping everyone stay calm, including yourself, is very important. The victim might be injured further if someone got excited and did the wrong thing or was so upset that they did nothing.

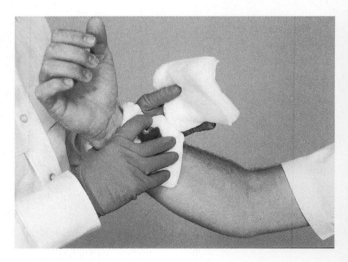

FIGURE 7–1
Wear gloves during first aid to prevent contamination from body fluids.

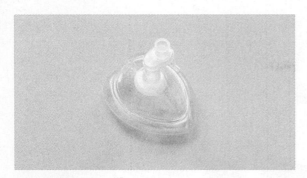

FIGURE 7-2
A pocket face mask.

For example, an untrained person might try to move an injured victim to a more comfortable place, and in doing so cause further injury. One of the most important rules of first aid is not to move the victim unless it is absolutely necessary to protect him or her from further danger.

Once you begin first aid, you are in charge until someone more qualified relieves you. As the first person to act, you are more likely to have the victim's confidence. Keep curious bystanders away. The more people who gather, the more chance there is that someone will do the wrong thing.

Emergency Assessment

When you come upon the scene of an emergency, you must assess the situation before you take action. *Assess* means to examine or evaluate. During the assessment, you will be gathering information that will determine your response. You will need to assess the scene of the incident and the seriousness of the victim's injuries or illness.

Assessing the Scene

The first priority is to determine if there are any dangerous elements to consider. You will need to know if the victim is at risk of further injury and if it is safe for you to help. For example, an accident victim lying in the middle of a busy highway is in an unsafe situation that must be made safe before first aid can begin. As soon as you have determined that you can safely assist the victim, you can proceed with the assessment.

Assessing the Victim

Your first responsibility in assessing the victim is to check for life-threatening conditions. These are situations in which the victim might die if help is not given immediately. Life-threatening situations include

- *Cardiac arrest* (the heart stops beating)
- *Respiratory arrest* (breathing stops)
- *Hemorrhage* (severe bleeding)
- Smoke inhalation
- Shock
- Drowning
- Poisoning

You will also need to check for wounds and broken bones. An extremity that is twisted or in an unusual position may be broken. Do not move the extremity because you could cause further injury. These injuries can become life-threatening and should be assessed carefully.

Activate the EMS System

If a life-threatening condition exists, EMS (Emergency Medical Services) must be called. In most areas of the United States, EMS is activated by dialing 911. The caller will be expected to give the following information:

- The location (with the name of the nearest cross street)
- The telephone number from which the call is made
- The type of emergency
- The number of persons needing help
- The first aid that is being given

When emergency personnel arrive, they will take over and relieve you of your responsibility. In the health care facility, the nurse will make the decision to call EMS or their own emergency team.

Basic Life Support

The American Heart Association recently revised the guidelines for basic life support. The aim of the revisions is to improve resuscitation outcomes by providing techniques that are easier to learn, remember, and perform. Because of these changes, individuals who were previously trained in cardiopulmonary resuscitation (CPR) must be retrained when their current certification expires.

Several of the AHA revisions involve emergency procedures for lay rescuers (people who are not trained medical personnel). However, this chapter does not address those changes. It focuses on guidelines and procedures that you will need to learn as a part of your nursing assistant training.

The ABCs of Emergency Care

Assessment of heart and lung function is called the ABCs of emergency care.

- **A = Airway** (breathing passage). The airway must be open or air cannot enter the lungs. If the airway is blocked by an object, the object must be removed. If it is blocked by the tongue, repositioning the head and chin may open the airway.

■ **B = Breathing.** Check *respirations* (breathing). If the victim is not breathing, you will need to *ventilate* (supply the lungs with air).

■ **C = Circulation.** Check for a *pulse* (heartbeat). If there is no heartbeat, circulation will have to be artificially initiated by chest compressions.

Airway Obstruction

The airway involves the structures of the respiratory system through which air enters and leaves the body. Airway obstruction means that something is partially or completely blocking the airway.

Partial Airway Obstruction

A partial airway obstruction occurs when an object is caught in the throat but does not totally block the airway. Symptoms include coughing, difficulty in breathing, making high-pitched sounds, and *cyanosis*—a bluish color of the skin due to lack of oxygen. Encourage the victim to continue coughing, which may bring up the obstruction. Do **not** hit the person on the back to dislodge the object as that action is more likely to

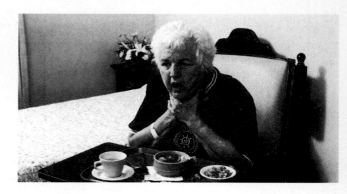

FIGURE 7–3
Clutching the throat with the hands is the universal sign of choking.

cause further blockage. As long as the person is coughing or talking, do not intervene or take emergency measures. Do not leave the victim alone, because the obstruction might become complete.

Complete Airway Obstruction

If the airway is completely blocked, the condition must be relieved quickly to prevent death. The victim will be unable to cough or speak, and the skin will gradually become cyanotic. The victim may clutch her throat with her hands. This is referred to as the "universal sign of choking" (Figure 7–3).

Procedure for the Heimlich Maneuver

1. Determine if there is partial or complete obstruction and ask "Are you choking?". Offer assistance.
2. Stand behind the victim and wrap your arms around the waist, keeping your elbows out, away from the victim's ribs. (Figure 7–4A).
3. Make a fist with one hand and place the thumb side of the fist against the midline of the abdomen, slightly above the naval.

4. Grasp your fist with the other hand with your thumbs toward the victim (Figure 7–4B).
5. Press your fist into the abdomen with a quick inward and upward thrust. Deliver rapid inward and upward thrusts until the airway is cleared or the victim loses consciousness.

A. Stand behind the victim and wrap your arms around the waist, keeping your elbows out and away from the victim's ribs.

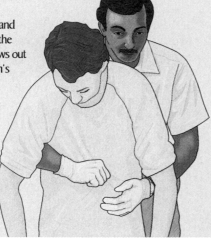

B. Grasp your fist with the other hand with your thumbs toward the victim.

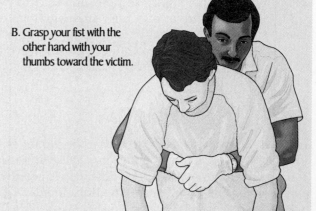

FIGURE 7–4
The Heimlich Maneuver

Procedure for Care of the Unconscious Person with an Airway Obstruction

1. Determine unresponsiveness by shaking gently and asking, "Are you okay?"
2. If there is no response, call for help and activate EMS.
3. Kneel beside the unconscious person and open the airway by using the head tilt/chin lift method. Tilt the head back with one hand while you lift the chin with the other.
4. Place your cheek close to the victim's face. Take three to five seconds to look at the victim's chest while you listen and feel for air movement against your cheek (Figure 7–5A).
5. If there is no air movement, give two ventilations. If the air will not enter, reposition the head in order to open the airway and attempt two additional ventilations.
6. If air still does not enter the airway, kneel and straddle the victim's thighs.
7. Place the heel of one hand on the abdomen, slightly above the navel, at the midline. Place your other hand on top of the first hand. Your fingers should point toward the victim's chest (Figure 7–5B).
8. With your shoulders directly above your hands, press inward and upward for up to five abdominal thrusts.
9. Open the victim's mouth using the tongue–jaw lift and perform a finger sweep. Insert the index finger of your other hand into the victim's mouth and sweep it along the inside surfaces to the base of the tongue. Hook your finger slightly to dislodge and remove any object you find (Figure 7–5C).
10. Attempt ventilation again.
11. Repeat the series of five abdominal thrusts, finger sweep, and attempts to ventilate.

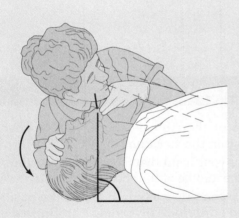

A. Use the head tilt/chin lift method to open the airway. Look, listen, and feel.

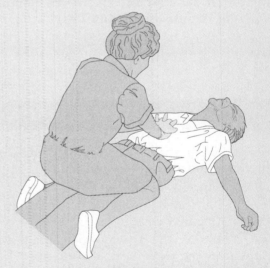

B. Place the heel of one hand on the abdomen slightly above the navel, at the midline. Place your other hand on the top of the first hand and give up to 5 abdominal thrusts.

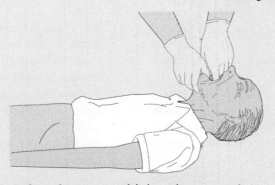

C. Perform a finger sweep to dislodge and remove any objects.

FIGURE 7–5 Care of the unconscious patient with an obstructed airway.

Causes of Airway Obstruction

The most common cause of airway obstruction in a conscious person is food. Anyone can choke, but children and the elderly are at increased risk. A decrease in the gag reflex causes many elderly people to have difficulty swallowing. Missing teeth, loose teeth, or dentures contribute to the problem. Small children put all kinds of objects in their mouths that can block the airway. Grapes, popcorn, and pieces of hot dog can cause a small child to choke. Laughing and talking while eating can cause *aspiration* (choking due to inhaling food or fluid into the airway).

The Conscious Victim with a Complete Airway Obstruction

The immediate first aid for a complete airway obstruction is called the *Heimlich maneuver* (a procedure performed to dislodge a foreign body from the airway). The maneuver pushes the diaphragm upward, which forces air from the lungs. The sudden burst of air should move the obstruction and expel it out the mouth. (See Figure 7–4.)

The Unconscious Victim with an Airway Obstruction

If the victim with an airway obstruction loses consciousness, you will need to help lower him or her to the floor. Perform the procedure explained in Figure 7–5. CPR may be necessary.

Emergency Care for Cardiopulmonary Arrest

Earlier in this chapter you learned the ABCs of emergency care—airway, breathing, and circulation. Opening the airway will not be enough to save the victim's life if the respiratory and circulatory systems have stopped functioning. This situation is called cardiac arrest, and the emergency care necessary is *cardiopulmonary resuscitation* (*CPR*).

Procedure for One-Rescuer CPR

1. Determine unresponsiveness by gently shaking the victim and asking, "Are you okay?"
2. Call for help and activate the EMS system.
3. Open the airway by using the head tilt/chin lift method. (Figure 7–6A).
4. While holding the airway open, place your cheek near the victim's mouth and nose. Look at the victim's chest, while you listen and feel for air movement against your cheek (Figure 7–6B).
5. Provide two breaths (1½ to 2 seconds each) into the victim's airway. If the air will not enter the lungs, reposition the head and try again. Use a pocket face mask if one is available.
6. Check for circulation by feeling the carotid pulse, which is located in the groove between the "Adam's apple" and the large muscle of the neck. This should take 5 to 10 seconds (Figure 7–6C).
7. If no pulse is present, use the index and middle finger of the hand nearest the victim's feet to locate the compression site. Follow the
edge of the rib cage to the notch where the ribs join the sternum (Figure 7–6D).
8. Place your hand that is nearest the victim's head on the middle of the chest over the sternum.
9. Place the other hand on top of the positioned hand. Interlock or extend the fingers of the top hand in order to lift all fingers off the chest. Begin compressions and compress the chest 1½ to 2 inches (Figure 7–6E).
10. Deliver compressions at the rate of 100 per minute.
11. Alternate 15 compressions with two ventilations, and repeat this sequence for four full cycles. Do not lift your hands from the chest during compressions.
12. Finish the four cycles with two ventilations before rechecking the pulse. If the pulse is still absent, continue the cycles of chest compressions and ventilations, beginning with chest compressions. Check the pulse every few minutes thereafter. Do not interrupt CPR for more than 5 seconds.

Procedure for One-Rescuer CPR (cont.)

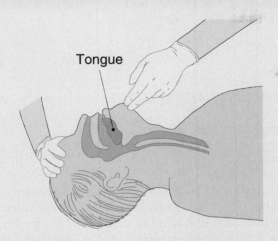

Tongue

A. Use the head tilt/chin lift method to open the airway.

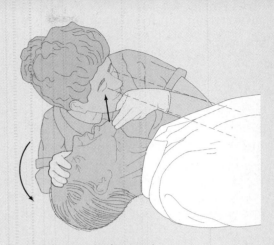

B. Look, listen, and feel for breathing.

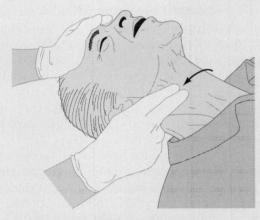

C. Check for circulation by feeling the carotid pulse on either side of the neck.

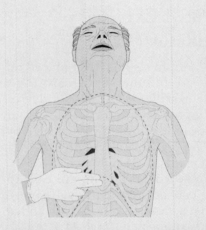

D. Locate the compression site by following the edge of the rib cage to the notch where the ribs join the sternum.

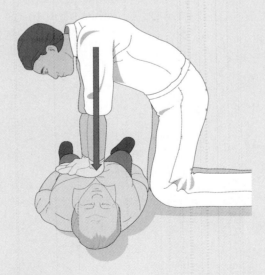

E. Position your hands and begin chest compressions.

FIGURE 7–6
One-rescuer CPR.

The principle of CPR is to bring oxygen into the body and circulate it to the cells. The quicker the procedure begins, the better the victim's chance of survival. A person can live only four to six minutes without oxygen. Once you begin CPR, you must continue until one of the following occurs:

■ You become exhausted and cannot continue.
■ A qualified person takes over for you.
■ The victim is resuscitated.
■ The victim is declared dead.

Before beginning CPR, the victim must be positioned on a hard surface, so that the heart can be compressed between the sternum and the spine. (See Figure 7–6.)

Automated External Defibrillator (AED)

Increased emphasis has been placed on the use of defibrillators in emergency care. An automated external defibrillator (AED) is a device about the size of a laptop computer. It delivers an electrical shock that is used to correct heart rhythm problems. An AED can be lifesaving to victims of sudden cardiac arrest. (See Figure 7–7.)

Automated defibrillators are easy to use. Even laypeople can be taught to use them. After determining that a victim has no breath and no pulse, adhesive pads connected to the AED are placed on the victim's chest. When the AED is turned on, it detects and analyzes heart rhythm and tells the operator what to do. The device automatically delivers an electrical shock at the right moment as needed to stabilize the heart's rhythm.

Emergency Care for Hemorrhage

Hemorrhage is severe bleeding and is a life-threatening condition. The severity of the problem depends on how fast the blood is flowing, where it is coming from, and how much blood has already been lost. You will need to determine if bleeding is from a vein or an artery. Arterial blood is bright red, flows rapidly or spurts with each heartbeat, and creates the most serious threat.

Follow standard precautions and wear gloves or use a waterproof barrier over the wound when caring for a victim who is bleeding. Blood transports many pathogens that can cause disease, such as AIDS and hepatitis B. When a victim is hemorrhaging, their pulse and respiratory rates increase, consciousness decreases, and their blood pressure may drop quickly. Emergency care must be prompt if the victim is to survive.

The goal of first aid for hemorrhage is to stop the bleeding. With your gloved hand, apply pressure directly to the wound (see Figure 7–8). Use a sterile pad or dressing if one is available. Maintain pressure on the wound while continuing to add pads. If the bleeding is from an extremity, elevating the limb above the level of the heart may help. If bleeding continues, you must next apply pressure with the fingers of your other hand to the pressure point of the artery that supplies blood to the area of the injury (see Figure 7–9). Prompt and correct response can make the dif-

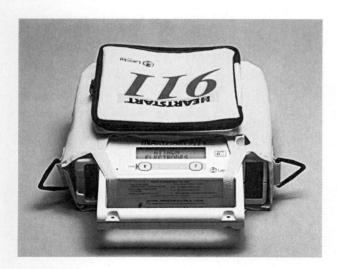

FIGURE 7–7
An automated external defibrillator.

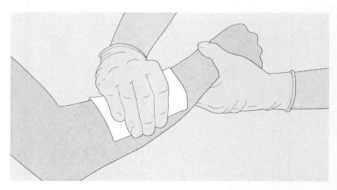

FIGURE 7–8
Apply pressure directly to the wound.

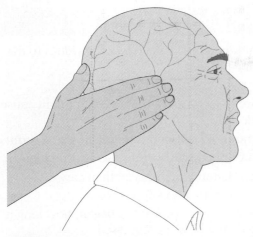

A. Temporal Artery

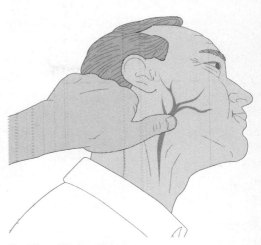

B. Mandibular Artery

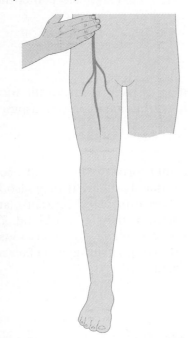

C. Femoral Artery

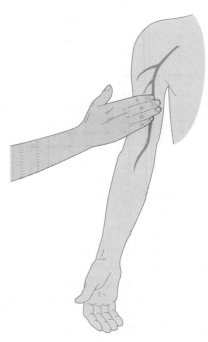

D. Brachial Artery

FIGURE 7–9
Location of pressure points.

ference between life and death to a victim who is hemorrhaging.

*E*mergency Care for Shock

Shock is the body's reaction to the failure of the circulatory system to provide enough food and oxygen to the cells. People are often unaware of the danger of shock, but if it is not treated promptly, death can result.

Signs and Symptoms of Shock

Signs and symptoms of shock include:

- Altered mental status (confused or disoriented)
- Pale, cool, clammy skin
- Nausea and vomiting
- Tremors and nervousness
- Dilated pupils of the eyes
- A weak, rapid pulse
- Rapid, shallow respirations
- A drop in blood pressure

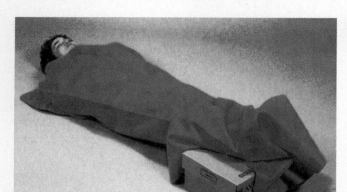

FIGURE 7–10
To prevent or relieve shock, lay the patient down with the feet and legs elevated.

Guidelines for Seizures

- If standing or sitting, lower the victim to the floor.
- Stay with the victim and call for help.
- Move objects out of the way that might cause injury.
- Do not hold the victim down or use restraints.
- Do not put anything into the victim's mouth.
- Keep visitors and other patients away.
- Remain calm and supportive.
- Observe when the seizure began, how long it lasted, and how it progressed.
- Allow the victim to rest or sleep after the seizure is over.

Infants and Children

Shock in infants and children is more critical and must be treated immediately. They have less blood volume and can be in critical condition before symptoms appear.

Care of the Victim in Shock

The first response in treating shock is to look for the cause. For example, shock can result from a hemorrhage. The shock will not improve until the bleeding is stopped. Elevate the legs and feet higher than the rest of the body, if there is no sign of leg, hip, spinal, or head injury (Figure 7–10). Cover the victim with a blanket to help maintain body heat. Do not give food or fluids to the person in shock. Reassure the victim frequently and help the victim to remain calm. If there is bleeding or vomiting from the mouth, position the victim on the side to prevent aspiration.

Fainting

Fainting is a mild form of shock that occurs when blood vessels suddenly dilate. It may also be caused by a sudden change in blood pressure, stress, bad news, an accident, or the sight of blood. The victim may feel faint or completely lose consciousness. The victim who is standing or sitting in a chair may fall to the floor and be injured.

Emergency Care for Seizures

A *seizure* (convulsion) is a sudden contraction of muscles that is caused by abnormal brain activity. The length and severity of the seizure varies. A small seizure might only involve rapid blinking of the eyes, while in a more severe seizure the victim may fall to the floor. Regardless of the length of the seizure, the victim will be unconscious and unable to respond.

Emergency Care for a Stroke

A stroke is the common name for a cerebrovascular accident (CVA), and it can be a life-threatening situation. Blood circulation in the brain is interrupted by a clot or the bursting of a blood vessel. The guidelines in Figure 7–11 will help you know how to care for the victim until help arrives.

Guidelines for Fainting

- Help the victim to sit or lie down.
- Stay with the victim and call for help.
- Help the victim to bend forward and lower the head between the knees or lie down with the feet higher than the head. The goal is to increase blood flow to the brain.
- Loosen the clothing.
- Keep the victim quiet with the head lowered for several minutes.
- Provide reassurance and emotional support.
- Help the victim to sit up gradually.
- Take vital signs as directed by your supervisor.

Guidelines for Emergency Care for a Stroke

- Call for help or activate EMS immediately.
- Maintain the victim's airway and be prepared to provide CPR.
- Keep the victim at rest and protect all paralyzed limbs.
- Position the victim so that the head and shoulders are slightly elevated. Turn the head to the side to allow drainage from the mouth (Figure 7–11).

- Keep the victim warm but do not overheat.
- Measure pulse, respirations, and blood pressure.
- Do not administer anything by mouth.
- Keep bystanders away.
- Provide emotional support.

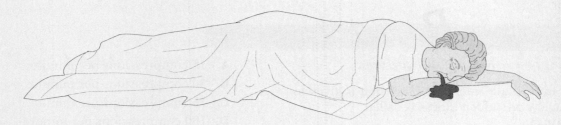

FIGURE 7–11
Turn the head to the side to allow drainage from the mouth.

Review

Read each sentence and fill in the blank with the vocabulary term that best completes the sentence.

1. In _____, the heart stops beating.
2. _____ is the medical term for severe bleeding.
3. The heartbeat is called the _____.
4. _____ is choking due to inhaling food or fluid into the airway.
5. The emergency procedure performed to dislodge a foreign body from the airway is called the _____.

Remember

1. First aid is the immediate care that is given for injury or sudden illness.
2. If an injury or sudden illness occurs to a patient at work, stay with the patient and call for help.
3. Following standard precautions will help to protect you from infection while you are providing emergency care.
4. Helping everyone, including yourself, to stay calm is very important.
5. Do not move the victim unless it is absolutely necessary.
6. The ABCs of emergency care include airway, breathing, and circulation.
7. Clutching the throat with the hands is the universal sign of choking.
8. Perform the Heimlich maneuver if the victim has a complete airway obstruction.
9. Initiate CPR if respiratory and cardiac arrest occur.
10. First aid for hemorrhage is to apply pressure directly to the wound.
11. Keeping the victim warm and lying down help to prevent shock.
12. The fainting victim should lower the head to increase blood flow to the brain.
13. Protect the seizure victim from injury.
14. Call for help or activate EMS immediately if you suspect a victim has had a stroke.

Reflect

Read the following case study and answer the questions.

Case Study

Crystal works as a nursing assistant at a long-term care facility. When she enters a room she finds a patient, Mrs. Swenson, lying on the floor with her body jerking. Crystal remembers that the patient has a history of seizures. Mrs. Swenson's roommate is standing by her bed looking frightened. Crystal turns on the emergency light and runs out of the room to get help.

1. Did Crystal properly summon help? Explain your answer.
2. List three actions Crystal should have taken after summoning help.
3. List two observations Crystal should be able to report to the nurse.
4. Should Crystal have taken the other patient with her when she left to summon help? Explain your answer.

Respond

Choose the best answer for each question.

1. The immediate emergency care that is given for an injury or sudden illness is called
   A. CPR
   B. Heimlich maneuver
   C. First aid
   D. Critical care

2. What is the nursing assistant's responsibility if a patient is injured or becomes suddenly ill?
   A. Stay with the patient and notify the nurse.
   B. Notify the nurse and call 911.
   C. Call the doctor and the family.
   D. Go to the nurse's station and call for help.

3. Which of the following is a life-threatening situation?
   A. A broken arm
   B. Fainting
   C. Headache
   D. Cardiac arrest

4. The emergency device that delivers an electrical shock to the heart is called
   A. An autoclave
   B. A defibrillator
   C. A generator
   D. A carburetor

5. The ABCs of emergency care are
   A. Assessment, breathing, and collapse
   B. Assignment, beating, and coronary
   C. Automatic, bathing, and cleansing
   D. Airway, breathing, and circulation

6. What is the correct chest compression rate in one-rescuer CPR?

A. 15 compressions per minute
B. 50 compressions per minute
C. 75 compressions per minute
D. 100 compressions per minute

7. Which of the following is a sign or symptom of shock?
   A. Hot, flushed skin
   B. A weak, rapid pulse
   C. Constricted pupils of the eye
   D. A rise in blood pressure

8. What is the best emergency response to a patient who complains of feeling faint?
   A. Lower the head between the knees.
   B. Elevate the head.
   C. Turn the victim on the side.
   D. All of the above.

9. What is the best emergency response to a patient who is having a seizure?
   A. Restrain the victim's arms.
   B. Insert a spoon between the teeth.
   C. Move objects that might injure the patient during the seizure.
   D. Hold the victim down to protect her from injury during the seizure.

10. You find a patient unconscious on the floor and she is bleeding from the mouth. How should you position her head?
    A. Elevate the head.
    B. Lower the head by elevating the feet.
    C. Turn the head to the side.
    D. Position the head between two pillows.

Chapter Eight

Communication Skills

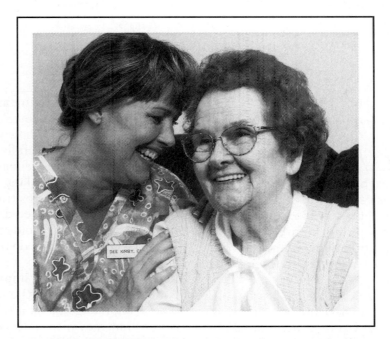

After studying this chapter, you will be able to

1. Explain the importance of communication in the health care facility.

2. Give two examples each of verbal and non-verbal communication.

3. Identify three guidelines for effective communication.

4. List six guidelines for age-specific communication.

5. Explain four guidelines for communicating with people from diverse cultures.

6. Identify four communication blocks.

7. List four guidelines each for communicating with vision-, hearing-, and speech-impaired patients.

8. List four guidelines for communicating with the confused patient.

9. List three ways to communicate with a developmentally disabled patient.

10. Explain the importance of communication with visitors.

11. Explain the correct way to answer the telephone in the health care facility.

aphasia   A loss of speech.

communication impairment   A disability that interferes with communication.

communication block   Anything that interferes with communication.

communication   The exchange of thoughts, information, and ideas.

disoriented   Confused as to time, place, and/or person.

nonverbal communication   The exchange of information without using words.

rapport   Mutual trust.

verbal communication   The exchange of thoughts, ideas, and information, using words.

Communicating in the Health Care Facility

Communication is the exchange of thoughts, information, and ideas and is essential to quality health care. Communication is necessary to keep information flowing smoothly among members of the health care team. Open communication promotes understanding among patients, family members, and health care workers.

The ability to communicate well is a valuable skill for a nursing assistant to develop. Health care is person-to-person work, and communication skills are part of the "tools of the trade." Communication is the basis for all human interactions and good communication is at the center of good nursing care.

The Communication Process

The three basic elements of the communication process are a sender, a receiver, and a message. The sender is the communicator and the receiver is the person to whom the message is directed. The receiver must also interpret the meaning of the message. Communication is an ongoing process with sending, receiving, and interpreting going on at the same time.

Forms of Communication

There are two forms of communication—verbal and nonverbal. Talking is actually only a small part of the communication process.

Verbal Communication

Verbal communication is communication using words. The words may be either spoken or written.

You use verbal communication when introducing yourself to the patient. You also use it to explain what you are going to do and how you can help the patient. Choose your words carefully because certain words can indicate negative feelings, like anger or frustration. Avoid the use of slang and vulgar terms. You want to communicate positive feelings of caring and respect. Use ordinary, everyday language that the patient understands and avoid medical terms or abbreviations. Speak clearly and do not whisper or mumble.

It may be necessary to write messages to patients who are hearing impaired. Speech-impaired patients may need to write their needs on a pad or board. Sign language is a type of verbal communication that may also be used with people who are speech or hearing impaired.

Reading to patients is another example of verbal communication. Read slowly and carefully, observing punctuation and placing proper emphasis on important words. Ask permission before reading personal mail to the patient and remember to respect confidentiality. (See Figure 8–1.)

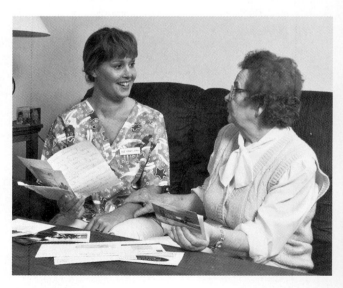

FIGURE 8–1
Reading a letter to a patient is an example of verbal communication.

Nonverbal Communication

Nonverbal communication is communication without words. Just as words can be positive or negative, so can nonverbal communication. What messages are you communicating as you go about your daily duties? If you come rushing into the patient's room with a frown on your face, you are communicating that you are in a hurry and expect the patient to hurry also. Observe the patient's nonverbal communication as well. The patient may not be able to tell you what is wrong or may not want to complain. However, a patient who is clutching her side and grimacing with tear-filled eyes is probably communicating that she is in pain. Examples of nonverbal communication include:

- Gestures
- Facial expressions
- Smiling
- Body language
- Posture
- Listening
- Touch

Most of the time, we use a combination of verbal and nonverbal communication. For instance, you are describing an experience on a recent fishing trip. You extend your hands to show the size of the fish and indicate how you moved the fishing rod. Your eyes light up, and you smile widely as you describe what a thrill it was to catch a fish of that size. You are sending a message that you had a wonderful time, are thrilled, and a bit proud of your accomplishment. The message was communicated through a combination of words, facial expressions, voice tones, gestures, and body language. (See Figure 8–2.)

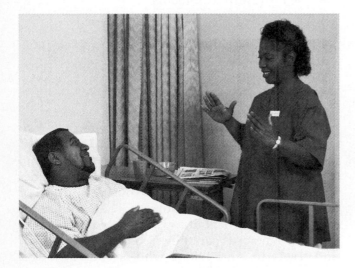

FIGURE 8–2
Most of the time we use a combination of verbal and nonverbal communication.

In order for this combination to work, the words must agree with the nonverbal communication. Confusion can result if your verbal and nonverbal communication does not agree. When you send mixed messages, your nonverbal communication is more likely to be believed. For example, suppose that you go into the room of a patient who has had a bowel movement in bed. The patient is embarrassed and starts apologizing. You wrinkle your nose, get a distasteful look on your face, and say to the patient "That's all right, I really don't mind." The patient will probably not believe what you say, because your nonverbal communication always speaks louder than your words.

Manner of Communication

Paying attention to your manner of speaking will help you to become a better communicator. The tone of your voice as well as how loudly, softly, or quickly you speak all play a role in how easy it is for listeners to understand you. Try and listen critically to yourself. Is the tone of your voice demanding, bossy, or soothing? Are you speaking loudly or softly? Are you sending a mixed message that leaves the receiver wondering what you really mean?

Patients should be addressed formally (Mr. Brown or Mrs. Smith, for example). Do not call a patient by his or her given name unless the patient has given you permission to do so. Never use terms such as "honey" or "sweetheart." Not only do these terms indicate lack of respect, their use might also be considered sexual harassment. Avoid "talking down" or talking "baby talk" to elderly or confused patients. All adult patients should be spoken to as adults, regardless of age or mental status. Communication can also be restorative. Using a comment such as "May I help you get out of bed?" in place of "I'm going to get you out of bed." helps the patient maintain dignity and independence.

Interpersonal Skills

Develop your interpersonal skills. These are the skills that are used to deal successfully with other people and include courtesy, respect, tact, patience, and empathy. Using the holistic approach, consider how your words and actions will affect the whole person. Will they understand the message? How will it make them feel? Will it boost their self-esteem or bring on sadness? Can you get the message across in a gentler manner? Think before you speak.

Listening

Listening involves paying attention to what you are hearing. It is an active process—you have to work at it. A good listener encourages the speaker to continue. Responses such as "Go on," "I see," and "Oh, yes" indicate that you are not only listening, but you are thinking about what has been said. Sometimes a smile or a nod of the head will have the same effect.

There are some problems that interfere with listening. Some people listen selectively—that is, they hear only what they want to hear or what they think the message is going to be. Unfamiliar words can interfere with concentration and understanding. Prejudice can affect listening because you concentrate on the person instead of the ideas.

Listening can be a healing process. We all have a need to express ideas and a need to be heard. It is important to listen to your patients. Being sick and confined in a health care facility can be very stressful. Take time to listen to the patient's problems, his pains, and his joys. The patient will be reassured that you cared enough to listen. (See Figure 8–3.)

Touch

Touch often communicates when other methods have failed. It can involve a handshake, a pat on the shoulder, or a warm hug. The feel of a cool hand on a fevered brow communicates hope and consolation. Throughout this text, you will find references to the value of touch in communicating caring concern.

Be aware that culture may determine the effectiveness of touch. For example, in many Latin cultures, touch is an essential part of communication. These people are constantly touching, patting, and hugging one another. They may extend the warmth and touching to you and other staff members. However, many other cultures use a more formalized method of communication that does not include a lot of touching. Observe their interactions with others and take your cue from their behavior.

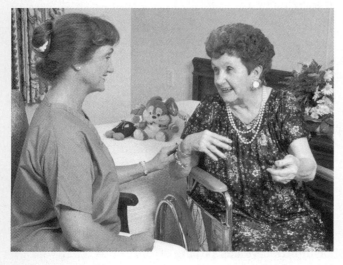

FIGURE 8–3
Listening can be a healing process.

Effective Communication

Effective communication is communication that works—the sender and the receiver both understand the message. The sender includes feelings, beliefs, and intentions in the message. The receiver interprets the message in the same manner. The intent of the message must be understood as well as the actual words. Otherwise, there will be confusion or conflict. For example, you say to a friend, "I really like the way you are wearing your hair." Your friends replies, "What was wrong with it before?" You intended to pay a compliment but she interpreted it as a criticism. Try to make the intention of your message as clear as possible. The following list of guidelines will help you to communicate more effectively. The more you practice this technique, the easier it will become.

Guidelines for Effective Communication

- Introduce yourself and show interest.
- Make eye contact with the other person.
- Lean forward and pay attention.
- Try to build *rapport* (mutual trust).
- Organize your thoughts before you speak.
- Allow others to express their ideas.
- Listen attentively.
- Be respectful and considerate.
- Be warm and caring.
- Develop a positive, willing attitude.
- Make sure verbal and nonverbal communications agree.
- Use restorative comments.
- Make your message as clear as possible.

Age-Specific Communication

Age must be taken into consideration when communicating. Would you use the same words or manner when speaking to a 2-year-old, your best friend, or your grandmother? Of course not. Most toddlers have a limited vocabulary, so you would need to choose your words carefully. You might speak easily and freely to your friend who is your own age. However, your grandmother comes from a different time when language was more formal. You adjust your manner according to the person's age. This is what is meant by age-specific communication. The following guidelines focus on two age groups—the elderly and children.

Guidelines for Communicating with the Elderly

- Address elderly persons by their titles or names they prefer.
- Avoid terms of relationship such as "Granny" or "Uncle" unless you are related to the person.
- Show respect and courtesy.
- Be aware of generational differences.
- Speak to them as adults regardless of behavior or confusion.
- Be aware of sensory impairments such as hearing loss.
- Encourage and assist with the use of eye-glasses and hearing aids when needed.
- Repeat the person's name frequently.
- Encourage them to talk about themselves and their families.

Guidelines for Communicating with Children

- Consider the age level.
- Remember that regardless of age, each child is unique.
- Use appropriate language the child can understand.
- Do not "talk down" to the child or use "baby talk."
- Avoid using commands or words that sound threatening.
- Explain what you are going to do, simply and clearly.
- Call the child by name and be respectful.
- Tell the truth whenever possible.
- Talk to infants whether they can answer you or not. Infants respond to sound.
- Keep your voice tones soft and comforting. Loud talking may frighten or startle the infant.
- Observe the infant's sounds and movements to determine needs.
- Touch the infant, hold it against your chest, and rock it to communicate caring and security. (See Figure 8–4.)

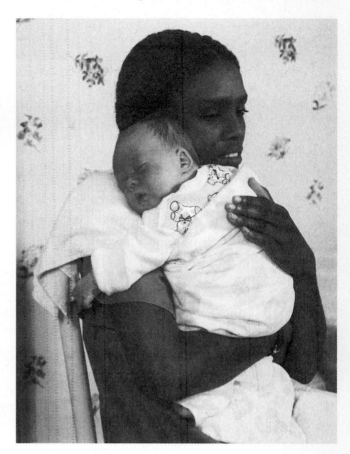

FIGURE 8–4
Holding and rocking the infant communicates caring and security.

Communicating with People from Different Cultures

As a health care worker, you must be able to communicate effectively with patients, visitors, and co-

Guidelines for Communicating with People from Different Cultures

- Learn about other cultures, particularly those in your own community.
- Be accepting and nonjudgmental.
- Remember that gestures may be interpreted differently.
- Be aware that touch and personal space are cultural issues.
- Speak slowly and choose your words carefully.
- Avoid using slang or uncommon terms.
- Verify that the listener has understood your message.
- Listen carefully and verify your interpretation of the message you are being given.
- Ask for help from the nurse if necessary.

workers from diverse cultural backgrounds. Their expectations, understanding, and communication tactics may be different from your own. You may not even share a common language. Patients have a right to receive information in a language they can understand. This may involve providing an interpreter. However, most of the time it means using consideration and common sense before you speak. The guidelines on page 97 will be helpful.

Communication Blocks

A *communication block* is something that interferes with the exchange of information and ideas. It may prevent the receiver from listening or understanding. Examples of communication blocks include:

- Giving pat answers—"Everything will be all right."
- Being judgmental—"That's not right."
- Daydreaming.
- Hearing, sight, or speech loss.
- Changing the subject.
- Giving your opinion.
- Talking too much.
- Failing to listen.
- Using medical terminology with patients.
- Cultural and language differences.

Communication Impairments

A patient who has difficulty communicating because of a disability is said to have a *communication impairment*. The impairment or disability may include a problem with vision, hearing, or speech. A patient might also have a mental condition that affects communication. Included in this group are patients who are confused and those who are comatose. Some developmentally disabled patients also have difficulty communicating.

The Vision-Impaired Patient

The term "vision-impaired" means that something is affecting the patient's ability to see. Patients who lose their sight tend to rely more heavily on other senses. They use the senses of hearing, smell, and touch to assist in communication. Do not be surprised if the patient with a vision impairment calls you by name when you walk in the room. He or she heard your footsteps and recognized your walk. Some vision-impaired patients use touch to identify people and objects. The patient who is blind may ask to feel your face with her hands in order to "see" you. (See Figure 8–5.)

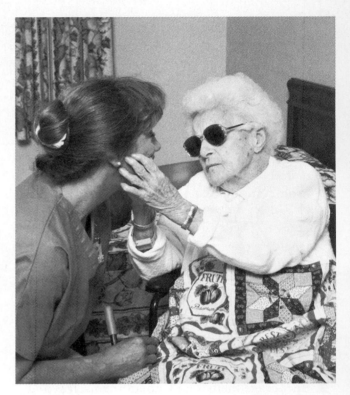

FIGURE 8–5
The blind patient may feel your face with her hands in order to "see" you.

Communicating with vision-impaired patients requires special skills. Always speak to the patient when you enter the room. Do not touch the patient until you have identified yourself. It can be irritating or frightening to have someone touch you before you know who is there. Have you ever had someone come up behind you, put their hands over your eyes, and say "Guess who?" How did you feel?

Pay close attention to what you say. Comments like "It's right in front of you" or "It's over there on

Guidelines for Communicating with the Vision-Impaired Patient

- Identify yourself before approaching or touching the patient.
- Face the person with whom you are talking.
- Encourage and respect the patient's independence.
- Be specific in your explanations.
- Use the clock method to describe the location of items.
- Talk in a normal tone of voice.
- Encourage the patient's use of hearing, smell, and touch.
- Let the patient know when you leave the room.

the dresser" have little meaning to a patient who cannot see. Try to be specific in giving information, and watch your nonverbal communication carefully. The blind patient listens closely, not just to your words but to the tone and volume of your voice.

The clock method is used to identify the location of objects or the location of food at meal times. The following example will help you to understand the clock method.

> You are assisting Mrs. Marshall, who is blind, to brush her teeth. She is sitting up in bed with the overbed table in front of her. You have placed the supplies for brushing her teeth on the table. You tell her that a glass of water is at 12 o'clock, her toothbrush is at 3 o'clock, an emesis basin is at 6 o'clock, and the toothpaste is at 9 o'clock. These instructions will make it easier for her to brush her teeth independently.

The Hearing-Impaired Patient

The hearing-impaired patient has trouble understanding words or sounds. Hearing impairment can range from a slight hearing loss to total deafness. Communicating with hearing-impaired patients can be difficult. Move in front of and face the hearing-impaired patient before touching to avoid startling him or her. Facing the person also helps hearing-impaired patients who depend on lip reading. These patients watch your mouth and lip movements to identify the sounds you are making. The use of key words can be helpful when communicating with the hearing-impaired patient. This technique involves emphasizing the most important words in the message.

Guidelines for Communicating with the Hearing-Impaired Patient

- Approach the hearing-impaired patient so that you can be seen.
- Face the patient with whom you are speaking and look directly at him or her.
- Avoid mumbling or looking at the floor.
- Keep instructions simple and use key words.
- Remind the patient to wear a hearing aid, if required.
- Check the hearing aid batteries and volume. (See Figure 8–6.)
- Lower the pitch of your voice but do not shout.
- Eliminate or reduce background noises, such as radios and televisions.

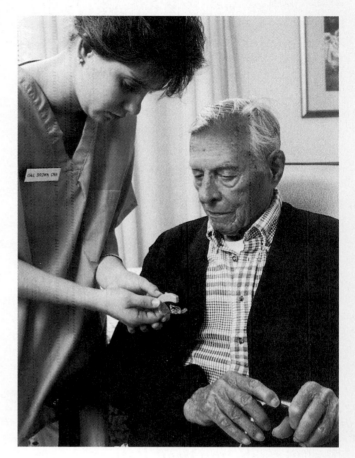

FIGURE 8–6
Check the hearing aid batteries and volume.

Hearing Aid Care

A hearing aid is a device used to amplify sound. Although they come in various sizes and shapes, most hearing aids include a microphone, amplifier, ear mould, battery, and volume control. (See Figure 8–7.) The ear mould is custom-made to fit each individual. The hearing aid will make a whistling noise if the ear mould does not fit snugly into the ear. Some

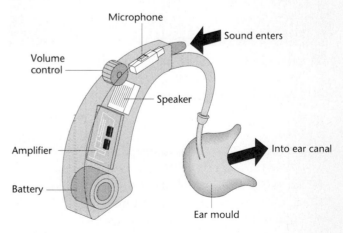

FIGURE 8–7
Basic parts of a hearing aid.

Guidelines for Hearing Aid Care

- Turn the volume on low and assist the patient to place the hearing aid into the ear.
- If whistling occurs, reposition the hearing aid until it fits snugly.
- Adjust the volume to a range that is comfortable for the patient.
- To remove the hearing aid, turn it off and pull it gently toward you.
- Check the patient's ear and ear mould for wax buildup.
- Wipe the hearing aid with a clean, dry tissue after each wearing.
- Clean the ear mould with soap and water. Never put the body of the hearing aid in water.
- Check the battery at regular intervals.
- When not in use, store the hearing aid away from heat or cold.

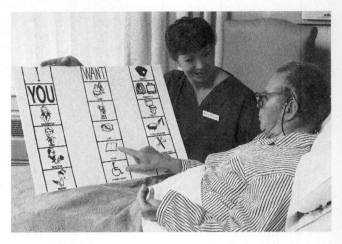

FIGURE 8–8
A picture board may be helpful for the speech-impaired patient.

patients may need assistance to insert, adjust, remove, and care for their hearing aids.

The Speech-Impaired Patient

The speech-impaired patient has difficulty using language. The problem may involve speaking, reading, or writing. The medical term for loss of speech is *aphasia* ("a" means lack of or without and "phasic" means speech). There may be difficulty with retrieval (finding the right word to use). This can be very frustrating to the patient who knows the right word but keeps saying the wrong word.

A picture board has pictures that indicate common items and needs. Patients who are unable to speak can point to pictures that best describes their needs. This piece of equipment may be a magnetic board with a variety of items that can be changed as needed. However, a picture board can be made with a piece of cardboard and a marking pen, or pictures can be cut out and pasted on it. (See Figure 8–8.)

Communicating with Confused or Mentally Impaired Patients

The confused or mentally impaired patient may be able to see, hear, and speak normally, but still have

Guidelines for Communicating with the Speech-Impaired Patient

- Stand in front of the patient so that you can be seen.
- Create a calm, quiet environment.
- Allow time for response and avoid rushing the patient.
- Do not finish sentences too quickly for the patient.
- Keep explanations short and simple.
- Make sure that the patient understands.
- Acknowledge the patient's frustration.
- Use a picture board if necessary.

Guidelines for Communicating with the Confused Patient

- Get the patient's attention. Make eye contact and touch the patient gently.
- Identify yourself and the patient. Some confused patients are not sure of their own identity.
- Keep directions simple, one step at a time.
- Be patient and empathetic.
- Offer frequent general reassurance. "You're okay" or "I'll take care of you."
- Try not to rush the patient.
- Develop rapport. Build a trusting relationship with the patient.
- Watch your nonverbal communication. Confused patients usually understand actions better than words.
- Listen carefully and try to understand the patient's message.
- Use touch. A hug or pat on the shoulder speaks for itself.

difficulty communicating. The degree of confusion is important. Is the patient mildly or severely confused? Does the confusion come and go, or is it constant? Is the patient *disoriented* (confused as to time, place, and person)? The patient may be able to communicate clearly one time and be confused the next. Because there are so many levels and types of confusion, it is difficult to develop techniques that will always work. The guidelines on page 100 will be helpful in most situations.

Communicating with Developmentally Disabled Patients

Developmentally disabled patients are individuals who have not developed normally due to disease, injury, or a birth defect. Many of these patients have mental impairments and difficulty communicating.

The Comatose Patient

Talk to the comatose patient as you would any other patient. Introduce yourself and explain what you are going to do. For example, tell the patient, "I am going to turn you on to your right side, now. The side rail is up, so you won't fall." Think how frightening it would be if someone suddenly started moving your body in the bed, and you had no idea what was going to happen. Assume that the patient can hear your voice and feel your touch. Do not talk across the bed to someone else as though there was no one in the bed. Patients

have awakened from a coma (an unconscious state) and recalled hearing conversations that took place over them.

Communicating with Visitors

Family members and friends play an important role in the patient's quality of life. Their love and concern can affect the patient's response to treatment and desire to live. When we focus on the patient as a whole person, we must include family and friends.

Sometimes family members may be irritable or angry out of anxiety and concern for the patient. Because the nursing assistant provides so much of the patient's direct care, you may become the target of that anger. Listen quietly until the person has finished talking. (See Figure 8–9.) Do not interrupt, argue, or become defensive. Remember, they are not really mad at you—you just got in the way of an angry outburst. Refer the person to the nurse and return to your duties. Do not just point in the direction of the nurses' station. Either escort the person to the desk or go get the nurse. Let the nurse know immediately if a visitor threatens you or becomes violent.

If family members or other visitors ask questions about the patient's care or treatment, refer them to the nurse. However, there are things you can say that do not risk confidentiality. Your comment that the patient "ate all of his breakfast this morning," if that is true, can be very reassuring to

Guidelines for Communicating with the Developmentally Disabled Patient

■ Treat the patient with respect and dignity.
■ Be aware of the patient's limitations.
■ Communicate at the patient's level of understanding. Talk to adults in an adult manner.
■ Position yourself at the patient's eye level, especially if the patient is in a wheelchair.
■ Include the patient in your conversation.
■ Offer praise and encouragement.
■ Provide adaptive equipment such as a picture board if needed.

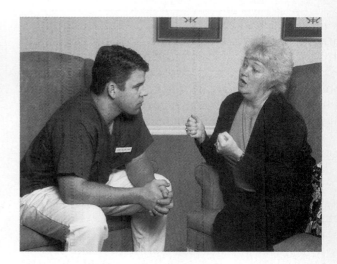

FIGURE 8–9
Anxiety and concern for the patient may cause a family member to be irritable or angry.

Guidelines for Communicating with Visitors

- Be pleasant, courteous, and respectful to all visitors.
- Be helpful and friendly.
- Be aware of cultural diversity.
- Listen carefully and do not interrupt.
- Refer questions about the patient's condition or treatment to the nurse.
- Maintain confidentiality.
- Avoid getting involved in family affairs or disagreements.
- Never argue with visitors.
- Don't take a visitor's anger personally.
- Refer angry visitors to the nurse.
- Report visitor's threats or violence immediately.

Guidelines for Using the Telephone

- Answer the telephone promptly.
- Speak slowly and clearly. Be aware of your tone of voice.
- Be polite and respectful.
- Identify yourself promptly by giving your name, title, and work area.
- If you must transfer a call, be sure it is answered.
- Ask permission before putting the caller on hold.
- Write down the information immediately when taking a message. (See Figure 8–10.)
- Verify the accuracy of the message by reading it back to the caller.
- Never use the business telephone for personal calls.

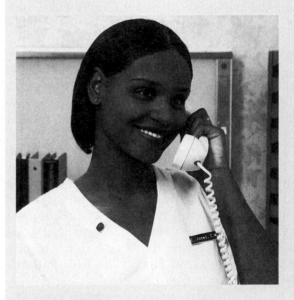

FIGURE 8–10
Write down the information immediately when taking a telephone message.

the family. Follow facility policy regarding questions about vital signs or other procedures that you have performed.

Families do not always agree and get along with one another. If there is a quarrel, either the patient or a family member may want you to take sides. **Do not** get involved in family affairs or disagreements. If the patient gets upset or seems stressed during a visit, report this information to the nurse immediately.

Using the Telephone

A telephone call is often the first communication a person has with a health care facility. The manner in which the call is handled can leave a lasting impression. If the person answering the telephone is polite, if information is given promptly, and if the voice communicates caring concern, the caller is likely to have a positive impression of the facility.

Identify yourself to the caller, giving your name, title, and unit or area. If you are asked to take a message, write down the information as you receive it. Include the name of the person for whom the message is intended, the name and telephone number of the caller, and the message. Add your name, the date and time of the call. To be certain you have the message correct, read it back to the caller. If a doctor is calling, quickly identify yourself as an aide and state that you will get a nurse. Nursing assistants are not allowed to take doctor's orders.

Never use the business telephone for personal calls. Ask your family to call only in an emergency. When you tie up the line for personal calls, doctors and other health care providers cannot get through to check on their patients.

Review

Read each sentence and fill in the blank with the vocabulary term that best completes the sentence.

1. _____ is the exchange of thoughts, information, and ideas.
2. Building _____ (mutual trust) is important for effective communication.
3. A patient who has difficulty communicating because of a disability is said to have a _____.
4. The medical term for loss of speech is _____.
5. A patient who is _____ is confused as to time, place, and person.

Remember

1. Open communication promotes understanding among patients, family members, and health care workers.
2. It is important that your words agree with your nonverbal communication.
3. Listening is an active process—you have to work at it.
4. Touch is one of the most valuable methods of communication.
5. Effective communication occurs when both the sender and the receiver understand the message.
6. It is important to adjust your manner of speaking to the patient's age.
7. Be aware that touch, personal space, and gestures are cultural issues.
8. A communication block interferes with the exchange of information and ideas.
9. Identify yourself before touching the vision-impaired or the hearing-impaired patient.
10. Never put the body of a hearing aid in water. Clean the ear mould with soap and water.
11. Do not interrupt or quickly finish sentences for the speech-impaired patient.
12. Make eye contact and touch the confused patient before attempting to communicate.
13. Communicate at the developmentally disabled patient's level of understanding. Talk to adults in an adult manner.
14. Assume that the comatose patient can hear your voice and feel your touch.
15. Communicate with visitors in a courteous, respectful manner.
16. Answer the telephone promptly and politely to give a positive impression of the facility.

Reflect

Read the following case study and answer the questions.

Case Study

Helen Washington is a 90-year-old patient in a nursing home. She is confused, hearing impaired, and in a wheelchair. When Bob enters her room, she is looking down at the floor and mumbling softly to herself. Bob says, "Good morning Granny. I'm Bob, your nursing assistant for today, and I'm here to help you get ready to go to the dining room." Mrs. Washington does not look up or answer. Bob raises his voice and shouts, "Helen, can you hear me?" Pam, another nursing assistant, enters the room and Bob says to her, "Helen is really out of it today. She's acting crazy." Pat steps in front of the wheelchair and squats down until she is at eye level with Mrs. Washington. She places her hand on Mrs. Washington's arm and says clearly, "Mrs. Washington. It's Pam. Let's go eat." Mrs. Washington looks up at Pam, smiles, and says, "Okay, Pam."

1. Was Bob's greeting appropriate when he first came into Mrs. Washington's room? Why or why not?
2. List three other mistakes Bob made while trying to communicate with Mrs. Washington.
3. How could Bob have gotten Mrs. Washington's attention after his first comment failed?
4. Name three things Pam did that aided effective communication.

Respond

Choose the best answer for each question.

1. The three basic elements of the communication process are
   A. Sender, receiver, and message
   B. Sender, interpretation, and message
   C. Receiver, message, and rapport
   D. Talker, writer, and sender

2. You should use medical terminology when speaking to a patient.
   A. True
   B. False

3. An example of nonverbal communication is
   A. Gestures
   B. Facial expressions
   C. Body language
   D. All of the above

4. What is the correct way to greet a new, elderly patient whose name is Edward B. Mason?
   A. "Good morning, Edward."
   B. "Good morning, Pops."
   C. "Good morning, Mr. Mason."
   D. All of the above.

5. Skills used to deal successfully with other people are called
   A. Interpersonal skills
   B. Activity skills
   C. Interrelated skills
   D. Procedural skills

6. Which of the following comments is the best way to communicate with a 7-year-old child about lunch?
   A. "Hi, Jimmy. Would you like to eat now?"
   B. "Here's your food tray, Mr. Smith."
   C. "Be sure you eat all the food on this tray."
   D. "If you don't eat, I'll tell your Mom."

7. Which of the following are guidelines for communicating with the vision-impaired patient?
   A. Touch the patient before you speak.
   B. Face the patient you are talking to.
   C. Talk in a very loud voice.
   D. Use a picture board to help the patient understand.

8. What is the correct way to clean a hearing aid?
   A. Soak the entire hearing aid in warm, soapy water.
   B. Clean the hearing aid with Betadine.
   C. Avoid getting water on any part of the hearing aid.
   D. Clean the ear mould with soap and water.

9. What is the best response to a developmentally disabled adult patient who wants to go home to her mother?
   A. "Don't be silly. You can't go home to your mother."
   B. "Your mother left you here to stay."
   C. "Your mother will be here to visit this evening."
   D. "Your mother has been dead for years."

10. A visitor is very angry and accuses you of neglecting his mother. What is the best response?
    B. "It's not my fault. I do the best I can."
    B. "Your mother is not even one of my patients."
    C. "You get tough with me and I'll call security."
    D. "I can see you're upset. Let me get the nurse."

Chapter Nine
Communicating *with* Co-Workers

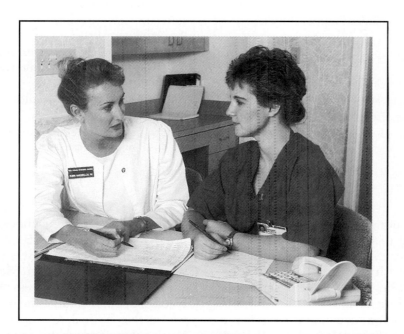

OBJECTIVES

After studying this chapter, you will be able to

1. Explain the importance of observation.

2. Explain the difference between objective and subjective observations.

3. Give two examples of objective reporting.

4. Demonstrate the proper way to correct a written error.

5. List six guidelines for recording patient information.

6. Identify two items that are included in the care plan.

7. Identify four basic components of a computer.

8. Recognize examples of a word root, a prefix, and a suffix.

9. Divide medical terms into their elements.

10. Recognize and identify the meaning of commonly used abbreviations.

Glossary

abbreviation A shortened form for writing a word or phrase.

care plan A written document outlining the care of an individual patient.

central processing unit (CPU) The "brain" or controlling part of a computer.

glossary A collection of specialized terms with the meaning of each term.

hardware The physical equipment used by a computer to process data.

objective observations Information that can be observed by seeing, hearing, smelling, or touching.

observation The process of noticing facts and events.

prefix The element of a medical term found at the beginning of the word.

recording Writing information on the correct form; also called charting or documenting.

reporting The act of communicating information to the proper person.

root The element of a medical term that represents the foundation of the word.

software The programs or sets of instruction that make the computer work.

subjective observations Information that cannot be observed but must be communicated and described by the person experiencing it.

suffix The element of a medical term found at the end of the word.

vital signs Measurements of temperature, pulse, respirations, and blood pressure.

Communication among members of the health care team is vital to the safety and quality of care in a health care facility. This chapter focuses on ways that health care workers communicate with each other. It begins with the observation, reporting, and recording of patient information. *Observation* means noticing facts and events. It is a method of collecting information about the patients. *Reporting* is communicating information to the proper person. *Recording* is writing information about the patient on the correct form. This may also be called "charting" or "documenting." Observation, reporting, and recording are important responsibilities of the nursing assistant.

The chapter also provides an introduction to computers—a modern, efficient way to communicate. Understanding and using computers is an important skill in today's world. The final section addresses medical terminology, the language of medicine. Learning to understand medical terms is an important part of your nursing assistant training.

The Importance of Observation

As a nursing assistant, you spend more time with the patient than any other member of the health care team. Because you provide direct hands-on care every day, you have more opportunity to notice changes in a patient's condition. You may be the first one to see a reddened area on the skin or to smell an odor coming from under a cast. You may

be the one the patient chooses to talk with about problems and concerns. Because of the unique role you play in patient care, it is necessary that you develop skills in observation. (See Figure 9–1.)

Observation is a process that must focus on the whole person, including the psychosocial concerns as well as the physical. An important part of observation involves knowing what is normal and what is not normal. In Chapter 10, you will study normal body structure and the changes of aging. This information will help you to understand normal versus abnormal.

Observation also includes an awareness of changes in the patient's usual condition. Observing

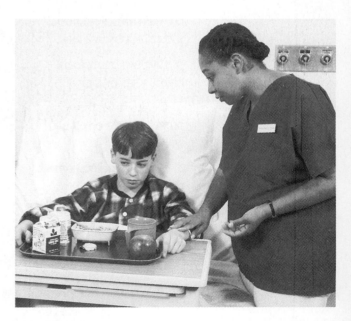

FIGURE 9–1
The nursing assistant observes and records the patient's food intake.

these changes requires that you know what the person's usual condition is. The term "usual" rather than "normal" is used because it more accurately describes the information. For example, a patient might usually have a blood pressure of 180/100 (an above normal reading). However, if the same patient's blood pressure reading was 110/64 (a normal reading), that measurement indicates a change in the patient's condition and should be reported.

One of the best times for patient observation is at bath time. During the bath you are able to see the patient's entire body. You can observe breathing patterns, skin conditions, and body movements. It is also important to listen to the patient. Pay close attention to complaints and concerns that the patient may communicate. Assisting the patient in bathing, dressing, and grooming takes a considerable amount of time. Use this time to communicate, to listen, and to observe the patient. Observations may be either objective or subjective.

Objective Observations

Objective observations are things that you can see, hear, smell, and touch. You observe them with your eyes, your ears, your nose, and the touch of your fingertips. As you give the patient a bath, you might see a reddened area on the skin or the skin might feel hot when you touch it. You hear the patient cough, or you smell a peculiar odor. These are all examples of objective observations. A list of objective observations is included in Figure 9–2.

Subjective Observations

Subjective observations are things that the patient must tell you and cannot be objectively observed. Complaints of pain, nausea, and dizziness are examples of subjective observations. Even though you may observe signs of pain, you cannot be sure that it really exists. A patient wanting sympathy might groan and grimace as though in terrible pain, when in fact there is no pain. On the other hand, a patient trying to be brave might be in real pain without showing it. A subjective observation usually involves sensations that only the patient can experience. The following patient comments are examples of subjective observations that should be reported to the nurse immediately:

- "I have pain in my right leg."
- "I feel nauseated. I think I am going to be sick."
- "I have a headache."
- "My throat is sore."
- "My chest hurts."
- "I don't feel good."

Reporting

As a nursing assistant, you will report your observations to the nurse. Always include the patient's full name and room number to avoid confusion. It will be helpful to carry a small note pad in your pocket so you can write down the facts. This practice will also help you to report and record accurately.

Objective Reporting

Objective reporting is reporting only the facts that you are able to observe. Vague reports that are incomplete or influenced by your own opinion can delay patient care and may not be accurate. An objective report should give the nurse enough information to take action. The following examples indicate the correct way to report objectively.

Right: "Jane Bragg in 204A has a reddened area on her left ankle that is about the size of a dime."

Wrong: "Janie's skin is starting to break down again."

Right: "Mr. Chen in 346B says he has a sharp pain in his right shoulder that started right after lunch."

Wrong: "Mr. Chen wants a pain pill."

Right: "Billy King in crib 16 drank eight ounces of formula and is crying."

Wrong: "That baby boy in the last crib on the left is still hungry. We need to change his formula."

The best way to objectively report a complaint or comment from a patient is to use the patient's exact words. Repeating the information back to the patient will help you get the message right.

Report any abnormal or unusual observations to the nurse promptly and accurately. (See Figure 9–3.) Do not wait until the end of the shift to report. The nurse needs to be aware of your observations as soon as possible. If you are unsure about reporting an observation, the safest action would be to report it and let the nurse decide its importance. It is always better to report an observation unnecessarily than to fail to report something important. Examples of observations that should be reported to the nurse include the following:

- Any change in the patient's physical condition
- Behavior and personality changes
- Skin injuries, rashes, reddened or discolored areas
- A change or abnormal reading in *vital signs* (temperature, pulse, respiration, and blood pressure)
- Edema (swelling of a body part with fluid)
- Coughing and other breathing problems

Objective Observations

Observations You Can See

- Activities of daily living such as eating, drinking, walking, dressing, and toileting
- Body posture and movement
- Skin color, injuries, and swelling
- Breathing depth and difficulty
- Bowel movement consistency, color, amount, frequency, and control
- Urine consistency, color, amount, frequency, and control
- Drainage color, consistency, and amount
- Vomitus
- Bleeding
- Facial expressions

Observations You Can Hear

- Breath sounds, coughing, sneezing
- Cracking and popping of joints or bones
- Bowel sounds
- Crying or moaning
- Patient response
- Blood pressure

Observations You Can Smell

- Breath odors
- Poor hygiene
- Urine or bowel movement
- Drainage or vomitus
- Any unusual odor

Observations You Can Feel

- Skin temperature and texture
- Pulses
- Response to touch

FIGURE 9–2
Objective observations are things you can see, hear, smell, and touch.

- Dizziness or weakness
- Abuse or suspicion of abuse
- Safety hazards
- Defective equipment

Shift Report

Each shift in a health care facility begins with a report that includes information about the patients and the work area. Changes in a patient's care or condition are discussed, as well as events that took place on that shift. The report may include all the nursing staff or only selected nurses. Nursing assistants do not always receive the entire report. The nurse may give each nursing assistant a report as assignments are distributed. The assignment sheet contains information that you need to provide care for each of your patients.

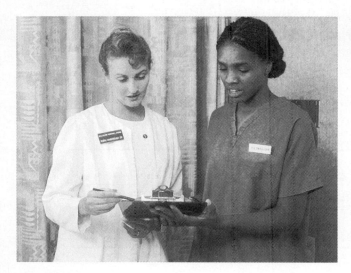

FIGURE 9–3
Report observations promptly to the nurse.

Guidelines for Recording Patient Information

- Write with ink. Never use a pencil.
- Use correct grammar and spelling.
- Use abbreviations that are approved by your facility.
- Be brief and accurate.
- Write neatly and clearly.
- Chart in order of occurrence.
- Record the date and time of each entry.
- Sign your name and title to each entry.
- Do not leave empty spaces or lines.
- Do not chart a procedure until you have completed it.
- When charting what a patient said, use the exact words in quotation marks.
- Correct errors properly.
- Chart objectively. Don't draw conclusions or judge.

Recording

One of the purposes of recording or charting is to provide a written record of the patient's care. Members of the health care team can refer to the chart to see what happened on other shifts. The doctor uses the chart to check, record, and plan the patient's treatment and care. The doctor's orders are influenced by information that other members of the health care team have recorded. Always record neatly and accurately. The chart is a legal document and can be used in court to prove what actions were or were not taken. (See Figure 9–4.)

It is important to maintain the confidentiality of patient information. Do your charting in the proper area and return the chart or form to the nurses' station when you are finished. If a patient or family member asks for information that you have observed, refer the person to the nurse.

Correcting an Error

Remember that the chart is a legal document. Never scribble through, erase, or use correction fluid on a recorded entry. Try to avoid errors on the chart, but if you do make a mistake, correct it properly. Draw a single line through the error (so it can still be read), write "error" and "mistaken entry" above the error, and the correct information. Sign it with your name and title (Figure 9–5).

Graphic Sheets

The graphic sheet is used to record observations, measurements, and activities of the patient. It may

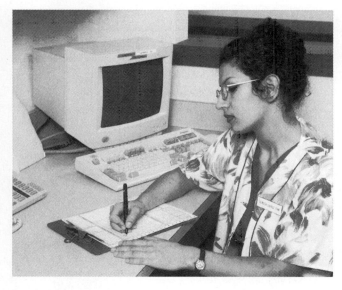

FIGURE 9–4
Always record neatly and accurately.

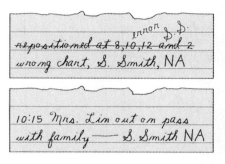

FIGURE 9–5
Examples of corrected errors.

ACTIVITIES OF DAILY LIVING CHECKLIST

Self   Done by patient
Assist   Patient assisted by nursing staff
Total   Done by nursing staff
✔   Check procedure performed
           Include time if appropriate

DATE															
DIET	B'fast	Dinner	Supper	B'fast	Dinner	Supper	B'fast	Dinner	Supper	B'fast	Dinner	Supper	B'fast	Dinner	Supper
Ate all food served															
Ate approx. 1/2 food served															
Refused to eat															
PROCEDURE	11-7	7-3	3-11	11-7	7-3	3-11	11-7	7-3	3-11	11-7	7-3	3-11	11-7	7-3	3-11
A.M. or H.S. Care															
Oral hygiene															
Bath-Bed bath complete															
Bed bath partial															
Shower															
Tub															
Self care															
Back care															
Bed made															
ELIMINATION															
Bowel movement															
Involuntary B.M.															
Voided															
Incontinent															
Foley catheter															
Sitz bath @															
ACTIVITY															
Bed rest complete															
Dangle															
Bed rest–B.R.P.															
Up in chair															
Up in room															
Walk in hall															
Ambulatory															
POSITION CHANGED															
Flat in bed															
Semi-Fowler's															
Deep breathe, cough															
Range of motion															
Turn from side to side															
Side rails–Up															
Down															
Fresh water @															
SIGNATURE & TITLE															

FIGURE 9–6

A sample activities of daily living (ADL) sheet.

include measurements of vital signs, height, and weight. Space is usually provided to note the patient's appetite, fluid intake and output, and bowel movements. In some facilities this form may be called a flow sheet or an activities of daily living (ADL) sheet (see Figure 9–6).

Facility policy determines whether or not you will be allowed to handle the patient's chart. You may be instructed to record on your assignment sheet or on a form that will be added to the chart later. In other facilities, you may record directly in the patient's chart. Regardless of where you chart, you should always follow the guidelines for recording patient information.

*C*are Plans

The *care plan* is a written document outlining the patient's plan of care. An individualized plan is written and reviewed regularly for every patient by nurses and other members of the health care team. Ideally, the care plan should be used by each member of the team who provides care for that patient.

The care plan starts with a list of patient problems and needs. Each problem is studied, and a goal or expected outcome for improvement is set. Actions are listed to resolve each problem. At regular intervals the care plan is evaluated. As a problem is resolved, it is deleted from the care plan. If a problem is not resolved, the plan will be reviewed and revised as needed throughout the patient's stay in the facility.

As a nursing assistant, you may be the one who identifies a problem or the one to devise a solution. You can use the care plan to help provide quality patient care. Check the care plan daily for each of your assigned patients, and make a note of any actions that are your responsibility. Let the nurse know if you observe anything during your shift that might affect the patient's care plan.

*U*sing Computers

More and more, health care facilities are using computers to store information that can easily be retrieved. A computer is fast, accurate, and useful in many ways, such as the following:

▪ Exchange of information between departments and facilities.

▪ Storage of patients' records.

▪ Inventory of supplies.

▪ Storage of billing information.

▪ Ordering of supplies, equipment, and medication.

▪ Printout of assignments.

▪ Monitoring of body changes and vital signs.

Basic Computer Components

Although there are many different kinds of computers, they all work the same way and provide the same functions. These functions include the input, processing, and output of information. Input is data or information that is entered into the computer, which processes or changes the data and prepares it to be stored or output where it can be retrieved as needed. (See Figure 9–7.) The basic components (parts) of a computer can be divided into two groups—hardware and software.

Hardware

Hardware is the physical equipment used by a computer to process data, the parts you can see and touch. Basic computer hardware includes the central processing unit (CPU), monitor, keyboard, mouse, and printer. The *central processing unit (CPU)* is the "brain" or controlling part of the computer. Everything that happens on the computer goes through the CPU before you see it or hear it.

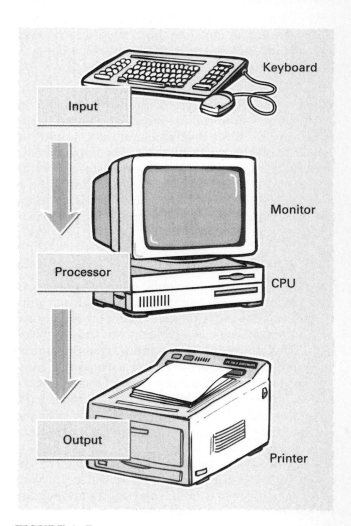

FIGURE 9–7
Basic computer components.

The monitor is the screen that allows you to see what is happening. It looks and works much like a television screen. The keyboard is used to enter data and commands for the computer. It looks and works like a typewriter keyboard. A mouse or ball is a hand-operated device that is used to move things around on the computer screen and to give commands to the computer. The printer provides hard copy output of information.

Software

Software includes the programs or sets of instruction that make the computer work. There is software available to perform thousands of different tasks. The heath care facility will provide training to use specific software programs.

Memory

Memory is a data storage device where information and files are stored. The two types of computer memory are RAM (random access memory) and ROM (read-only memory). RAM temporarily stores data that is lost when the file is closed. ROM data is stored on a disk and may be retrieved later, even after the file is closed or the computer shut down.

Disk Drives

The hard disk is inside the computer. It is called the "C drive" and stores all the information used to run the computer. Both programs and information can be stored on the hard disk drive. The floppy disk or diskette is a flat, square piece of plastic that is inserted into a slot on the front of the computer. It provides portable storage space for data. A floppy disk may be taken from one computer and used in another.

Security and Confidentiality

The same legal rules of confidentiality apply to all patient information. Computerized records require special security precautions. It is important that patient information be available only to those persons authorized to use it. A password is usually required before accessing information on a computer. Most systems are equipped to keep track of the number of entries into a file. Regardless of electronic safeguards, confidentiality is best protected by individuals who are careful and guarded with patient information.

You may work in a facility that allows you the opportunity to use a computer. It will be to your advantage to learn as much as you can about computers. In fact, basic computer skills are a requirement of many nursing assistant programs. As more and more facilities turn to cross-training, computer knowledge and skill may soon be an essential job skill.

The Language of Health Care

A whole new world is opening to you when you enter the health care field. It even has its own language called medical terminology. Learning to use and understand this language is an important part of your nursing assistant training. Medical terminology is used in developing care plans, charting in the patient record, giving reports, and preparing your assignment.

This textbook is designed to help you become familiar with medical terminology. Each chapter contains a list of key words that will help you understand the material. The key words are italicized and defined in the text. Refer to the glossary in the back of the textbook for words that are not defined in the text. The *glossary* is a collection of specialized terms with their meanings. Some of the words you may already know. Medical terms such as arthritis and diarrhea are commonly used by the public. Television shows and movies featuring health care settings have made people even more aware of medical terms.

Medical terms may refer to body parts, treatments, measurements, and directions. Many of these terms are derived from either the Greek or Latin language. Once you learn the basics, it will be easier to understand new terms.

Word Elements

Medical terms are composed of word elements (parts of words). These word elements are called roots, prefixes, and suffixes. The basic meaning of the word is the *root*. The element that is placed at the beginning of a word is the *prefix*, and the element placed at the end of the word is the *suffix*. Medical terms are composed of combinations of these elements. Learning the meanings of some commonly used elements eliminates the need to memorize each new term. It is important to learn to recognize word roots, prefixes, and suffixes. It is also necessary to know how to combine these parts to form medical terms. (See Figure 9–8.)

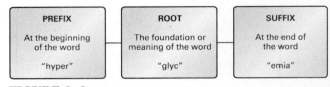

FIGURE 9–8
The root contains the basic meaning of the word. A prefix is placed at the beginning and a suffix at the end of the word.

Roots

The root contains the meaning of a word and forms the word's foundation. A root is usually combined with a prefix, a suffix, or another root to form a medical term. A combining vowel, usually an "o" may be inserted between word elements to make the word easier to pronounce. The following list contains commonly used roots, the combining vowels, and the meanings.

Root & Vowel	Meaning	Root	Meaning
abdomin(o)	abdomen	hyster(o)	uterus
aden(o)	gland	mam(o)	breast
arteri(o)	artery	my(o)	muscle
arthr(o)	joint	nephr(o)	kidney
cardi(o)	heart	neur(o)	nerve
cerebr(o)	brain	ocul(o)	eye
cephal(o)	head	orth(o)	straight
col(o)	colon	oste(o)	bone
cost(o)	rib	ot(o)	ear
crani(o)	skull	path(o)	disease
cyst(o)	bladder, cyst	ped(o)	child, foot
cyt(o)	cell	phleb(o)	vein
dent(o)	tooth	proct(o)	rectum
derm(a)	skin	pulm(o)	lung
enter(o)	intestine	rhin(o)	nose
gastr(o)	stomach	septic	infection
geront(o)	old age	stomat(o)	mouth
gloss(o)	tongue	therm(o)	heat
gyn(o)	woman	uter(o)	uterus
glyc(o)	sugar	vas(o)	vessel
hem(a)	blood	ven(o)	vein
hepat(o)	liver	vertebr(o)	spine

Prefix

A prefix is placed at the beginning of a word and cannot be used alone. It must be combined with another element to become a word. Common prefixes and their meanings include

Prefix	Meaning	Prefix	Meaning
a, an	without, not	hyper	high, above normal
ab	away from	hypo	low, below normal
ad	toward	inter	between
ante	before	intra	within
anti	against	macro	large
arterio	arteries	micro	small
auto	self	muco	mucous membrane
bi	double, two	neo	new
bio	life	neuro	nerves
brady	slow	non	not
cardio	heart	patho	disease
circum	around	per	through, by way of
contra	against	peri	around
derma	skin	poly	many
dys	difficult, abnormal, or painful	post	after, behind
endo	inside	pre	before, in front
epi	on top of, over	retro	backward, in back of
endo	inside	semi	half
eryth	red	sub	under
ex	out, away from	supra	above
gastro	stomach	tachy	rapid, fast
hemi	half	trans	across, through

Suffix

A suffix is placed at the end of a word and must be combined with another element. A combining vowel is sometimes placed between the root and the suffix. Common suffixes and their meanings include

Suffix	Meaning	Suffix	Meaning
algia	pain	ectomy	surgical removal
centesis	puncture and aspiration	emia	blood
gram	record	otomy	cutting into
ism	condition	pathy	disease
itis	inflammation of	phasia	speaking
lysis	destruction of	phobia	fear
megaly	enlargement of	plegia	paralysis
meter	measuring	pnea	to breathe
ology	study of	rrhea	profuse flow
oma	tumor	scope	examining instrument
ostomy	surgical opening	uria	condition of the urine

Identifying Medical Terms

Breaking down a word into its elements will help you to understand its meaning. As you may have noticed in the list of roots, prefixes, and suffixes, some word elements have the same meaning as others. Many word elements have more than one definition. For example, "ped" can mean either child or foot. You will need to choose the definition that fits each situation best.

When translating or identifying medical terms, it is easier to begin with the suffix. For example, in the word "hysterectomy," the suffix is "ectomy," which means "removal of." The root "hyster" means uterus, so the term "hysterectomy" means removal of the uterus. Once you have learned some common suffixes, medical terminology will seem much simpler. The list below includes some common medical terms that have been divided into their elements.

Word Combinations

Medical Term	Prefix	Root	Suffix	Meaning
antiseptic	anti	septic		against infection
antitoxin	anti	toxin		against poison
apnea	a	pnea		absence of breathing
arthritis		arthr	itis	inflammation of the joints
cardiology		cardi	ology	study of the heart
colostomy		col	ostomy	surgical opening into the colon
dermatitis		derma(t)	itis	inflammation of the skin
dyspnea	dys	pnea		difficult breathing
gastrostomy		gastr	ostomy	surgical opening into the stomach
hemiplegia	hemi	plegia		paralysis of half (one side) of the body
hepatitis		hepat	itis	inflammation of the liver
hyperglycemia	hyper	glyc	emia	high blood sugar
intravenous	intra	venous		within the vein
microscope	micro	scope		instrument to measure very small objects
nephrectomy		nephr	ectomy	surgical removal of the kidney
osteoarthritis		osteo arthr	itis	inflammation of the bones and joints
polyuria	poly	uria		a large amount of urine
prenatal	pre	natal		before birth
tachycardia	tachy	cardia		rapid heartbeat
tracheostomy		trache(o)	ostomy	surgical opening into the trachea
transdermal	trans	dermal		through the skin

Abbreviations Suggestions

An abbreviation may

▣ Use the first letter of each word (VS = vital signs).

▣ Use the first and last letter of the word (ht = height).

▣ Use three of four letters of a word (amb = ambulate).

▣ Use a chemical symbol that includes a numeral (O_2 = oxygen; H_2O = water).

Remember that

▣ The letter "q" usually means "every" (qd = every day), or

▣ it may indicate four (qid = four times a day).

▣ The letter "h" usually means hour (qh + every hour).

It helps to

▣ Associate ac with am (ac = before meals, am = before noon) and pc with pm (pc = after meals, pm = after noon).

▣ Think of bid, tid, and qid as 2 in a day, 3 in a day, and 4 in a day.

FIGURE 9–9
Use these suggestions to help you recognize medical abbreviations.

Abbreviations

An *abbreviation* is a shortened form of a word or phrase. The use of abbreviations saves time and provides a method of quick communication in the health care facility. Your assignment may contain abbreviations, and you will use them when you are charting. The chart in Figure 9–9 contains some suggestions that will help you to recognize abbreviations.

There are hundreds of abbreviations that may be used in a health care facility. Each facility will have a list that contains approved abbreviations. Do not use abbreviations that are not included on the list. If you are not sure if the abbreviation is correct or acceptable, write out the word or phrase in full. Commonly used medical abbreviations and their meanings are found in the following list.

Abbreviation	Meaning	Abbreviation	Meaning
abd	abdomen	B&B	bowel and bladder training
ac	before meals	bid	twice a day
ADL	activities of daily living	BM	bowel movement
ad lib	as desired	BP	blood pressure
A.D.O.N.	assistant director of nurses	BR	bedrest/bathroom
am	morning	BRP	bathroom privileges
amb	ambulate	BS	blood sugar
amt	amount	BSC	bedside commode
AP	apical pulse	c̄	with
approx	approximately	Ca	cancer
aqua	water	CBC	complete blood count
ASAP	as soon as possible	CBR	complete bed rest

Abbreviation	Meaning	Abbreviation	Meaning
cc	cubic centimeter	lt or L	left
CCU	coronary care unit	LVN	licensed vocational nurse
CHF	congestive heart failure	LTC	long-term care
CNA	certified nursing assistant	meds	medications
c/o	complains of	MD	medical doctor
COPD	chronic obstructive pulmonary disease	MI	myocardial infarction
CPR	cardiopulmonary resuscitation	min	minute
CS	central supply	ml	milliliter
CXR	chest X-ray	NA	nursing assistant
CVA	cerebrovascular accident/stroke	N/G tube	nasogastric tube
dc	discontinue/discharge	noc	night
DNR	do not resuscitate	NPO	nothing by mouth (nil per os)
DON	director of nurses	N/V	nausea/vomiting
Dx	diagnosis	OB	obstetrics
F	Fahrenheit	O_2	oxygen
FBS	fasting blood sugar	OJ	orange juice
Fx	fracture	OOB	out of bed
gal	gallon	OR	operating room
GI	gastrointestinal	ord	orderly
gtts	drops	os	mouth
GU	genitourinary	OT	occupational therapy
Gyn	gynecology	oz	ounce
H_2O	water	$\bar{p}$	after
HOB	head of bed	PAR	post anesthesia room
HOH	hard of hearing	pc	after meals
hr, h	hour	Peds	pediatrics
hs	hour of sleep/bedtime	per	through, by way of
ht	height	pm	afternoon
I&O	intake and output	po	by mouth (per os)
ICU	intensive care unit	postop	post operative, after surgery
in	inch	preop	preoperative, before surgery
Irr	irregular	prep	preparation
Isol	isolation	prn	when necessary/as needed
IV	intravenous	pt	patient or pint
L or l	liter	PT	physical therapy
lab	laboratory	q	every
lb	pound	qam	every morning
liq	liquid	qd	every day
LPN	licensed practical nurse	qh	every hour

Abbreviation	Meaning	Abbreviation	Meaning
q2h, q3h, q4h, etc.	every 2 hours, every 3 hours, every 4 hours, etc.	spec	specimen
qhs	every night at bedtime	SSE	soapsuds enema
qid	four times a day	stat	at once/immediately
qod	every other day	STD	sexually transmitted disease
qs	quantity sufficient/enough	Surg	surgery
qt	quart	Tbsp or T	tablespoon
R	rectal	tid	three times a day
Rm	room	TLC	tender loving care
RN	registered nurse	TPR	temperature, pulse, and respirations
ROM	range of motion	tsp or t	teaspoon
rt or R	right	VS	vital signs
Rx	prescription	U/A	urinalysis
s̄	without	WBC	white blood cells
S&A	sugar and acetone test	w/c	wheelchair
SOB	shortness of breath	wt	weight

Review

Read each sentence and fill in the blank with the vocabulary term that best completes the sentence.

1. Another term for charting or documenting is _____.
2. _____ are things that you can see, hear, smell, or touch.
3. A written document outlining the care of an individual patient is called a _____.
4. The _____ is the "brain" or controlling part of the computer.
5. The element of a medical term found at the end of the word is the _____.

Remember

1. It is necessary that the nursing assistant develop observation skills.
2. Objective observations are things you can see, hear, smell, or touch. Subjective observations are things the patient tells you.
3. Report your observations to the nurse promptly.
4. Objective reporting involves reporting only the facts that you are able to observe.
5. One of the purposes of recording is to provide a written record of the patient's care.
6. Never scribble through, erase, or use correctional fluid when correcting a charting error.
7. An individualized care plan is written for each patient.
8. It will be to your advantage to learn as much as you can about computers.
9. The central processing unit (CPU) is the controlling part of the computer.
10. Learning to use and understand medical terminology is an important part of nursing assistant training.
11. The use of abbreviations saves time and provides a quick method of communication.

Reflect

Read the following case study and answer the questions.

Case Study

You are caring for Gladys Jones this morning. On your assignment sheet you read the following order: "pt OOB & amb TID." Mrs. Jones says she doesn't feel like getting up this morning. Her face is pale and she is breathing heavily. Her skin feels cold and damp with perspiration. When you ask her what's wrong, she says, "I've had this pain in my right side all night and I'm worn out." You respond, "You'll probably feel better if you get up and move around. I'll tell the nurse as soon as I get you up and dressed."

1. What does the order "pt **OOB** & amb **TID**" mean?
2. List the objective observations you could make about Mrs. Jones.
3. What subjective observations can you make?
4. Was the response to Mrs. Jones appropriate? What would have been more appropriate?

Respond

Choose the best answer for each question.

1. Which of the following is a subjective observation?
   A. Dark, cloudy urine
   B. A rapid pulse
   C. A patient's complaint of pain
   D. A peculiar odor of the breath

2. Which is the best example of objective reporting?
   A. "Mr. Brown has a reddened area the size of a dime on his left hip."
   B. "Mr. Brown has a bedsore on his hip."
   C. "Mr. Brown wants a pain pill."
   D. "Mr. Brown is complaining about his hip again."

3. When recording patient information you should
   A. Use a pencil so you can erase mistakes.
   B. Use a pen and ink.
   C. Wait until the end of your shift to chart.
   D. Tell the nurse so you won't have to chart.

4. How would you chart that a patient walked 25 feet with help?
   A. Patient walked 25 ft with help.
   B. Pt walked 25 ft with help.
   C. Pt amb 25 ft with help.
   D. Pt amb 25 ft c̄ help.

5. The patient's care plan is used to
   A. Identify problems and needs.
   B. Determine goals and outcomes.
   C. Evaluate actions and treatments.
   D. All of the above.

6. Computer software includes
   A. A monitor
   B. A keyboard
   C. Programs
   D. Printers

7. Which of the following is the best measure to protect the confidentiality of computerized records?
   A. Require a password to gain access.
   B. Turn the computer off.
   C. Save the data to a floppy disk.
   D. List the people who are allowed access.

8. Which of the following is NOT a prefix?
   A. Anti
   B. Dys
   C. Ectomy
   D. Hyper

9. What is the meaning of the medical term "hysterectomy"?
   A. Removal of the tonsils
   B. Removal of the uterus
   C. Slow heart rate
   D. Surgical opening into the colon

10. The abbreviation "ac" means
    A. Morning
    B. Afternoon
    C. Before meals
    D. After meals

Chapter Ten

Anatomy *and* Physiology

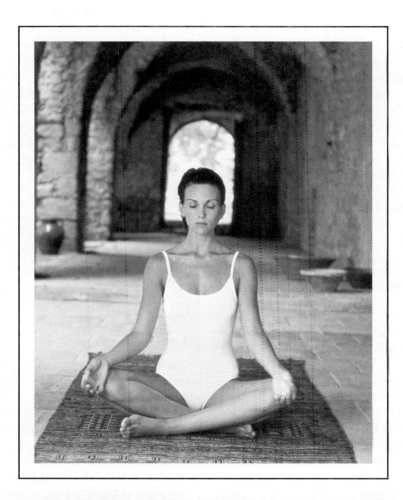

OBJECTIVES

1. Describe the basic structure of cells, tissues, organs, and systems.

2. Identify the structures and functions of each body system.

3. Identify two changes of aging in each system of the body.

After studying this chapter, you will be able to

4. Identify and describe the special senses of the body.

5. Describe the interdependence of the body systems.

Glossary

anatomy   The study of body structure.

cell   The unit of structure of all animals and plants; the smallest unit of the body that performs all vital life functions. The basic building block of the body.

chromosomes   Structures found in the nucleus of a cell that contain information that controls heredity.

defecation   The process of eliminating solid waste from the body through the anus.

diastole   The stage of the cardiac cycle during which the heart is relaxing and filling with blood.

digestion   The process of physical and chemical breakdown of food so that it can be used by the body.

feces   The solid waste products that remain after the body has absorbed all nutrients and water from ingested food.

hormones   Chemicals secreted by the endocrine glands directly into the bloodstream. These chemicals regulate and control the functions of other organs and glands.

integument   The anatomical name for the skin.

menstruation   The periodic discharge of the lining of the uterus when fertilization of the egg does not occur.

metabolism   The combination of processes of physical and chemical change within the cell that produces energy for growth and repair.

organ   A group of similar tissues that work together to perform a particular function.

peristalsis   The wavelike muscular contractions of the digestive system that propel food through the digestive tract.

physiology   The study of body function.

system   A group of organs that work together to perform one or more functions.

systole   The stage of the cardiac cycle during which the heart is contracting and pumping blood out through the blood vessels.

tissue   A group of similar cells that work together to perform a specific function.

Over the centuries, man has invented many wonderful machines, but nothing equals the marvel of the human body. All of its many parts work together in a smooth, steady rhythm. *Anatomy* (the study of body structure) and *physiology* (the study of body function) can be fascinating as well as informative.

This chapter offers you basic information on how the body is constructed and how it works. Changes that take place in the body with aging are identified to help you make observations as to what is normal and what is not normal. Emphasis is placed on the relationship of body systems. It explains how the systems affect one another and how they all work together to operate the body. An understanding of this material will help you to care for your patients safely and effectively.

Basic Body Structure

Cells

The *cell* is the basic building block of the body. It is the smallest unit that performs all vital life functions. The basic structure of a cell includes the cell membrane, cytoplasm, and nucleus (see Figure 10–1). The cell membrane is the outer protective covering. It controls the entry of food, water, and oxygen, as well as the exit of waste material. Cytoplasm is the material inside the cell. The nucleus—the control center of the cell—contains *chromosomes*, the part of the cell that controls heredity (the physical and mental characteristics passed from generation to generation).

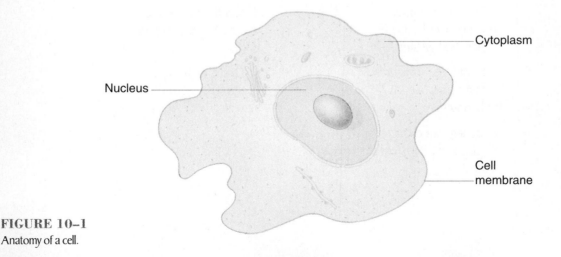

Cytoplasm

Nucleus

Cell membrane

FIGURE 10–1
Anatomy of a cell.

Cells require food, water, and oxygen to function and reproduce. Deprived of any of these three essential elements, the cells will die. The food you eat, the water you drink, and the air you breathe determine the health of cells, and healthy cells produce a healthy body. Although each cell is capable of performing many functions, most cells do not work alone. They combine with other cells that are alike in size, shape, and function.

Tissues

A *tissue* is a group of similar cells that work together to perform a particular function. The four main types of tissue are epithelial, connective, muscle, and nerve tissue.

Organs

An *organ* is a group of similar tissues that work together to perform a particular function. Organs vary in size and shape. You may be familiar with the shape of the heart or the kidneys, but did you know that the largest organ in the body is the skin? See Figure 10–2 for some of the major organs of the body.

Systems

A group of organs that work together to perform one or more functions is called a *system*. The systems of the body include the following:

- Integumentary system
- Skeletal system
- Muscular system
- Respiratory system
- Circulatory system
- Digestive system
- Urinary system
- Nervous system
- Endocrine system
- Reproductive system

Each system performs certain functions, but no system works totally independently. A change in any one of the systems will affect the others. Although you will study the systems separately, remember that a healthy body requires the combined functioning of all the systems, called interdependence. The chart in Figure 10–3 briefly summarizes the major structure and function of each system.

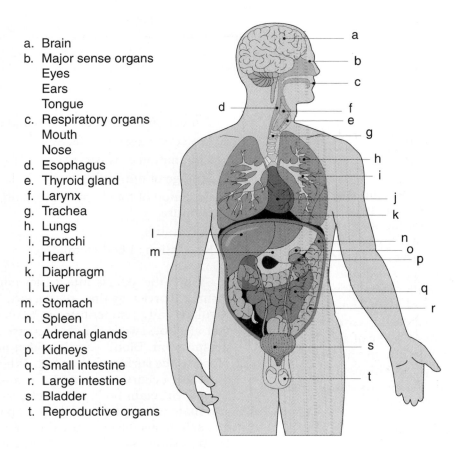

a. Brain
b. Major sense organs
   Eyes
   Ears
   Tongue
c. Respiratory organs
   Mouth
   Nose
d. Esophagus
e. Thyroid gland
f. Larynx
g. Trachea
h. Lungs
i. Bronchi
j. Heart
k. Diaphragm
l. Liver
m. Stomach
n. Spleen
o. Adrenal glands
p. Kidneys
q. Small intestine
r. Large intestine
s. Bladder
t. Reproductive organs

FIGURE 10–2
Major organs of the body.

SYSTEM	STRUCTURE	FUNCTION
Integumentary	Skin and appendages	Protects against infection Protects internal organs Regulates body temperature and eliminates wastes Provides awareness of environment
Musculoskeletal (combination of muscular and skeletal systems)	Bones, joints, muscles, tendons, and ligaments	Provides structure and framework Produces movement Protects internal tissues and organs Maintains posture and body temperature
Respiratory	Nose, pharynx, larynx, trachea, bronchi, lungs, and alveoli	Brings oxygen into the body and removes carbon dioxide
Circulatory	Heart, blood, and blood vessels	Carries food, water, and oxygen to the cells and waste products away from the cells Maintains fluid balance
Digestive	Mouth, pharynx, esophagus, stomach, small intestine, and large intestine	Prepares food for the body's use and eliminates waste products
Urinary	Kidneys, ureters, bladder, and urethra	Filters wastes from blood, produces urine, and eliminates waste products from the body
Nervous	Brain, spinal cord, and nerves	Controls and coordinates body activities
Endocrine	Pituitary, thyroid, thymus, parathyroid, and adrenal glands; pancreas and gonads	Secretes hormones that regulate and coordinate body functions
Reproductive	**Female:** Ovaries, fallopian tubes, uterus, and vagina **Male:** Testes, scrotum, penis, seminal vesicles, and prostate gland	Reproduction of the species

FIGURE 10–3
Summary of systems, structure, and function.

The Integumentary System

Structure

The integumentary system is composed of the skin and its appendages (nails, hair, sweat glands, and oil glands). The correct anatomical name for skin is *integument*. The thin outer surface of the skin is called the epidermis. It gives skin its color and helps protect against sun rays. Cells in the epidermis slough off and are replaced by new cells from the dermis or inner layer of skin. The dermis contains blood vessels, nerve endings, sweat glands, oil glands, and hair roots. A layer of subcutaneous fatty tissue attaches the skin to the underlying structures. This fatty layer cushions and protects deeper tissue. It also provides insulation against heat and cold. (See Figure 10–4.)

Function

The functions of the integumentary system include:

- Protection of internal tissues and organs
- Protection against infection
- Elimination of waste
- Storage of nutrients
- Detection of touch, pressure, pain, and temperature
- Lubrication
- Regulation of body temperature

When the skin is intact (not cut or broken), it forms a barrier against pathogens. The skin helps regulate body temperature in several ways. When you are hot, sweat glands increase the amount of perspiration. Blood vessels widen and bring more blood to the surface for cooling. When you are cold, shivering occurs to create heat, and blood vessels narrow to retain body heat. Perspiration also helps eliminate waste products through pores in the skin. The skin helps the body use the sun to make vitamin D. An awareness of the environment is provided by nerve endings, which allow sensations such as pressure, pain, pleasure, and temperature to be experi-

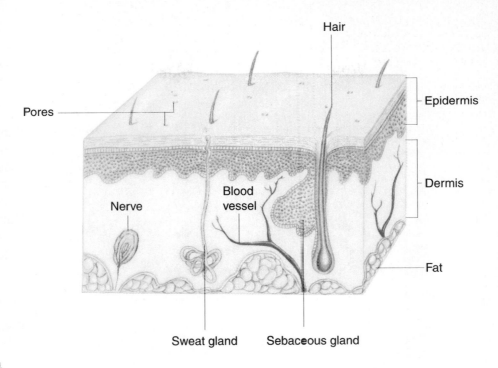

FIGURE 10–4
Structure of the skin.

enced. Oil glands provide lubrication to keep the skin and hair soft.

Changes of Aging

With aging, the skin becomes thinner and more fragile (easily damaged). It loses its elasticity (ability to stretch), causing wrinkles and sagging. The skin dries and may become scaly. It pales, becomes more sensitive to sun, and brown spots (sometimes called liver spots) may develop. Vitamin D production is reduced, and skin repairs itself more slowly. The subcutaneous fat layer that provides padding becomes thinner, leaving the skin with less protection and less insulation. One of the reasons the elderly person complains of feeling cold is the loss of this insulating layer. As a result of decreased sensitivity of nerve endings, the elderly person is less able to identify sensations or temperatures. This lack of sensation can lead to burns and cold damage. Hair color fades, and hair may turn gray or white. The hair thins and partial or total baldness may result. Fingernails and toenails become thick and tough.

The Musculoskeletal System

The musculoskeletal system is a combination of two systems, the muscular and the skeletal. However,

because they share many structures and functions, it is easier to study them together. (See Figure 10–5.)

Structure

The skeletal system is composed of bones and joints. The muscular system is composed of muscles, tendons, and ligaments. Joints are areas where bones connect with one or more other bones. (See Figure 10–6.) Ligaments are tough, fibrous cords that connect one bone to another, and tendons are elastic structures that attach muscle to bone.

There are three types of muscle tissue: skeletal muscle, smooth muscle, and cardiac muscle. Skeletal muscles are attached directly or indirectly to bones. They move the body by pulling on bones. Smooth muscles are located in the respiratory, circulatory, digestive, and reproductive systems. They push food and fluids through body passages. Cardiac muscle is found only in the heart. Muscles may be voluntary (controlled at will) or involuntary (work automatically). When you move your legs to walk, you are using voluntary muscles. Involuntary muscles help you to breathe and digest food.

Groups of muscles may work together to produce motion, or they may work against each other. For example, when you flex (bend) your arm a muscle in the front of the arm contracts (shortens),

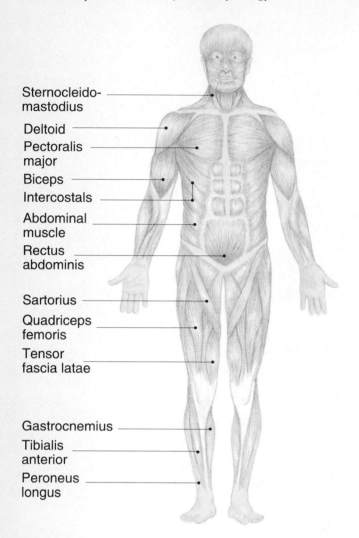

Sternocleido-
mastodius

Deltoid

Pectoralis
major

Biceps

Intercostals

Abdominal
muscle

Rectus
abdominis

Sartorius

Quadriceps
femoris

Tensor
fascia latae

Gastrocnemius

Tibialis
anterior

Peroneus
longus

FIGURE 10–5A
The muscular system.

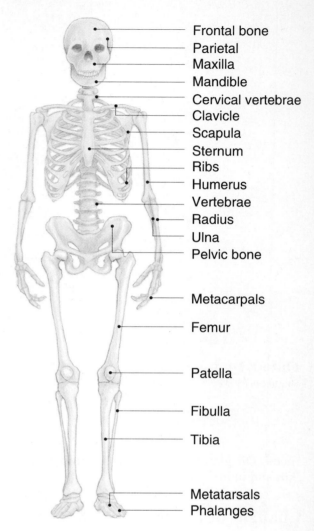

Frontal bone
Parietal
Maxilla
Mandible
Cervical vertebrae
Clavicle
Scapula
Sternum
Ribs
Humerus
Vertebrae
Radius
Ulna
Pelvic bone

Metacarpals

Femur

Patella

Fibulla

Tibia

Metatarsals
Phalanges

FIGURE 10–5B
The skeletal system.

while the one in the back relaxes (lengthens). (See Figure 10–7.)

Function

The functions of the musculoskeletal system include the following:

■ Provide structural support and framework for the body

■ Produce movement

■ Protect tissues and organs

■ Produce blood cells in bone marrow

■ Maintain posture and body position

■ Maintain body temperature

Changes of Aging

With age, strength and endurance decrease while body movements slow. These changes of aging in the musculoskeletal system can interfere with body movement. Muscles weaken, become smaller, and lose elasticity. Muscle tone that keeps muscles tense and firm decreases. Muscle weakness can affect any system of the body. For example, a weak heartbeat or shallow breathing may be the result of weak muscles.

Joints become stiff as cartilage deteriorates and tissue hardens. Bones become thin and brittle and can be easily broken. Changes in the spinal column and the bony structure that supports the spinal column can result in stooped posture and a loss of height.

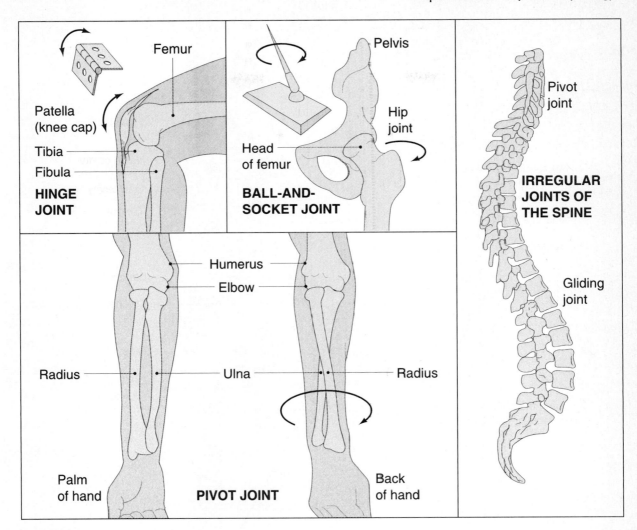

FIGURE 10–6
Moveable joints.

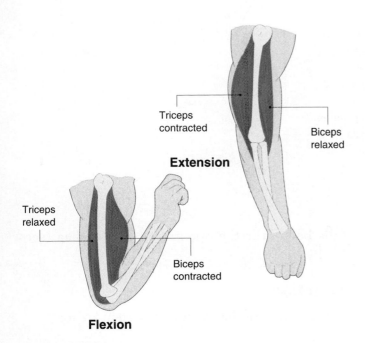

FIGURE 10–7
Coordination of muscles.

The Respiratory System

Structure

Structures of the respiratory system include the nose, pharynx, larynx, trachea, bronchi, lungs, and alveoli (see Figure 10–8).

Air enters the body through the nose and pharynx (throat), where it is filtered, warmed, and moistened. After leaving the pharynx, air passes through a narrow opening called the glottis. The glottis is surrounded by the larynx, which contains the vocal chords, or the "voice box." From there, air goes into the trachea (windpipe). The trachea divides into the left and right bronchi. The bronchi branch out into smaller tubes, called bronchioles, which lead to small air sacs in the lungs called alveoli. Blood vessels in the alveoli exchange oxygen for carbon dioxide (waste gases from the body).

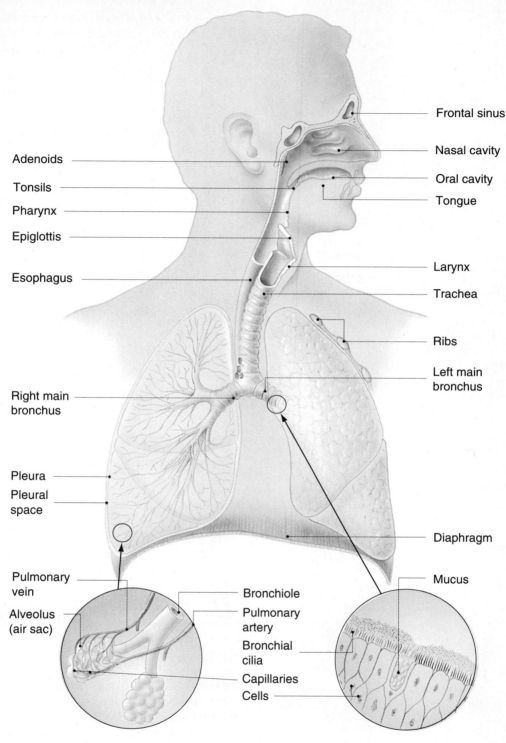

FIGURE 10–8
The respiratory system.

The respiratory system shares some structures with the digestive system. Both food and air enter through the mouth and the pharynx. The body has a unique method of keeping food and fluids from entering the trachea. A small piece of cartilage called the epiglottis protects the opening to the trachea. During respiration (breathing), the epiglottis opens and allows oxygen to enter the airway. When food or fluids are swallowed, the epiglottis closes and falls back over the opening of the trachea (see Figure 10–9).

Function

The functions of the respiratory system are to:

■ Bring oxygen into the body
■ Remove carbon dioxide from the body

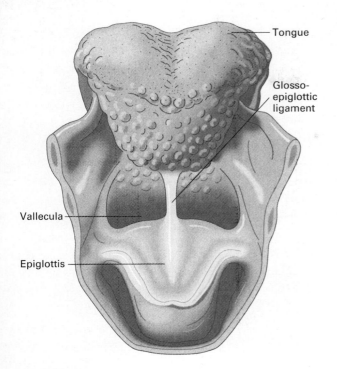

FIGURE 10–9
The epiglottis opens and closes to protect the airway.

- Allow communication through speaking and making other sounds

Each cell of the body needs oxygen to survive. The process of exchanging oxygen and carbon dioxide is accomplished by respiration (breathing). One respiration consists of an inhalation (breathing in) and an exhalation (breathing out). These movements push air in and out of the lungs. Contractions of the diaphragm enlarge the chest cavity and draw air containing oxygen into the lungs. Relaxation of the diaphragm decreases the size of the chest and forces air containing carbon dioxide out of the lungs. Other respiratory muscles assist in this process. The center that controls respiration is in the brain.

Normal breathing occurs automatically. Although it is possible to temporarily change respiratory patterns, you cannot decide to stop breathing for very long. If you hold your breath long enough, you will lose consciousness and protective reflexes will cause breathing to resume. Sneezing and coughing are other examples of reflexes that help protect the respiratory system.

Changes of Aging

Changes of aging in the respiratory system are affected by the slowing of blood circulation and weakening of muscles. Because the rib cage becomes more rigid and lung tissue loses elasticity, full ex-

pansion of the lungs and chest is limited. The result of these changes is a decrease in the exchange of oxygen and carbon dioxide. This in turn can affect all the other body systems.

The Circulatory System

Structure

The structures of the circulatory system include the heart, blood, and blood vessels. It may also be called the cardiovascular system. (Cardio means heart and vascular refers to the blood vessels.) This system is the body's transportation system because it transports substances to and from the cells.

Function

The functions of the circulatory system are to:

- Carry food, water, oxygen, and other vital substances to the cells
- Collect waste products and carry them away from the cells
- Help regulate body temperature
- Protect the body against disease
- Maintain fluid balance (See Figure 10–10.)

The Heart

The heart is a pear-shaped organ about the size of your fist that is composed of cardiac muscle and is located in the chest slightly to the left of the midline. The sternum and ribs help protect it from injury. The heart is divided into four chambers that are separated by thick muscular walls. The two upper chambers are the right and the left atria, and the two lower chambers are the right and left ventricles. The atria receive blood coming into the heart, while the ventricles pump blood out of the heart to other parts of the body.

The Cardiac Cycle

The heart moves blood through the body in a continuous one-way direction because of valves that prevent backflow. The blood travels through the right side of the heart to the lungs where it receives oxygen. From the lungs, this oxygenated blood returns to the left side of the heart and is pumped out to all parts of the body.

Blood enters the right atrium through large veins called the inferior and the superior vena cava. This blood coming from body tissues is low in oxy-

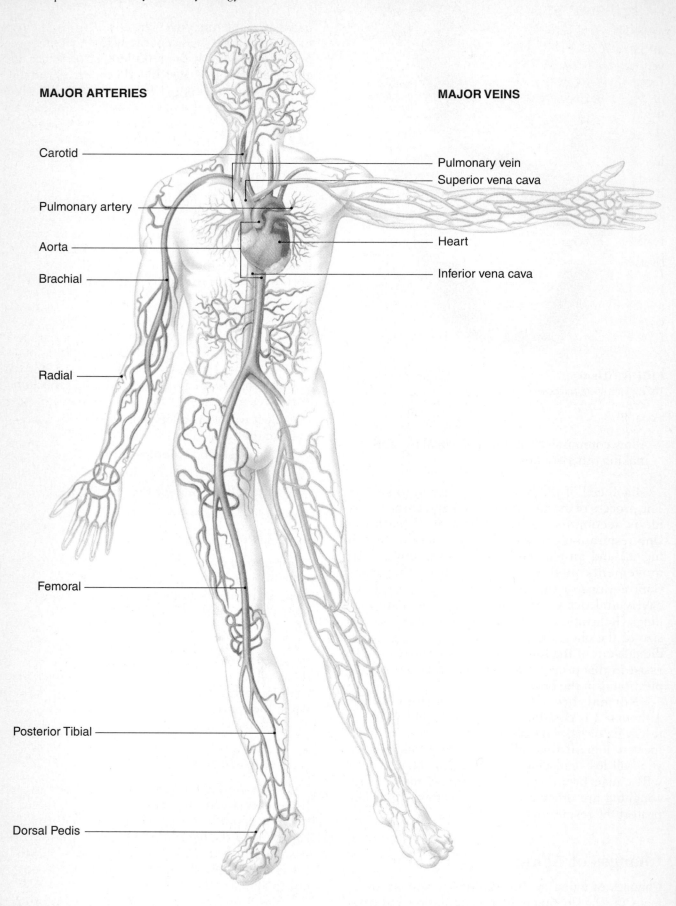

MAJOR ARTERIES

MAJOR VEINS

Carotid

Pulmonary vein

Superior vena cava

Pulmonary artery

Aorta

Heart

Brachial

Inferior vena cava

Radial

Femoral

Posterior Tibial

Dorsal Pedis

FIGURE 10–10
The circulatory system.

gen and high in carbon dioxide. From the right atrium, blood flows through a valve into the right ventricle, which contracts and pumps blood through the pulmonary artery into the lungs. The exchange of carbon dioxide for oxygen takes place in the alveoli of the lungs. The oxygenated blood returns from the lungs to the left atrium through the pulmonary veins. The blood then flows through a valve into the left ventricle. Contraction of the left ventricle pumps blood into the aorta (the largest blood vessel in the body). The blood circulates through a series of blood vessels to all parts of the body.

This continuous, coordinated movement of blood is called the cardiac cycle. The cardiac cycle is divided into two stages: diastole and systole. *Diastole* is the stage of the cardiac cycle when the heart is resting and filling with blood. *Systole* is the stage when the heart is contracting and pumping out the blood. Look at Figure 10–11 and trace the flow of blood through the heart.

The Blood

Blood is the fluid that carries oxygen, food, waste products, and other substances. It travels through a network of blood vessels and is kept in constant motion by contractions of the heart. The three main types of blood cells are red blood cells, white blood cells, and platelets. Red blood cells carry oxygen to the cells and give blood its red color. White blood cells help protect the body from infection and are a part of the body's immune or defense system. Platelets help the blood to clot.

The Blood Vessels

The three major types of blood vessels are arteries, veins, and capillaries. Arteries are the largest vessels and carry oxygen-rich blood away from the heart, except for the pulmonary artery, which carries oxygen-poor blood from the heart to the lungs. Veins carry oxygen-poor blood back to the heart, except for the pulmonary vein, which carries oxygenated blood from the lungs back to the heart. Veins are smaller and thinner than arteries and have valves to keep the blood flowing in one direction. Capillaries are tiny vessels that connect arteries and veins. Food, oxygen, waste, and other substances pass through the thin walls of the capillaries to and from the cells.

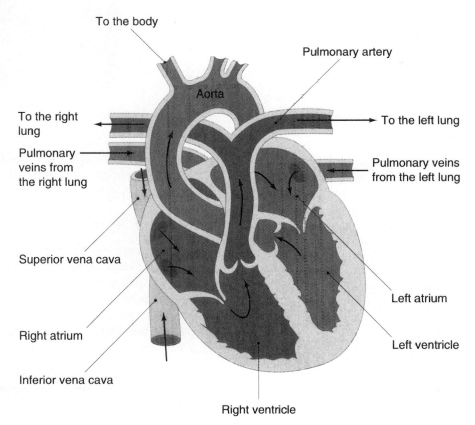

FIGURE 10–11
The flow of blood through the heart.

Changes of Aging

Heart muscle weakens with age, causing the heart to pump with less force. Although the heart beats faster to keep the blood moving, it is less effective. With aging, blood vessels lose their ability to stretch and become hard and narrow. Fatty deposits and other substances may clog the narrowed vessels. Blood pressure may rise. All these changes result in a slowing of circulation, which causes problems in other systems of the body.

The Digestive System

Structure

The primary structures of the digestive system are the mouth, pharynx (throat), esophagus, stomach, small intestine, and large intestine. They form a long, continuous tube that extends from the mouth to the anus (the opening to the rectum). The accessory organs of the digestive system include the teeth, tongue, liver, pancreas, and gallbladder (see Figure 10–12).

Function

The functions of the digestive system are to prepare food for the body's use and to eliminate waste. The process of physically and chemically breaking down food for the body's use is called *digestion*. Food enters the mouth and is broken down into smaller pieces by the teeth. The salivary glands add chemicals and fluid to moisten the food. Once swallowing begins, digestion becomes automatic. Muscular actions of the tongue help move food to the back of the throat, where the swallowing reflex is located. Food passes from the throat through the esophagus into the stomach. Food moves through the digestive system by waves of muscular contractions called *peristalsis*.

The stomach churns and mixes the food with gastric juices secreted by the stomach walls. The stomach is a temporary storage area for the food, which may remain there for several hours. Nerve endings in the stomach wall signal when it is full. From the stomach, the food mixture enters the small intestine, where bile and other digestive juices from the gallbladder, liver, and pancreas are added. Digestion is completed in the small intestine, where projections, called villi, absorb the digested food particles and release them into the bloodstream. The rest of the food mass moves into the large intestine.

The large intestine includes the colon and the rectum. The function of the colon is to remove water from the food mass for the body's use. The material that remains forms a semisolid waste product called *feces*. Feces is stored in the rectum until it

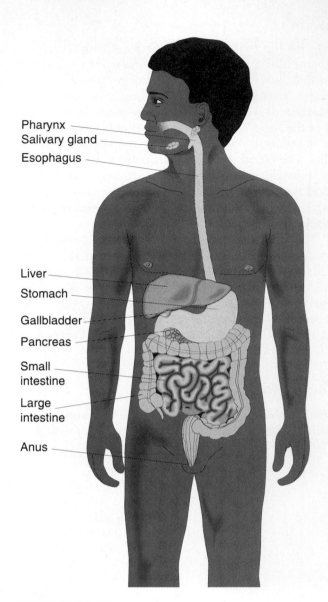

FIGURE 10–12
The digestive system.

leaves the body through the anus (opening to the rectum). The process of eliminating solid waste is called *defecation*.

Changes of Aging

Muscle tone decreases throughout the digestive system causing a slowing of peristalsis. A decrease in saliva and in the number of taste buds causes a decrease in appetite. Chewing and swallowing problems occur frequently. A decrease in digestive juices makes food, particularly fats, harder to digest.

The Urinary System

Structure

The primary structures of the urinary system are the kidneys, ureters, bladder, urethra, and urinary meatus. The two kidneys, shaped like lima beans, are located in the upper abdomen toward the back, one on each side of the spine. (See Figure 10–13.)

Function

The functions of the urinary system are to remove wastes from the bloodstream, eliminate waste products through urine, and help maintain the body's water and chemical balance. The major function of the kidneys is to filter and remove waste products from the blood. This is accomplished through a complicated filtration system of tubes and blood vessels. Filtration takes place in the nephrons (the basic cells of the urinary system), where waste products are filtered. The urine, containing waste products, drains out of the kidneys through the ureters to the bladder.

The bladder is a muscular, expandable sac. Urine, which is continuously produced by the kidneys, is held in the bladder until it is eliminated from the body. The average adult bladder can hold about one quart of urine. When the bladder is approximately one-third full, the brain sends a signal causing an urge to urinate. A tube from the bladder called the urethra leads to the outside of the body. Urine passes from the body through the urinary meatus, the external opening of the urethra.

Changes of Aging

The kidneys do not filter as efficiently in the elderly person due to fewer nephrons and slowed circulation. This can cause waste products and toxins (poisonous substances) to build up in the body. A decrease in the muscle tone of the bladder leads to a loss of elasticity. The bladder holds less urine for shorter periods of time and may not empty completely. The muscle that keeps urine in the bladder weakens and may allow urine to escape involuntarily.

The Nervous System

Structure

The nervous system is composed of the brain, the spinal cord, and the nerves. Nerves connect the organs of the nervous system with each other and with other systems of the body. The central nervous system (CNS) consists of the brain and spinal cord. The brain coordinates most body activities, and each part of the brain controls specific functions. The right side of the brain controls the left side of the body and the left side of the brain controls the right side of the body. Intelligence, memory, and emotions are under the control of the central nervous system. The brain is protected by the skull, and the spinal cord is protected by the vertebral (spinal) column. (See Figure 10–14.)

The peripheral nervous system includes both the 12 cranial nerves and the 31 spinal nerves. The basic unit of the nervous system is the neuron (nerve cell). There are billions of neurons transmitting messages throughout the body.

Function

The nervous system controls and coordinates body activities and provides sensations from the environment. The nervous system is the body's communica-

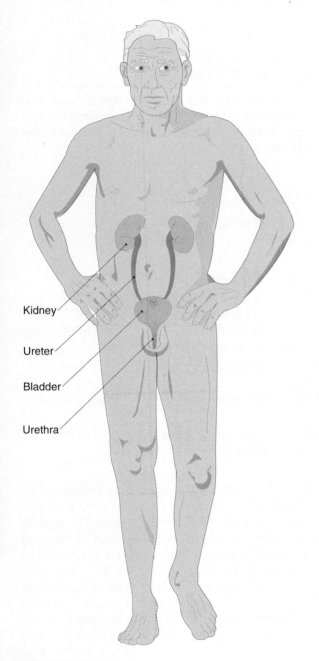

Kidney

Ureter

Bladder

Urethra

FIGURE 10–13
The urinary system.

Central nervous system

Brain

Spinal cord

Peripheral nerves

Peripheral nervous system

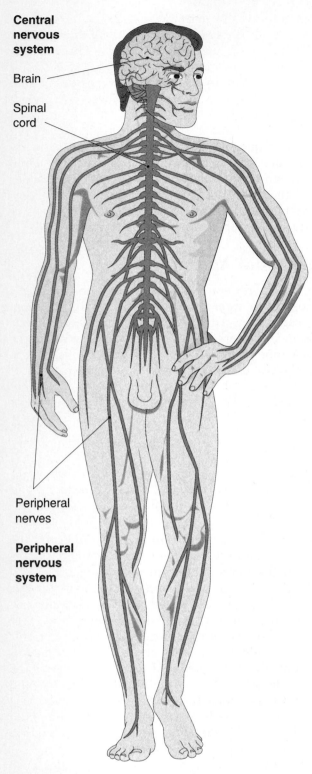

FIGURE 10–14
The nervous system.

tion center. Nerves carry information into the nervous system from both inside and outside the body. The brain processes this information and sends instructions by way of the nerves to all parts of the body.

Changes of Aging

The number of neurons decreases with aging. Unlike other body cells, nerve cells in the CNS are not replaced by new cells if they are destroyed. Transmission of messages is delayed, resulting in slower responses and reflexes. Reaction time and performance slow as well.

Short-term memory loss may occur. Elderly persons may forget information such as names, dates, telephone numbers, or items on lists. A decrease in the sensitivity of nerve endings in the skin may interfere with the ability to handle small objects. The sense of touch is not as accurate, and sensitivity to heat and cold may be reduced.

The Special Senses

The five senses are sight, hearing, smell, taste, and touch. Receptors (specialized nerve endings) in certain parts of the body transmit received information to the brain.

The Eye

The eye is the sense organ for vision. The structure of the eye includes the following:

- Eyeball: The globe-shaped part of the eye
- Orbit: The cavity in the front of the skull that contains and protects the eyeball
- Muscles: Tissue that connects the eye to the orbit and allows it to move
- Eyelids: Skin folds that protect the eye from injury
- Conjunctiva: Mucous membrane that protects the eyeball
- Optic nerve: Band of nerve tissue that carries sight messages to the brain

The outer layer of the eyeball is composed of the sclera (the white part of the eye) and the cornea, which helps to focus light rays. The middle layer contains the iris (the colored part of the eye) and the pupil, a round, dark opening that changes size to control the amount of light that can enter the eye. Located against the back wall of the eyeball is the lens, which focuses light images onto the retina. The retina contains sight receptors called rods and cones. Light passes through the cornea, the pupil, and the lens. The retina receives and transmits these images through the optic nerve to the brain. (See Figure 10–15.)

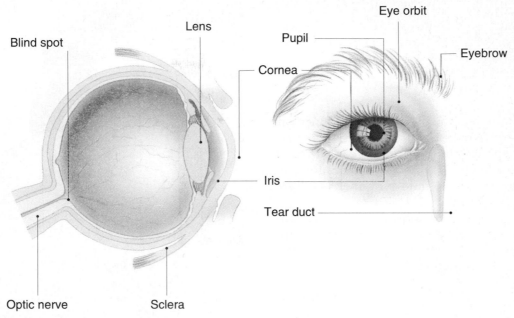

FIGURE 10–15
The eye.

The Ear

The ear is responsible for hearing and balance. It is divided into three areas: the external or outer ear, the middle ear, and the inner ear. The external ear is composed of the pinna, or auricle, and the auditory canal. The pinna is the projecting part of the outer ear that surrounds the opening to the auditory canal. The auditory canal ends at the tympanic membrane (ear drum), which separates the external ear and the middle ear. The middle ear includes the eustachian tube and three small bones called the malleus, the incus, and the stapes. The eustachian tube equalizes air pressure between the ear and the throat. The inner ear contains the semicircular canals filled with fluid and nerve receptors that aid in balance. (See Figure 10–16.)

Sound vibrations are picked up by the pinna, which directs them through the auditory canal to the eardrum, causing it to vibrate. The bones in the middle ear amplify these sound vibrations and transmit them to the semicircular canals of the

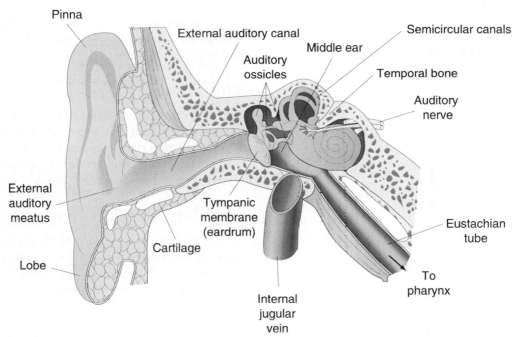

FIGURE 10–16
The ear.

inner ear. Nerve receptors change the vibrations to electrical impulses, which travel to the brain by way of the auditory nerve. The brain interprets the nerve impulses as sound.

Balance

The fluid in the semicircular canals in the inner ear also contains nerve receptors for balance. These receptors sense changes in the position of your head and move accordingly. The nerve impulses for balance are initiated by this fluid movement and are transmitted to the brain.

The nose, tongue, and skin also provide sensory stimulation. Nerve receptors for smell are located in the nose, taste receptors are on the tongue, and touch receptors are under the surface of the skin.

Changes of Aging

All of the special senses are affected by aging. The eyes take longer to adjust to changes in light, distance, and direction. The visual field narrows and interferes with the ability to see objects off to the side. More light is required to see, causing night vision to decrease. The ability to tell colors apart declines (blues, greens, and violets tend to look alike). Vision decreases for close-up work, and small print becomes hard to read, requiring eyeglasses in order to see well.

The hearing receptors become less sensitive, causing sound to be distorted. The number of smell receptors in the nose decreases and affects the accuracy of smell. A decrease in the number of taste buds on the tongue causes taste to become less distinctive. The sense of touch may be changed due to a decrease in the sensitivity of receptors in the skin.

The Endocrine System

The endocrine system secretes chemicals called *hormones* directly into the bloodstream to regulate and control body organs and glands. The major endocrine glands are as follows:

- Pituitary gland
- Thyroid gland
- Parathyroid glands
- Thymus
- Adrenal glands
- Pancreas (islets of Langerhans)
- Gonads (testes in the male; ovaries in the female) (See Figure 10–17.)

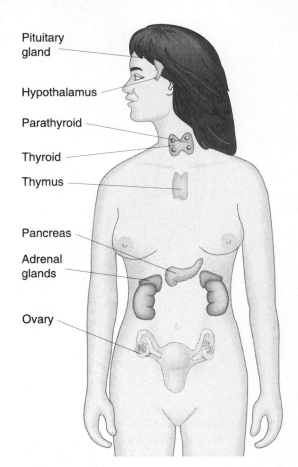

FIGURE 10–17
The major endocrine glands.

The Pituitary Gland

Located in the brain, the pituitary gland is called the master gland because it regulates the function of the other glands. It produces nine important hormones, which regulate growth, water balance, and reproduction.

The Thyroid Gland

The thyroid gland, located in the neck, secretes hormones that affect body growth and development. This gland also regulates *metabolism* (the combination of processes that produces energy in the body, allowing cells to grow and repair).

The Parathyroid Glands

Two pairs of parathyroid glands are located on the back of the thyroid gland and secrete a hormone that regulates calcium in the body. Calcium levels affect nerve and muscle function.

The Thymus

The thymus is in the chest, just behind the sternum. It assists in the immune process, which helps the body resist pathogens and disease. White blood cells called "T-cells," which regulate the immune function, also develop in this gland.

The Adrenal Glands

There are two adrenal glands, one on top of each kidney. These glands produce hormones that help to regulate water balance and the metabolism of some foods. Small amounts of sex hormones are also secreted by the adrenals. Hormones such as epinephrine, which control the body's response to stress, are produced here. Epinephrine (adrenalin) allows the body to quickly produce great amounts of energy in an emergency situation.

The Pancreas

The pancreas is located behind the stomach and near the beginning of the small intestine. Clusters of cells in the pancreas, called "the islets of Langerhans," produce insulin and glucagon. These hormones are needed to convert sugar to energy. The pancreas also secretes substances into the small intestines to assist in digestion.

The Gonads

The gonads control human reproduction and male and female sexual characteristics. In the male, the testes produce testosterone. The ovaries of the female produce estrogen and progesterone.

The Exocrine Glands

Exocrine glands secrete substances into organs or outside the body, **not** directly into the bloodstream. The sweat glands, oil glands, and parotid glands are examples of exocrine glands.

Changes of Aging

Changes of aging in the endocrine system affect the level of hormones in the body. Decrease in the production of most hormones occurs. Some hormones, such as insulin, become less effective. There is also a decrease in the response of body cells to hormones. Changes in hormone levels result in a decrease in the endocrine system's ability to regulate body activities.

The Reproductive System

All living things must have a method to reproduce themselves. The human species has survived for thousands of years through the activities of the reproductive system. A mature male and a mature female have special cells, organs, and hormones that work together during the sexual act to produce an infant human being.

The Female Reproductive System

The major structures of the female reproductive system are the ovaries, fallopian tubes, uterus, and vagina. The breasts are also considered part of this system. See Figure 10–18A for the location of the structures of the female reproductive system.

The ovaries are located on each side of the uterus in the pelvic cavity. The major function of the ovaries is to produce ova (eggs), the female reproductive cells, and to secrete the female hormones—estrogen and progesterone. Fallopian tubes carry the ovum from the ovary to the uterus. The uterus is a hollow, muscular organ in the pelvic cavity, above the bladder and in front of the rectum. The functions of the uterus are to protect and nourish the fetus (unborn baby) during pregnancy and to expel the fetus during childbirth.

The vagina acts as a passageway for birth of the baby and for *menstruation* (the discharge of the unused lining of the uterus). It is also a receptacle for the male penis during sexual intercourse. During intercourse, sperm (the male reproductive cells) enter through the vagina into the uterus and the fallopian tubes. If the sperm unites with an ovum (egg), pregnancy occurs, and the fertilized ovum passes from the fallopian tube to the uterus. If pregnancy does not occur, the ovum will die and be discharged from the body with the menstrual flow.

The Male Reproductive System

The major structures of the male reproductive system are the testes, scrotum, penis, seminal vesicles, and prostate gland. The functions of the testes are to produce sperm and secrete the male hormone testosterone. The scrotum contains two sacs, each containing one testicle, and is located behind the penis. The penis becomes enlarged and erect when sexually stimulated. Semen, the fluid that contains the sperm, is released through the penis during sexual intercourse. The seminal vesicles and the prostate gland both secrete fluids that become part of the semen. See Figure 10–18B for the location of the structures of the male reproductive system.

Changes of Aging

In women, menstruation ends with menopause, and natural pregnancy can no longer occur. A decrease in the production of estrogen leads to a loss of calcium, causing the bones to become more brittle, and to a thinning and drying of the vaginal walls. Weakened supporting muscles cause the breasts to sag. In men, there is a change in hormone levels and a decrease in

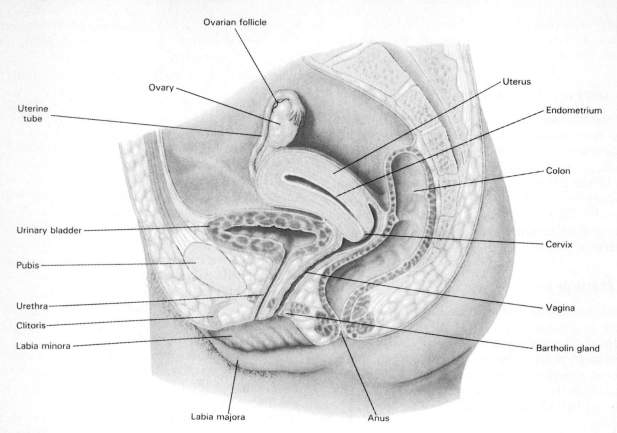

FIGURE 10–18A
The reproductive system.
A. The female reproductive system.

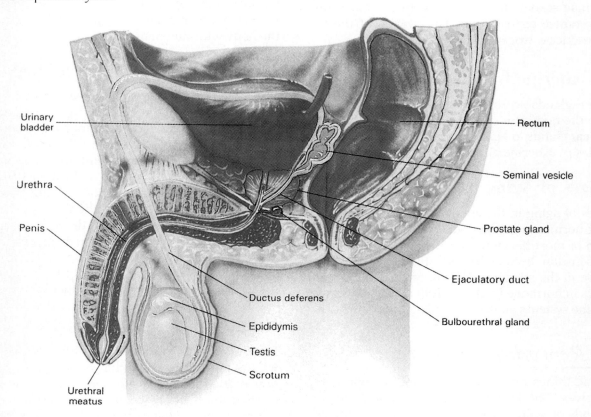

FIGURE 10–18B
The reproductive system (continued).
B. The male reproductive system.

sperm. The prostate gland can enlarge and harden, causing pressure on the urinary urethra.

Summary of the Systems

Now that you have studied each system, you should have a better understanding of how each system functions and how they all work together. Remember that all body systems tend to slow and weaken with aging. A summary of the physical changes of aging in all systems of the body is provided in Figure 10–19. For more detailed anatomy and physiology illustrations refer to the anatomy supplements on pages xxx–xxx.

Physical Changes of Aging

Integumentary System

- Dry, thin, fragile skin
- Wrinkles and liver spots
- Loss of fatty tissue
- Decrease in feeling
- Hair thins and loses color
- Thick, tough nails

Musculoskeletal System

- Muscles weaken and lose tone
- Body movements slow
- Stiff joints
- Thin, brittle bones
- Changes in height and posture

Respiratory System

- Rib cage more rigid
- Respiratory muscles weaken
- Lung tissue less elastic
- Voice weakens

Circulatory System

- Heart muscle weakens and heartbeat less effective
- Blood volume decreases
- Blood vessels become hard, stiff, and narrow

Digestive System

- Peristalsis slows
- Decreased saliva and number of taste buds
- Difficulty chewing and swallowing

Urinary System

- Decreased kidney function
- Decreased bladder muscle tone

Nervous System

- Decrease in the number of neurons
- Delayed transmission of messages
- Slowed response and reflexes
- Short-term memory loss
- Decreased sensitivity of nerve endings

Sensory Changes

- Decreased vision
- Hearing loss
- Smell and taste less accurate
- Touch less sensitive

Endocrine System

- Decrease in hormones
- Decrease in body's response to hormones

Reproductive System

- Menopause occurs in women
- Thinning and drying of the female vaginal walls
- Weakened supporting muscles cause the breasts to sag
- Hormone levels decrease in the male
- Enlargement of male prostate gland

FIGURE 10–19
Summary of changes of aging.

Review

Read each sentence and fill in the blank with the vocabulary term that best completes the sentence.

1. _____ is the study of body structure.
2. The basic building block of the body is a _____.
3. _____ is the stage of the cardiac cycle when the heart is contracting and pumping blood.
4. Chemicals secreted by the endocrine glands that regulate and control body functions are called _____.
5. The combination of processes of physical and chemical change within the cell that produce energy is called _____.

Remember

1. The basic building block of the body is the cell.
2. The body systems are interdependent and work together.
3. The major function of the skin is protection.
4. The musculoskeletal system provides body movement.
5. The respiratory system brings oxygen into the body and removes carbon dioxide.
6. The circulatory system carries food, water, and oxygen to the cells and assists in the elimination of waste.
7. The digestive system breaks down food for the body's use and eliminates waste.
8. The urinary system removes waste products from the blood and helps maintain fluid balance.
9. The nervous system controls and coordinates body activities.
10. Sight, hearing, smell, taste, and touch are the five senses.
11. The endocrine system secretes hormones that regulate and control body organs and glands.
12. A decrease in the production of sex hormones can lead to changes in both males and females.
13. All body systems tend to slow and weaken with aging.

Reflect

Read the following case study and answer the questions.

Case Study

Sarah Barton is an 82-year-old patient who is being treated for a urinary tract infection. She has difficulty moving around because she says her joints are stiff and her muscles are weak. She wears eyeglasses and uses a hearing aid.

1. List the major structures of the urinary system.
2. List the functions of the musculoskeletal system.
3. What changes of aging might you expect to observe in Mrs. Barton's skin?
4. What changes of aging in vision might require Mrs. Barton to wear eyeglasses?

Respond

Choose the best answer for each question.

1. Physiology is the study of
   A. Body structure
   B. Body function
   C. Body hygiene
   D. Body changes
2. The control center of a cell is the
   A. Cytoplasm
   B. Membrane
   C. Nucleus
   D. Trachea
3. The correct anatomical name for the skin is
   A. Integument
   B. Nucleus

C. Trachea

D. Urethra

4. Which of the following are types of muscle tissue?

A. Skeletal

B. Smooth

C. Cardiac

D. All of the above

5. The exchange of oxygen and carbon dioxide takes place in the

A. Alveoli

B. Bronchi

C. Pharynx

D. Larynx

6. The stage of the cardiac cycle when the heart is resting and filling with blood is called

A. Respiration

B. Pulse

C. Diastole

D. Systole

7. Where does most of food digestion and absorption take place?

A. In the mouth

B. In the stomach

C. In the small intestine

D. In the large intestine

8. Which systems control and coordinate all body functions?

A. Skeletal and muscular

B. Respiratory and circulatory

C. Nervous and endocrine

D. Digestive and urinary

9. The ear controls hearing and

A. Vision

B. Mobility

C. Touch

D. Balance

10. The urethra is a major structure of which body system?

A. Urinary

B. Respiratory

C. Circulatory

D. Endocrine

Chapter Eleven

Care *of* Patients *with* Common Health Problems

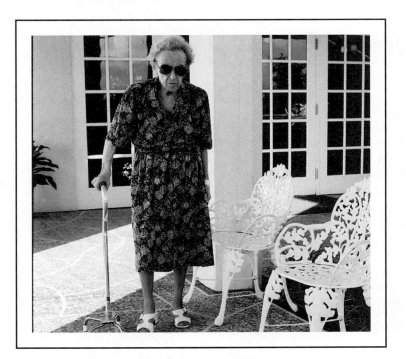

OBJECTIVES

After studying this chapter, you will be able to

1. Describe the three categories of illnesses.

2. Explain how culture influences health care.

3. List five guidelines for prevention of a pressure ulcer.

4. List three guidelines for care of the patient with arthritis.

5. List six guidelines for care of the patient with respiratory problems.

6. List two guidelines for care of the patient with circulatory problems.

7. List two guidelines for care of the patient with digestive problems.

8. List five guidelines for care of the patient with urinary problems.

9. List six guidelines for care of the patient who has had a stroke.

10. List four guidelines for care of the patient with diabetes mellitus.

11. List three guidelines for care of the patient with reproductive problems.

12. List three guidelines for care of the patient with cancer.

acute illness   An illness that begins suddenly and continues for a short period of time.

amputation   Surgical removal of all or part of an extremity.

chronic illness   An illness that progresses slowly, or gradually, over a long period of time.

contracture   Shortening and wasting of muscle tissue due to lack of use.

dyspnea   Difficulty breathing or labored breathing.

flaccid   A condition of having little or no muscle tone; limp or flabby.

fracture   A break in a bone.

hemiplegia   The condition of paralysis of one side of the body.

hyperglycemia   A condition of abnormally high glucose levels in the blood; high blood sugar.

hypertension   A condition of consistently elevated blood pressure above 140/90; high blood pressure.

hypoglycemia   A condition of abnormally low glucose levels in the blood; low blood sugar.

inflammation   The body's response to injury or disease, evident by the presence of redness, swelling, heat, and pain.

obese   Condition of excess fat resulting in the individual being more than 20% to 30% over ideal body weight.

paraplegia   The condition of paralysis of the lower half of the body.

pressure ulcer   A breakdown of skin tissue caused by the interrupted blood flow to the area.

quadriplegia   The condition of paralysis of both arms and legs.

terminal illness   An illness in which recovery is not expected.

There are many diseases and health problems identified by the global health care community. This chapter focuses on the ones with which you will most likely come into contact in you role as a nursing assistant. Understanding the nature, cause, and treatment of these conditions will help you provide quality care.

Guidelines for patient care are provided throughout the chapter. The first guideline in caring for a patient is to follow the patient's plan of care. All patients are unique individuals with their own needs, who respond to disease in their own way. Therefore, it will be necessary to adapt the guidelines to fit each individual patient.

Cultural Aspects of Care

It is important to be aware of the variety of cultural values and beliefs that influence health care behavior. A patient's response to medical treatment and nursing care may depend on culture. Some of the health problems discussed in this chapter occur more frequently within certain ethnic groups. For example, diabetes and hypertension are more common in Hispanics, Native Americans, African Americans, and Filipinos.

It is not necessary to thoroughly understand each culture. The first step is to recognize that cultural differences do exist and that your patient's culture may differ from your own. The differences may include health care practices, gender roles, religious rituals, and communication styles. Dietary preferences and the symbolism of food are important areas. Remember, however, there may be great variations among individuals within a culture. Avoid making assumptions based on ethnic identification.

Types of Illnesses

Illnesses can usually be divided into three categories—acute, chronic, and terminal. An *acute illness* is an illness that begins suddenly and continues for a short period. This type of illness, while it can be severe, can often be successfully treated and cured. Appendicitis is an example of an acute illness.

A *chronic illness* is an illness that progresses slowly, or gradually, over a long period of time. The person who has a chronic illness may not be sick all the time. Although most chronic illnesses are incurable, many can be controlled by treatment. Diabetes is an example of a chronic illness. A *terminal illness* is an illness in which recovery is not expected. AIDS is an example of a terminal illness.

Integumentary System

Considering that the skin is the largest organ in the body, it has fewer serious problems than most other organs. Skin does not wear out, nor does it fail with aging. A patient may die of kidney failure or heart failure, while the skin is still intact and functioning.

Dermatitis

Dermatitis is inflammation of the skin. ("Derma" means skin and "itis" means inflammation of). One type of severe dermatitis is eczema. Dermatitis can be caused by any chemical or natural compound that ir-

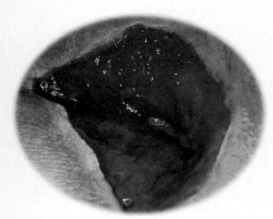

FIGURE 11–1
A pressure ulcer is a breakdown of skin tissue that occurs when blood flow to the area is interrupted.

ritates the skin. Examples of common irritants include plants, fruits, vegetables, soaps, cleaning solutions, cosmetics, and insect bites. Symptoms include redness, rash, swelling, oozing, and scaling. Pain and itching may also occur.

Skin Injuries

A skin injury, commonly called a wound, interferes with the skin's primary function—protection. Pathogens can enter through a break in the skin and cause infection. Bruises, lacerations, and incisions are examples of skin injuries. A bruise is an injury that discolors, but does not break, the skin. A laceration is a ragged tear in the skin that might be caused by a piece of torn metal. Bleeding will occur if a blood vessel is cut. An incision is a clean, smooth skin cut that is usually caused by a sharp object, such as a knife or a piece of broken glass. Incisions usually bleed freely, and if the cut is very deep, hemorrhage may occur.

Pressure Ulcer

A *pressure ulcer* is a breakdown of skin tissue that occurs when blood flow to an area is interrupted. Each cell of the body needs oxygen, fluid, and food in order to live. It also needs to rid itself of waste products. This is accomplished through blood circulation. When blood flow is interrupted, tissues die and an ulcer forms. A pressure ulcer may be called a pressure sore, a decubitus, or more commonly, a bedsore. Patients who are elderly, bedbound, paralyzed, comatose (unconscious), very thin, or *obese* (very fat) are at greater risk of developing pressure ulcers. (See Figure 11–1.)

Cause of Pressure Ulcers

The major cause of a pressure ulcer is pressure that interferes with the circulation of blood. This pressure may be caused by:

- Lying or sitting too long in one position
- Wrinkled clothing or bed linen
- Crumbs or other small objects left in the bed
- Poor nutrition
- Inadequate fluid intake
- Improper body positioning causing pressure over the bony prominences (places where bones are near the surface of the skin)

Shearing is another cause of pressure ulcers. Shearing occurs when one layer of skin tissue is pulled in a direction opposite another layer. This causes blood vessels to stretch or kink and interferes with the circulation of blood. Shearing results when a patient slides down in the bed or chair. Shearing can be reduced by using a pull sheet (a small sheet that is placed under the patient). A pull sheet may also be called a draw sheet, lift sheet, or turning sheet.

Stages of a Pressure Ulcer

Pressure ulcers are classified by the depth of tissue destruction. The deeper the ulcer goes into skin tissue, the more serious the problem and the more difficult it is to heal. Figure 11–2 describes the four stages of pressure ulcers.

Guidelines for the Prevention of Pressure Ulcers

- Follow each patient's care plan.
- Turn or change the patient's position at least every two hours.
- Keep the skin clean and dry and free of urine or feces.
- Make sure that bed linens are clean, dry, and free of wrinkles.
- Remove crumbs and small objects from the bed or chair.
- Make sure that shoes and clothing are not too tight.
- Check the edges of casts and braces for pressure.
- Position the patient's body and limbs to reduce pressure over bony prominences.
- Apply lotion to keep the skin lubricated.
- Encourage exercise to promote circulation.
- Encourage the patient to drink fluids and eat a proper diet.
- Make use of pressure-relieving equipment.

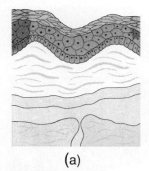

Inflammation or redness of the skin that does not return to normal after 15 minutes of removal of pressure. Edema is present. It involves the epidermis. Skin may or may not be broken.

(a)

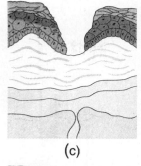

Skin blister or shallow skin ulcer. Involves the epidermis and dermis. Looks like a shallow crater. Area is red, warm, and may or may not have drainage.

(c)

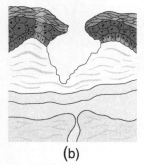

Full-thickness skin loss exposing subcutaneous tissue, may extend into next layer. Edema, inflammation, and necrosis present. Drainage present, which may or may not have an odor.

(b)

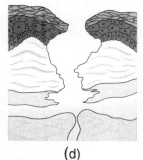

Full-thickness ulcer. Muscle and/or bone can be seen. Infection and necrosis are present. Drainage present, which may or may not have an odor.

(d)

FIGURE 11–2
Stages of pressure ulcers.

Prevention of Pressure Ulcers

Curing a pressure ulcer is more stressful and time consuming than preventing one. Preventing skin breakdown depends upon careful observation and your commitment to restorative care. While you are giving the patient a bath, assisting with toileting, and other activities of daily living (ADLs), observe the skin carefully. Check for change in skin temperature, texture, and color. Make sure that the patient is clean and dry. Report any skin injuries or changes to the nurse immediately. Check the patient's care plan for the use of equipment that is designed to relieve pressure on the patient's skin. (See Figure 11–3.)

Musculoskeletal System

Diseases and injuries of the musculoskeletal system often interfere with the patient's mobility. Decreased mobility can result in physical, mental, and emotional problems, affecting even the patient's attitude and motivation. A common complication of limited activity is a *contracture* (a wasting and shortening of a muscle due to lack of use). Contractures are discussed in more detail in Chapter 18. (See Figure 11–4.)

Osteoporosis

Osteoporosis is a disease in which loss of bone tissue causes bones to become brittle. The disorder may cause pain, loss of height, or a *fracture* (broken bone). Accidental injuries may occur when a hip bone breaks and causes a fall or the brittle bone breaks during a fall. Osteoporosis is more common in women because of hormonal changes and a loss of calcium that occurs after menopause.

Fractures

A fracture may be of the open or closed type. In an open fracture (also called a compound fracture), the skin is broken and sometimes the bone protrudes through the skin. In a closed fracture, the bone is broken but the skin is intact or closed. At the hospital, a fractured bone must be put back into alignment and immobilized (kept from moving) until it heals. A cast or traction may be used to immobilize the bone. Cast care is discussed in Chapter 24.

Amputation

Amputation is the removal of all or a part of an extremity, usually by surgery. Amputation may be the result of a severe injury, a tumor, or a circulatory problem. Most amputees wear a prosthesis, such as an artificial leg. Rehabilitation will be necessary to teach the patient how to use the prosthesis and maintain independence.

Arthritis

The two most common types of arthritis are osteoarthritis and rheumatoid arthritis. Both diseases

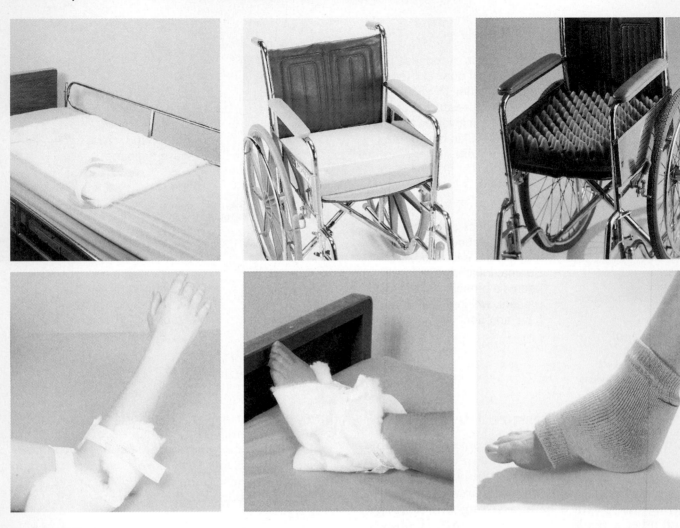

FIGURE 11-3
Use pressure-relieving equipment to help prevent pressure ulcers.

cause *inflammation* (redness, swelling, heat, and pain) of the joints.

Osteoarthritis

Osteoarthritis is one of the most disabling conditions of the elderly. It is caused by the wearing away of the cartilage that covers the ends of bones at the joint. This loss allows the bones in the joints to grind against each other, causing pain and inflammation. Because movement causes pain, people who have this condition may be less active.

Rheumatoid Arthritis

Rheumatoid arthritis can affect people of all ages, including children. The disease can cause severe disability and crippling of the hands or feet. Rheumatoid arthritis, like many chronic diseases, comes and goes in intensity. Severe arthritic attacks may be followed by long periods in which the patient is symptom free.

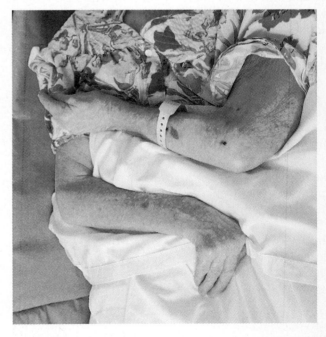

FIGURE 11-4
The patient with arthritis is at risk of developing contractures.

Treatment of Arthritis

Medications will be ordered to treat the pain and inflammation of arthritis. Heat or warm soaks may be used on inflamed joints, and regular exercise is recommended. However, patients with rheumatoid arthritis need frequent periods of rest, and at times complete bedrest may be ordered. Patients should eat well-balanced meals. There is no cure for arthritis. Treatment is aimed at reducing pain and improving joint function. Arthritic joints may be surgically replaced by a prosthesis (an artificial body part). Hip or knee replacements can be successfully performed on patients of all ages.

Nursing Care of the Patient with Arthritis

Patients suffering from arthritis who have difficulty performing ADLs (activities of daily living) may need your assistance. Encourage the patient to be as independent as possible. Caring for oneself provides exercise, helps maintain independence, and raises self-esteem.

Exercise is an important part of the care of the patient with arthritis. Exercise helps to maintain joint movement. Patients may avoid movement because the joints are painful. Inactivity actually causes more pain and places the patient at risk for a contracture. Exercise helps to maintain motion, increase overall strength, improve circulation, and provide a sense of well-being.

Limited mobility and stiffness cause the arthritic patient to be more at risk of accidents such as falls. The patient with arthritis may be slow and unable to move quickly out of the path of danger. Encourage the use of adaptive equipment, such as canes and walkers. Allow the patient plenty of time in moving or performing tasks.

Guidelines for the Care of the Patient with Arthritis

- Follow each patient's care plan.
- Assist with ADLs as necessary.
- Provide adaptive equipment as needed.
- Help the patient to avoid fatigue.
- Allow time for the patient to move at his or her own speed.
- Protect the patient's safety.
- Provide exercise and range of motion as ordered.
- Encourage activity.
- Encourage and promote independence.

A loss of mobility affects independence and self-esteem. Feelings of frustration and anger are common, and depression may occur. Encourage patients to attend activities. Many of the programs that are provided help to maintain joint movement as well as offer social interaction.

Respiratory System

Chronic obstructive pulmonary disease (COPD) is a progressive and irreversible condition in which the airway is obstructed. Symptoms may include *dyspnea* (difficult breathing), coughing, wheezing, and fatigue.

Emphysema

Emphysema is a chronic respiratory disease in which lung tissue loses its elasticity, and the alveoli remain expanded. Mucus obstructs or plugs the bronchi and bronchioles, making it difficult to get air in and out of the lungs. As a decrease in the exchange of oxygen and carbon dioxide occurs, the patient with emphysema breathes harder and faster in an attempt to get more air. The patient with emphysema is constantly struggling to breathe. Wheezing may occur and coughing may bring up secretions from the lungs. The skin is usually pale or there may be cyanosis (a blue color caused by a lack of oxygen). Although there is no cure for emphysema, treatment can relieve symptoms and slow the progression of disease.

Bronchitis

Bronchitis is an inflammation of the bronchial tubes to the lungs. Although it may occur as an acute illness, it may also become chronic. Bronchitis can be caused by a natural or chemical compound and is often part of an upper respiratory infection that results from a common cold. Bronchitis can be serious or even fatal in small children, the elderly, and patients with weakened immune systems. Symptoms of bronchitis include fever, chills, aching muscles, sore throat, and cough. Dyspnea may be present, and the patient may develop spasms of coughing. Coughing spasms can become continuous and, if unrelieved, can lead to death. Acute attacks can be very frightening.

Pneumonia

Pneumonia is an acute infection of the lungs. Symptoms may include chills, fever, chest pain, cough, headache, and weakness. If diagnosed and treated early, bacterial pneumonia can usually be successfully treated with antibiotics. A vaccine to prevent some types of pneumonia is available.

Aspiration pneumonia is caused by food, fluid, or secretions in the lower airway. Aspiration can happen to someone who is not alert and oriented, to a patient who is vomiting, to a patient who has difficulty swallowing, or to a patient who has a feeding tube. **Hypostatic pneumonia** can result from lying in one place too long. Because of gravity, fluid tends to accumulate in the lungs, leading to infection. Bedridden patients or those recovering from surgery are at risk for hypostatic pneumonia.

Pneumonia is often the actual cause of death in patients who have AIDS or some other life-threatening disease. Patients recovering from surgery, especially the elderly, may also develop pneumonia. Preventing pneumonia in these patients may mean the difference between life and death.

Caring for the Patient with Respiratory Problems

Patients with respiratory problems may be too weak to eat or care for themselves and will need assistance with ADLs. The mouth may have an unpleasant odor that affects taste, smell, and appetite. Assist the patient to a sitting or upright position that allows maximum lung expansion. (See Figure 11–5.) Assist bedbound patients in changing position at least every two hours. Encourage surgical patients to follow postoperative instructions regarding deep breathing and leg exercises. Emotional stress may increase respiratory rate and the need for more oxygen. Provide emotional reassurance to help relieve stress and fear.

Some patients with respiratory problems may have oxygen administration ordered. Follow the rules of oxygen safety presented in Chapter 6. Care of the patient receiving oxygen is discussed in Chapter 24.

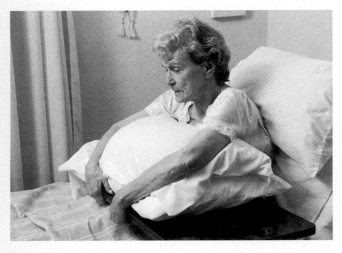

FIGURE 11–5
An upright position allows maximum lung expansion and helps the patient breathe easier.

> ## Guidelines for the Care of the Patient with Respiratory Problems
>
> ■ Follow each patient's care plan.
> ■ Position the patient for easier breathing.
> ■ Assist the patient in changing position every two hours.
> ■ Encourage fluids and proper nutrition.
> ■ Provide frequent rest periods.
> ■ Provide skin care as needed.
> ■ Provide mouth care every two hours or more often, if needed.
> ■ Keep clothing and bed linens clean and dry.
> ■ Provide emotional support.
> ■ Observe closely and report changes to the nurse immediately.
> ■ Follow safety rules if oxygen is being used.
> ■ Follow standard precautions.

Circulatory System

Heart disease is a leading cause of death worldwide in people over the age of 60. Diseases of the heart and blood vessels can range from mild to severe and may involve all age groups. Some people are born with heart disorders.

Coronary Artery Disease

Coronary artery disease (CAD) causes a narrowing of the coronary arteries supplying blood to the heart muscle. Arteriosclerosis (hardening of the arteries) causes the blood supply to the heart muscle to be reduced. The heart muscle requires more oxygen than the hardened blood vessels can supply. Many health problems such as high blood pressure and heart attacks may result from CAD.

Angina

Angina is chest pain that occurs when narrowed blood vessels do not allow enough oxygenated blood to reach the heart muscle. Attacks may be triggered by exercise, eating, or an emotional experience. An angina attack may begin with sudden intense chest pain that radiates down the left arm or up into the neck and jaw. The pain usually lasts only a few minutes and is usually relieved by rest and medication. Attacks may vary in frequency from several in a day to symptom-free intervals of weeks or months.

Myocardial Infarction

A myocardial infarction (MI) occurs from an abrupt decrease in coronary blood flow to a portion of the heart muscle. It may be caused by a blood clot or other material blocking the blood vessel. The first symptom of an MI is often a sudden, severe, crushing pain in the chest with pain radiating to the back, jaw, or left arm. The skin may become pale, cyanotic, or cold. The patient may be sweating and experiencing dyspnea. Nausea and vomiting may occur. With all these symptoms occurring, fear and anxiety may be high. An MI is a life-threatening situation that requires immediate medical attention, because death can occur suddenly.

Congestive Heart Failure

Congestive heart failure (CHF) occurs when the heart muscle weakens and fails to pump efficiently. One of the first symptoms observed in CHF is edema of the hands and feet. (See Figure 11–6.) Since the lungs are congested (filled with fluid), breathing is labored and the pulse may be fast and irregular. Urine output is usually decreased because the body is holding fluid.

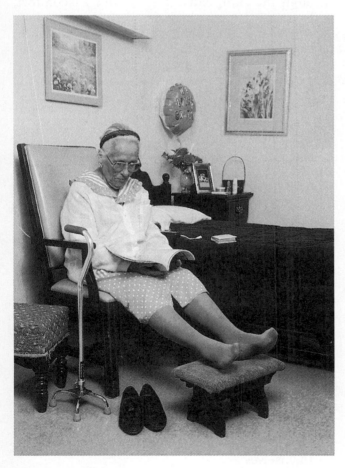

FIGURE 11–6
Edema can be a complication of congestive heart failure.

Guidelines for the Care of the Patient with Circulatory Problems

- Follow each patient's care plan.
- Provide emotional support.
- Observe the patient carefully and report changes promptly.
- Encourage the patient to follow diet restrictions.
- Measure and report vital signs accurately.

Pain, nausea, vomiting, a wet cough, and dyspnea may be present. An acute episode of CHF can result in death. CHF is treatable with medication that strengthens the pumping action of the blood.

Hypertension

Hypertension is the medical term for high blood pressure. Diagnosis is made when a person's blood pressure is consistently higher than normal. The upper limit of normal blood pressure in adults is 140/90. Although the cause of hypertension is not always known, factors that contribute to it include heredity, diet, weight, and lifestyle. Hypertension is common in heart disease and diabetes and can lead to other complications.

Caring for the Patient with Circulatory Problems

The safest way to care for the patient with a circulatory problem is to follow the individual care plan. Many circulatory problems are life-threatening, so patients will need close observation and emotional support.

Digestive System

Problems of the digestive system can involve the digestion of food or the elimination of waste products. Elimination problems are discussed in Chapter 23.

Gallbladder Disease

The gallbladder is located on the under surface of the liver and secretes bile, a substance necessary for digestion of fats. Problems with this organ can include inflammation, spasms, or gallstones (for-

Guidelines for the Care of the Patient with Digestive Problems

- Follow each patient's care plan.
- Encourage the patient to follow dietary restrictions.
- Provide frequent mouth care.
- Report the amount and frequency of vomiting.
- Report complaints of pain promptly to the nurse.
- Observe and report abnormal stools.

mations of hard, rocklike material). Any one of these conditions may restrict the flow of bile and interfere with digestion.

Symptoms may include severe abdominal pain, nausea, and vomiting. There may be fever and a yellowing of the skin. Pain usually appears about an hour after eating. Treatment may include a low-fat diet that is high in protein and carbohydrates. Conservative treatment with diet, rest, and medication is usually ordered. If that is not effective, surgery may be recommended. Gallbladder disease is more common in women over 40, particularly those who are overweight.

Urinary System

Problems of the urinary system can interfere with elimination of fluids and wastes from the body. Aside from the two disorders of the kidney discussed in this chapter, other problems of the urinary system are addressed in Chapter 23.

Kidney Stones

The body sometimes creates "stones" made of a hard, rocklike material. These stones may get into

Guidelines for the Care of the Patient with Urinary Problems

- Follow each patient's care plan.
- Measure fluid intake and output accurately.
- Encourage the patient to follow fluid restrictions.
- Encourage the patient to follow the proper diet.
- Measure vital signs accurately.
- Provide frequent mouth and skin care.
- Report any changes promptly.

one of the narrow tubes in the kidney and block the tube. Stones may also be found in the urinary bladder. Kidney stones vary in size from small gravel to very large stones. Small, round, smooth stones may pass through the urinary system unnoticed. Pain occurs when a large, irregular-shaped stone enters a ureter (a tube that leads from the kidney to the bladder). The pain begins in the back or hip area and radiates into adjoining organs. Nausea and vomiting may occur, along with heavy perspiration. Chills and shock are not unusual. The attack may last for hours, and soreness may linger for days. Treatment depends on the size of the stones. Pain medication may be necessary during the attack. If the person is not able to pass the stone, surgery may be required.

Nephritis

"Nephr" means kidney, and "itis" means inflammation of, so nephritis is inflammation of the kidney. Nephritis can result from an infection or a circulatory problem. Symptoms include hypertension and edema, resulting from a decrease in urinary output. Toxins (poisons) can build up in the blood, resulting in mental confusion and irritability if these toxins reach the brain. Toxins may also be secreted through the skin, causing irritation, discomfort, and odor. Treatment includes bedrest and a low-sodium diet. Fluid intake and output will need to be measured. Vital signs are measured on a regular basis. Treatment may include kidney dialysis, the process of filtering waste products from the blood by a machine that functions as an artificial kidney.

Nervous System

Diseases of the brain, spine, or nerves may interfere with thinking, talking, and moving. Mental disorders, such as Alzheimer's disease, are addressed in Chapter 27.

Multiple Sclerosis

Multiple sclerosis (MS) is a progressive disease that affects the brain and spinal cord. Gradual destruction of myelin, the substance that coats and insulates nerve fibers, interferes with the transmission of nerve impulses. Signs and symptoms may include numbness, tremors, loss of balance and coordination, staggering gait, weakness, and paralysis. Speech problems are common in advanced disease. The patient may be mentally and emotionally unstable, although intelligence is usually not affected. Eventually, patients with MS may be unable to care for themselves.

Onset of MS is usually between 20 and 40 years of age. Although the person's condition progressively gets worse, there may be periods when the disease symptoms level off or seem to disappear. There is no cure for MS, and it can eventually lead to total deterioration and death.

Parkinson's Disease

Parkinson's disease is a chronic CNS disorder that affects control of motor function. It is commonly called "shaking palsy." The onset of disease is after the age of 40, and it frequently affects older age groups. Common symptoms include slow movements, muscular stiffness, tremors, and a shuffling walk. The face becomes masklike, and the mouth tends to hang open. There may be difficulty speaking, swallowing, and handling oral secretions. Intelligence is generally not affected. Medication and/or surgery may help the symptoms of Parkinson's disease.

Epilepsy

Epilepsy is a disease in which convulsive seizures occur. A seizure is a sudden spasm of muscle caused by abnormal brain activity. Most patients are completely normal between attacks. The cause of epilepsy is not always known.

A seizure may take many forms, ranging from grand mal (very large) to petit mal (very small). The seizure may be preceded by an aura (a light, sound, or smell sensation experienced by the patient), which warns of the attack. A typical grand mal seizure begins with a cry, loss of consciousness, falling, and contractions of the muscles of the arms, legs, trunk, and head. The attack may last from two to five minutes, although it seems much longer to an observer. After the seizure, the patient may go into a deep sleep. Petit mal seizures may be so slight that they go unnoticed. There may be rapid blinking of the eyes or the patient seems to go into a brief "trance."

Epilepsy is treated with medications aimed at controlling the frequency of attacks. These patients will need compassion and emotional support. Years ago, patients with epilepsy were placed in insane asylums, and, even today, epileptics may experience discrimination or ridicule. The major issue in caring for the patient having a seizure is safety. Review emergency care for seizures in Chapter 7. Epileptics are often barred from jobs that require driving or operating machinery. This can restrict their social lives as well as work roles.

Bell's Palsy

Bell's palsy is a neurological disorder caused by infection or injury to a nerve. It affects the facial muscles, usually on one side only. Physical symptoms include facial muscle weakness or paralysis, with an overall droopy appearance. The eye on the affected side of the face droops and sometimes will not blink or close. There may be difficulty speaking, eating, and drinking, and the patient may drool. Hearing and smell may also be affected. Emotional damage can be as severe as the physical effects. Radical changes in facial appearance can lower self-esteem and lead to problems with communication and social interactions. The sudden onset of disease leaves no time to adjust to all the changes. The duration and quality of recovery may depend on the severity of the condition.

Nervous System Injuries

Injuries of the brain or spinal cord result in a large number of severe disabilities and deaths each year. These injuries may be caused by falls, vehicle accidents, sports accidents, or bullet wounds. An injury to the nervous system may result in *hemiplegia* (paralysis of one side of the body), *paraplegia* (paralysis of the lower half of the body), or *quadriplegia* (paralysis of both arms and legs).

Symptoms of a brain injury will depend on the location and severity of the damage. There is usually loss of consciousness immediately after the injury. Dyspnea, weakness, headache, spasms, or seizures may occur. Vision and hearing problems are common. Mental changes may include irritability, restlessness, confusion, or amnesia (loss of memory). Partial or complete paralysis may result. The person with a brain injury may be comatose and unable to respond.

Symptoms of spinal cord injuries depend on whether the spinal cord is damaged or severed (cut in two). If the cord is damaged, there may be weakness, spasms, or paralysis. If the spinal cord is severed, the result will be total paralysis of body structures below the injury. Paralysis can result in the inability to control urine or bowel movements.

In recent years there has been an increase in research on spinal cord injuries. One of the goals of this research is to reverse the effects of paralysis, even in patients whose paralysis was considered permanent in the past.

Transient Ischemic Attack

Transient ischemic attacks (TIAs) are caused by a temporary interruption in blood flow to a part of the brain. They are sometimes called "mini strokes." The attack lasts only a brief time, and may go unnoticed or thought to be a "fainting spell."

The person experiences a sudden feeling of numbness, tingling, or weakness on one side of the body. There may be slurred speech or loss of speech, but the person usually remains conscious. It is very important to report these attacks to the nurse, because a TIA is sometimes a warning of a major stroke. Treatment is aimed at preventing a stroke from occurring.

Cerebrovascular Accident

A stroke is the common name for a cerebrovascular accident (CVA). It is the result of an interruption in blood flow in the brain, causing brain cells to die from lack of oxygen. A stroke is frequently caused by a blood clot or ruptured (broken) blood vessel in the brain. A stroke patient may be able to do a complex task such as balancing the checkbook and not be able to do a simple task like buttoning his shirt. A minor stroke may cause minor, temporary symptoms, while a major stroke can cause severe, permanent damage or death.

Signs and symptoms depend on the area of the brain that is involved and the amount of tissue that is damaged. Damage on one side of the brain affects the opposite side of the body. A stroke on the left side of the brain will cause weakness or paralysis on the right side of the body. There may be partial or permanent paralysis of the right face, arm, and leg. Aphasia (loss of language) may occur, involving speaking, understanding, reading, and writing. The patient may be very slow and cautious in behavior. (See Figure 11–7.)

A stroke in the right side of the brain will cause damage on the left side of the body. There may be partial or complete paralysis of the left face, arm, and leg. Thought processes, memory, and the ability to tell time may be affected. There may be difficulty

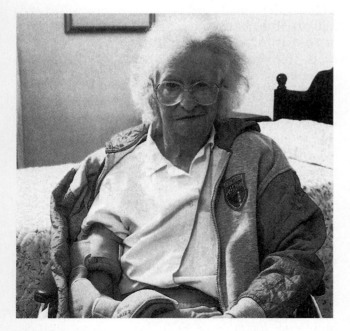

FIGURE 11–7
A stroke in the left side of the brain may cause weakness or paralysis in the right side of the body.

in estimating distance and movement. Judgement may be affected and the patient may act impulsively and inappropriately. (See Figure 11–8.)

Physical Complications

Physical complications of a stroke may include the following:

- Respiratory difficulties
- Weakness
- Paralysis
- Hemiplegia
- Contractures
- Spasm (involuntary contraction of muscles)
- Muscles that are drooping or *flaccid* (limp)
- Aphasia
- Incontinence
- Difficulty swallowing
- Coma

Emotional and Behavioral Complications

The emotional impact of a stroke can be as strong as the physical effects. Memory loss can be minor or severe and long-lasting. It is difficult to judge how the patient feels, because he or she may have little emotional control. Angry outbursts and sudden tears seem to come from nowhere. Depression is common, and the patient may express a wish to die. There may be intense anger, aimed at anyone who crosses the patient's path. Family members and caregivers are the target of much of this anger. If the patient lashes out in anger, try to remember that the patient is not really angry at you, he or she is angry and frustrated at the situation. Early attempts at independence may be extremely difficult.

Any emotion may trigger frequent and intense inappropriate crying or laughing. The patient may cry when he is happy, cry when he is sad, or cry for no reason at all. Do not ask the patient why he is crying because he probably does not know. Your question is a reminder of how little control he actually has.

Family members may be frustrated, angry, confused, and embarrassed. There are times when nothing they do or say seems to help, and they are concerned that they have somehow upset the patient. The needs of family members may be almost as great as those of the patient.

The patient may undergo personality and behavior changes. Increased irritability is common. There may be difficulty expressing emotions. Strong or negative emotions, such as anger, are easier to express. The patient may curse, use abusive language, or make inappropriate sexual remarks and gestures.

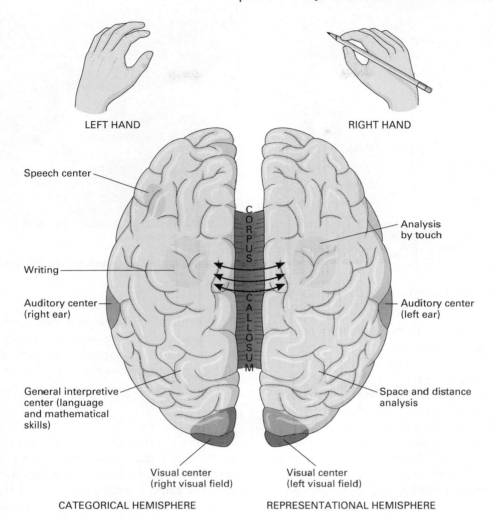

LEFT HAND   RIGHT HAND

Speech center

Analysis
by touch

Writing

Auditory center
(right ear)

Auditory center
(left ear)

CORPUS CALLOSUM

General interpretive
center (language
and mathematical
skills)

Space and distance
analysis

Visual center
(right visual field)

Visual center
(left visual field)

CATEGORICAL HEMISPHERE   REPRESENTATIONAL HEMISPHERE

FIGURE 11–8
Functional differences between the left and right cerebral hemispheres of the brain.

Often these actions are the total opposite of previous behavior patterns for that person. Patients may appear rude or self-centered. The stroke patient may have to relearn social skills just as he may have to relearn to walk or feed himself.

Nursing Care of the Patient with a Stroke

A stroke is a very serious and frightening condition. It often strikes without warning and leaves the person unconscious. The first concern is survival of the patient. During the acute stage, immediately after the stroke, the patient will probably be in the hospital. If

Guidelines for the Care of the Patient Who Has Had a Stroke

- Follow each patient's care plan.
- Encourage activity. There is often a decrease in energy and initiative.

- Allow time. It may take the patient a long time to perform even a simple task.
- Provide a calm environment. Patients can be easily distracted or overstimulated.
- Encourage decision making, but limit choices. Too many choices may cause frustration.
- Dress the patient on the affected side first. Undress the unaffected side first. (See Figure 11–9.)
- Feed on the unaffected side of mouth.
- Show patience and understanding.
- Encourage self-care.
- Be empathetic with family members.
- Use simple language and say what you mean.
- Provide physical reassurance through touch.
- Remind the patient and family that recovery takes time.
- Observe and report changes in the patient's condition.

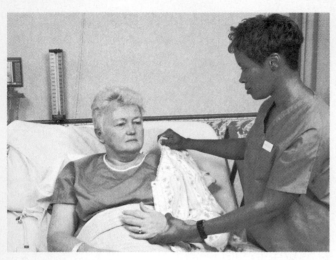

FIGURE 11–9
Dress the stroke patient on the affected side first.

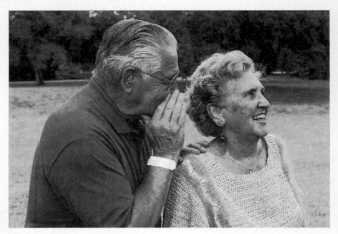

FIGURE 11–10
Conduction hearing loss may be helped by a hearing aid, which makes sounds louder.

the stroke was very severe, the patient may be comatose and in an intensive care unit. Your responsibilities in caring for the stroke patient during the acute period include monitoring vital signs, performing range of motion, providing frequent oral care and skin care, and turning and repositioning at least every two hours. You may also need to apply and remove elastic stockings or provide urinary catheter care. Your observations are very important during this stage. Observe and report changes in vital signs, level of consciousness, breathing patterns, mobility, and skin condition.

*S*ensory *Organs*

Loss of vision or hearing are common problems of the sensory organs. Either of these losses can interfere with the patient's independence and quality of life.

Eyes

Children and adults of all ages may have vision problems. They may be nearsighted (can see things that are near, but distant vision is poor) or farsighted (can see things that are far away but have difficulty with close vision). Gradual vision impairment usually begins in middle age or later years. Sometimes vision may be corrected by eyeglasses, contact lenses, or surgery.

Cataracts

A cataract is a clouding of the lens of the eye. There is a progressive, painless loss of vision. The degree of loss depends on the location and severity of the clouding. Some people with cataracts have problems with bright lights, and night driving becomes difficult. In the early stage of cataract development, corrective eyeglasses or contact lenses help main-

tain vision. When these methods cease to be effective, the diseased lens may be surgically removed and a new lens implanted. Cataract surgery can be done on an outpatient basis quickly and safely.

Glaucoma

Glaucoma is a disorder in which pressure within the eye gradually increases. As the disease progresses, symptoms may include headaches and blurred vision. The pupil remains dilated and the eyeball appears sunken. The patient may complain of seeing "halos," rings of lights around objects. However, in early glaucoma there may be no symptoms at all. The damage can range from slight vision impairment to total blindness. Although the cause is unknown, heredity, high blood pressure, and diabetes are related factors. Glaucoma is treated with eye drops that decrease pressure and improve vision. Surgery is helpful in some types of glaucoma.

Ears

Hearing loss may affect one or both ears and can range from slightly hard-of-hearing to total deafness. It can be caused by disease, years of exposure to loud noise, injury, or the changes of aging. Treatment depends on the type of hearing loss. Conduction hearing loss may be helped by a hearing aid, which makes sounds louder. Neural hearing loss is not usually helped by a hearing aid. (See Figure 11–10.)

*E*ndocrine *System*

The most common problem of the endocrine system is diabetes mellitus. This disease can affect men, women, and children of all races and nationalities.

Diabetes Mellitus

Diabetes mellitus is a disease that affects the body's ability to use carbohydrates (starches and sugars). It is primarily the result of a lack of insulin or the failure of the body to use insulin properly. Insulin is a hormone produced in special cells of the pancreas and used by the body to convert sugar to energy. If the body is not able to use sugar for energy, it will use fat. The breakdown of fat for energy produces substances called ketones or acetone. The ketones and unused sugar build up in the blood and spill over into the urine. The most common types of diabetes are Type 1 and Type 2. Most diabetics have Type 2 diabetes.

Type 1 diabetes includes patients who are insulin dependent. Because the body produces little or no insulin, it must be given by injection. Type 1 used to be called juvenile diabetes. **Type 2 diabetes** includes patients who produce a decreased or normal amount of insulin, which the body is unable to use. These patients are not insulin dependent. Their disease can usually be controlled by diet, exercise, and oral medication. Insulin is used only when other methods fail.

Although the exact cause of diabetes is not known, certain factors such as heredity, obesity, and age contribute to the development of the disease. The symptoms of untreated diabetes include excessive urination, thirst, weight loss, and hunger. Fatigue and vision problems may occur, and sores take a long time to heal. Women may complain of vaginal itching. On examination, tests show a high level of sugar in the blood.

Although there is presently no cure for diabetes, proper treatment may prevent complications. Treatment for diabetes includes diet, exercise, oral medication, and insulin. Treatment begins with an individually planned diet and exercise program. Oral medications are effective for some diabetics, while others may need insulin injections. The goal is to keep the patient's blood sugar level within a normal range.

Complications of Diabetes Mellitus

There are many short-term and long-term complications of diabetes. *Hyperglycemia* occurs when the amount of sugar in the blood is abnormally high. It can result from eating too much, not taking enough medication, not exercising enough, stress, or illness. High blood sugar may lead to diabetic coma. *Hypoglycemia* occurs when the amount of sugar in the blood is abnormally low. It can be caused by not eating enough, too much medication, or too much exercise. Low blood sugar may lead to insulin shock. Because either of these reactions can result in coma or death, it is important that you know the symptoms of hyperglycemia and hypoglycemia (see Figure 11–11). Long-term complications of diabetes include cardiovascular disease, vision problems, leg ulcers, and nerve damage. These chronic conditions account for more episodes of blindness, kidney disease, and lower leg amputations than any other disease. Diabetic complications can seriously impair the patient's quality of life.

Care of the Patient with Diabetes Mellitus

The diabetic patient will be on a special diet to maintain correct blood sugar levels. The daily diet is divided between three meals and snacks. The diabetic must eat at regular intervals to keep the blood sugar at normal levels. Although the patient should avoid foods that are not included in the dietary plan, do not argue or take food away from the patient. The patient has the right to refuse dietary restrictions or any treatment. Let the nurse know if there is a problem. The diabetic diet is discussed in more detail in Chapter 22.

	Hyperglycemia (High Blood Sugar)	Hypoglycemia (Low Blood Sugar)
Behavior	Sluggish	Irritable, excited, dizziness, coma
Skin	Hot, dry, flushed	Cold, clammy, pale
Breathing	Deep, fruity odor	Shallow
Pulse	Slow to normal	Rapid, thready
Speech	Slurred	Normal
Urine	Glucose and acetone present	No glucose or acetone
Possible Causes	Overeating, infection, vomiting, not enough insulin	Not eating enough, excessive exercise or activity, too much insulin
Complications	Diabetic coma	Insulin shock

FIGURE 11–11
Hyperglycemia and hypoglycemia.

One of the most important ways to prevent complications is to control blood glucose levels (the amount of sugar in the blood). This requires frequent testing followed by appropriate treatment. Glucose levels can be obtained by testing urine or blood. Since blood testing is more accurate, it is the preferred method.

Nursing assistants may be responsible for diabetic urine testing and in some areas are allowed to perform the procedure for testing blood for glucose levels. In other areas, this procedure is considered a responsibility of the nurse. It is important that you know what the policy is where you work. The procedure is discussed in Chapter 24.

Observing and reporting are important responsibilities of the nursing assistant. Report any signs or symptoms of hyperglycemia or hypoglycemia. Note any change in the patient's appetite, mood, behavior or personality. Watch for skin problems and signs of infection. Report the results of sugar and acetone testing promptly and accurately.

Special Foot Care

Slowed circulation and nerve damage place the feet and legs of the diabetic patient at risk for injury, infection, and gangrene. Examine the feet carefully, observe for discoloration or injury, and report abnormal observations immediately. Wash the feet daily and dry them thoroughly, especially between the toes. Use moisturizing lotion to keep the skin soft and supple, but do not use lotion between the toes. Toenails must be carefully trimmed. Although you may not be allowed to perform this procedure, let the nurse know if the toenails need trimming. Prevent pressure on the feet or toes from bed linens, shoes, or socks. (See Figure 11–12.)

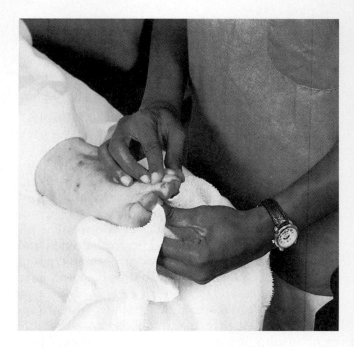

FIGURE 11–12
Carefully examine the feet of the diabetic patient and report abnormal observations immediately.

Reproductive System

Vaginitis

Vaginitis is an infection of the female vagina. Sexual intercourse with an infected person may cause vaginitis. Frequent vaginal irrigations (douches) may contribute to vaginitis by washing away normal flora that protect the area from infection. Treatment is aimed at curing the infection. A vaginal irrigation may be ordered to cleanse the area. Guidelines for giving a vaginal irrigation are located in Chapter 24. Wear gloves and follow standard precautions, because vaginal secretions may contain bloodborne pathogens.

Enlarged Prostate

The prostate gland is located below the bladder and surrounds the male urethra. Enlargement of the prostate gland is a common problem in men over 50 years old. Symptoms include a decrease in the stream of urine, difficulty starting to urinate, and frequency of urination. If the bladder does not completely empty, a urinary tract infection may develop. As long as symptoms remain mild, the patient may not seek treatment. However, as the gland continues to enlarge, problems increase. Surgery is often required for this condition. A urinary catheter may be inserted into the bladder to drain urine. You will be responsible for providing catheter care. This procedure is described in Chapter 23.

Guidelines for the Care of the Patient with Diabetes Mellitus

- Follow each patient's care plan.
- Encourage the patient to follow dietary guidelines.
- Serve meals on time.
- Observe and report dietary and fluid intake.
- Encourage exercise and activity.
- Provide good skin care.
- Report sugar and acetone test results promptly and accurately.
- Report changes in the patient's condition immediately.
- Provide special foot care.

Guidelines for the Care of the Patient with Reproductive Problems

- Follow each patient's care plan.
- Wear gloves and follow standard precautions if contact with body fluids is possible.
- Provide catheter care when necessary.
- Measure fluid intake and output accurately, if ordered.
- Assist the patient in performing proper hygiene.
- Report changes in the patient's condition promptly.

*C*ancer

Cancer (CA) is a disease that can affect any system of the body at any age. Cancer cells grow and divide rapidly and may group to form tumors. A malignant (cancerous) tumor may metastasize (spread to other body tissues). As the cancer cells grow and spread, they interfere with normal body functions. Although the cause of cancer is not known, certain factors are believed to be involved.

Seven Warning Signs of Cancer

- **C** — **C**hange in bowel or bladder habits.
- **A** — **A** sore that doesn't heal.
- **U** — **U**nusual bleeding or discharge.
- **T** — **T**hickening or lump in the breast or elsewhere.
- **I** — **I**ndigestion or difficulty in swallowing.
- **O** — **O**bvious changes in a wart or mole.
- **N** — **N**agging cough or hoarseness.

FIGURE 11–13
The warning signs of cancer.

These factors include viruses, diet, smoking, and a family history of cancer.

Cancer may be treated by surgery, radiation, chemotherapy, or a combination of methods. Treatment may cause side effects such as weakness, nausea, diarrhea, and hair loss. Some cancers, such as breast cancer, may be successfully treated and cured if the disease is identified early. For many types of cancer, early diagnosis and treatment can mean the difference between life and death. Figure 11–13 identifies the early warning signs of cancer according to the American Cancer Society.

Nursing Care of the Cancer Patient

One of the most important aspects of caring for cancer patients is pain control. Listen carefully to complaints of pain and ask about location, intensity, and duration of the pain. Observe for signs and symptoms of pain or discomfort in patients who cannot or do not verbalize their feelings. Report all observations about pain to the nurse promptly. The nursing care of the patient with cancer will depend on the location of the disease and the type of treatment used. The following guidelines apply in most situations.

Guidelines for the Care of the Patient with Cancer

- Follow each patient's care plan.
- Provide emotional support and encourage expression of fears.
- Encourage a proper diet.
- Provide good skin care.
- Encourage exercise as tolerated.
- Report complaints of pain immediately.
- Report changes in the patient's condition.
- Provide assistance with ADLs as needed.
- Promote self-care and independence.

*R*eview

Read each sentence and fill in the blank with the vocabulary term that best completes the sentence.

1. An illness that begins suddenly and continues for a short period of time is a/an _____.

2. A _____ is a wasting or shortening of a muscle due to lack of use.

3. _____ of a joint means that it is red, swollen, hot, and painful.

4. The medical term for difficult breathing is _____.

5. _____ occurs when the amount of sugar in the blood is abnormally low.

Remember

1. In order to provide quality care, you will need to have a basic understanding of common medical problems.

2. It is important to be aware of the variety of cultural values and beliefs that influence health care behavior.

3. The major cause of a pressure ulcer is pressure that interferes with circulation.

4. Patients who have arthritis may need your assistance with ADLs.

5. Patients with respiratory disorders may need to assume a position that makes breathing easier.

6. Heart disease is a leading cause of death worldwide in people over 60 years of age.

7. Patients with digestive problems should be encouraged to follow dietary restrictions.

8. Problems of the urinary system usually interfere with the elimination of fluids from the body.

9. The patient who has had a stroke can have many physical and emotional problems.

10. Loss of vision or hearing are common problems of the sensory organs.

11. Diabetes mellitus is a disorder that affects the body's ability to use carbohydrates.

12. Cancer can affect any system of the body at any age.

13. Everyone should be aware of the seven early warning signs of cancer.

Reflect

Read the following case study and answer the questions.

Case Study

Mr. Cordone is a 71-year-old patient admitted to the hospital in a diabetic coma. He has Type 2 diabetes mellitus and coronary artery disease. You observe that his skin is dry and flaky, and that there are several bruises on his left foot. His wife, who doesn't speak English well, seems to resent that you are providing nursing care for her husband. One time she yelled at you in Spanish but you couldn't understand her.

1. What might have caused the hyperglycemia that resulted in diabetic coma?

2. What are the symptoms of hyperglycemia?

3. What special foot care would you need to provide for Mr. Cordone?

4. What might be causing Mrs. Cordone's behavior?

Respond

Choose the best answer for each question.

1. Diabetes is an example of what kind of illness?
   A. Acute
   B. Chronic
   C. Terminal
   D. Occasional

2. A pressure ulcer that is blistered and involves the epidermis and dermis layers of skin is a
   A. Stage I
   B. Stage II
   C. Stage III
   D. Stage IV

3. What type of fracture has broken skin with the bone sometimes protruding?
   A. An open fracture
   B. A closed fracture
   C. An aligned fracture
   D. All of the above

4. A pneumonia that results from lying too long in one place is called
   A. Viral pneumonia
   B. Aspiration pneumonia
   C. Hypostatic pneumonia
   D. Chronic pneumonia

5. Inflammation of the kidney is called
   A. Dermatitis
   B. Gastritis
   C. Neuritis
   D. Nephritis

6. A chronic CNS disease that affects control of motor function and is commonly called shaking palsy is
   A. Parkinson's disease
   B. Multiple sclerosis
   C. Epilepsy
   D. Hypertension

7. A clouding of the lens of the eye is a sign of
   A. A cataract
   B. A stroke
   C. Glaucoma
   D. Nephritis

8. The medical term for high blood sugar is
   A. Hypertension
   B. Hypotension
   C. Hyperglycemia
   D. Hypoglycemia

9. What gland frequently causes urinary problems in elderly men?
   A. Pituitary gland
   B. Prostate gland
   C. Thyroid gland
   D. Thymus gland

10. Which of the following are warning signs of cancer?
    A. A change in bowel habits
    B. A sore that doesn't heal
    C. Changes in a wart or mole
    D. All of the above

Chapter Twelve

Life Cycle

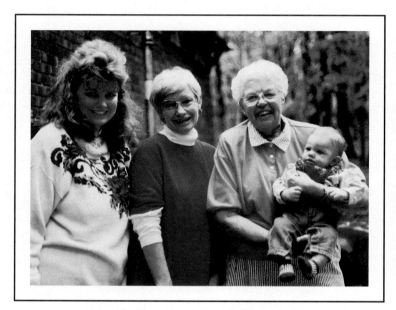

O B J E C T I V E S

After studying this chapter, you will be able to

1. Identify the major developmental task of the infant.

2. Explain the cause of much of the difficult behavior of the toddler.

3. Explain why play is so important for preschoolers.

4. Identify the major developmental task of school-age children.

5. Briefly describe the physical growth and development of the teenager.

6. Identify the major developmental task of the young adult.

7. Explain the meaning of midlife crisis.

8. Briefly describe the developmental task of old age.

9. Identify the major goal of the "very old" age group.

10. List four characteristics of centenarians.

Glossary

adolescence   The period of life from puberty to adulthood.

initiative   The power or right to take independent action in a situation.

integrity   The state of being whole or complete.

intimacy   A personal relationship involving love or affection.

menarche   A female's first menstrual period.

menopause   The period of life when menstrual periods cease.

neonate   An infant in the first six weeks of life.

peers   Those who have equal standing in age or rank.

psychosocial   Related to emotional, mental, spiritual, sexual, and social factors.

puberty   The developmental period of life in which secondary sex characteristics appear and reproduction can occur.

L ife cycle includes the series of stages and changes through which an individual passes between birth and death. There are changes in physical form and in functional activities. Since the early twentieth century the life cycle in the United States has changed significantly. Life expectancy has increased dramatically as people live longer lives. Recent studies also indicate that girls are maturing at an earlier age than ever before. There are not yet enough reliable studies to establish if this is also true in other parts of the world.

We do know that racial, ethnic, and cultural factors affect the life cycle. Social and spiritual variations may be very obvious, but there are some physical differences as well. People with dark skin do not wrinkle as much as those with lighter skin, and brunettes become gray sooner than blondes. Expectations of the various age groups also differ. For example, some cultures believe that small children should be allowed to express themselves freely. Good behavior is not expected at an early age. To you, they may seem spoiled, and your attempts to help the child adjust to illness may seem harsh to the parents. Remember that their cultural wishes must always be respected and they should be followed whenever possible.

Although each person is a separate and unique individual, we share many similarities. This chapter addresses the changes and similarities of normal, healthy people at different stages of life. As appropriate, each section describes physical development, psychosocial development, developmental tasks, and basic needs. The term *psychosocial* refers to emotional, mental, social, spiritual, and sexual considerations. Meeting the basic needs of individual patients is discussed in later chapters.

As a nursing assistant, you may care for a variety of patients of all ages. People are individuals and do not always fit what we describe as "normal." For example, while the "terrible two's" really do exist, all two-year-olds are not terrible. It is difficult to fit human beings into neat categories. However, knowing what to expect of people at certain ages will help you

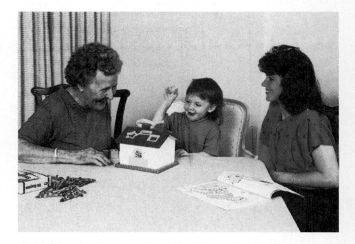

FIGURE 12–1
Knowing what to expect of people at certain times will help you to understand your patients.

to better understand and care for your patients. (See Figure 12–1.)

Developmental Stages and Tasks

Erik Erikson, an American psychologist, outlined an eight-stage life cycle process. According to his theory, human development is a lifelong process in which the individual faces certain tasks during each stage of life (see Figure 12–2). Each life stage builds on the one before it and adds to a higher level of development. Erikson believed that failure to accomplish a developmental task would interfere with normal, healthy development.

For example, the developmental task of the infant is to develop trust. An infant who is neglected or mistreated may not learn to trust people. In later life, that inability to trust may interfere with the individual's ability to maintain a long-term relationship.

Erikson's Life Stages and Developmental Tasks	
Stage	Developmental Task
1. Infancy	Develop trust
2. Early childhood	Develop independence and self-direction
3. Play age	Develop initiative
4. School age	Develop competence
5. Adolescence	Develop self-identity
6. Early adulthood	Develop intimacy and love
7. Middle adulthood	Develop concern for others and continue productivity
8. Old age	Develop integrity

FIGURE 12-2
Erik Erikson's life stages and developmental tasks.

The Infant (0-2 Years)

Growth and Development

A baby grows rapidly during the first two years of life. Weight doubles in the first six months, and the infant triples its birth weight by the end of the first year. At one year old, the seven-pound baby will weigh about 21 pounds. The baby does not grow evenly, in every direction. At times the body seems to be out of proportion, with the head too big and the legs too short. In fact, the newborn's head makes up about 25 percent of the body length.

A baby's bones are fairly soft and pliable at birth. The bone-hardening process begins before birth and continues into the late teens. A baby has soft spots in the skull called fontanelles. The fontanelles at the back of the skull harden at three or four months, while those in the front of the skull may not close until 18 months. "Baby" teeth start appearing at about seven months. Growth and development in the second year continue at a less rapid pace.

Motor Development

The baby is called a *neonate*, or newborn, for the first six weeks of life. During this period, many of the baby's movements are reflexes. The rooting reflex helps the baby find the nipple of the bottle or the mother's breast. The sucking reflex is necessary for eating. The grasping reflex closes the fingers around an object. A sudden movement or loud noise will cause the startle reflex, in which the infant's arms and legs open wide and the back and neck arch. These reflexes gradually disappear as the nervous system develops and the infant gains control over muscular movements.

An infant is able to lift its head and chest off the bed by the second or third month. There is more ability to control the head. The infant may roll over by four months. It will hold and move an object (like a small rattle) and put it into its mouth. The infant plays with its hands and feet and is able to sit alone at seven or eight months. Crawling starts about the same time. At about 10 months the baby will use the thumb and finger to pick up objects. By 12 months the baby may pull up on the furniture or stand with assistance. (See Figure 12–3.) By 15 months the baby can stand and walk alone. Motor activity depends on growth and development, rather than on practice or experience.

Psychosocial Development

For the first few months of life, babies smile at everyone. By six months they can usually recognize familiar faces and voices. They know the difference between a smile and a frown, a pleasant or unpleasant sound, and a friendly or angry gesture. At eight or nine months, infants tend to cling to their mothers or primary caregivers. They recognize and smile at people they are used to and show fear of strangers. Speech patterns are fairly similar in most babies during the first year, while later speech development is affected by the people around them and by their environment.

Developmental Tasks of Infancy

The primary developmental task of infancy is learning to trust. Relationships with a warm, loving family who make every effort to meet the baby's needs help the infant develop trust. Bonding (the develop-

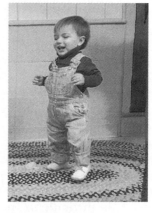

FIGURE 12–3
By 12 months of age, the infant may pull up on the furniture.

ment of a close, loving relationship) between a baby and its mother is necessary for developing trust. Bonding is not automatic, and situations that separate the mother from the baby during the first few hours or days of life can interfere with bonding.

Basic Needs

An infant is completely dependent on someone else to meet all of its needs. The physical needs of the infant include oxygen, food, water, sleep, elimination, and temperature control. The need for sleep gradually decreases during the first year. A baby's heartbeat and respirations are more rapid than adults'. Episodes of shallow, irregular breathing are normal. A fairly even temperature, neither too hot nor too cold, is best for babies.

Infants have psychosocial needs as well as physical ones. The need for love and caring is present throughout the life cycle. Infants like to be talked to, held, and cuddled. Contact with other children and adults helps to provide social interaction. Meeting the needs of infants is addressed in Chapter 30.

The Toddler Age (2–3 Years)

Growth and Development

The average 3-year-old is about 38 inches tall and weighs about 32 pounds. The temporary teeth are usually all in place, allowing the toddler to eat regular adult food. Vital signs are more stable. Heart and respiratory rate slow, while blood pressure increases. Muscle strength, energy, and stamina are increasing.

Motor Development

By three years old, the average child can run, jump, and climb stairs. Reaching, handling, and moving items become a favorite pastime. Most children are able to feed themselves and perform more finger and thumb skills.

Psychosocial Development

The 2-year-old is walking, talking, and ready to explore the world. The child is beginning to feel the power he has over the environment. Things can be picked up, moved, and thrown. He tastes Mother's perfume and moves Daddy's papers. He chases the cat and pulls the dog's ears. Because the 2-year-old has learned that he can do things alone—without the help of an adult—safety becomes an important factor. The toddler has little concept of danger and is able to move quickly. He may run onto a busy highway or jump into the deep end of the swimming pool. Toddlers enjoy playing games, talking, and interacting with other children. Sharing is not yet understood, and, while toddlers are very happy to take, they are not so willing to give.

Communication takes on increased importance at this age. The child's vocabulary is growing and the ability to understand words increases. The two-year-old can speak, understand, and think. However, there is little concept of what adults call "right or wrong behavior." In the first year of life and well into the second, most infants are allowed to do pretty much as they please. Somewhere around the age of two, certain restrictions are imposed. Suddenly, it seems, the child is being told to be quiet, sit still, and stop making a mess. No wonder the two-year-old rebels! His world has been turned upside-down!

Toilet training is a major issue. By the age of three, most children have achieved bowel and bladder control. The path to success can be a rocky one for the child and the parents.

Developmental Tasks of Toddlers

Gaining independence is the major developmental task for toddlers. That task, combined with curiosity, gets the toddler into a lot of trouble. The period from two to three years of age has been called the "terrible two's." The toddler's vocabulary seems to consist of only one word—"No!" The toddler does not want to eat, go to bed, get up, get dressed, or do anything else that is requested. This negative attitude often focuses on eating, and the dining area may become a war zone.

Most of this difficult behavior is an effort to gain independence. It requires patience and understanding to care for the 2-year-old. It helps to remember that this is a temporary, but necessary, phase of development in the child's life. If allowed to make choices and assert independence, the child will eventually learn that self-control is a part of being independent. If the child does not master these tasks, it will be difficult to move through the rest of the childhood tasks of gaining confidence, competence, and self-esteem. (See Figure 12–4.)

Basic Needs

The toddler has basic needs such as food, water, and sleep, but other more complex needs are also now present. The toddler wants to be with mother or the primary caregiver most of the time. The child may cry at any separation. The growing need for independence seems to conflict with the fear of separation. The toddler may cry and cling to mother to prevent her from leaving, and then answer "No!" when she says "Would you like to go with me?"

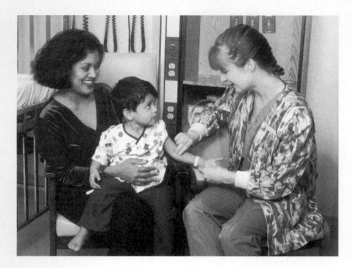

FIGURE 12-4
It takes patience and understanding to care for toddlers.

Meeting the challenging needs of the toddler is discussed in Chapter 30.

The Preschool Age (3-6 Years)

Growth and Development

There is a great deal of difference between the 3-year-old and the 6-year-old. Growth is seen in height more than in weight. The upper parts of the body grow slowly, while the legs grow rapidly. The child stands straighter, and, by the age of six, body proportions look more normal. Six-year-old boys are usually taller and more muscular than girls. The bones in the body have grown harder, and the brain has reached 90 percent of its adult weight. Muscular development is rapid during the fifth and sixth year. There is more control over body movements, an increase in strength, and a decrease in fatigue.

A large 3-year-old may be taller and heavier than a small 6-year-old. Keep in mind, however, that the younger child may be bigger but is not necessarily more mature.

Motor Development

Physical growth slows during this period, while motor skills increase. The child becomes more coordinated, and simple athletic activities such as throwing and catching are possible. Hand coordination improves, and over the three-year period, the child progresses from drawing circles to writing words. By 5 years old, most children can tie their shoes, button buttons, and dress themselves without help.

Psychosocial Development

Language and social skills increase during this three-year period. The child's focus gradually shifts from mother to playmates as the world expands beyond the home. Lifelong personality traits become evident at this age.

Vocabulary increases as new words are questioned and imitated. Sentences become longer and more complex. The 3-year-old questions everything. The toddler's "No!" becomes the preschooler's "Why?" By the age of 4, most children can sing simple songs, count, and repeat letters of the alphabet. The five-year-old can take part in adult conversations. The preschooler gradually learns to follow rules and accept some responsibility. A basic understanding of right and wrong behavior develops. Preschoolers are eager to please and respond well to praise.

Social skills are gained through play. The child learns to play with others, to share, and to cooperate. Proper manners and polite behavior start to emerge.

Developmental Tasks

The major task of preschoolers is to develop initiative. *Initiative* means taking an independent action to try something new or different. Preschoolers are also learning how to play and get along with others. Learning occurs by observing and imitating family members. Dressing up in Mommy's or Daddy's clothes and playing house are favorite activities of this age group. Preschoolers should be encouraged to ask questions and explore, because that is how they learn.

Basic Needs

Because physical growth has slowed, preschoolers need less food. It is important to see that the child gets proper nutrition. Most 5-year-olds would rather fill up on potato chips and candy than eat a well-balanced meal.

It is necessary to provide opportunities for the preschooler to play. Play serves several purposes and is not just a way to have fun. Play provides an outlet for physical energy. A child who is not allowed to expend this energy through play may become cranky or destructive. Play allows an opportunity to practice new skills. Motor skills, like those necessary for running and jumping, are strengthened this way. The child practices behavior during play. Play also provides opportunities to learn communication skills. How successful the child is in developing these various skills can affect schooling, job performance, and interaction with others in later years. (See Figure 12-5.) Meeting the needs of preschoolers is discussed in Chapter 30.

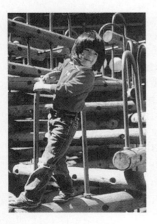

FIGURE 12–5
Preschoolers learn through play.

School Age (6-12 Years)

The school-age years cover a six-year period. Although this age group shares many similarities, six years is a wide range, and there is a lot of variation and overlap.

Growth and Development

Growth changes in build occur during this period and are the result of lengthening arms and legs. The school-age child's body is proportioned more like that of an adult. Muscle tissue increases, and the child grows stronger. Up until 10 or 11, boys are usually taller and heavier than girls. From 10 to 15 the opposite is true, and girls are usually bigger than boys. Sex differences become increasingly obvious with boys having more muscle tissue, and girls more fatty tissue.

The period between the ages of nine and twelve is called preadolescence. In some children of this age, certain body changes take place that indicate the approach of puberty. *Puberty* is the period when adult sex characteristics appear and the reproductive organs begin to function. In girls, the pelvis widens, fat appears on the chest and hips, and breasts begin to form. Boys show fewer changes of sexual maturity at this age. It is within this age group that researchers have noted an earlier onset of puberty in some girls. Problems arise when emotional and mental maturity does not match physical maturity.

At about age six, the child starts losing the first teeth, and by age 12, most of the permanent teeth have emerged. Most of the bones have hardened as well. Because they are no longer soft and pliable, the 12-year-old child's bones are easier to break than those of the 6-year-old. Variations of general body types, such as tall and slender or short and stocky, start to appear.

Motor Development

Muscle strength and coordination improve, and increasingly complex motor skills are possible. It was once thought that boys were naturally more skilled in athletic activities. In recent years, as more girls are encouraged to participate in sports, it appears that athletic skill is not as related to sex as it is to physical ability, personal interest, and opportunity.

Psychosocial Development

School-age children have more awareness of others, of themselves, and of their bodies. They are more able to communicate their thoughts and feelings. They are concerned about the world beyond their homes because their world now includes school.

Entering school requires a major adjustment in a child's life. For some, it is the first separation from mother, and the task of reducing dependency must also begin. For school-age children, two new pressures appear—teachers and *peers* (equals, belonging to the same age group). The child learns that acceptance must be earned from teachers and peers. Peer group acceptance becomes important to the child's self-esteem, and rejection can have long-term effects. At this age, girls usually play with girls, and boys with other boys. They learn to play with special friends and in groups. (See Figure 12–6.)

Developmental Tasks

The major developmental task for school-age children is to gain competency in such intellectual skills as reading, writing, and speaking correctly. However, the competencies learned in school include more than learning to read, write, and do arithmetic. Students develop the ability to set long-term goals and to postpone immediate reward for greater reward in the future. They also learn the moral standards that are necessary for acceptance.

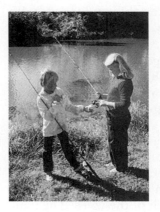

FIGURE 12–6
Peer group acceptance becomes important to school-age children.

Basic Needs

School-age children need a well-balanced diet to provide for the growth that takes place, particularly during the preadolescent years. They also need to achieve balance in school work, rest, and play, because all three are necessary to development. They need support and encouragement as they learn new competencies. Parents and family members must be aware that they are setting examples for their children. Many of the behavior problems encountered at this age are the child's attempt to imitate adult actions. As children enter preadolescence, they need basic sex information. If this information is not offered at home, the children will learn from their peers. Young people are maturing earlier today, and they need accurate information before they become sexually active. Meeting the needs of school-age children is discussed in Chapter 30.

The Teenage Years (13-19 Years)

The teenage years, between 13 and 19, are known as *adolescence*, the period from puberty to adulthood. During this time, the individual changes from a child to an adult. Many physical changes take place in the body that create psychosocial changes as well. It is a difficult time for the children and their families.

Growth and Development

There is a sudden increase in height and weight over a short period during adolescence. Individuals vary greatly in growth, development, and maturity. Girls begin the growth period at about 11 or 12 years old and by 14 have usually reached adult height and weight. Boys mature later, with rapid growth occurring between 13 and 16. The average girl grows about six inches, while boys may grow eight inches or more. After this sudden growth spurt, growth slows, and by the end of adolescence growth has usually stopped.

Body proportions change with the approach of puberty. Puberty begins with the *menarche* (the first menstrual period) in girls, and the development of pubic hair (hair in the genital area) in boys. Changes take place in the reproductive system as the secondary sex characteristics appear. Girls develop breasts, pubic hair, and underarm hair. The secondary sex characteristics for boys include the growth of pubic, underarm, facial, and body hair, and the lowering of the pitch of the voice. The male reproductive organs, the testes and scrotum, and the penis grow to adult size. The sex hormones—estrogen in females and testosterone in males—play a major role in teenage growth and development.

At the onset of puberty, the adolescent may be capable of sexual intercourse and reproduction. The young male starts producing sperm and is able to maintain an erection of the penis. About every 28 days in females, the menstrual cycle occurs. The ovaries release eggs (ova or ovum) during the ovulation phase. During sexual intercourse, if sperm come into contact with an ovum, pregnancy can occur.

Motor Development

The teenager develops adult muscular control and strength. While experiencing periods of rapid growth, the young person may appear awkward and clumsy. However, as growth slows and almost stops in the late teens, the adolescent becomes more coordinated.

Psychosocial Development

Psychosocial development during adolescence is as intense as physical growth. How well the teenager adjusts to those changes will affect life as an adult. Within a brief time span, teenagers must learn to deal with sexuality, prepare for a job, separate from parents, assume adult responsibilities, and develop values and morals. As if those pressures aren't stressful enough, teenagers receive mixed messages from adults. No wonder they are confused. In fact, the awkwardness we observe in teenagers is as much from psychological confusion as it from rapid physical growth.

Teenagers are concerned about personal appearance. Rapid growth and developmental changes can be embarrassing or even frightening. The child who is slow to mature may feel especially insecure. Choices of clothing and hairstyle are frequently a source of conflict between teenagers and their parents. The influence of parents begins to decrease as the teenager becomes more concerned with peer approval than parental approval. The average teenager wants to conform and be "just like everybody else my age."

Most teenagers mature sexually during this time period. However, society expects them to avoid expressing this new-found sexuality. Dating starts during adolescence, and most teenagers experiment with sex. This often results in mixed feelings of guilt and resentment. Teenage pregnancy is a serious problem today.

Rapid changes in growth and development often result in poor emotional control. Teenagers can be pleasant and agreeable one minute, and angry and rebellious the next. Depression is not uncommon, and teenage suicide continues to rise at an alarming rate.

Developmental Tasks

The major developmental task of adolescence is to gain self-identity. Much of the assessment process is done by comparison. Teenagers compare themselves with their peers, their parents, and other people they admire.

Another task for teenagers is to separate from parents and develop independence. Some parents are reluctant to give up control and may stand in the way of their teen's independence. They are afraid something bad may happen to their child, and indeed it may. This striving for independence is at the root of most child/parent conflicts during the teenage years. (See Figure 12–7.)

Basic Needs

Healthy teenagers are usually capable of meeting their own physical needs. What they do need is acceptance, understanding, education, and training to help them to make wise choices. They need guidance to avoid the many problems that confront the adolescent. The most common problems of adolescence are teenage pregnancy, drug and alcohol abuse, juvenile delinquency, and criminal activities. Falling into any one of these traps can alter their lives forever. Meeting the needs of teenagers is discussed in Chapter 30.

The Young Adult (20-35 Years)

There is not much physical growth after adolescence. By this time, body systems are usually fully developed and functioning. Young adults are concerned with completing their education and preparing for employment. Today, it is very clear that education and economic security are closely related. The more education a person has, the greater the likelihood of financial independence.

Many young adults marry, establish a home, and start a family during this period. (See Figure 12–8.) They raise their children while they are young and are reaching middle age when the children are ready to leave home. For the last 20 years there has been a trend toward marrying later and postponing parenthood. This trend could change lifestyles during middle age and early old age, because many of these people will still be raising children. It is too early to tell what effects, if any, this trend will have on children who are being raised by older parents. Some couples elect not to have children.

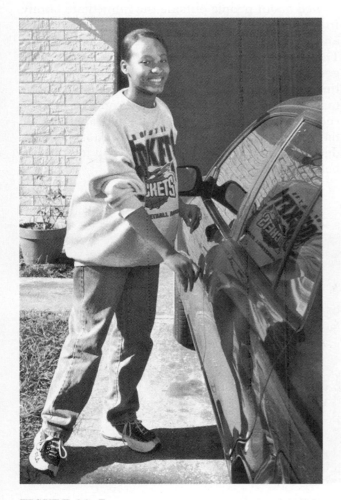

FIGURE 12–7
Increased independence brings increased responsibility during the teenage years.

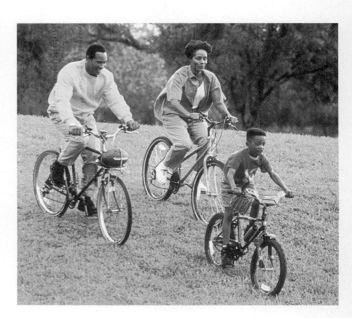

FIGURE 12–8
Many young adults marry and start a family.

Some young adults remain single during this period or for a lifetime. There are increasing numbers of people today who are choosing not to marry for many complex reasons. Certainly one reason is the increased financial and social independence of women.

Developmental Tasks

According to Erikson, the major developmental task for young adults is to establish intimacy. *Intimacy* is a close personal relationship involving love or affection. The young adult searches for a life partner. Dating and building relationships are part of the process of selecting a mate. Building a trusting relationship that will last is not easy. Couples must learn how to communicate and to share. Developing a loving, satisfying sexual relationship is also important.

Failure to Achieve Developmental Tasks

There are some young adults who have not completed the developmental tasks of adolescence. They remain home with their parents and do not prepare for employment. They are either unemployed or take low-paying jobs to obtain spending money. This situation may be the result of an immature young adult, a parent who will not let go, or a combination of the two. It is not a very satisfactory arrangement for anyone and may cause major conflict in the home.

Middle Age (35–55 Years)

People who are middle-aged are just what the name suggests—they are in the middle, neither young nor old. They often begin thinking about old age and death. Grandchildren are born, a further reminder that the middle-aged individual is getting older. The body starts showing signs of aging. Hair grays, wrinkles appear, and speed, strength, and endurance decline.

During these years most women experience *menopause*, the cessation or end of menstruation. The loss of the ability to reproduce may cause a woman to question her attractiveness and her sexuality. Usually, the children grow up and leave home during these years. The parents whose lives have been wrapped up in their children may feel alone and abandoned. This is often referred to as the "empty nest syndrome."

Men or women may experience what is called a midlife crisis. They may feel confused and uncertain. There is a feeling that time is running out for them—it is now or never. Despair and depression may result. They deny old age and try to recapture their youth by changing their hair, clothing, and sometimes lifestyle. Divorce is not uncommon during this unsettled period.

Midlife crisis does not have to occur. Many people find that middle age includes the best years of their lives. They accept life's changes and feel satisfied with themselves. They have more time for themselves and are in a better position financially to do some of the things they never had time or funds for before. With the children gone, husbands and wives have more time for each other. (See Figure 12–9.)

Developmental Tasks

The developmental task of middle age is to achieve productivity. While the focus is on establishing and guiding the next generation, it involves being concerned about people outside the immediate family. Interest moves beyond meeting one's own needs and comfort into caring for society as a whole. The goal is to help make the world safe for future generations. Productivity can be accomplished through employment or community service. If this task is not accomplished, the person can become self-absorbed, and the tasks of old age may be harder to complete. People who do not meet the developmental task of middle-age tend to grow old before their time.

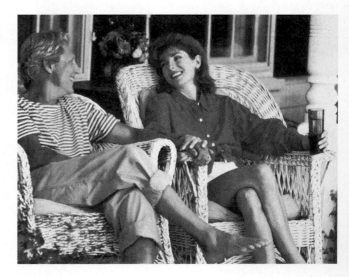

FIGURE 12–9
Middle-aged couples have more time for each other.
Ariel Skelley, The Stock Market

Early Old Age (55-65 Years)

Today, people are living longer and healthier lives. The majority of people between 55 and 65 are still a part of the workforce and do not consider themselves old. Many are back in school, learning a new skill or adding to ones they already have.

There is great variation in the way individuals deal with this period of life. Some become depressed and see the end as near, while others age gracefully. Physical changes of aging that began in middle age become more obvious. A decrease in vision and hearing occurs, physical strength and endurance are lessened, and fatigue may occur more frequently. However, the majority of Americans in early old age are in good health. Today, this age group has better health, higher education, and more financial security than ever before in history.

Many people look forward to this time of life, when some of the stresses of young and middle age are resolved. Establishing a home, raising children, and building a career have been accomplished. They are ready to sit back and relax. However, for many, a new challenge arises—the care of elderly parents. Some people have a child still at home or in college and are also caring for an elderly parent. This group is sometimes referred to as the "sandwich generation," because they are caring for both the young and the old. This can be a very stressful time.

Developmental Tasks

The developmental task of old age does not really fit this group because it involves looking back at life and letting go of occupational identity. However, there are tasks to be accomplished. Retirement may occur during this period. One of the tasks of early old age is to finalize and adjust retirement plans.

The death of a spouse or significant other may take place during these years. For both men and women, losing a life partner is difficult. Women frequently encounter financial difficulties. Widowers may have a difficult time socially. Traditionally, women take care of social contacts, and, when the wife dies, the husband may lose his support system as well. Today, many people do not meet the traditional description of widowhood. There are widows and widowers who are still active in their careers, their families, and their communities. They are happy, manage their own homes, and are financially secure.

One of the joys of this age is grandchildren. Grandchildren provide the same satisfaction as children, but without the responsibility. We see many changes in the traditional roles of grandparents, too. Grandmother is not always at home baking cookies. She may be working, dating, and traveling. Grandfather may be at work or on the golf course. However, these changes do not mean they cannot play an important role in the lives of their grandchildren. Many grandparents may raise their grandchildren due to death, illness, or other problems experienced by their children.

Old Age (65-85 Years)

Traditionally, old age starts at 65. The selection of this particular age was influenced by Medicare and Social Security regulations. For many years, 65 was the magical age of retirement from work, the start of Medicare coverage and Social Security benefits.

During the 20 years between 65 and 85, retirement becomes a reality for most people. There are several types of retirement, however. Some people fully retire, change their lifestyle, and move to another location. Others continue to work on a part-time schedule that allows more leisure time, while providing extra income. There are also those people who retire from one job to take on another. (See Figure 12–10.)

Successful retirement often depends on how well the person has planned for it. Usually, there is more time and less money available. Retirement income is frequently fixed, meaning the same amount comes in monthly regardless of changes in the cost of living. Some people retire to a different part of the country, such as Florida or Arizona, leaving behind friends and family. If there is sickness or

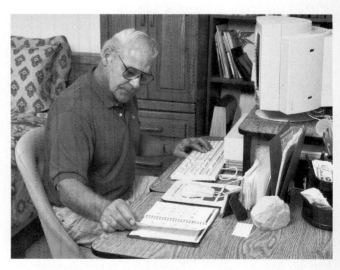

FIGURE 12–10
The retired professional may decide to continue working out of his home.

death, the usual support may be too far away to be helpful.

Time can become a major problem during retirement. After a lifetime of schedules, going to school and to work, leisure time looks inviting. And, indeed, it is for those people who have interests and hobbies to occupy all that available time. For those who were always absorbed in their work, leisure time may soon become a burden.

Changes of Aging

The physical changes of aging become more obvious in this age group. Although aging is very individualistic, some general changes do occur in most people over 65. Body systems slow down and a progressive decline in heart and lung function occurs. Energy and endurance decrease, and the body is less able to defend itself against disease. Problems with hearing and eyesight are common. However, normal changes of aging do not usually interfere with the ability to care for oneself. A detailed explanation of changes of aging is presented in Chapter 10.

Developmental Tasks

According to Erikson, the major task of old age is the development of integrity. *Integrity* is the state of being whole or complete and is achieved by looking back over one's life and examining experiences. People who feel good about their pasts usually find peace in old age and have less fear of death. Inner strength and wisdom develop. This age group must also prepare for their own deaths.

The Very Old (85 and Older)

The fastest growing age group in America today include those people who are 85 years of age or older. The majority are women. One characteristic they all seem to share is adaptability. They have adapted to the empty nest, retirement, and the death of a spouse. In short, they are survivors.

Many people over the age of 85 need assistance physically, emotionally, or financially. They are frail and more susceptible to disease and accidents. Many have one or more chronic illnesses. Vision problems are common, even with the help of eyeglasses. Musculoskeletal problems interfere with ac-

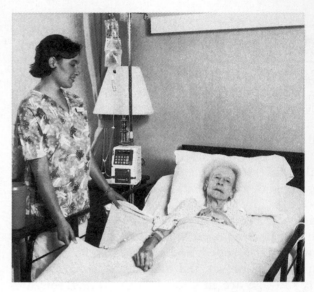

FIGURE 12–11
Many of the very old are frail and in need of assistance.

tivity and mobility. They fatigue easily and must choose activities carefully.

Some live with their children, grandchildren, or other family members; few live alone. Approximately five percent live in nursing homes. The major goal of this age group is to maintain independence. This is not easy, and most are at least partially reliant on others. (See Figure 12–11.)

Centenarians

Centenarians, those people who are 100 years of age or older, used to be scarce but their numbers are on the increase today. Many studies have been done to determine how and why some people manage to live past the century mark. Although centenarians differ in many ways, they seem to have some things in common. Characteristics of centenarians include:

- A strong attachment to freedom and independence
- Ambition and adaptability
- Regular physical activity
- A positive and optimistic attitude
- A sense of humor
- A strong religious faith
- A desire to learn
- Concern for others
- Many social contacts

Review

Read the sentence and fill in the blank with the vocabulary term that best completes the sentence.

1. A newborn is called a _____ for the first six weeks of life.
2. The teenage years, between 13 and 19, are known as _____.
3. Puberty begins with the _____, the first menstrual period.
4. _____ is a close personal relationship involving love or affection.
5. _____ is the cessation or end of menstruation.

Remember

1. Knowing what to expect of people at a certain age will help you to understand and care for your patients.
2. Racial, ethnic, and cultural factors affect the life cycle.
3. According to Erik Erikson, an individual must complete certain developmental tasks during each stage of life.
4. The primary developmental task of infancy is learning to trust.
5. Gaining independence is the major developmental task of toddlers.
6. The major task of preschoolers is to develop initiative.
7. The major developmental task for school-age children is to gain competency.
8. The major developmental task of adolescence is to gain self-identity.
9. The major developmental task for young adults is to establish intimacy.
10. A developmental task of middle age is to establish and guide the next generation.
11. One of the tasks of early old age is to finalize retirement plans.
12. The major task of old age is to develop integrity.
13. The major task of the very old is to maintain independence.

Reflect

Read the case study and answer the questions.

Case Study

You are assigned to care for Gene, a 2-year-old boy and Lisa, a 5-year-old girl. Gene refused to take a bath this morning and feeding him was a chore. He played around in his food and threw food at you. Lisa follows you around all day, asking one question after another. Lisa's mother is a single parent who works long hours and is impatient and cranky during her visits. Gene's elderly grandmother speaks very little English but it's obvious that she thinks Gene's throwing food at you is cute.

1. What developmental task for toddlers may be causing Gene's difficult behavior?
2. What is the major developmental task of a 5-year-old and how might it influence Lisa's behavior?
3. What developmental task of young adults might Lisa's mother have failed to achieve?
4. What factors might account for the grandmother's attitude?

Respond

Choose the best answer for each question.

1. The developmental task of the infant is to develop
   A. Intimacy
   B. Trust
   C. Independence
   D. Competence
2. The soft spots on a baby's skull are called the
   A. Fontanelles
   B. Alveoli

C. Meatus

D. Bronchi

3. The major developmental task of toddlers is to develop
   A. Integrity
   B. Trust
   C. Initiative
   D. Independence

4. The major developmental task of preschoolers is to develop
   A. Intimacy
   B. Trust
   C. Initiative
   D. Independence

5. The period when sexual characteristics appear and reproductive organs begin to function is called
   A. Puberty
   B. Menarche
   C. Menstruation
   D. Menopause

6. The major developmental task of adolescence is to develop
   A. Identity
   B. Integrity
   C. Initiative
   D. Independence

7. Some adults have trouble making loving, satisfying relationships because they fail to achieve which developmental task?
   A. Competence
   B. Initiative
   C. Integrity
   D. Intimacy

8. The term "empty nest syndrome" may occur as a result of what circumstance?
   A. The children leave home
   B. The birth of grandchildren
   C. Caring for children and elderly parents
   D. Retirement

9. Looking back over one's life and examining experiences helps to achieve which developmental task?
   A. Initiative
   B. Integrity
   C. Intimacy
   D. Independence

10. The fastest growing age group in America is/are
    A. Infants
    B. Teenagers
    C. 25 to 35
    D. Over 85

Chapter Thirteen

Basic Needs *of* Patients

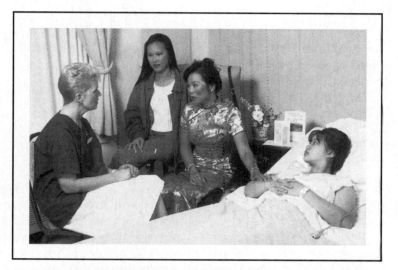

OBJECTIVES

1. Identify and describe the basic human needs of patients in their order of importance.

2. List four guidelines for dealing with cultural diversity.

3. List three guidelines for assisting patients with psychosocial needs.

4. Identify two ways the nursing assistant can assist patients in meeting their social needs.

After studying this chapter, you will be able to

5. Briefly explain pet therapy.

6. List three guidelines for assisting patients to meet spiritual needs.

7. Explain the best way to handle sexually aggressive patients.

8. Describe three common behaviors that may occur when basic needs are not met.

hygiene   The observance of rules for health and cleanliness.

prejudice   A dislike or hatred of a particular culture, race, or group of people.

rapport   The development of a mutually trusting relationship.

self-actualization   To prove oneself as real or worthy; self-fulfillment.

spirituality   The relationship with one's self, nature, and a supreme being.

The concept of quality health care is centered around identifying and assisting patients in meeting their basic needs. This chapter addresses those needs, gives examples, and suggests ways that you, as a nursing assistant, can contribute. Although all human beings share some basic needs, it is important to treat each patient as an individual.

Basic Human Needs

The psychologist Abraham Maslow arranged human needs in their order of importance with the most basic needs forming the foundation of a pyramid (see Figure 13–1). According to Maslow, the basic needs at the bottom of the pyramid must be satisfied before those at the top can be met. The basic needs include:

- Physiological (physical)
- Security and safety
- Belonging and love
- Self-esteem
- Self-actualization

Physical Needs

Physical needs are the most basic of all human needs and include oxygen, water, food, rest and sleep, elimination, and *hygiene* (cleanliness). The physical needs must be satisfied before a person can meet higher needs, like love and self-esteem. For example, a man who has not eaten for several days is not interested in giving or receiving love. He wants food, and only when he has eaten will he be concerned with higher needs.

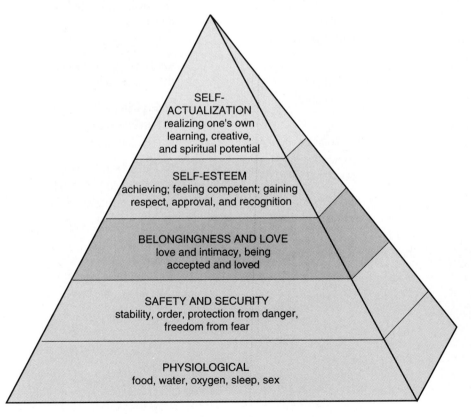

FIGURE 13–1
Maslow's pyramid of basic human needs.

Assisting with Physical Needs

Much of this textbook is concerned with meeting patients' physical needs. Procedures, guidelines, and suggestions are provided for your convenience. As a nursing assistant, you help patients meet many of their physical needs. You assist patients in bathing, dressing, and performing personal hygiene. You assist them to the bathroom and provide whatever is needed for elimination. You prepare a clean, neat bed that allows for proper rest and sleep. Offering fluids and encouraging patients to eat well-balanced meals helps them to meet their physical needs. You help with exercise and mobility when necessary. By assisting patients to meet physical needs, you help them to maintain health and well-being.

Security and Safety Needs

Safety and security needs include a place to live, appropriate clothes to wear, and shelter from the weather. Patients also need to feel safe from harm and secure that we will protect them from infection and injury while they are in our care.

Assisting with Security and Safety Needs

Safety features in health care facilities include handrails, safety bars, and emergency signals. It is your responsibility to encourage patients to use these safety features. You protect the safety of patients by using side rails and restraints correctly. Answering call signals promptly not only protects patients from injury, but it also makes them feel more secure. Following standard precautions and other aseptic practices helps prevent the spread of infection. Using correct body mechanics and transfer techniques protects you and the patient from injury. Following safety guidelines presented in earlier chapters of this text will help keep the environment safer for everyone.

Belonging and Love Needs

Love takes many forms and is both physical and emotional. It involves intimacy and a caring relationship. Sexual relationships, marriage, and family are expressions of love. Love and belonging needs may also be met by a pet such as a cat, a dog, or a bird.

Assisting with Belonging and Love Needs

Assisting patients to participate in group activities helps meet the need for belonging. Encourage involvement with the family, church, and community. Treating patients with compassion and kindness shows that you care. Remember that touch is a way of showing concern, and a pat on the hand or shoulder can sometimes be more meaningful than words.

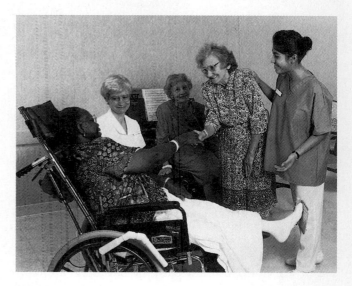

FIGURE 13–2
Introducing patients helps them get acquainted with one another.

Introducing patients helps them to get acquainted with one another. (See Figure 13–2.) Older patients who come from a more formal era may find it difficult to meet new people. Patients who share a room for several days may become friends and support each other. This is particularly true in nursing homes where patients may remain in the facility for a long time.

Self-Esteem Needs

Self-esteem is the opinion one has of oneself. A high degree of self-esteem contributes to the quality of life and well-being. Independence and the ability to care for oneself improves self-esteem. Although self-esteem comes from inside oneself, it is affected by other people's statements and opinions.

Assisting with Self-Esteem Needs

One of the best ways to help patients meet their need for self-esteem is by promoting independence. The more people are able to do for themselves and the more decisions they are allowed to make, the better they will feel about themselves. Give positive feedback and praise all the patient's efforts. Helping patients to be clean and neat improves their self-esteem. Just as you feel better when you are neat and clean, so do your patients.

Self-Actualization Needs

Self-actualization or self-fulfillment means proving oneself. Accepting challenges and meeting goals help to meet the need for self-actualization. Patients do this frequently as they attempt to recover from an illness or an injury. For example, stroke patients may need to learn how to walk or talk again. The rehabilitation team sets goals and so do the patients. Reaching goals helps the patient meet the need for self-actualization.

Assisting with Self-Actualization

Asking questions and listening to the patient helps you to understand his or her self-actualization needs. The care plan contains some of this information. Encouraging and assisting a patient with the goals on the care plan will help him or her achieve self-actualization.

Remember, basic needs must be met in their order of importance. Love can be offered and received but will have little value if physical needs are not met first. Be familiar with the patient's care plan and refer to it as you plan your daily tasks. This helps to ensure that the basic needs of each individual patient are being met.

Cultural Diversity

Culture is the shared customs, beliefs, and values of a group of people. The term cultural diversity means a variety of cultures. Certain cultural groups may also be called ethnic groups. Cultural differences can involve race, nationality, customs, and religion. The United States has been culturally diversified from the very beginning. It received and welcomed immigrants from all over the world, and today, America truly is a "melting pot" of different cultures. (See Figure 13–3.)

Every person has a right to be treated with courtesy and respect. However, sometimes *prejudice* (a dislike or a hostile attitude toward a specific culture or group of people) may occur. Prejudice is usually caused by lack of knowledge and understanding.

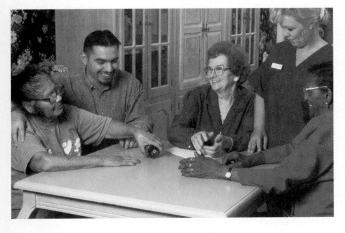

FIGURE 13–3
America is a "melting pot" of different cultures.

Guidelines for Dealing with Cultural Diversity

- Learn about other cultures.
- Develop understanding and acceptance.
- Appreciate the talents of others.
- Keep an open mind.
- Be flexible and adaptable.
- Treat every person with respect.
- Develop effective communication skills.
- Identify and manage cultural conflicts.

Dealing with Cultural Diversity

The key to dealing with cultural diversity is to obtain knowledge and develop understanding of other cultures. Be accepting and nonjudgmental about the cultural differences in patients and co-workers. Learn to identify and manage cultural conflicts. Treat each person as an individual and judge the person, not the culture. The patient population is culturally diverse and so is the workforce. Therefore, it is important that you learn how to get along with people from cultures other than your own.

Caring for Culturally Diverse Patients

Following these guidelines will help you to care for patients of all cultures. You will also need to know how communication styles differ and how people from different cultures react to illness. Culture influences our behavior and our needs. For example, recent immigrants to the United States may hold on to their own traditional beliefs about health care and have difficulty relating those beliefs to American health care delivery. You will need to think and act in ways that are culturally sensitive as you provide care.

Communication between people who speak different languages can be difficult. Slang, local expressions, or regional accents can also be confusing. In some cultures, it is considered rude to say "No." These patients may appear to agree with everything you say, regardless of their feelings. You have to listen carefully for nonverbal clues to be sure that you understand the patient and that the patient understands you.

Reaction to illness varies among cultures. For example, Native Americans are taught not to cry or show emotion, so you must observe very carefully to know when the patient is uncomfortable. Hispanics, on the other hand, are expected to cry and become emotional. They are often more accepting of your concern and attempts to help. You will need to be skilled in communication, observation, and reporting in order to care for patients of diverse cultures.

*P*sychosocial *Needs*

The psychosocial needs are the emotional, mental, social, spiritual, and sexual needs. They include love and belonging, self-esteem, and self-actualization, which form the upper part of the basic needs pyramid. The psychosocial needs are closely related, and when you meet one need you will probably satisfy others as well. For example, walking in the garden with a loved one can meet the need for love, social involvement, spirituality, and sexuality. (See Figure 13–4.) When you take time to listen to a patient, you are showing love, building self-esteem, and perhaps helping the patient to meet the need for self-actualization.

The psychosocial needs are even more important when a person is ill. The patient in a health care facility is separated from home, family, and other loved ones. At a time when they are least able to change, patients must adjust to a new environ-

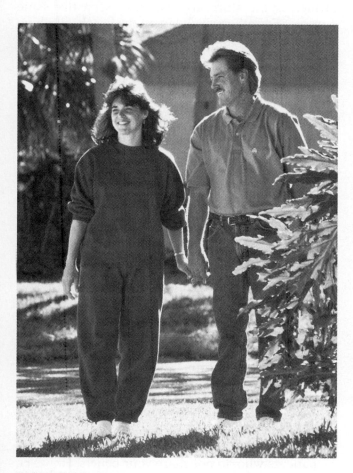

FIGURE 13–4
Walking in the garden with a loved one can help meet psychosocial needs.

Guidelines for Assisting Patients with Psychosocial Needs

■ Promote independence.
■ Use praise and encouragement.
■ Encourage choices and decisions.
■ Listen and observe.
■ Be sensitive to feelings.
■ Ask for and respect the patient's opinion.

ment, a lack of privacy, and being cared for by strangers.

Emotional stress is common, with feelings of fear and anxiety. Patients must adjust to new routines and schedules. Identity is threatened with the loss of control, status, and self-esteem.

Meeting the Psychosocial Needs

It is often more difficult to help patients meet psychosocial needs than it is to help with physical needs. It is fairly easy to determine when a patient needs a bath or a bed needs changing, but you must be a very careful observer to be aware of psychosocial needs. By returning as much control as possible to the patient, you can help to restore confidence and self-esteem.

*S*ocial *Needs*

We all have a need to interact and be socially involved with others. Illness interferes with the ability to socialize, and admission to a health care facility reduces social contacts even further. Patients who have suffered an illness or injury may not be able to socialize independently. For example, a patient who is recovering from a stroke may not be able to move without a wheelchair or walker. The hearing-impaired patient may need a hearing aid to participate in conversations with others.

You can help patients meet socialization needs by encouraging the patient's family members and friends to visit. Do your best to make their visits pleasant and comfortable. Sometimes health care workers make visitors feel as if they are unwelcome and in the way. (See Figure 13–5.)

Encourage patients to take part in activities and social events. Let your patients know if an activity is scheduled that might interest them. Assist patients as needed with eyeglasses, hearing aids, walkers, and other equipment. A volunteer might be available to spend time with patients who have few visitors. Let the charge nurse know if one of your patients seems lonely.

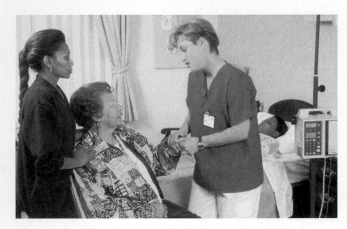

FIGURE 13–5
Do your best to make family visits pleasant and comfortable.

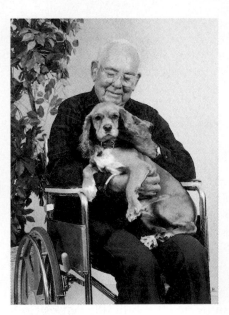

FIGURE 13–6
Pets may be able to get through to patients who have stopped interacting with other humans.

Pet Therapy

Pets help patients meet their need for love and social interaction. Although cats and dogs are the pets most commonly seen, birds, fish, rabbits, and other animals may also be used. Some facilities have a pet or pets "in residence." Fish tanks are common in health care facilities, and some facilities have a bird that talks or sings.

Some dogs are handled by pet therapists who work with the health care team. The dogs are trained to approach patients carefully and gently. They make some type of brief physical contact, such as brushing against the patient's body, touching the patient's hand with their nose, or offering a paw in a handshake. The dog is taught to respond and react to the patients' moves and messages.

Patients who have stopped interacting with other people may be able to form emotional attachments to pets. Patients who hesitate to talk to other people will often talk to a cat or dog. The pet listens attentively and does not care if the patient's words are unclear or even if they make sense. Pets give love and receive love unconditionally. (See Figure 13–6.)

Spirituality

Spirituality means nourishing the inner spirit. It refers to a person's relationship to self, nature, and a supreme being. Spirituality involves a search for the meaning and purpose of life. Religion helps meet the spiritual needs for many people. A group of people with similar beliefs may join together to form an organized religion. Belonging to a religious group has advantages that go beyond spirituality. It provides social interaction, emotional support, and improved self-esteem. However, religion may be practiced through personal beliefs without any formal organization.

Religion is not the only way to express spirituality. Keep in mind that the definition of spirituality is to nourish or feed the inner spirit. For some, the enjoyment of literature, art, and music serve that same purpose. For others, walking on the beach, climbing a mountain, or strolling through a garden can be spiritually uplifting.

Some people express spirituality by caring for or serving others. Volunteer work with a hospital or other health care organization helps meet their spiritual needs. Creative activity such as needlework, gardening, or painting offers spiritual outlet for many people.

Assisting Patients to Meet Spiritual Needs

You will need to know how the patient normally meets spiritual needs. Encourage patients to express their feelings and listen carefully to what they say. Sometimes people find it difficult to talk about spiritual matters. You must first develop rapport with your patients. *Rapport* is a mutually trusting relationship. That means you can trust each other. If patients feel that you really care and want to help, and that you will protect their confidentiality, they will be more willing to share their feelings and needs with you.

Be aware of how your own spirituality affects your behavior and communication. Statements such as "I'll pray for you" may be appreciated even by patients who do not share your beliefs. However, it is never appropriate to try to force your own beliefs on patients or visitors.

Guidelines for Assisting Patients to Meet Spiritual Needs

■ Encourage expression of feelings.

■ Listen carefully.

■ Protect confidentiality.

■ Develop rapport.

■ Help patients to attend religious services of their choice.

■ Provide privacy for spiritual visits and practices.

■ Do not criticize or belittle a person's individual expression of spirituality.

Sexuality

Everyone has sexual needs. Sexuality is both physical and emotional and includes affection, love, and belonging. Sexual needs are individualistic and met in a variety of ways. There is more to sex than the physical act of intercourse. Touching, caressing, and kissing are sexually satisfying. Sometimes just being with the person you love is all that is necessary. (See Figure 13–7.)

Sexuality provides an opportunity for expressing one's sexual identity. Sexual identity is usually formed early in life. Children usually pattern themselves after the parent of the same sex. Most little girls learn from their mothers how to be women, while boys learn to be men from their fathers and other male role models. Some people grow up uncertain of their sexual identity.

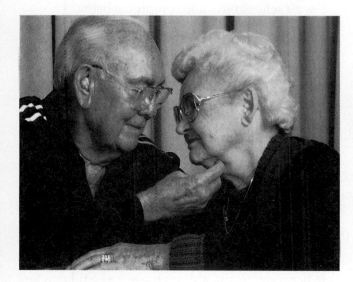

FIGURE 13–7
Sexuality includes touching the person you love.

Illness and injury can affect a patient's sexuality. Patients who have cardiac problems may be concerned that sexual activity may worsen their condition. Diabetes can interfere with the male's ability to participate in intercourse, and medication can also alter sexual performance. A stroke or spinal injury can contribute to sexual difficulties. Sexual needs do not disappear when a patient enters a health care facility.

Sexual Aggression

Some patients may flirt, make sexual remarks, or touch staff members inappropriately. Illness and medication may cloud the patient's judgment and cause this kind of behavior. The patient may also be responding to your warm, caring attitude. Whatever the reason, you must deal with sexual advances in a professional manner. Firmly tell the patient to stop the objectionable behavior. Remain calm and explain that these actions are not acceptable. Do not scold, embarrass, or shame the patient.

Some patients may make sexual advances to other patients. Health care workers have a responsibility to protect patients from this kind of unwanted behavior. If the patient becomes sexually aroused in front of others, the patient should be removed to a private area.

Assisting Patients with Sexual Needs

Before you can help the patient, you must first get in touch with your own feelings about sexuality. You may be embarrassed or offended by public displays of affection. While you have a right to your own feelings and opinions, you cannot impose your beliefs on others. Remember that patients have as much right to express sexuality as they do to show spirituality or any other need. The following guidelines may help you to assist patients in meeting their sexual needs.

Guidelines for Assisting Patients with Sexual Needs

■ Get in touch with your own feelings.

■ Assist patients with hygiene and grooming.

■ Protect patient privacy and maintain confidentiality.

■ Accept displays of affection as normal and healthy.

■ State clearly when behavior is not acceptable.

■ Protect helpless patients from sexually inappropriate advances from other patients.

*W*hen Basic Needs Are *Not Met*

When physical needs are not met, the results are very noticeable. The patient may lose weight, become dehydrated, or develop an illness. Infection and accidents occur when safety needs are not met. The results are not as obvious when psychosocial needs are not met. What is usually noticed is that behavior or personality changes. These changes are frequently cries for help. Some common behavioral reactions include anger, depression, withdrawal, or demands for attention. Patients who use the call signal frequently may have unmet needs. Anxiety is often the cause of this type of behavior. It may take all your observation skills to identify their needs if patients are not able to express themselves adequately. When you suspect that the patient's behavior is due to unmet needs, you must focus on meeting those needs. Let the nurse know if there is a problem that you are not able to resolve. When providing patient care, remember the concept of the "whole person," which is concerned with all the patient's needs.

*R*eview

Read each sentence and fill in the blank with the vocabulary term that best completes the sentence.

1. _____ means proving oneself and is often accomplished by meeting personal goals.
2. A dislike or hostile attitude toward a specific culture or group of people is called _____.
3. _____ is the development of a mutually trusting relationship.
4. The observance of rules for health and cleanliness is _____.
5. _____ is the relationship of oneself, nature, and a supreme being.

*R*emember

1. In order to meet patients' needs, you must treat each patient as an individual.
2. Basic human needs include physical, safety and security, love and belonging, self-esteem, and self-actualization needs.
3. Physical needs are the most basic and must be met first.
4. Basic needs must be satisfied in their order of importance.
5. Prejudice is caused by lack of knowledge and understanding.
6. It is important that you learn how to get along with people from cultures other than your own.
7. One of the best ways to help patients meet psychosocial needs is by promoting independence.
8. Pet therapy involves the use of pets to help patients meet the need for love and social interaction.
9. Spirituality refers to a person's relationship with self, nature, and a supreme being.
10. Before you can help the patient with sexual issues, you must first get in touch with your own sexuality.
11. A behavior change frequently occurs when basic needs are not met.

*R*eflect

Read the following case study and answer the questions.

Case Study

Mrs. McQueen is an elderly woman who was admitted to the nursing home yesterday. She has used the call signal four times in your first hour of duty. Each time you answer the signal, she has some minor complaint. You notice that the signal light is on outside her room again, although you just left her a few minutes ago. You feel like ignoring her, but you know that is not the professional way to respond. This time she wants to know if her daughter has called this morning like she promised. You tell her that you will find out and let her know. Then you report her behavior to the nurse.

1. What could be causing Mrs. McQueen's behavior?

*R*espond

Choose the best answer for each question.

1. Which of the following is the best way to report on a patient?
   A. "The gallbladder in 202 is complaining of pain."
   B. "The old woman in 202 is complaining of pain."
   C. "Mrs. Green in 202 is complaining of pain."
   D. "Mary in 202 is complaining of pain."

2. The most basic of all human needs is
   A. Physical needs
   B. Safety needs
   C. Self-esteem needs
   D. Self-actualization needs

3. Safety and security needs include
   A. Food, water, and rest
   B. Protection from infection and injury
   C. Intimacy and a caring relationship
   D. Independence and self-esteem

4. Self-actualization needs are best met by
   A. Provision of food and water
   B. Protection from infection and injury
   C. Provision of personal hygiene and rest
   D. Accepting challenges and meeting goals

5. The term cultural diversity refers to
   A. Latin cultures
   B. American culture
   C. The same culture
   D. A variety of cultures

2. Frequently using the call signal is often a sign of what emotion?

3. What is your best response to this type of behavior?

4. Was it necessary to report this behavior to the nurse? Why or why not?

6. The emotional, social, spiritual, and sexual needs are called the
   A. Psychosocial needs
   B. Physiological needs
   C. Safety needs
   D. Physical needs

7. Spirituality needs can be met only by
   A. Organized religion
   B. Religious people
   C. Nourishing the inner spirit
   D. Nourishing the physical body

8. A male patient, sitting in the hallway in a wheelchair, has unzipped his pants and exposed himself. What is your best response?
   A. "Mr. Meadows, that's not very nice."
   B. "Mr. Meadows, I'm going to tell your wife."
   C. "Mr. Meadows, I'll take you to your room."
   D. "Mr. Meadows, you're a real comedian."

9. A patient has been very irritable and demanding today. What might you suspect?
   A. She has unmet needs.
   B. She is a mean person.
   C. She wants to get you in trouble.
   D. She doesn't like you.

10. Which of the patient's needs should concern the nursing assistant?
    A. The physical needs
    B. The safety needs
    C. The psychosocial needs
    D. All of the above

Chapter Fourteen

Rehabilitation *and* Restorative Care

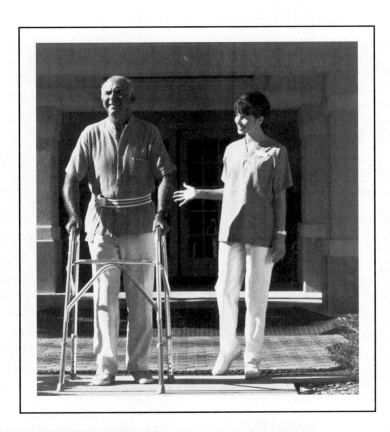

OBJECTIVES

After studying this chapter, you will be able to _____

1. Explain the relationship of restorative patient care to quality of life.

2. Briefly describe the roles of two members of the rehabilitation team.

3. List three safety rules for using special equipment.

4. Describe four restorative care guidelines.

5. Briefly explain the concept of wellness.

Glossary

prosthesis   A device that replaces or assists the function of a body part.
rehabilitation   Process of restoring the patient to as nearly normal function as possible.

restorative care   Type of nursing care that assists patients in meeting their needs as independently as possible.

Promoting quality of life is the focus of health care today. Quality of life can be defined as the ability to gain enjoyment and satisfaction from life. Although individual patients differ in their needs and wants, certain factors are almost always considered. Love, security, comfort, and dignity are essential. Autonomy (being in control of one's life) and independence are equally important. The best way to promote quality of life is through restorative care using the holistic approach. As a nursing assistant you will have the opportunity to provide restorative patient care. You will also have the satisfaction of knowing that you have made a difference in the patients' lives.

The Omnibus Budget Reconciliation Act (OBRA) recognizes the importance of restorative care in helping patients maintain independence. OBRA mandates that this type of care be provided in all health care settings. Learning to use restorative measures and equipment will prepare you for a career in the health care field.

Rehabilitation is the process of restoring the patient to as nearly normal function as possible. *Restorative care* is the nursing care that assists patients in meeting their needs as independently as possible. Most people want to be independent—to take care of themselves and to make decisions. They want to make choices and maintain control of their lives whenever possible. This chapter provides a foundation for the many restorative measures and programs included in the text. (See Figure 14–1.)

The Rehabilitation Team

The center of the rehabilitation team is the patient. Other members of the team may include doctors, nurses, family members, nursing assistants, physical therapists, occupational therapists, speech therapists, social workers, activity directors, and clergy. Anyone who provides care in a restorative manner is considered part of the team. Nursing assistants are important members of the rehabilitation team because they have so many opportunities to provide restorative care.

Physical Therapy Team

The physical therapy team uses special training and equipment to assist patients in regaining or maintaining muscle strength and mobility. Members of this team help patients who have been immobilized by injury or disease regain physical independence. (See Figure 14–2.) They measure, fit, and teach patients how to use canes, crutches, walkers, and other prosthetic devices.

Occupational Therapy Team

The occupational therapist is trained to assist patients in performing ADLs such as bathing, grooming, dressing, and feeding as independently as possible. The occupational therapy team also helps patients learn new homemaking or occupational skills to overcome problems caused by weakness or disability. All members of the rehabilitation team work together to help patients meet their needs.

Special Equipment

Special equipment is available to help the patient function independently. This equipment may be

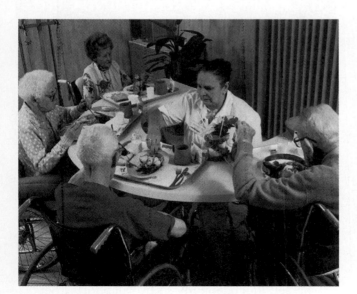

FIGURE 14–1
Restorative dining programs help patients maintain independence.

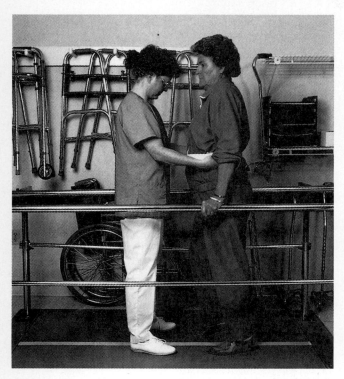

FIGURE 14–2
The physical therapist helps patients regain muscle strength and mobility.

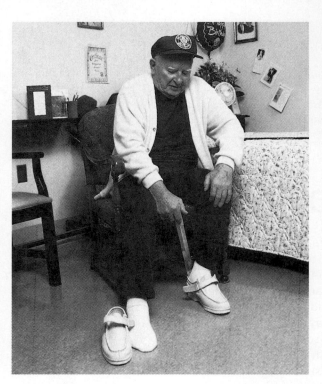

FIGURE 14–3
Special equipment is available to help the patient function independently.

used to assist the patient with mobility, eating, or performing personal care activities. Canes, crutches, and walkers help patients with walking. Other special equipment needed by the patient will be listed in the care plan. (See Figure 14–3.) One type of special equipment is called a *prosthesis* (a device that replaces or assists the function of a body part). Eyeglasses, false teeth, and artificial limbs are examples of prosthetic devices.

Safety Rules for Using Special Equipment

When special equipment and prosthetic devices are not used correctly, they can be dangerous. The following safety rules will help protect you and the patient from injury:

- Check the patient's care plan for special equipment.
- Do not use any device that you have not been trained to use.
- Do not use a device for anything other than its intended purpose.
- Be sure that the patient is using the device correctly.
- Inspect all devices for defects, such as broken or loose parts.
- Report any defective device to the nurse immediately.

Restorative Measures

The following guidelines include measures and techniques that you can use to provide restorative care.

Guidelines for Restorative Care

- Use the holistic approach. Consider all the needs of the person, not just the physical needs.
- Use the humanistic approach. Respect each person's individuality.
- Follow each patient's plan of care. This ensures consistent care on all shifts.
- Consider the patient's abilities and disabilities. Encourage the patient to be as active as possible.
- Be sensitive and empathetic. Empathy is the ability to share another person's point of view and understand their feelings.
- Be patient and do not rush the patient. Relearning takes time.
- Encourage the patient to do for himself or herself independently. Praise all efforts. (See Figure 14–4.)

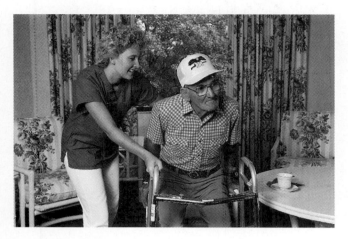

FIGURE 14–4
Encourage the patient to do as much as possible for himself.

- Know how to use the special equipment that has been ordered. Check with the nurse if you are not sure.
- Know when to offer assistance. Watch for signs of fatigue or frustration.
- Maintain a positive attitude. If you are going to convince a patient of the importance of a restorative measure, you must first believe in it yourself.

Promotion of Health and Wellness

Health and wellness are not always the same thing. The World Health Organization (WHO) defines health as: "A state of complete physical, mental, and social well-being, not merely absence of disease and infirmity." Wellness involves functioning at the highest level, regardless of circumstance. Even the patient who has a chronic illness can find a level of wellness and live the best life possible with the disease. (See Figure 14–5.)

The primary goals of wellness are dignity and quality of life. Many factors, such as lifestyle, nutrition, and exercise, affect wellness. The ability to handle stress and adapt to change is essential. Wellness is being able to function at the highest possible level and successful adaptation to change. Restorative care promotes wellness. A high level of wellness is possible when emphasis is placed on promotion of independence and autonomy. The way you treat the patient has a direct affect on the patient's level of wellness.

You are also responsible for achieving your own wellness. Personal wellness requires motivation, self-control, and accountability. It would be helpful to review the sections of Chapter 2 that deal with taking care of yourself.

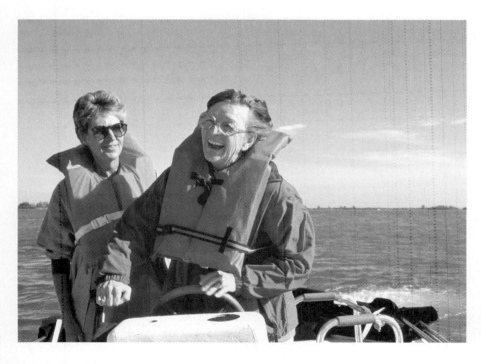

FIGURE 14–5
Wellness is living the best life possible.

Review

Read each sentence and fill in the blank with the vocabulary term that best completes the sentence.

1. The process of restoring the patient to as nearly normal function as possible is called _____.
2. _____ is the nursing care that assists patients in meeting their needs as independently as possible.
3. _____ is being in control of one's life.
4. A device that replaces or assists the function of a body part is a _____.
5. _____ is a state of complete physical, mental, and social well-being, not merely absence of disease or infirmity.

Remember

1. Quality of life is the ability to gain enjoyment and satisfaction from life.
2. The best way to promote quality of life is through restorative care.
3. Nursing assistants are important members of the rehabilitation team.
4. The physical therapy team assists patients with muscle strength and mobility.
5. The occupational therapy team assists patients to perform ADLs independently.
6. Special equipment is available to help patients function independently.
7. Restorative measures that help promote independence should be used whenever providing patient care.
8. Wellness means living life to the fullest.

Reflect

Read the following case study and answer the questions.

Case Study

Jenna Ward is a 24-year-old patient recovering from a motorcycle accident. A severe head injury resulted in mental confusion and muscle weakness. Her left arm and leg are in casts because of fractures. She frequently gets upset and angry with people. Physical therapy and occupational therapy are included in the many health care services she receives.

1. Where will you check to identify any special equipment needed in Jenna's care?
2. What part of Jenna's care will occupational therapy focus on?
3. How should you respond if Jenna yells at you in anger?
4. How can you help Jenna achieve wellness?

Respond

Choose the one best answer for each question.

1. The ability to gain enjoyment and satisfaction from life is called
   A. Autonomy
   B. Empathy
   C. Quality of life
   D. Quality of health care

2. The major function of the physical therapy team is to help patients
   A. Regain muscle strength and mobility
   B. Perform ADLs independently
   C. Perform hygiene and grooming
   D. Handle financial problems

3. The major function of the occupational therapy team is to help patients
   A. Regain muscle strength and mobility
   B. Perform ADLs independently
   C. Handle spiritual problems
   D. Get along with other patients

4. Nursing assistants are important members of the rehabilitation team.
   A. True
   B. False

5. Which of the following are prosthetic devices?
   A. Walkers
   B. Eyeglasses
   C. Artificial limbs
   D. All of the above

6. A patient's hand splint has a broken strap. What should you do?
   A. Report it to the nurse and do not apply it.
   B. Apply it and report it to the nurse.
   C. Tape the strap in place and apply it.
   D. Put it away and do not apply it.

7. The ability to share another person's point of view is called

   A. Autonomy
   B. Empathy
   C. Mobility
   D. Independence

8. You are assisting a patient who is relearning to dress himself. Which of the following is a restorative measure?
   A. Remind him to finish quickly.
   B. Dress him yourself.
   C. Be patient and respectful.
   D. All of the above.

9. Functioning at the highest level regardless of circumstances is known as
   A. Health
   B. Autonomy
   C. Empathy
   D. Wellness

10. Which of the following can help promote your own health and wellness?
    A. Proper nutrition
    B. Regular exercise
    C. Reducing stress
    D. All of the above

Chapter Fifteen

The Patient's Unit

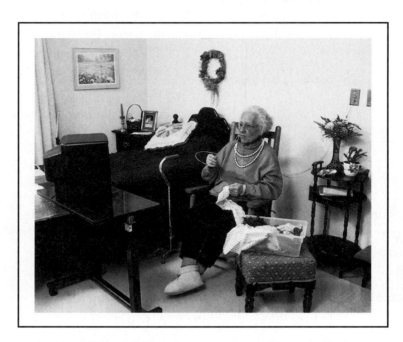

OBJECTIVES

After studying this chapter, you will be able to

1. Identify three factors that contribute to a comfortable environment in the patient's unit.

2. List four pieces of furniture and equipment that the patient's unit might contain.

3. List five guidelines for cleaning equipment.

4. Explain how to help prevent waste and help contain health care costs.

5. Identify three guidelines for maintaining the patient's unit.

emesis Vomitus.

emesis basin A small, kidney-shaped pan used for oral care, spitting, or vomiting.

motivation The internal feeling or external stimulus causing one to take action.

urinal A container into which male patients urinate.

The patient's unit is the room or area that contains the patient's furniture and belongings. The size and layout of the unit depend on the type of health care the patient is receiving. For example, the patient's unit in an acute care hospital might be rather small and bare, while a unit in a long-term care facility would be more personal and homelike. At home, the patient's unit might be a bedroom or a section of the living room. Keep in mind that the patient's unit is a private, personal area that serves as the patient's temporary home.

The Environment

It is important that the patient's unit be as safe, comfortable, and private as possible. This type of environment contributes to the patient's health and well-being.

Safety

Protecting the patient's safety is at the center of all health care delivery. A safe unit is one that is arranged to prevent accidents. All furniture and equipment are in proper working order and the call signal is within the patient's reach. The area is neat and uncluttered. Safety bars and emergency call signals are provided in the bathroom. The bed is positioned close to the floor with the wheels locked and side rails raised, when appropriate. The unit is kept clean and sanitary to prevent the spread of pathogens.

Comfort

The room temperature in the patient's unit is climate-controlled, allowing the patient to be warm in winter and cool in summer. Extra blankets and pillows are available when needed. It helps promote comfort if patients are able to adjust the temperature in their own units to meet individual needs. Good lighting is provided with night lights available. A comfortable chair with a lamp nearby provides a spot for reading or visiting. Regular cleaning routines prevent objectionable odors. Noise is kept to a minimum. Employees are instructed to be quiet in the hallways and not gather outside a patient's door. Whenever possible, noisy equipment is operated during the daylight hours to allow unbroken sleep during the night.

Privacy

Window blinds and drapes help provide privacy for patients. Privacy curtains can be pulled around each patient's bed when a room is shared. Each unit contains a closet and furniture for the patient's clothes and other belongings. Staff members are instructed to knock on the patient's door and wait for a response before entering. Respecting the patient's privacy is one of the principles of good nursing care and is mandated by law.

Restorative Environment

A restorative environment promotes independence and self-care. It increases the patient's self-esteem and *motivation* (an inner feeling that causes a person to take action). In the long-term care facility where residents may stay for long periods, efforts are made to create a homelike environment. Wall treatments and furniture are designed to look less institutional. Residents are encouraged to bring their own clothing, photographs, and other personal belongings as space permits. (See Figure 15–1.)

It is more difficult to maintain a restorative environment in an acute care setting. While the units are neat and clean, they are seldom warm and homelike. However, these patients need a restorative environment as much as patients in other settings. You will need to be creative to help make these units more personal and inviting.

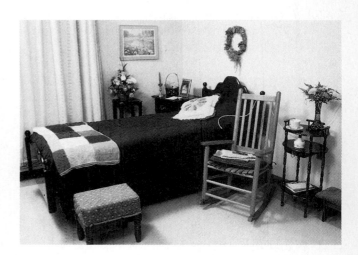

FIGURE 15–1
A homelike environment is important in a long-term care facility.

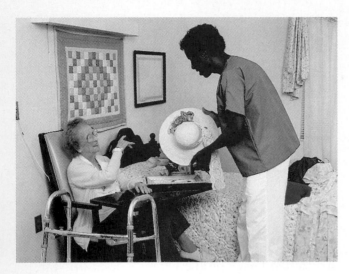

FIGURE 15–2
You can help make the patient's unit more personal and inviting.

Personal Belongings

Patients enter a health care facility with a variety of personal belongings. Usually, they bring grooming and toiletry items such as a comb, brush, toothbrush, and toothpaste. Pajamas, gowns, robes, and slippers are often included. A patient in a long-term care facility may have personal clothing, pictures, furniture, and mementoes from home. Always handle the patient's personal belongings with care and respect. This indicates that you respect the patient as well. (See Figure 15–2.)

Furniture and Equipment

Each unit contains furniture and equipment to meet the individual patient's needs. Basic furniture includes a bed, overbed table, bedside stand, and a chair. Some units may include a dresser, desk, and extra chairs. In many pediatric units, a daybed or couch is provided for the comfort of family members. In the long-term care facility, some of the furniture may belong to the resident.

The Overbed Table

The overbed table base slides under the bed, and the top is adjustable. The patient may use the table for eating, writing, or other activities. Staff members may use it for treatments and personal care procedures. The overbed table is considered a clean area, so do not place contaminated (soiled or exposed to germs) items on it.

The Bedside Stand

The bedside stand provides storage for personal care equipment. The patient's personal belongings,

such as combs, makeup, shaving equipment, and eyeglasses are usually placed in the top drawer for easy access. Wash basins and bedpans are placed in the lower drawers or cabinet. The top of the stand provides space for the telephone, tissues, and water pitcher. Avoid clutter on the top of the bedside stand. You are responsible for keeping the bedside stand neat and tidy.

The Call System

A call signal is provided for each unit to allow the patient to call for assistance. The call signal is usually connected to a light above the door and to the nurses station. When the patient pushes a button, a light goes on, and sometimes an alarm will sound. The nurse may be able to respond from the desk through an intercom. Staff members must be alert for the patient's signal and answer all lights promptly. The patient must be shown how to use the call signal when he or she is first admitted to the unit. In the home, a tap bell may be used.

Some facilities provide a bathroom in each room. If the room is not a private room, the bath will be shared by the patients who occupy that room. In other facilities, the bathroom may be located between two rooms. Other bathrooms may be located off the main hallways for patients who are out of their rooms. The bathroom usually contains a toilet, washbasin, mirror, and shower.

Standard Equipment

Each unit usually contains a washbasin, bedpan, *urinal* (a container the male patient uses for urination), and an *emesis basin* (a small kidney-shaped pan for oral care, spitting, or vomiting). The term *emesis*

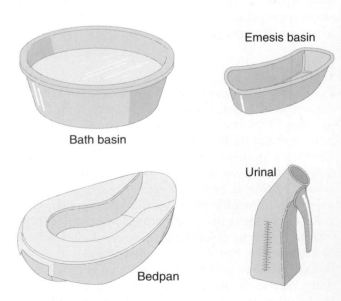

FIGURE 15–3
Examples of standard equipment issued to patients

means vomitus. These items are used for personal care and toileting. A water pitcher and glass may also be furnished. Liquid soap is provided in dispensers, and lotion is available for those who need it. Although most people bring their own toothbrush, comb, brush, and other personal care items, these supplies are available when needed. (See Figure 15–3.)

Special Equipment

Special equipment may be located in the unit as needed to administer oxygen, feedings, or fluids, or perform suction. Special equipment is frequently used in rehabilitation programs. Wheelchairs, walkers, canes, and crutches may be needed to assist with mobility. Restorative equipment used in personal care or dining may be left in the patient's unit. Sometimes the equipment is the patient's personal property. You will need to know which equipment belongs to the patient and which is the property of the facility. Check with the charge nurse if you are not sure. (See Figure 15–4.)

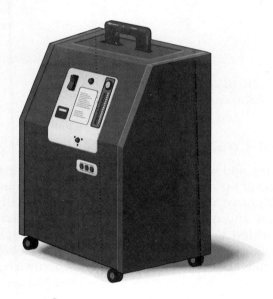

Oxygen concentrator

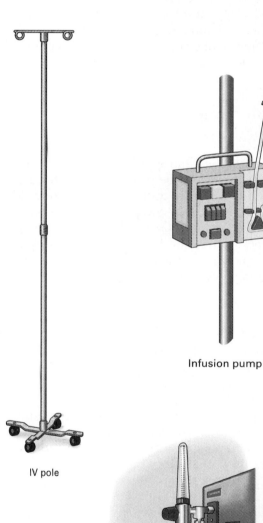

IV pole

Infusion pump

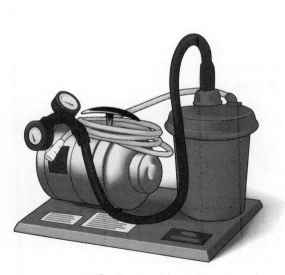

Suction machine

Wall oxygen outlet

FIGURE 15–4
Examples of special equipment

Care and Use of Equipment

It is important that you learn how to use and care for medical equipment and supplies. Correct care and use of equipment protects both you and the patient from injury or infection and helps prevent waste. The correct method for using equipment is usually found in the procedure book. This book gives step-by-step instructions on how to perform procedures that take place in the facility. It includes information about using and cleaning certain pieces of equipment. The manufacturer's instructions may also be included. If you still do not know how to use a piece of equipment after reading the instructions, ask the nurse to explain.

Disposable Supplies and Equipment

Some of the supplies and equipment you will use are disposable and are to be thrown away after use. Items such as latex gloves and gauze pads are used once and discarded, while equipment such as wash basins, bedpans, and urinals may be used by the patient for a period of time before being discarded. Disposable equipment must be discarded in the proper container according to facility policy.

Nondisposable Equipment

Not all equipment is disposable. Wheelchairs, bedside commodes, and blood pressure cuffs are examples of nondisposable equipment. These items must be cleaned, disinfected, or sterilized before reuse. Although proper cleaning reduces the number of microorganisms on the equipment, some items must be further disinfected or sterilized.

Disinfection is the use of chemicals to destroy pathogens. Although this process reduces the risk of infection, it does not kill all microorganisms. An object that is sterile is free from all microorganisms. Surgical instruments and equipment, as well as supplies needed for dressing changes, must be sterile. A patient who has been severely burned may require sterile linens and equipment. Regardless of whether disinfectant or sterilization is used, the item must be cleaned first. It is your responsibility to know whether an item is to be disinfected or sterilized.

Check carefully to make sure that equipment is not defective or damaged. Using defective equipment can cause accidents or injuries. Report defective equipment to the nurse immediately. (See Figure 15–5.)

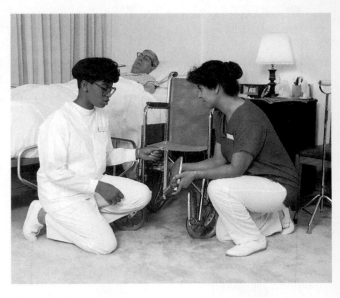

FIGURE 15–5
Report defective equipment to the nurse.

Cost Containment

Buying and replacing expensive medical equipment is one of the reasons that health care costs so much. Equipment used correctly and carefully will last longer and need fewer repairs. Use only what you need and avoid wasting supplies. If a package comes with more than one item, close the package carefully to protect the unused items. Return equipment and supplies to their proper places where they will be available for others.

Guidelines for Cleaning Equipment

- Wear gloves and follow standard precautions.
- Rinse equipment in cold water.
- Wash with soap and hot water.
- Rinse and allow to dry thoroughly.
- Disinfect or sterilize as needed.

Maintaining the Patient's Unit

Although the housekeeping department regularly cleans each unit, it is up to the nursing assistant to see that the unit remains neat and clean.

Remember, this is the patient's room, and it contains many of the patient's belongings. Do not become so concerned with neatness that you forget the patient's rights and preferences.

Guidelines for Maintaining the Patient's Unit

- Clean up after yourself each time you provide care.
- Put away equipment and supplies as soon as you finish using them.
- Keep the unit neat and tidy.
- Pick up and discard trash.
- Ask permission before touching the patient's personal belongings.
- Handle the patient's belongings with care and respect.

Review

Read each sentence and fill in the blank with the vocabulary term that best completes the sentence.

1. The internal feeling that causes a person to take action is called _____.
2. A _____ is a container that the male patients uses for urination.
3. A small, kidney-shaped basin for oral care, spitting, or vomiting is an _____.
4. _____ is the medical term for vomitus.
5. An object that is _____ is free from all microorganisms.

Remember

1. The patient's unit is a private, personal area.
2. The patient's environment should be as safe, comfortable, and private as possible.
3. It is important to keep the call signal within the patient's reach and to answer lights promptly.
4. Using equipment correctly prevents injury to the patient and yourself.
5. If you do not know how to use a piece of equipment, ask the nurse to explain.
6. Always discard disposable equipment in the proper container.
7. Immediately report equipment that is defective or damaged.
8. Using equipment correctly and carefully saves money and prevents waste.
9. Be considerate of the patient's rights and preferences.
10. It is the responsibility of the nursing assistant to help keep the patient's unit neat and tidy.

Reflect

Read the following case study and answer the questions.

Case Study

Mary is assigned to care for Mr. Billie, who is recovering from abdominal surgery. After helping him with his bath, she begins to straghten his hospital unit. On his bedside stand are some objects made of beads and feathers. When Mary starts to pick them up, Mr. Billie gets very upset. Mary politely explains that the top of the bedside stand must be kept clean for his surgical supplies. He says they are religious objects that she must not touch. When she asks him to put them away himself, he refuses. Mary grabs the objects, throws them in the drawer, and hurriedly leaves the room.

1. Did Mary do the right thing? Explain your answer.
2. What should Mary have done when Mr. Billie got upset?
3. How should Mary have handled this situation?
4. What patient's rights did Mary violate?

Respond

Choose the best answer for each question.

1. What is the safest way to position the bed when you have completed providing care?
   A. Position the bed in the highest position from the foor.
   B. Position the bed with the side rails down.
   C. Position the bed in the lowest position, close to the floor.
   D. Position the bed crossways in the room.

2. Which of the following will help keep the patient's unit comfortable?
   A. Providing good lighting.
   B. Keeping noise to a minimum.
   C. Adjusting the room temperature as the patient desires.
   D. All of the above.

3. Which of the following help provide privacy in the patient's unit?
   A. Opening the window blinds.
   B. Opening the privacy curtains.
   C. Knocking before entering.
   D. All of the above.

4. What is the best way to treat the patient's personal belongings?
   A. Handle them with care and respect.
   B. Don't handle them at all.
   C. Handle them as quickly as possible.
   D. Ask the patient to care for his own belongings.

5. Which of the following items should be placed on the overbed table?
   A. Bedpan
   B. Urinal
   C. Clean linens
   D. Used linens

6. You have just removed a pair of gloves in the patient's unit. What should you do with them?
   A. Put them in your pocket.
   B. Place them on the bedside stand.
   C. Wash them and hang them in the bathroom.
   D. Dispose of them in the proper container.

7. The use of chemicals to destroy pathogens is called
   A. Sterilization
   B. Disinfection
   C. Contamination
   D. Suffocation

8. You have used one lemon glycerine swab out of a package of three. What should you do with the other two swabs?
   A. Close them up carefully in the package.
   B. Throw them all away.
   C. Leave the package open for convenience.
   D. Sterilize the other 2 swabs.

9. You observe that the patient's walker has one of the tips missing. What should you do?
   A. Report it to the nurse immediately.
   B. Tell the patient to be careful using the walker.
   C. Get another patient's walker for the patient's use.
   D. Do nothing, it's not your problem.

10. Which of the following is your responsibility in maintaining the patient's unit?
    A. Go through the patient's closet daily.
    B. Put away supplies as soon as you finish using them.
    C. Remove everything from the top of the bedside stand.
    D. Discard and replace the patient's bedpan daily.

Chapter Sixteen

Bedmaking

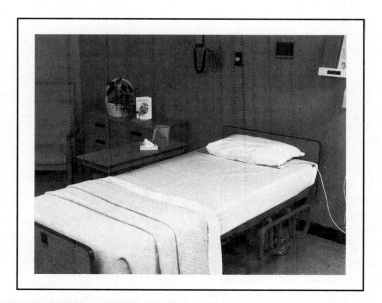

OBJECTIVES

1. Explain the importance of a well-made bed.

2. List six guidelines for bedmaking.

3. List three guidelines for using correct body mechanics while making beds.

After studying this chapter, you will be able to

4. Demonstrate the procedures described in this chapter.

body alignment   Positioning the body in correct anatomical position.

closed bed   A method for making a bed in which the blanket and bedspread cover the sheets.

gatch handle   Crank handle located at the foot of a hospital bed, used for changing bed positions.

occupied bed   A method of bedmaking in which the linens are changed while the patient remains in the bed.

open bed   A method of bedmaking in which the top linens are turned down for a patient who will be returning to the bed soon.

surgical bed   A method of bedmaking in which the top linens are folded to the side of the bed to accommodate the patient's return from surgery.

Rest and Sleep

Adequate rest and sleep are essential to health and well-being. Sleep disorders can result in severe disturbances in activities of daily living (ADLs). Many patients in health care facilities have difficulty sleeping. They may be uncomfortable or in pain. Sometimes just being in a different bed away from home can interfere with sleep.

As a nursing assistant you can help patients with rest and sleep. Keep the unit as pleasing and comfortable as possible by following the guidelines given in the previous chapter. One of the most important things you can do is to provide a well-made bed. (See Figure 16–1.)

A well-made bed offers a pleasing, professional appearance. It indicates that the person who made the bed is also a professional. A well-made bed is one in which the linens are kept clean and free of wrinkles. Sheets are tucked in neatly, with seams turned away from the patient's skin.

Linens are applied correctly and straightened as necessary.

Basic Bedmaking

Some considerations you will need to be concerned with while making beds include safety, infection control, and patient comfort. Safety is always a major concern. Procedures must be performed in a manner that will protect the patients and yourself from injury. Patient comfort and safety are at the center of all health care delivery. A well-made bed not only provides comfort but it also helps to protect the patient from complications such as pressure ulcers.

Infection Control

It is important to use aseptic techniques and follow standard precautions when making beds. According to the latest Centers for Disease Control and Prevention (CDC) guidelines, all used linen is considered contaminated and should be handled carefully. Wear gloves and any other necessary protective gear as needed when handling linen that is contaminated with blood or other body fluids. Handwashing may be necessary several times during the bedmak-

FIGURE 16–1
A well-made bed helps the patient with rest and sleep.

Guidelines for Handling Dirty Linen

- Wear gloves and protective equipment when required.
- Wash your hands after removing gloves and after handling dirty linen.

- Keep dirty linen away from your uniform.
- Avoid shaking dirty linen.
- When stripping a bed, roll the dirty linen away from you with the side that touched the patient inside the roll.
- Do not place dirty linen on the overbed table nor on the floor.
- Place dirty linen directly in the dirty linen container.
- Keep the dirty linen container covered.

Guidelines for Handling Clean Linen

- Wash your hands before handling clean linen.
- Hold clean linen away from your uniform.
- Place clean linen on a clean surface such as the overbed table.
- Take only the linen you need into the patient's unit. Unused linen in the patient's unit is considered contaminated and should be placed in the dirty linen container.
- Avoid shaking or handling clean linen unnecessarily.
- Keep the linen cart covered.
- Do not return unused linen to the clean linen cart.

ing procedure. The following guidelines will help protect you and the patients from infection.

Body Mechanics

Always use correct body mechanics while you are making a bed to help protect yourself from back strain or other injury. Before beginning the bedmaking procedure, raise the bed to a height that is comfortable for you to avoid back fatigue.

Stand with your feet apart, your back straight, and your weight evenly distributed. Move your body as one unit and avoid twisting it. Bend your knees and point your feet in the direction you are working. These are all basic guidelines for body mechanics that were discussed in Chapter 6. It would be helpful to review those guidelines again.

Types of Beds

Standard hospital beds are either electric or manual (operated by hand). Usually, there are three controls. One raises and lowers the entire bed. The second handle operates the head of the bed, and the third control operates the foot of the bed. An electric bed has controls that allow the patient to change position independently.

Always check to see that the wheels are locked if a patient is in the bed or preparing to get into the bed. If you unlock the wheels to move a bed, make sure you lock them when you are finished.

Side Rails

Hospital beds come equipped with side rails for patient safety. There is a rail on either side of the bed that may be raised or lowered as needed. Never fasten or tie things to the side rails. For example, a restraint or drainage bag attached to a side rail would go up and down every time the rail was raised or lowered and could cause injury. Side rails can be considered a restraint and are not routinely raised on all patient's beds. Check with the nurse or the patient's care plan if you are not sure about raising the side rails.

Organizing Your Work

Plan the procedure before you begin making the bed. You will need to know if the patient can get out of bed. If not, you will make an occupied bed. Make arrangements before you begin if you will need help. Determine the supplies and equipment that you need. Some facilities use protective pads on the bed.

Most facilities use draw sheets, also known as pull sheets or turning sheets. A draw sheet is a small sheet that is placed across the middle of the bottom sheet. It extends from the patient's shoulders to the knees. When the draw sheet is tucked in, it helps keep the bottom linens clean, in place, and wrinkle-free. Untucked, it can be used to turn and reposition the patient. If a draw sheet is not available, you can make one by folding a full sheet in half.

Organize the linen you will need in a way that will save time and effort. Collect the linen in the order in which it will be used. The mattress pad, if you are using one, will be on the bottom of the stack. Then pick up a bottom sheet, draw sheet,

Guidelines for Bedmaking

- Reposition the bedbound patient at least every two hours.
- Place the patient in correct *body alignment* (normal or correct anatomical position).
- Keep linens smooth and free of wrinkles, crumbs, and small objects.
- Make sure that seams and rough edges of linen do not touch the patient's skin.
- Change a wet or soiled bed immediately.
- Avoid using plastic that might come into contact with the patient's skin.
- Change protective pads as soon as they become wet or soiled.
- Return the bed to its lowest position when you leave the room.
- Fold the *gatch handle* (a crank located at the foot of the bed, which is used to change the position of the bed) out of the way when not in use. (See Figure 16–2.)
- Be sure the call signal is within the patient's reach.
- Follow correct body mechanics.
- Make as much of one side of the bed as you can before going to the other side to finish.
- Raise the side rail on the opposite side of the bed when you are working with the patient.
- Raise the side rails when you leave, if appropriate.
- Use aseptic technique and follow standard precautions.
- Wash your hands before you begin, after handling soiled linen, and when you are finished.

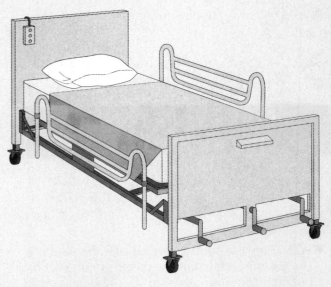

FIGURE 16–2
Gatch handles are used to change the position of the bed.

top sheet, blanket, bedspread, and pillow case. Take the linen to the patient's unit. Place one hand on top of the linen, turn the entire stack over, and place the linen on a clean surface. It will now be arranged in the order in which it will be used. The mattress pad will now be on top and the pillow case will be on the bottom. (See Figure 16–3.)

*B*edmaking *Procedures*

This chapter contains the basic bedmaking procedures for a closed bed, an open bed, an occupied bed, and a surgical bed. It also provides a procedure for stripping a bed. Remember to follow the rules of safety and infection control when making any kind of bed.

Stripping a Bed

Dirty linen must be stripped from the patient's bed before you can begin to make up the bed with clean linen. Check carefully for personal items such as jewelry, glasses, or dentures that the patient may have left in the bed. Patients sometimes put these items under their pillows, and they may be lost or ruined if they go through the laundry.

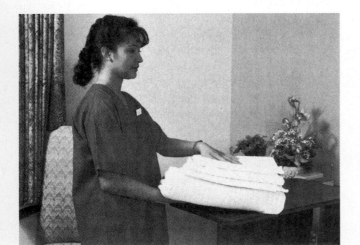

FIGURE 16–3
Stack the linen you will need in a way that will save time and effort.

Procedure for Stripping a Bed

Beginning Steps

■ Collect necessary equipment and supplies.
■ Wash your hands and use standard precautions.
■ Use correct body mechanics.

1. Raise the bed to a comfortable working height. Adjust the bed as flat as possible.
2. Loosen the linen all around the bed and remove the pillow from the pillow case.
3. If the bedspread and blanket are soiled, roll them up with the rest of the linen. If they are to be reused, fold them separately, using the following steps.

   a. Grasp the bedspread at the top center edge and the corner nearest you. Fold it by bringing the top edge of the spread to the bottom edge of the spread.

   b. Grasp the center of the folded edge with one hand and the corner nearest you with the other hand. Fold the bedspread again by bringing the folded edge to the bottom edge of the spread.

   c. Fold the spread by grasping the edges nearest you and bringing these edges to the edges of the spread on the other side of the bed.

   d. Fold the spread over the back of the bedside chair.

   e. Repeat the steps for the blanket.

4. Roll or fold the rest of the linen away from you with the side that touched the patient inside the roll (see Figure 16–4).
5. Place the soiled linen in a plastic bag and take it to the soiled linen hamper when you are finished or place it directly in the hamper.
6. Wipe the mattress with disinfectant and observe it for damage.

Ending Steps

■ Lower the bed to the floor.
■ Wash your hands.

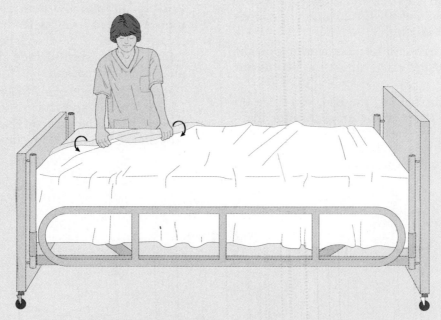

FIGURE 16–4
When stripping a bed, roll the soiled linen away from you, with the contaminated side inside the roll.

A Closed Bed

A *closed bed* is fully made with a blanket and bedspread in place. It is made for the patient who is up for the day or when the bed will not be in use. A closed bed may be opened for a new admission. The patient is not in the bed, so you will not need to be concerned with side rails.

An Open Bed

An *open bed* is made with the linen turned down for a patient who will be returning to the bed soon or one who is being newly admitted. The linen is turned down, and the bed is ready for the patient.

An Occupied Bed

An *occupied bed* is a bed with a patient in it. The linens are changed with the patient in the bed. You might need to make an occupied bed if the patient is very ill or comatose (unconscious).

Safety is a major concern because you must perform this procedure with the patient in the bed. Check to see that the bed wheels are locked. Since you will be positioning the bed at a higher level, both side rails should be raised first. Lower the side

rail on the side where you are working. The side rail on the opposite side should be raised. If you have to leave the bedside, even for a moment, raise both side rails.

A Surgical Bed

A *surgical bed* is made for a patient who will be coming back from surgery. The top linens are positioned to accommodate the patient's return on a stretcher or gurney. They are usually folded lengthwise to the side of the bed. Extra blankets should be available. The stretcher is usually placed on the side of the bed nearest the door, and the top linen should be on the opposite side.

Procedure for Making a Closed Bed

Beginning Steps

■ Collect necessary equipment and supplies.
■ Wash your hands and use standard precautions.
■ Use correct body mechanics.

1. Stack the clean linen, in the order in which it will be used, on a clean surface in the patient's unit.
2. Raise the bed to a comfortable working height and lower the side rails. Adjust the bed as flat as possible.
3. If you have not stripped the bed, you must do so at this time (refer to the procedure for stripping a bed).

4. Slide the mattress to the top of the bed.
5. If a mattress pad is to be used, put the pad on the bed, even with the top of the mattress.
6. Place the bottom sheet in the center of the bed and unfold it lengthwise with the centerfold of the sheet in the center of the bed (see Figure 16–5).
7. Position the narrow hem of the sheet at the foot of the bed, even with the end of the mattress. The wide hem will be at the top. The hemstitching should face the mattress and away from the patient.
8. Pick up the sheet from the side, open it, and fanfold it toward the other side. (Fanfold means to fold the linen on itself and out of your way on the bed.) Smooth the side nearest you.

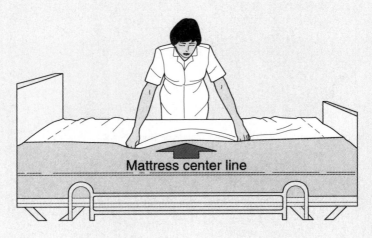
Mattress center line

FIGURE 16–5
Place the bottom sheet with the centerfold in the center of the bed.

Procedure for Making a Closed Bed (cont.)

9. Tuck the sheet under the top of the mattress at the head of the bed on the side nearest you.
10. Make a mitered corner (see Figure 16–6).
    a. Grasp the edge of the sheet 10 to 12 inches from the top of the bed and fold it onto the mattress (see Figure 16–6A).
    b. Tuck the part of the sheet that is hanging down under the mattress (see Figure 16–6B).
    c. Bring the folded part down over the edge of the mattress (see Figure 16–6C).
    d. Tuck the entire side of the sheet under the mattress (see Figure 16–6D).
11. If a draw sheet is to be used, place it on top of the sheet, about 12 inches from the top edge of the mattress (see Figure 16–7).
12. Tuck the draw sheet under the mattress on the side nearest you.

13. Place the top sheet on the bed and unfold it lengthwise with the centerfold of the sheet in the center of the bed.
14. Position the top sheet with the hemstitching facing up and the wide hem at the top, even with the top of the mattress.
15. Pick up the sheet from the side, open it, and fanfold it toward the other side.
16. Smooth the side of the bed nearest you. Do not tuck the bottom of the top sheet under the mattress yet.
17. Place the blanket over the top sheet as follows:
    a. Unfold and center it.
    b. The top of the blanket should be about 6 to 8 inches below the top edge of the top sheet.
    c. Smooth the blanket on the side nearest you.
    d. Fold the top sheet down over the top of the blanket to make a cuff.

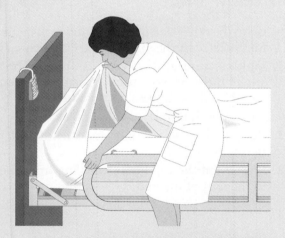

A. Grasp the edge of the sheet 10 to 12 inches from the top of the bed and fold the sheet onto the mattress.

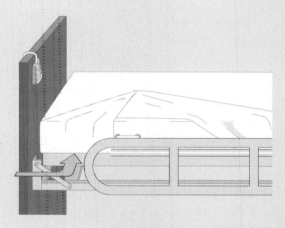

B. Tuck the part of the sheet that is hanging down under the mattress.

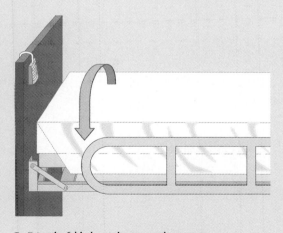

C. Bring the folded part down over the mattress.

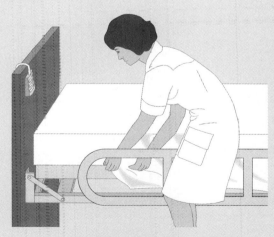

D. Tuck the entire side of the sheet under the mattress.

FIGURE 16–6
Making a mitered corner.

Procedure for Making a Closed Bed (cont.)

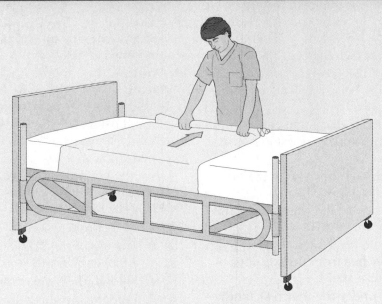

FIGURE 16–7
Place the draw sheet on top of the bottom sheet, about 12 inches from the top, and tuck it under the mattress.

18. Place the bedspread over the blanket as follows:
    a. Unfold and center it.
    b. Place the bedspread so that about 18 inches extends over the head of the bed (this will be used to cover the pillow).
    c. Smooth the bedspread on the side nearest you.
    d. Turn about 24 to 25 inches of the bedspread back from the head of the bed.
19. Tuck in the top sheet, the blanket, and the bedspread at the foot of the bed, on this side.
    a. Make a mitered corner.

20. Go to the other side of the bed and tuck in the bottom sheet at the head of the bed (see Figure 16–8).
21. Make a mitered corner and pull the bottom sheet tight as you tuck it under the entire length of the mattress on this side.
    a. Smooth it to remove wrinkles.
22. Pull the draw sheet tight and tuck it under the mattress.
23. Straighten the top linen, working from the top to the foot of the bed.

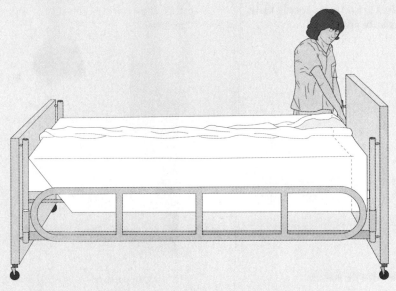

FIGURE 16–8
Tuck in the bottom sheet at the head of the bed on the other side.

Procedure for Making a Closed Bed (cont.)

24. Tuck the top linen under the foot of the mattress, smoothing and making it tight.
    a. Make a mitered corner.
25. Finish turning the top of the bedspread down about 24 to 25 inches. Turn the top of the sheet over the top of the blanket.
26. Place the pillow on the bed and put it into the pillowcase, using the following steps (see Figure 16–9):
    a. With one hand, grasp the pillowcase at the center of the seamed end (see Figure 16–9A).
    b. Turn the pillowcase back over that hand with your free hand (see Figure 16–9B).
    c. Grasp the pillow at the center of one end with the hand that is inside the pillowcase (see Figure 16–9C).
    d. Pull the pillowcase down over the pillow with your free hand (see Figure 16–9D).
    e. Straighten the pillowcase, making sure that the corners of the pillow are in the corners of the pillowcase. Line up the seams of the pillowcase with the edge of the pillow (see Figure 16–9E).
    f. Fold the extra material of the pillowcase under the pillow.
27. Place the pillow on the bed with the seam at the top and the open edge of the pillowcase facing away from the door.
28. Cover the pillow with the bedspread or finish according to facility policy.

Ending Steps

■ Lower the bed to its lowest position.
■ Place the call signal within the patient's reach.
■ Wash your hands.

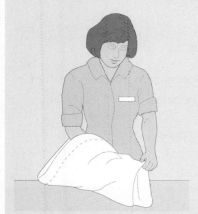

A. Grasp the pillowcase at the center of the seamed end with one hand.

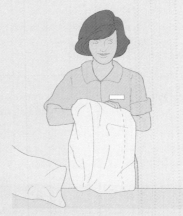

B. Turn the pillowcase back over that hand with your other hand.

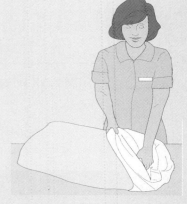

C. Grasp the pillow at the center of one end with the hand that is holding the pillowcase.

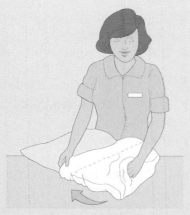

D. Pull the pillowcase down over the pillow with your free hand.

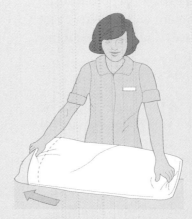

E. Straighten the pillowcase by lining up the seams of the pillowcase with the edges of the pillow.

FIGURE 16–9
Placing a pillowcase on a pillow.

Procedure for Making an Open Bed

Beginning Steps

- Collect necessary equipment and supplies.
- Wash your hands and use standard precautions.
- Use correct body mechanics.

1. Make a closed bed.
2. Grasp the top linen in both hands and fold it to the foot of the bed (see Figure 16–10A).

3. Fold the bedding back onto itself toward the head of the bed, forming a wide cuff (Figure 16–10B).
4. Smooth the hanging sheets on the sides.

Ending Steps

- Lower the bed to its lowest position.
- Place the call signal within the patient's reach.
- Wash your hands.

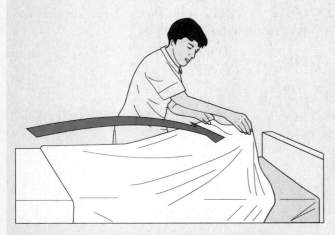

A. Grasp the top linen in both hands and fold the linen to the foot of the bed.

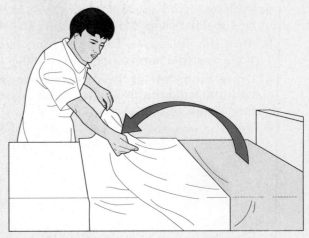

B. Form a wide cuff by folding the linen back onto itself toward the head of the bed.

FIGURE 16–10
Making an open bed.

Procedure for Making an Occupied Bed

Beginning Steps

- Identify the patient and explain the procedure.
- Collect necessary equipment and supplies.
- Wash your hands and use standard precautions.
- Protect the patient's privacy.
- Use correct body mechanics.

1. Place the clean linen, in the order in which it will be used, on a clean surface in the patient's room.
2. Pull the curtain around the bed and close the door.
3. Raise the side rails, raise the bed to a comfortable working height, and lock the wheels.
4. Lower the head of the bed, being sure to maintain a height that is safe and comfortable for the patient.

5. Lower the side rail on the side of the bed nearest you. Keep the rail up on the opposite side of the bed.
6. Loosen the top linen at the foot of the bed.
7. Remove the blanket.
   a. If it is dirty, remove it by rolling or folding it away from you, with the side that touched the patient inside the roll.
   b. If it is to be reused, fold it over the back of the chair.
8. Cover the patient with a bath blanket, using the following steps:
   a. Unfold the bath blanket and place it over the top sheet.
   b. Ask the patient to grasp the top of the bath blanket or tuck the top edge under the patient's shoulders to keep it in place (see Figure 16–11).

Procedure for Making an Occupied Bed (cont.)

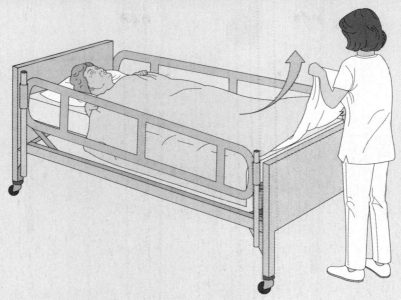

FIGURE 16–11
Slide the top sheet out from under the bath blanket without exposing the patient's body.

   c. Grasp the sheet under the bath blanket and slide it out at the foot of the bed, rolling it with the side that touched the patient on the inside. Place it with the dirty linen.

   d. If you do not have a bath blanket, leave the top sheet in place over the patient or use a clean top sheet. The patient must be kept covered for warmth and privacy.

 9. Help the patient to turn away from you to the far side of the bed.

   a. Help the patient to maintain correct body alignment.

   b. Adjust the pillow as needed.

   c. Be sure the patient is not too close to the side rail.

10. Loosen the bottom linen on this side of the bed and fold it to the patient's body (see Figure 16–12).

   a. Tuck it under the patient's body.

11. If a mattress pad is to be used, put the pad on the bed, even with the top of the mattress.

12. Place the bottom sheet in the center of the bed, with the centerfold of the sheet next to the patient.

13. Position the narrow hem of the sheet at the foot of the bed, even with the end of the mattress. The wide hem will be at the top. The hemstitching should face the mattress.

14. Pick up the sheet from the side, open it, and fanfold it toward the patient. Smooth the side nearest you.

15. Tuck the sheet under the top of the mattress at the head of the bed and make a mitered corner.

16. If a draw sheet is to be used, place it on top of the sheet, about 12 inches from the top edge of the mattress.

17. Tuck the draw sheet under the mattress.

18. Fold the clean linen toward the patient, next to the dirty linen (see Figure 16–13).

19. Assist the patient to turn toward you to the clean side of the bed.

   a. Explain that the patient will roll across the folded linen.

   b. Be sure the patient is not too close to the rail.

   c. Adjust the pillow.

20. Raise the side rail on this side.

21. Go to the opposite side of the bed.

22. Lower the rail on this side.

23. Loosen the used bottom linen and roll it away from you with the side that touched the patient on the inside.

   a. Place it with the other dirty linen.

24. Unfold the clean linen that is in the center of the bed.

25. Straighten the bottom sheet and tuck the top in at the head of the bed.

   a. Make a mitered corner.

26. Tuck the side of the sheet under the mattress while pulling it tight.

27. Straighten the draw sheet and tuck it under the mattress while pulling it tight (see Figure 16–14).

Procedure for Making an Occupied Bed (cont.)

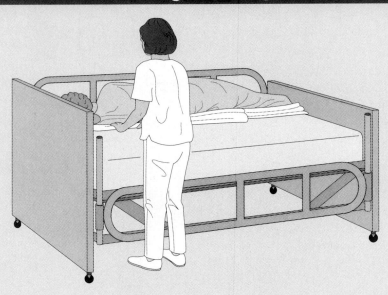

FIGURE 16–12
Loosen the bottom linen and fold it to the patient's body.

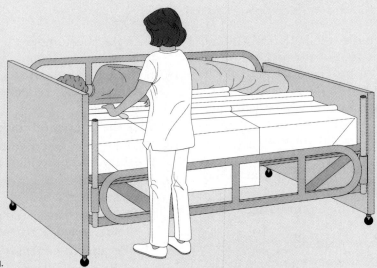

FIGURE 16–13
Fold the clean linen toward the patient, next to the dirty linen.

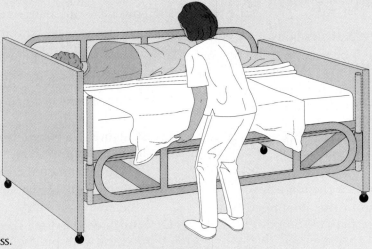

FIGURE 16–14
Straighten the draw sheet, pull it tight, and tuck it under the mattress.

Procedure for Making an Occupied Bed (cont.)

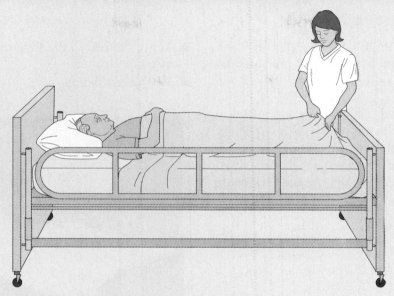

FIGURE 16–15
Loosen the top linen over the patient's feet.

28. Assist the patient to a comfortable position.
29. Place the top sheet in the center of the bed, with the centerfold of the sheet next to the patient.
30. Position the narrow hem of the sheet at the foot of the bed, even with the end of the mattress. The wide hem will be at the top. The hemstitching should face up, away from the patient.
31. Pick up the sheet from the side, open it, and fanfold it toward the patient.
32. Smooth this side of the bed. Do not tuck the bottom of the top sheet under the mattress yet.
33. Place the blanket over the top sheet as follows:
    a. Unfold and center it.
    b. The top of the blanket should be about 6 to 8 inches below the top edge of the top sheet with the top sheet folded down over it.
    c. Smooth the blanket on this side.
34. Ask the patient to hold the clean top sheet and blanket as you remove the bath blanket by pulling it from under the clean linen at the foot of the bed. Roll the dirty linen with the side that touched the patient to the inside.
    a. If the patient cannot hold the sheet, you may tuck it beneath the shoulders.
    b. Place it with the dirty linen that has already been removed.
35. Tuck the top linen under the bottom of the mattress on this side of the bed.
    a. Make a mitered corner.

36. Put the side rail up on this side of the bed.
37. Go to the other side of the bed and lower the side rail.
38. Complete the bed by straightening the top linen and tucking it in at the bottom of the mattress.
    a. Make a mitered corner.
39. Raise the side rail.
40. Check the tightness of the linen over the patient's feet. Loosen it by pulling up on the top linen (see Figure 16–15).
41. Place the pillow on the bed and put it into the clean pillowcase.
42. Position the pillow under the patient's head with the seam at the top and the open edge of the pillowcase facing away from the door.
43. Place the soiled linen in the dirty linen hamper.

Ending Steps

- Check to see that the patient is comfortable.
- Lower the bed to the floor and raise the side rails if appropriate.
- Place the call signal within the patient's reach.
- Wash your hands.
- Report and record your observations.

Procedure for Making a Surgical Bed

Beginning Steps

■ Collect necessary equipment and supplies.
■ Wash your hands and use standard precautions.
■ Use correct body mechanics.

1. Make a closed bed. (Do not tuck top linens under the foot of the mattress.)
2. Fanfold the top linen lengthwise to the side of the bed (see Figure 16–16).
3. Place the pillow upright against the headboard to protect the patient's head during the transfer.

Ending Steps

■ Leave the bed in the high position for the stretcher transfer.
■ Wash your hands.

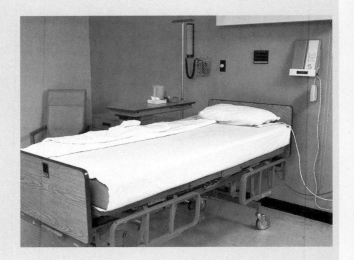

FIGURE 16–16
To prepare a surgical bed, fold the top linen lengthwise to the side of the bed.

Review

Read each sentence and fill in the blank with the vocabulary term that best completes the sentence.

1. The _____ is a crank used to change the position of the bed.
2. Normal or correct anatomical position is called _____.
3. A/An _____ is a bed made with the top linens turned down for a patient's return to the bed.
4. If the patient was unable to get out of bed, you would need to make a/an _____.
5. You would make a/an _____ if there was no patient using the bed.

Remember

1. A well-made bed helps the patient get a good night's sleep.
2. Follow the standard precautions.
3. Wash your hands frequently during bedmaking.
4. Never place dirty linen on the overbed table or on the floor.
5. Raise the bed to comfortable height and use correct body mechanics.
6. Change a wet or soiled bed immediately.
7. Stack the clean linen in the order in which it will be used.
8. Handle the patient gently and position him in the correct body alignment.
9. Make as much of the bed as you can from one side before going to the other side to finish.
10. Raise the side rails when appropriate.
11. Protect the patient's privacy while making the bed.
12. Leave the call signal within the patient's reach.
13. Return the bed to its lowest position when you leave the room.

Reflect

Read the following case study and answer the questions.

Case Study

On her first day at work as a nursing assistant, Lena is assigned to make an occupied bed. She collects the linen and stacks it carefully. She enters Mr. Matthews's room and places the clean linen on the overbed table. She removes the top sheet from Mr. Matthews and places it on the floor at the foot of the bed. She rolls Mr. Matthews onto his side and removes all the soiled linen from under him. When Mr. Matthews tries to talk to her, Lena responds, "I can't talk now. I have to hurry and make your bed." She makes the bed with clean linens, rolling the patient from side to side as necessary. After finishing the bed, she returns it to its lowest position, pulls up the side rails, and places the call signal within reach.

1. How many times was handwashing necessary in the scenario above?
2. Did Lena properly protect Mr. Matthews's privacy during the procedure? Explain your answer.
3. What should Lena have done with the dirty linen?
4. Was Lena's response to Mr. Matthews's attempt at conversation appropriate? Explain your answer.

Respond

Choose the best answer for each question.

1. When should you wash your hands during the bedmaking procedure?
   A. Before handling clean linen
   B. After handling dirty linen
   C. After removing gloves
   D. All of the above

2. How should you carry clean linen that you will need to make a bed?
   A. On your right arm
   B. On your left arm
   C. Away from your uniform
   D. Close to your body

3. Where is the best place in the patient's room to place clean linen?
   A. On the bedside stand.
   B. On the overbed table.
   C. On the visitor's chair.
   D. On the other patient's bed.

4. You have taken an extra sheet into the patient's room. What should you do with it?
   A. Return it to the clean linen cart.
   B. Use it on the other patient's bed.
   C. Leave it on the overbed table.
   D. Place it in the dirty linen container.

5. Where is the best place to put dirty linen while you are making the bed?
   A. Directly into the dirty linen container
   B. On the floor until you are through
   C. On the visitor's chair until you are through
   D. On the overbed table until you are through

6. How is the best way to stand while making a bed?
   A. With back straight and knees bent
   B. With back straight and knees locked
   C. With knees locked and feet together
   D. With knees bent and feet together

7. Which of the following is a guideline for bedmaking?
   A. Keep seams and rough edges of linen away from patient's skin.
   B. Place the bed in the highest position when you leave.
   C. Use a plastic sheet to keep the bed dry.
   D. Shake linen to remove crumbs and small objects.

8. When collecting linen to make a bed, what should you pick up first?
   A. The bedspread
   B. The mattress pad
   C. The top sheet
   D. The pillowcase

9. The patient will be going back to bed when he returns from physical therapy. What kind of bed should you make for him?
   A. A surgical bed
   B. A closed bed
   C. An open bed
   D. An occupied bed

10. How can you protect the patient's privacy while making an occupied bed?
   A. Open the blinds and let the sun shine in.
   B. Cover the patient with a bath blanket while removing the top linen.
   C. Remove all the dirty linen before you begin the procedure.
   D. Leave the door open for ventilation.

Chapter Seventeen

Admission, Transfer, and Discharge

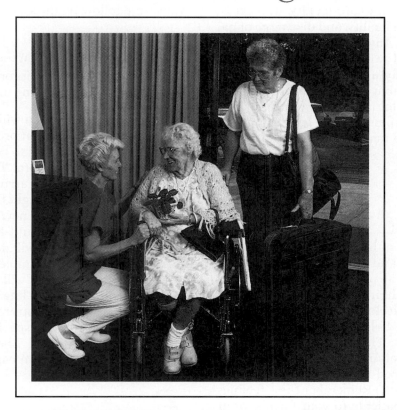

convalescence   The period of recovery after an illness or injury.

specimen   A sample of fluid or tissue from a person's body.

This chapter addresses three issues: admission of patients to a health care facility, transfer of patients within the facility, and discharge of patients from the facility. Any of these procedures can cause the patient and family stress and anxiety. Nursing assistants play a major role in all three processes. Remember that culture affects how people react to illness and to the delivery of health care. Be courteous and respectful and let the patient know that you want to make his or her stay in the health care facility as pleasant as possible.

The Admission Process

Admission to any kind of health care facility can be stressful for patients and their families. Patients may feel threatened or abandoned. Their health and independence, even their very lives, are at risk. Family members may feel guilt or fear. Certain cultural groups strongly believe in caring for their loved ones themselves. They view admission to a health care facility as failure. Just the fact that sickness may indicate a need for admission can cause anxiety. (See Figure 17–1.) Remember these feelings as you help to admit patients to your facility. Your empathy can make the admission process less threatening. Admission to the health care facility may be a well-planned event or a sudden emergency. Whether it begins in the admission office or

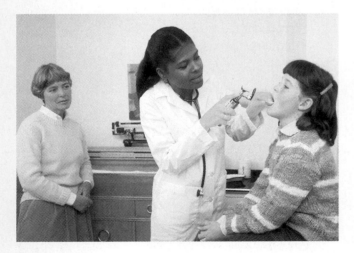

FIGURE 17–1
The possibility that sickness may indicate a need for admission to a health care facility can cause anxiety.

the emergency room, the admission process involves the following three stages:

- Collecting information.
- Admission to a room on the nursing unit.
- Orientation (receiving information and becoming familiar with the nursing unit and the facility).

As a nursing assistant you will be responsible for assisting with the admission process. You will need to get a report from the nurse before you can admit a patient to his or her room. The nurse will tell you how the patient will be arriving and if any specimens are needed. You might be required to collect a urine specimen from the new patient. A *specimen* is a sample of tissue or fluid from a person's body. How the patient arrives will determine how you will prepare the bed. For example, if the patient will be arriving by stretcher, you will need to prepare a surgical bed (folding the top linen to the side of the bed and raising the bed to stretcher height). You will also need to know if any special equipment, such as an IV pole will be needed. The procedure for admitting a patient is located on page 211.

Preadmission

The preadmission process involves collecting information and filling out all the many forms that admission requires before the patient is admitted to the facility. It may also include x-ray procedures and collection of specimens. A tour of the facility is sometimes part of the process, depending on the nature of the admission. Maternity units commonly include an extensive orientation to help prospective parents to be better prepared when they arrive for the actual birth of the baby. Check with the nurse to be sure what your responsibilities involve with the preadmitted patient.

Transferring a Patient

A patient may be transferred (moved) to another room, nursing unit, or facility. The patient may request the transfer or the decision may be made by the doctor and the facility. A patient may decide a private room would be better than a semiprivate and request a change. However, transfers are usually re-

Procedure for Admitting a Patient

Beginning Steps

- Identify the patient and explain the procedure.
- Collect necessary equipment and supplies.
- Wash your hands and use standard precautions.
- Protect the patient's privacy.
- Use correct body mechanics.

1. Assemble equipment on the overbed table.
2. Adjust the bed to the correct height and turn down the linen to open the bed.
3. Place the hospital gown or pajamas on the foot of the bed.
4. Introduce yourself to the patient and family. Call the patient by proper name and title unless directed to do otherwise ("Good morning, Mr. Smith").
5. Provide privacy and show the family where they can wait.
6. Assist the patient to change clothes if necessary.
7. Help the patient unpack. Inventory clothes and belongings according to facility policy.
8. Measure the patient's height and weight.
9. Assist the patient to the bed or a chair.
10. Measure the patient's vital signs.
11. Collect specimens if ordered.
12. Collect information and complete the admission checklist.
13. Provide water if allowed.
14. Orient the patient to facility routines such as mealtimes and visiting hours. Identify the location of the nurse's station, restrooms, and dining room. Demonstrate the bed controls and call signal. (See Figure 17–2.)
15. Identify and encourage the use of safety bars and rails.

Ending Steps

- Check to see that the patient is comfortable.
- Lower the bed and raise the side rails if appropriate.
- Place the call signal within the patient's reach.
- Wash your hands.
- Report and record your observations.

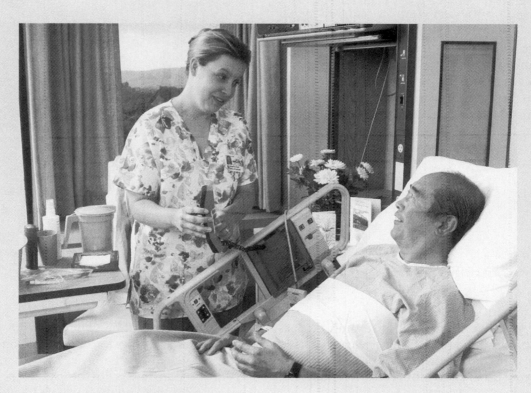

FIGURE 17–2
Demonstrate the bed controls and call signal to the new patient.

Procedure for Transferring a Patient

Beginning Steps

- Identify the patient and explain the procedure.
- Collect necessary equipment and supplies.
- Wash your hands and use standard precautions.
- Proect the patient's privacy.
- Use correct body mechanics.

1. Get a report by the nurse that includes the patient's destination and method of transport. Arrange for help if necessary.
2. Place the patient's belongings and supplies on a utility cart for transport. Check closets and drawers carefully.
3. Assist the patient to a wheelchair or stretcher. Sometimes the entire bed is transported with the patient in it. (See Figure 17–3.)
4. Acknowledge the patient's fears and distress while maintaining a positive attitude.
5. Transport the patient to the new unit.
6. Assist the patient to the bed or chair as needed.
7. Introduce the patient to the roommate and staff.
8. Put away the patient's belongings respectfully and carefully.
9. Demonstrate the bed controls and call signal. Make sure the patient is comfortable.
10. Report your observations to the nurse on the new unit when you have completed the transfer.
11. Return the wheelchair, utility cart, or other equipment to the storage area and return to your own unit.

12. Report to your supervisor and record your observations.
13. Strip the bed and remove supplies and equipment from the unit. In some facilities, this is the responsibility of the housekeeping staff.

Ending Steps

- Check to see that the patient is comfortable.
- Lower the bed and raise the side rails if appropriate.
- Place the call signal within the patient's reach.
- Wash your hands.
- Report and record your observations.

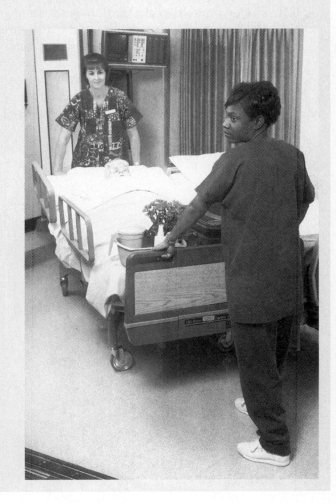

FIGURE 17–3
The patient may be transferred in the bed to another area in the facility.

lated to the patient's condition. For example, a patient might be admitted to the intensive care unit. As the patient's condition improves, he or she might be transferred to a progressive unit, and eventually to a private or semiprivate room.

Transferring can be physically and emotionally stressful. A move at any time takes planning and energy. The patient may feel satisfied with the care he or she is receiving and be unhappy about gathering up all belongings to move to another room. Long-term care residents must be given 24-hour notice if they are to be transferred. If the patient is being transferred to another facility, it will be handled much like a discharge. However, if the patient is being transferred to another area of the same facility, you will need to help the patient with the transfer.

Procedure for Discharging a Patient

Beginning Steps

- Identify the patient and explain the procedure.
- Collect necessary equipment and supplies.
- Wash your hands and use standard precautions.
- Proect the patient's privacy.
- Use correct body mechanics.

1. Help the patient get dressed.
2. Help the patient to pack. Check drawers and closets carefully. Place the patient's belongings on a utility cart.
3. Complete the inventory list according to facility policy.
4. Check with the nurse to make sure the patient has received discharge instructions.
5. Help the patient into a wheelchair.
6. Transport the patient to the discharge area (see Figure 17–4) and help him get into the discharge vehicle.

7. Make sure the patient is buckled in safely and comfortably.
8. Return the wheelchair and cart to the storage area.
9. Strip the bed and clean the unit unless this is the responsibility of the housekeeping staff.

Ending Steps

- Wash your hands.
- Report and record your observations.

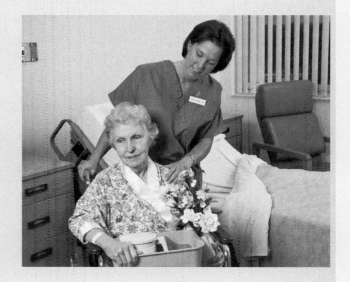

FIGURE 17-4
The nursing assistant may take the patient and her belongings to the discharge area.

Discharging a Patient

Discharge from a health care facility can be stressful. Many patients have mixed emotions about going home after an illness. They may fear not being able to care for themselves or getting sick in the middle of the night. Long-term care residents may be concerned about loneliness.

The Discharge Plan

Plans and arrangements for care of the patient after discharge begin on the patient's admission to the facility and follow through the patient's entire stay. The plan addresses each patient's physical, emotional, mental, social, cultural, and spiritual needs.

The discharge plan is of special importance because patients may leave the hospital sooner and spend more time convalescing at home. *Convalescence* is the period of time spent recovering from an illness or injury, and gradually regaining health. The discharge plan helps to prevent complications and readmission to a health care facility.

Discharge Instructions

The facility must provide the patient and family with discharge instructions. This form includes a summary of the discharge plan. You can assist in discharge planning by reinforcing what has been taught to the patient. Let the nurse know if the patient questions you about any of these instructions.

Review

Read each sentence and fill in the blank with the vocabulary term that best completes the sentence.

1. A/An _____ is a sample of tissue from a person's body.
2. Receiving information and becoming familiar with the nursing unit and the facility is called _____.
3. To prepare a _____, you would fold the top linen to the side of the bed and raise the bed to stretcher height.
4. To _____ is to move a patient from one place to another.
5. _____ is the period of time spent recovering from an illness or injury.

Remember

1. Admission to a health care facility can be stressful for patients and their families.
2. Remember that culture affects how people react to illness and to the delivery of health care.
3. Greet the patient by name and help to create a feeling of welcome.
4. List the patient's clothing and belongings on a special form.
5. Orient the new patient to the facility and introduce other patients and staff members.
6. A preadmitted patient may check in at admissions and then come directly to the room.
7. The patient who must transfer to another unit will need the emotional support of staff members.
8. Discharge planning begins upon admission and continues through the entire stay.

Reflect

Read the following case study and answer the questions.

Case Study

Mr. Cunningham, a nursing home resident, has shared a room with Mr. Long for two years. Mr. Cunningham's condition has deteriorated and he is to be transferred to another section of the facility. He is very upset about the move and tells Janet, the nursing assistant, that he isn't going to do it. Janet responds, "You have to move to another room because you're too sick to stay here. Besides, this unit is already assigned to another patient. If you refuse, I'll have to restrain you and take you anyway." Mr. Cunningham gets even more upset and says he is going home. He demands that Janet call his daughter and help him get ready for discharge. Janet tells him he can't leave until the doctor writes a discharge order.

1. Was Janet's response appropriate? What would have been more appropriate?
2. What should Janet have done when Mr. Cunningham demanded to be discharged?
3. Why do you think Mr. Cunningham was so upset?
4. What resident's rights were violated in the above scenario?

Respond

Choose the best answer for each question.

1. The patient's daughter is crying and says, "I feel terrible about admitting my mother to a nursing home." What is your best response?
   A. "You should be taking care of her at home."
   B. "You'll get over it. Everybody does."
   C. "I can see you're upset. Would you like to talk about it?"
   D. "She's confused and won't know the difference."

2. Which of the following will you need to know before admitting a new patient?
   A. How the patient will arrive
   B. If any specimens are to be collected
   C. What special equipment will be needed
   D. All of the above

3. Which of the following admission procedures are the responsibility of the nursing assistant?
   A. Measuring the patient's height and weight
   B. Ordering the patient's diet
   C. Performing an x-ray of the patient
   D. All of the above

4. Which is the best reason for transferring a nursing home patient to another room?
   A. The patient's condition changes.
   B. The room is needed for another patient.
   C. The room needs to be painted.
   D. The patient wants a nicer room.

5. Which of the following is NOT a correct step in the procedure for transferring a patient?
   A. Identify the patient and explain the procedure.
   B. Inform the nurse of the patient's reaction to the transfer.
   C. Discuss the patient's medications with the nurse.
   D. Introduce the patient to his or her roommate.

6. It is important to demonstrate the call signal in the new unit after the patient has been transferred.
   A. True
   B. False

7. Discharge is always a happy occasion for patients.
   A. True
   B. False

8. What is the primary reason for using a discharge plan?
   A. To speed up the discharge procedure
   B. To prevent complications and readmission
   C. To prevent telephone calls and visits to the doctor
   D. To make it easier on the staff

9. Which of the following is NOT part of the discharge procedure?
   A. Assist the patient to pack.
   B. Assist the patient to a wheelchair.
   C. Make sure the patient is safely buckled into the discharge vehicle.
   D. Make sure the patient gets home safely.

10. A confused nursing home patient is standing near the exit door and insists he has been discharged. What is your best response?
    A. "Let's go talk to the nurse about it."
    B. "You can't go home until the doctor says so."
    C. "Get away from the door before you get hurt."
    D. "Don't be silly. You're not going anywhere."

Chapter Eighteen

Moving *and* Positioning

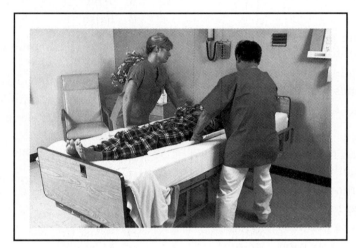

OBJECTIVES

After studying this chapter, you will be able to

1. List four complications of limited activity.

2. Describe four rules of body mechanics that are necessary when you are moving and positioning patients.

3. List two restorative devices that are used to help maintain body alignment.

4. Describe four basic body positions.

5. List two advantages of using a gait/transfer belt to transfer patients.

6. List three safety measures to implement when you are using a wheelchair.

7. Identify four guidelines for repositioning the patient in a wheelchair.

8. List two safety measures to be used when you are transferring a patient to and from a stretcher.

9. Demonstrate the procedures described in this chapter.

atrophy   A wasting and decrease in size of muscle tissue.

constipation   Infrequent, difficult defecation of hard, dry stool.

dangling   Sitting on the side of the bed with the feet hanging down.

fecal impaction   A large amount of hard, dry stool overloading the bowel.

Fowler's position   A sitting or semisitting position.

lateral position   Lying on either side.

prone position   Lying on the abdomen with the face downward or to the side.

supine position   Lying on the back with the face up.

The Importance of Activity

Staying active is important for children and adults of all ages. Exercise and activity benefit the whole person because it contributes to a healthy mind and body. Benefits of exercise and activity include the following:

- Increase muscle strength and tone.
- Maintain body flexibility and coordination.
- Improve respiratory function.
- Prevent pooling of fluid in the lungs.
- Improve circulation.
- Strengthen the immune system.
- Help maintain healthy skin.
- Promote effective elimination.
- Improve appetite and fluid intake.
- Aid digestion.
- Increase mental alertness.
- Relieve stress.

Complications of Limited Activity

Just as activity benefits the entire body, inactivity can cause problems. Some physical complications of limited activity include

- Pressure ulcers—a breakdown in skin tissue that occurs when blood flow to an area is interrupted
- Contractures—a wasting and shortening of a muscle due to lack of use (see Figure 18–1)
- Muscle *atrophy*—a wasting and decrease in the size of a muscle
- *Constipation*—hard, dry stool that is difficult to eliminate
- *Fecal impaction*—a large amount of hard, dry stool overloading the bowel

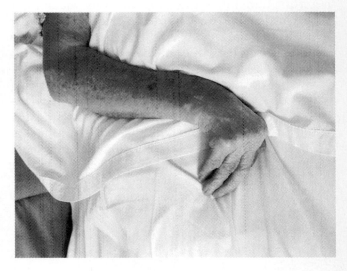

FIGURE 18–1
Contractures occur when the muscles are not used or exercised.

- Edema—swelling of a body part with fluid
- Blood clots or kidney stones
- Urinary tract infection or pneumonia

The Holistic Approach to Restorative Care

Assisting the patient to move and exercise gives you many opportunities for holistic, restorative care. Encourage the patient to move independently as much as possible. Give praise for every effort, no matter how slight. Remind the patient that activity strengthens and that rehabilitation takes time. Show pleasure in success and help the patient to build self-esteem. Treating each patient as an individual is very important when assisting with moving and positioning. Remember that every person does not react in the same manner to a disability or impairment.

Body Mechanics and Body Alignment

Body Mechanics

It is very important to use correct body mechanics when assisting the patient in moving and positioning. You will be performing procedures in which you could hurt yourself or the patient if you are not careful. Remember the rules of body mechanics that you learned in Chapter 6. Keep your back straight and stand with your feet apart. Bend your knees and use the large muscles of your legs when lifting.

When positioning a patient in bed or assisting with exercises, bring the bed to a comfortable working height for you. The bed should be as flat as the patient can tolerate. Keep the side rail up on the opposite side to prevent a fall. Use a turning sheet (draw sheet) when possible to protect the patient and yourself. Plan ahead and get help when necessary. These techniques will make your job easier and safer.

Body Alignment

It is important to position the patient in correct body alignment (placing the body in a normal or correct anatomical position). The trunk of the body should be in a straight line when the patient is lying down. Use pillows to support the extremities (arms and legs) as needed. When the patient is lying on the side, the upper arm and upper leg should be supported. Correct body alignment helps to prevent complications and makes the patient more comfortable.

The patient in a chair should sit up straight, with his lower back against the back of the chair. The feet should either touch the floor or be propped on a stool. Use pillows if necessary to prevent the patient from slumping over in the chair or leaning to one side. The back of the knees should not be touching the seat of the chair.

Restorative Equipment

Restorative equipment is designed to help the patient maintain correct body alignment and prevent complications. (See Figure 18–2.) Footboards and other foot supports keep the foot in a natural position and prevent foot drop. Hand splints are used to keep the hand from turning inward or outward in

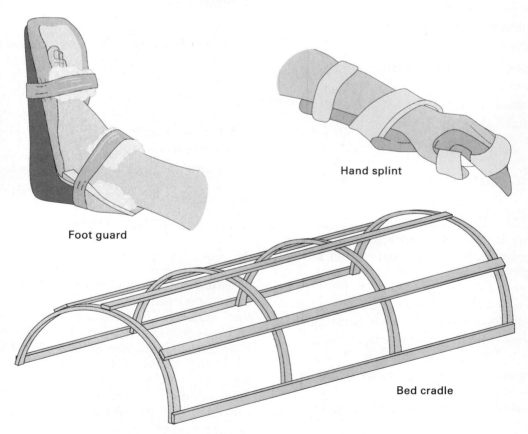

Foot guard

Hand splint

Bed cradle

FIGURE 18–2
Restorative equipment is designed to help the patient maintain correct body alignment.

an unnatural position. A bed cradle keeps the weight of the linen from pressing on the patient's body. These are only a few examples of restorative equipment used in positioning. It is important that you know how to use the equipment that has been ordered for the patient. Pillows and linen may also be used to help the patient maintain correct body alignment.

Assisting in Positioning and Turning

The patient should change position frequently when in bed or when sitting for any length of time. If the patient is not able to do this independently, you will need to assist. A patient who is comatose (unconscious) or dying needs to be turned at least every two hours. Because these patients are less likely to move independently, you must help protect their skin from pressure.

Basic Body Positions

Supine, prone, lateral, and Fowler's position are usually considered the four basic body positions. Other positions may be used in special circumstances to prevent complications.

The patient is lying on his or her back in the *supine position* (see Figure 18–3A). The head and shoulders are supported on a pillow, and if the patient's arms are at the sides, they may also be sup-

ported by pillows. A footboard or other support may be needed to keep the feet in a natural position.

The patient in the *prone position* is lying on the abdomen (see Figure 18–3B). The head may be turned to the side and supported by a small pillow, and the arms are at the sides or flexed upward by the head. The bed should be as flat as possible to promote comfort.

The patient in a *lateral position* is lying on the side (see Figure 18–3C). The upper arm and upper leg should be brought forward and supported on pillows. A pillow against the back may help the patient to maintain correct body alignment.

The patient in *Fowler's position* is in a sitting or semisitting position (Figure 18–3D). The head of the bed is elevated and the knees are raised slightly. The patient should sit straight with the head and arms supported by pillows, if necessary. A high-Fowler's or a semi-Fowler's position refers to the degree of elevation of the head of the bed. Patients with respiratory problems and those with feeding tubes may need to be in a Fowler's position. A foot support may be needed.

There are other positions that you may need to use in certain situations. To avoid pressure on bony areas, the patient may be placed in a semisupine or semiprone position (see Figures 18–4A and B). Sims' position is a lateral position with the lower arm behind the patient and the upper leg flexed toward the chest (see Figure 18–5A). This position is frequently used for bowel treatments. If the patient has difficulty assuming this position, a lateral position may be used.

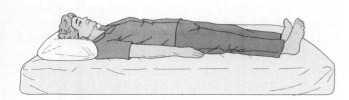

A. A Supine Position

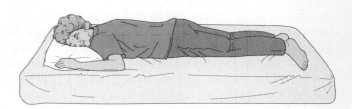

B. A Prone Position

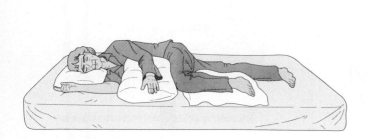

C. A Lateral Position

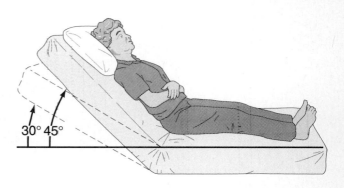

D. Fowler's Position

FIGURE 18–3 Basic body positions.

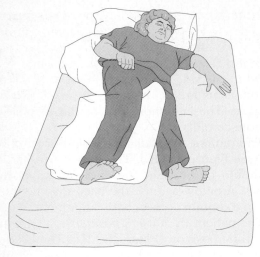

A. Semisupine Position

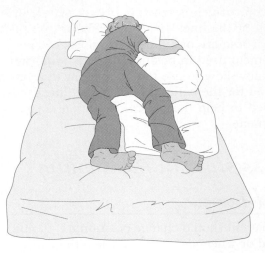

B. Semiprone Position

FIGURE 18–4 Positions to relieve pressure.

A patient assuming the orthopneic position sits straight up in bed, sometimes sitting on the edge of the bed, leans forward, and elevates the arms on a pillow or the overbed table (see Figure 18–5B). This position is frequently used by patients with respiratory problems. The object is to expand the chest and lungs in an effort to bring in more oxygen.

Assisting a Patient to Move Up in Bed

Patients tend to slide down in bed, especially when the head of the bed is elevated. The result is discomfort due to poor body alignment. Bedbound patients may need to be moved up in bed several times during a shift. Encourage the patient to do as much as possible independently. Sometimes you will be able to help the patient by yourself and other times you will need to get a co-worker to help you. A lift sheet makes the procedure easier for you and the patient.

It helps prevent friction against the patient's skin. The procedure for assisting the patient to move up in bed is located on page 221. The procedure for moving the patient up in bed with a lift sheet is on page 222.

Moving the Patient to the Side of the Bed

It may be necessary to move the patient to one side of the bed when you are turning the patient or getting the patient out of bed. This procedure brings the patient closer to you so you will not have to reach across the bed. Start from the top and move the patient's body in segments. Begin with the head and shoulders, next move the waist and thighs, and then move the legs and feet. If you use a lift sheet, you can pull the sheet to move the patient. Make sure the side rail is up on the opposite side. Get help from a co-worker, if necessary. This procedure is located on page 223.

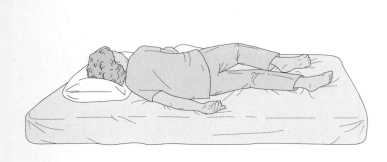

A. Sims' Position

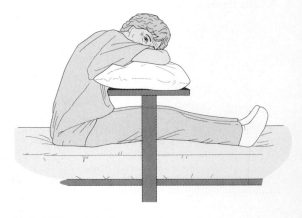

B. An Orthopneic Position

FIGURE 18–5 Special body positions.

Procedure for Assisting the Patient to Move Up in Bed

Beginning Steps

■ Identify the patient and explain the procedure.
■ Collect necessary equipment and supplies.
■ Wash your hands and use standard precautions.
■ Protect the patient's privacy.
■ Use correct body mechanics.

1. Make sure both side rails are up. Raise the bed to a comfortable working height and lock the brakes.
2. Adjust the bed to as flat a position as possible.
3. Lower the side rail on your working side.
4. Place the pillow against the headboard to avoid bumping the patient's head.
5. Stand with your feet apart (one in front of the other) and your toes pointed toward the head of the bed. Bend your knees.
6. Place one arm under the patient's shoulders and the other arm under his thighs (see Figure 18–6).
7. Ask the patient to bend his knees and brace his hands against the mattress. The patient may prefer to reach over his head and grab the headboard to assist.
8. On the count of three, shift your weight from one foot to the other as you lift and assist the patient to move up in bed.
9. Replace the pillow and straighten the linen.

Ending Steps

■ Check to see that the patient is comfortable.
■ Lower the bed and raise the side rails if appropriate.
■ Place the call signal within the patient's reach.
■ Wash your hands.
■ Report and record your observations.

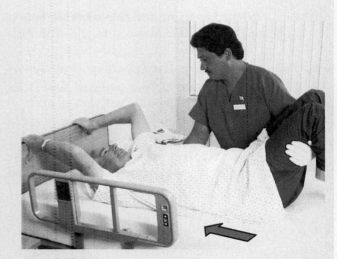

FIGURE 18–6
Assisting a patient to move up in bed.

Assisting the Patient to Turn

Many people prefer to be on their side when in bed. The lateral position relieves pressure on the bony areas of the back. You may either turn the patient away from you or toward you, whichever is appropriate. These procedures are located on pages 224 and 225.

Logrolling the Patient

A patient who has had a spinal injury or spinal surgery must be moved very carefully. The body must be in correct body alignment at all times and the back must be kept straight. Handling the spinal patient carelessly could result in further injury or paralysis. A procedure called logrolling is used to turn this type of patient. Logrolling means to turn the patient's whole body, as a unit, in one motion. Two or more people are required, depending on the size of the patient. A draw sheet makes this procedure easier and safer. (See Figure 18–11 on page 226.)

Assisting the Patient to a Sitting Position

This procedure is used in assisting the patient to sit up in bed. The procedure is a first step for many other procedures, such as assisting a patient out of bed. It may also be used to reposition the patient comfortably or to straighten the pillow and upper bed linen. (See Figure 18–12 on page 227.)

Assisting the Patient to Sit on the Side of the Bed (Dangle)

Dangling refers to sitting on the side of the bed with the feet hanging down. If the patient's feet do not reach the floor, you will need to provide a footstool. Patients are encouraged to dangle a few moments before getting out of bed. The sudden movement from lying down to standing may cause a patient to

Procedure for Moving the Patient Up in Bed with a Lift Sheet

Beginning Steps

- Identify the patient and explain the procedure.
- Collect necessary equipment and supplies.
- Wash your hands and use standard precautions.
- Protect the patient's privacy.
- Use correct body mechanics.

1. Make arrangements for a co-worker to assist you.
2. Raise the bed to a comfortable working height and lock the brakes. Make sure the side rails are up.
3. Adjust the bed to as flat a position as possible.
4. Lower the side rail on your working side. Your co-worker on the other side will do the same.
5. Place the pillow against the headboard to avoid bumping the patient's head.
6. Stand with your feet apart (one in front of the other) and your toes pointed toward the head of the bed.

7. Roll the lift sheet close to the side of the patient's body (see Figure 18–7). The lift sheet should extend from the patient's shoulders to the knees.
8. Grasp the lift sheet, with one hand at the patient's shoulder and the other hand at hip level.
9. On the count of three, shift your weight from one foot to the other as you and your co-worker lift and move the patient up in bed.
10. Replace the pillow, unroll the lift sheet, and straighten the linens.

Ending Steps

- Check to see that the patient is comfortable.
- Lower the bed and raise the side rails, if appropriate.
- Place the call signal within the patient's reach.
- Wash your hands.
- Report and record your observations.

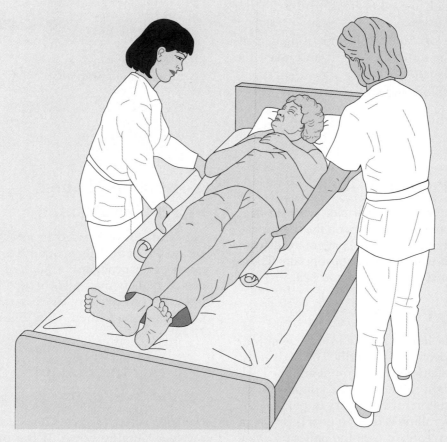

FIGURE 18–7
Roll the lift sheet close to the sides of the patient's body when you are repositioning.

Procedure for Moving the Patient to the Side of the Bed

Beginning Steps

■ Identify the patient and explain the procedure.
■ Collect necessary equipment and supplies.
■ Wash your hands and use standard precautions.
■ Protect the patient's privacy.
■ Use correct body mechanics.

1. Raise the bed to a comfortable working height and lock the brakes. Make sure the side rails are up.
2. Adjust the bed as flat as possible.
3. Lower the side rail on your working side. The side rail on the opposite side is raised.
4. Stand with your feet apart (one in front of the other), your knees bent, and your back straight.
5. Cross the patient's arms across the chest.
6. Place your arms under the neck and shoulders and move the upper section of the body toward you as you shift your weight from one leg to the other (Figure 18–8A).

7. Place your arms under the patient's waist and thighs and move the middle of the body toward you in the same manner (Figure 18–8B).
8. Place your arms under the patient's legs and move the lower part of the body toward you (Figure 18–8C).
9. Begin the positioning or transfer procedure or go on to the next step of this procedure.
10. If you are going to leave the patient in this position, reposition the pillow and straighten the linens.

Ending Steps

■ Check to see that the patient is comfortable.
■ Lower the bed and raise the side rails, if appropriate.
■ Place the call signal within the patient's reach.
■ Wash your hands.
■ Report and record your observations.

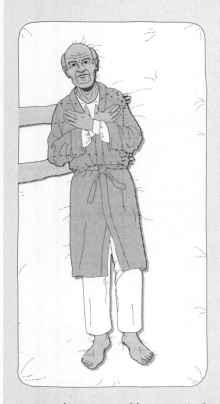

A. Move the upper part of the patient's body toward you.

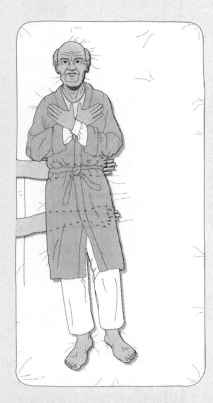

B. Move the middle part of the patient's body toward you.

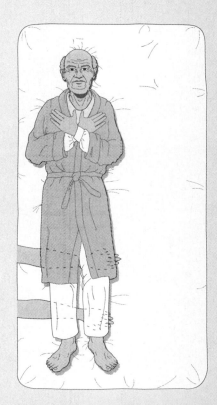

C. Move the lower part of the patient's body toward you.

FIGURE 18–8 Moving the patient to the side of the bed.

Procedure for Assisting the Patient to Turn Away from You

Beginning Steps

■ Identify the patient and explain the procedure.

■ Collect necessary equipment and supplies.

■ Wash your hands and use standard precautions.

■ Protect the patient's privacy.

■ Use correct body mechanics.

1. Raise the side rails and raise the bed to a comfortable working height and lock the brakes.

2. Adjust the bed as flat as possible and lower the side rail on your working side.

3. Move the patient to the side of the bed nearest you.

4. Flex the patient's farther arm next to the head and place the other arm across the chest. Cross the patient's leg that is nearer you over the other leg.

5. Place one hand on the patient's near shoulder and the other on the near hip. Turn the patient away from you onto the side (Figure 18–9A).

6. Reposition the pillow under the patient's head.

7. Place a pillow under the upper arm to support the elbow, wrist, and hand. Use a handroll, if necessary. Place a pillow under the upper leg supporting the knee, ankle, and foot (Figure 18–9B).

8. Raise the side rail on the side you have been working on.

9. Go to the other side of the bed and lower the side rail.

10. Adjust the bottom shoulder and hip and place a pillow at the patient's back for comfort and support. Raise the side rail.

Ending Steps

■ Check to see that the patient is comfortable.

■ Lower the bed and raise the side rails, if appropriate.

■ Place the call signal within the patient's reach.

■ Wash your hands.

■ Report and record your observations.

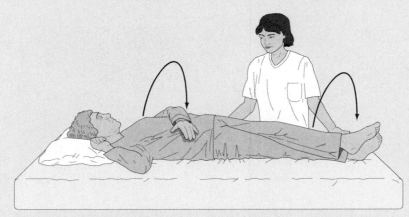

A. After placing the patient's arm and leg across her body, turn her away from you onto her side.

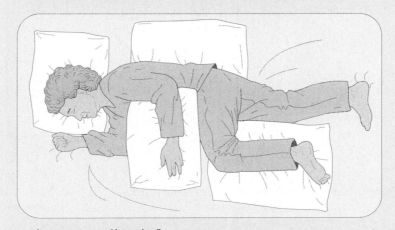

B. Support the upper arm and leg with pillows.

FIGURE 18–9 Turning the patient away from you.

Procedure for Assisting the Patient to Turn Toward You

Beginning Steps

■ Identify the patient and explain the procedure.
■ Collect necessary equipment and supplies.
■ Wash your hands and use standard precautions.
■ Protect the patient's privacy.
■ Use correct body mechanics.

1. Raise the bed to a comfortable working height and lock the brakes. Make sure both side rails are up first.
2. Adjust the bed as flat as possible and lower the side rail on your working side.
3. Move the patient to the side of the bed nearest you.
4. Raise the side rail that is nearer to you. Go to the other side of the bed and lower that side rail.
5. Flex the patient's nearer arm next to the head and place the other arm across the chest. Cross the leg that is farther from you over the other leg (Figure 18–10A).
6. Place one hand on the patient's far shoulder and the other on the far hip, and turn the patient toward you, onto the side (Figure 18–10B).
7. Reposition the pillow under the patient's head.
8. Place a pillow under the upper arm to support the elbow, wrist, and hand. Use a handroll, if necessary. Place a pillow under the upper leg, supporting the knee, ankle, and foot.

Ending Steps

■ Check to see that the patient is comfortable.
■ Lower the bed and raise the side rails, if appropriate.
■ Place the call signal within the patient's reach.
■ Wash your hands.
■ Report and record your observations.

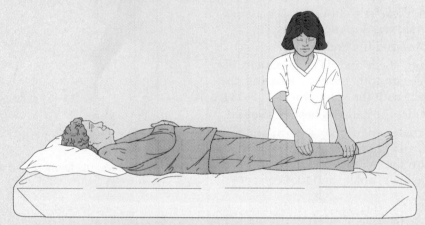

A. Place the patient's arm across her chest and cross the leg that is farther from you over the other leg.

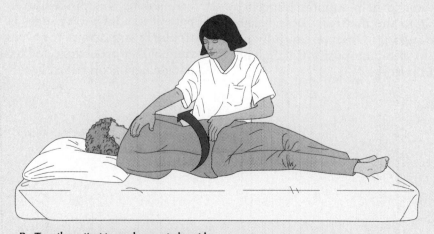

B. Turn the patient toward you onto her side.

FIGURE 18–10 Turning the patient toward you.

Procedure for Logrolling the Patient

Beginning Steps

■ Identify the patient and explain the procedure.
■ Collect necessary equipment and supplies.
■ Wash your hands and use standard precautions.
■ Protect the patient's privacy.
■ Use correct body mechanics.

1. Arrange for a co-worker to help.
2. Raise the side rails and raise the bed to a comfortable working height. Lock the brakes.
3. Keep the bed as flat as possible, and lower the side rail on your working side.
4. Roll the pull sheet up close to the patient's body and place a pillow between the patient's knees.
5. Grasp the pull sheet at the patient's shoulders and ask your co-worker to grasp the sheet at the thighs. Move the patient to the side of the bed.
6. Raise the side rail. Both you and your co-worker go to the other side of the bed and lower the side rail.
7. Stand near the patient's shoulders. Your co-worker stands near the patient's thighs.
8. Ask the patient to hold his body stiffly.
9. Grasp the turning sheet and roll the patient toward you in one smooth motion, keeping the head in alignment with the spine (Figure 18–11).
10. Place a pillow under the patient's head, if allowed.
11. Place a pillow under the upper arm to support the elbow, wrist, and hand. Use a handroll, if necessary. Make sure the pillow under the upper leg is supporting the knee, ankle, and foot correctly.

Ending Steps

■ Check to see that the patient is comfortable.
■ Lower the bed and raise the side rails, if appropriate.
■ Place the call signal within the patient's reach.
■ Wash your hands.
■ Report and record your observations.

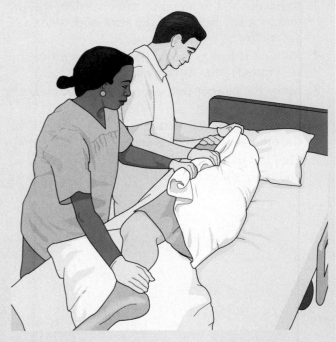

FIGURE 18–11
To logroll a patient, grasp the turning sheet and roll the patient toward you in one smooth motion.

lose balance or feel faint. Dangling helps patients to regain their balance and prevents dizziness. Encourage the patient to help support himself by pushing his hands into the mattress. Do not leave the patient alone dangling. Observe carefully and return the patient to a supine position if he complains of continued dizziness.

The dangling procedure may also be used as part of the procedure for getting a patient out of bed. Taking this procedure in two steps allows the patient to adjust to changes in position. This is particularly important for weak or frail elderly patients. The procedure for assisting the patient to dangle begins on page 228.

Procedure for Assisting the Patient to a Sitting Position

Beginning Steps

■ Identify the patient and explain the procedure.
■ Collect necessary equipment and supplies.
■ Wash your hands and use standard precautions.
■ Protect the patient's privacy.
■ Use correct body mechanics.

1. Raise the bed to a comfortable working height and lock the brakes.
2. Lower the side rail on your working side.
3. Stand facing the head of the bed, with your feet apart, your knees bent, and your back straight.
4. Place your arm under the patient's near arm and grasp his or her shoulder with your hand.
5. Ask the patient to grasp your shoulder (Figure 18–12A).
6. Place your free arm under the patient's neck and shoulders (Figure 18–12B).
7. On the count of three, assist the patient to a sitting position (Figure 18–12C).

8. Use the arm that was supporting the patient's neck and shoulders to straighten the linens and pillow while continuing to lock arms. Pull the pillow down so that the shoulders will be supported.
9. Continue the procedure
   a. If the patient wants to remain in this position for awhile, assure comfort and support.
   b. If the patient wants to return to the supine position, use the locked arm procedure to assist.

Ending Steps

■ Check to see that the patient is comfortable.
■ Lower the bed and raise the side rails, if appropriate.
■ Place the call signal within the patient's reach.
■ Wash your hands.
■ Report and record your observations.

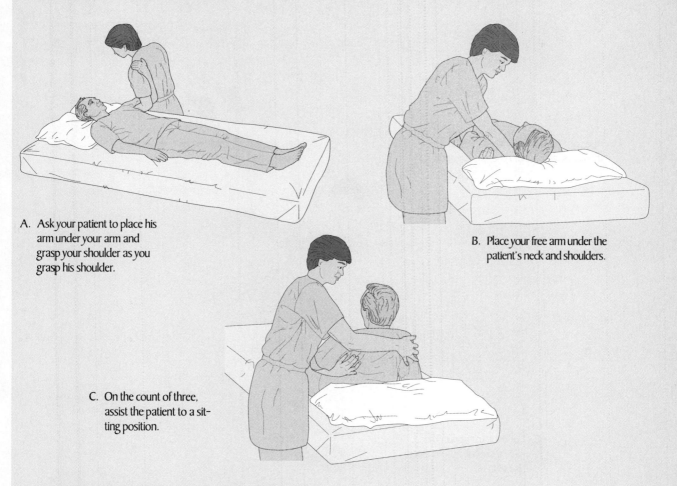

A. Ask your patient to place his arm under your arm and grasp your shoulder as you grasp his shoulder.

B. Place your free arm under the patient's neck and shoulders.

C. On the count of three, assist the patient to a sitting position.

FIGURE 18–12   Assisting the patient to a sitting position.

Procedure for Assisting the Patient to Sit on the Side of the Bed (Dangle)

Beginning Steps

■ Identify the patient and explain the procedure.
■ Collect necessary equipment and supplies.
■ Wash your hands and use standard precautions.
■ Protect the patient's privacy.
■ Use correct body mechanics.

1. Position the bed so that the patient's feet will either touch the floor or a footstool.

2. Lock the wheels and lower the side rails nearest you.
3. Assist the patient to a sitting position.
4. Place one arm behind the patient's neck and shoulders and place your other arm under the patient's knees (Figure 18–13A).
5. On the count of three, turn the patient toward you so that his legs hang over the side of the bed (Figure 18–13B).

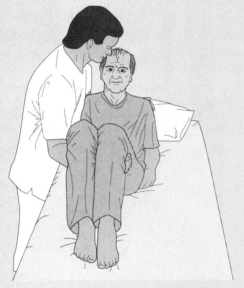

A. Place one hand behind the patient's neck and shoulders; place your other arm under his knees.

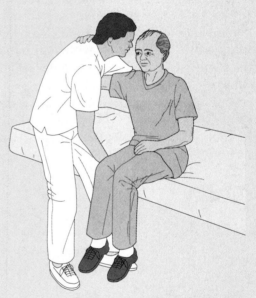

B. Turn the patient toward you so that his legs hang over the bed.

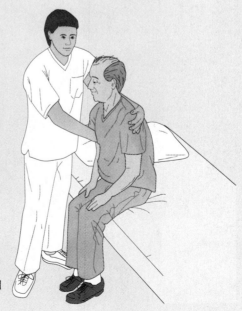

C. Continue to support the patient until he has regained his balance.

FIGURE 18–13 Assisting the patient to dangle.

Procedure for Assisting the Patient to Sit on the Side of the Bed (Dangle) (cont.)

6. Make sure the patient is sitting straight and in correct body alignment. Support the feet on a footstool, if necessary.
7. Ask the patient to push with his hands against the mattress to help maintain an upright position.
8. Keep your arm behind his neck and shoulders for support until you are sure the patient has regained balance (Figure 18–13C).
9. Check the pulse and respirations.
10. Allow the patient to dangle 15 to 20 minutes while you remain nearby.
11. Return the patient to bed by reversing the procedure.

Ending Steps

■ Check to see that the patient is comfortable.
■ Raise the side rails, if appropriate.
■ Place the call signal within the patient's reach.
■ Wash your hands.
■ Report and record your observations.

Assisting the Patient to Transfer

It is important that you learn to safely transfer patients from one place to another. You will need to understand basic anatomy, body mechanics, and body alignment. Take time to plan the transfer before you begin. Determine how much the patient will be able to do independently. Collect any special equipment needed and arrange for help, if necessary.

The patient may transfer from the bed to a chair, a wheelchair, or a stretcher and will also need to transfer back to the bed. Be sure that the wheels on beds, stretchers, and wheelchairs are locked during transfers. The patient or you may be injured if any of the equipment starts to roll.

The patient should always transfer in the direction of the strong side. This means that when the patient stands, weight bearing should be on the strong side first. It may help to remember that the "strong side leads." Place the chair on the patient's strong side when getting the patient out of bed.

Check your assignment sheet or the care plan for information that you will need to complete the transfer. The care plan indicates if the patient uses a cane or walker. It will also include any weakness or problems that would affect the transfer. However, careful patient observation is still necessary. A patient may not always need the same amount of assistance. Encourage the patient to be as independent as possible, while providing assistance as necessary.

Using a Gait/Transfer Belt

A gait/transfer belt is used to assist patients to ambulate or transfer. (See Figure 18–14.) It is useful for patients who are weak, unsteady, or prone to falling. The gait/transfer belt provides many safety advantages. It helps prevent falls and reduces the chance of injury to either the patient or the nursing assistant. The belt gives you more control and helps the patient feel more secure.

Apply the belt snugly around the patient's waist and over clothing. Make sure that it does not slip up over the ribs. Fasten the buckle slightly off-center in the front. Always explain that the belt is being used for the patient's safety and that it will be removed immediately after the procedure is complete.

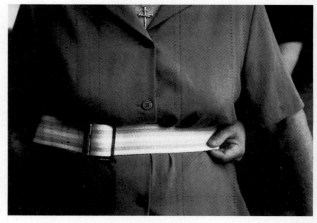

FIGURE 18–14
A gait/transfer belt is used to assist patients to ambulate or transfer.

Procedure for Assisting the Patient to Transfer from the Bed to a Chair or Wheelchair

Beginning Steps

- Identify the patient and explain the procedure.
- Collect necessary equipment and supplies.
- Wash your hands and use standard precautions.
- Protect the patient's privacy.
- Use correct body mechanics.

1. Position the chair on the patient's strong side.
2. Lock the wheels and fold the footrests out of the way if you are using a wheelchair.
3. Place the bed in its lowest position and lock the wheels.
4. Lower the side rail nearest you.
5. Put nonskid shoes on the patient and a robe if the patient is not already dressed.
6. Assist the patient to sit on the side of the bed and dangle for a few minutes.
7. Assist the patient to a standing position, using the following steps:
    a. Stand facing the patient, bend your knees, and keep your back straight.
    b. Place your arms around the patient's body, under the patient's arms.
    c. Brace your knees against the patient's knees and block his feet with yours (Figure 18–15A).
    d. If possible, the patient should brace with hands against the mattress and push up as you lift.
    e. On the count of three, straighten your knees as you bring the patient to a standing position (Figure 18–15B).
8. Ask the patient to take small steps as both of you turn toward the chair.
9. Ask the patient to back up until the back of the knees touch the front of the chair.
10. Ask the patient to grasp the arms of the chair, if possible. If not, the patient can place his hands on your forearms (Figure 18–15C).
11. On the count of three, bend your knees as you lower the patient into the chair (Figure 18–15D).

Ending Steps

- Check to see that the patient is comfortable.
- Lower the bed.
- Place the call signal within the patient's reach.
- Wash your hands.
- Report and record your observations.

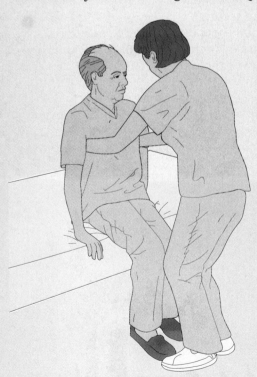

A. Brace the patient's knees and feet with your knees and feet.

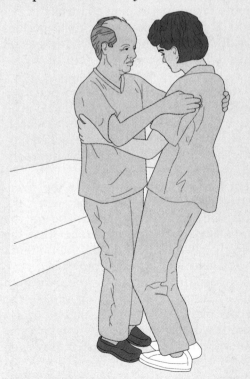

B. Bring the patient to a standing position.

FIGURE 18–15 Transferring the patient from the bed to a wheelchair.

Procedure for Assisting the Patient to Transfer from the Bed to a Chair or Wheelchair (cont.)

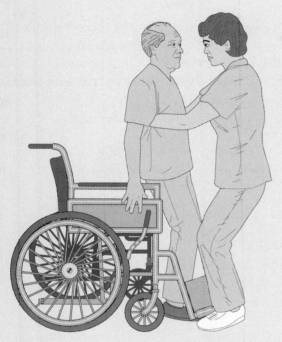

C. Ask the patient to grasp the arms of the chair or place his hands on your forearms.

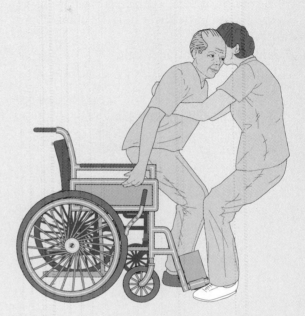

D. Bend your knees as you lower the patient into the chair.

FIGURE 18–15 Transferring the patient from the bed to a wheelchair (cont.).

Procedure for Using a Gait/Transfer Belt to Assist the Patient in Transferring from the Bed to a Chair or Wheelchair

Beginning Steps

■ Identify the patient and explain the procedure.
■ Collect necessary equipment and supplies.
■ Wash your hands and use standard precautions.
■ Protect the patient's privacy.
■ Use correct body mechanics.

1. Position the chair on the patient's strong side.
2. Lock the wheels and fold the footrests up if you are using a wheelchair.
3. Place the bed in its lowest position and lock the wheels.
4. Lower the side rail nearest you.
5. Put nonskid shoes on the patient and a robe if the patient is not already dressed.
6. Assist the patient to sit on the side of the bed and dangle for a few minutes.

7. Place a gait/transfer belt on the patient so that it fits snugly. Leave enough room for your fingers to slip under the belt. Fasten the buckle off-center, in the front (Figure 18–16A).
8. Assist the patient to a standing position, using the following steps:
   a. Stand facing the patient, bend your knees, and keep your back straight.
   b. The patient should brace with her hands against the mattress and push as you lift. If this is not possible, the patient's hands should be placed on your forearms.
   c. Grasp the gait/transfer belt from underneath at each side (Figure 18–16B).
   d. Brace your knees against the patient's knees and block her feet with your feet.
   e. On the count of three, straighten your knees as you bring the patient to a standing position.

FIGURE 18–16 Transferring the patient from a bed to a chair, using a gait/transfer belt.

Procedure for Using a Gait/Transfer Belt to Assist the Patient in Transferring from the Bed to a Chair or Wheelchair (cont.)

9. Assist the patient to move to the front of the chair.
10. On the count of three, bend your knees, as you assist the patient to lower into the chair (Figure 18–16C).
11. Remove the gait/transfer belt.

Ending Steps

■ Check to see that the patient is comfortable.
■ Lower the bed to the floor and raise the side rails if appropriate.
■ Place the call signal within the patient's reach.
■ Wash your hands.
■ Report and record your observations.

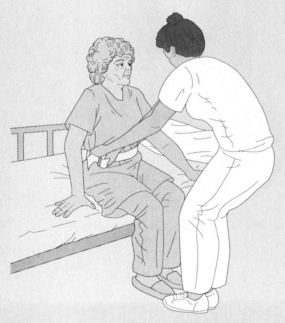

A. Place the gait/transfer belt on the patient so that it fits snugly, and fasten the buckle off-center in the front.

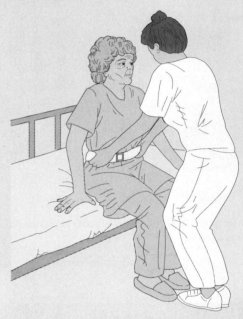

B. Grasp the gait/transfer belt from underneath at each side.

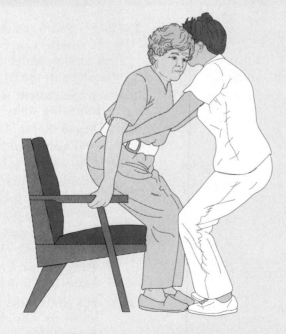

C. On the count of three, lower the patient into the chair.

FIGURE 18–16 Transferring the patient from a bed to a chair, using a gait/transfer belt.

A gait/transfer belt may not be appropriate for every patient. You would not use the belt with patients who have fractured ribs, have had abdominal surgery, or are having respiratory difficulties. Some confused patients might mistake the belt for a restraint and feel frightened.

Assisting the Patient to Transfer from the Bed to a Chair or Wheelchair

Patients are encouraged to get out of bed whenever possible. Even sitting up in a chair for a few minutes can be restorative. Bed rest for extended periods can cause many physical and psychosocial complications. Although it is safer to use a gait belt when getting the patient into or out of a chair, this method is not always appropriate. The procedure for assisting the patient to transfer from the bed to a wheelchair (not using a gait belt) begins on page 230. The procedure for using a gait belt to assist the patient in transferring from the bed to a wheelchair is located on page 231.

Assisting the Patient to Transfer from a Chair or Wheelchair to the Bed

The procedure for transferring the patient from a chair to the bed involves reversing the steps in the two previous procedures.

Using a Mechanical Lift

A mechanical lift helps protect you and the patient from injury. However, you must learn to use it carefully and safely. Operating the lift is safer with two people, one operating the lift and the other guiding the patient. The first few times you use the lift, get assistance from a co-worker who is experienced with that particular type of lift.

There are many different types available so the procedure varies. The following procedure describes the use of the type of lift shown in Figure 18–17. You will need to learn how to correctly operate the mechanical lifts used in your facility.

In this type, a sling is positioned flat under the patient. Chains hook into the sides of the sling and are attached to the lift. A hydraulic pump is used to raise and lower the sling. The pump may be operated by pumping a handle up and down or by pushing a button. The procedure for using a mechanical lift begins on page 234.

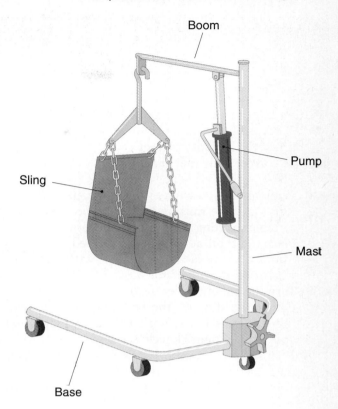

Boom

Pump

Sling

Mast

Base

FIGURE 18–17
A mechanical lift.

Using a Wheelchair

A wheelchair may be used to provide mobility for a patient who is unable to walk. A wheelchair may also be used by a patient who is recovering from surgery or an illness. Sitting upright in the wheelchair promotes normal body function and improves emotional outlook.

Wheelchairs are available in a variety of styles and sizes to accommodate individual needs. Some wheelchairs are lightweight and fold up for easy portability. Patients should be encouraged to operate the wheelchair independently whenever possible. A geri-chair (geriatric chair) is a special type of wheelchair that is well-padded and has a high back. It looks like a recliner chair and provides comfortable seating. The geri-chair is equipped with a tray that attaches to the front and may be used for eating and other activities. (See Figure 18–19 on page 236.)

Safety Measures with Wheelchairs

Check to see that the chair is in good repair before you use it. Make sure the wheels lock, the footrests work, and there are no sharp edges that might in-

Procedure for Using a Mechanical Lift

Beginning Steps

- Identify the patient and explain the procedure.
- Collect necessary equipment and supplies.
- Wash your hands and use standard precautions.
- Protect the patient's privacy.
- Use correct body mechanics.

1. Arrange for a co-worker to assist you.
2. Raise the side rails and raise the bed to a comfortable working height. Lock the brakes.
3. Place the chair at the head of the bed.
4. Stand on one side of the bed with your co-worker on the other side. Lower the side rails.
5. Turn the patient away from you onto his side.
6. Center the sling on the bed and fold it toward the patient's back, with the lower edge just above the patient's knees (see Figure 18–18A).
7. Turn the patient onto his side toward you, over the folded sling.
8. Your co-worker will straighten the sling on that side.
9. Turn the patient onto his back and make sure he is centered on the sling.
10. Raise the head of the bed and position the mechanical lift.
11. Pump the mechanical lift's handle or press the button that raises the boom, and with your co-worker guiding the chains or straps, position it over the patient (see Figure 18–18B).
12. Widen the base of the lift and lock the brakes.
13. Place the patient's arms over the chest and instruct him not to hold on to the chains or straps.
14. Attach the sling to the chains or straps. Make sure that the open ends of the hooks face away from the patient (see Figure 18–18C).
15. Pump the handle or press the button that raises the boom and the sling. Lift the patient clear of the bed (see Figure 18–18D).
16. Check again to see that the patient is centered on the sling before moving the patient off the bed.
17. Unlock the wheels and slowly move the lift away from the bed with the patient facing you. Your co-worker will guide the patient's legs off the bed.
18. Holding the steering handle with both hands, move the patient away from the bed toward the chair. Your co-worker will stabilize the patient's body and guide the chains or straps.
19. Position the lift with the patient's back toward the chair. Lock the brakes (see Figure 18–18E).
20. Lower the patient slowly into the chair with your co-worker guiding the patient's body into correct alignment. Leave the sling under the patient (see Figure 18–18F).

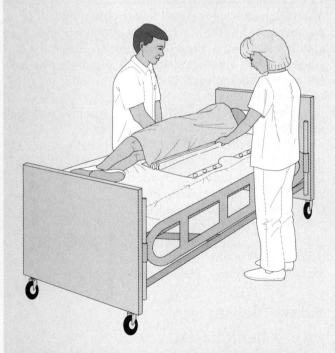

A. Center the sling and fold it toward the patient's back.

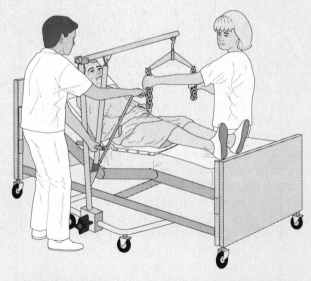

B. Raise the boom and, with your co-worker guiding the chain, position it over the patient.

FIGURE 18–18 Using a mechanical lift.

Procedure for Using a Mechanical Lift (cont.)

21. Lower the boom enough to detach the chains or straps. Unlock the brakes and move the lift away from the chair.
22. Pad the edges of the sling to protect the patient's skin.
23. Cover the patient's knees with a lap robe or bath blanket for warmth and privacy.
24. Return the mechanical lift to the storage area.

Ending Steps

- Report and record your observations.
- Check to see that the patient is comfortable.
- Lower the bed and raise the side rails if appropriate.
- Place the call signal within the patient's reach.
- Wash your hands.
- Report and record your observations.

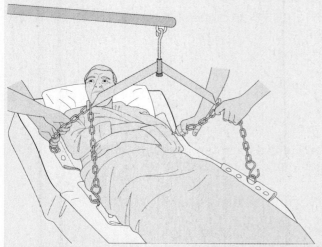

C. Make sure the open ends of the hooks face away from the patient.

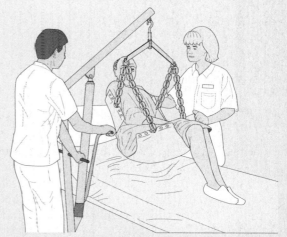

D. Pump the handle that raises the boom and the sling. Lift the patient clear of the bed.

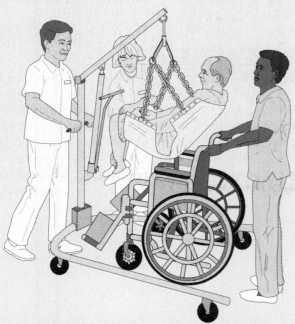

E. Position the lift with the patient's back toward the chair.

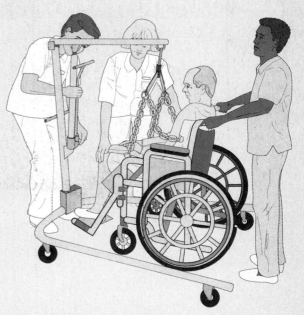

F. Lower the patient slowly into the chair with your co-worker guiding the patient's body into correct alignment.

FIGURE 18–18 Using a mechanical lift (cont.).

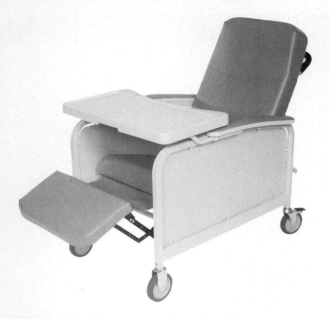

FIGURE 18–19   A geriatric (geri) chair.

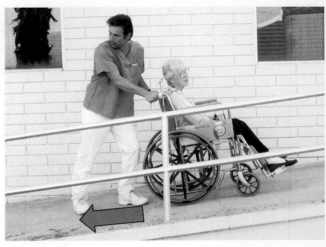

FIGURE 18–20   Turn the wheelchair around and back down the ramp.

jure the patient. Always lock the brakes when the wheelchair is stopped. Wheelchairs should be cleaned on a regular basis to prevent the spread of infection. The correct way to take a wheelchair down a ramp is to turn the wheelchair around and

back down the ramp. The same procedure is used to enter an elevator. (See Figure 18–20.)

Repositioning the Patient in a Wheelchair

The patient in a wheelchair should be repositioned at least every two hours. Repositioning may be needed more frequently if the patient slides down in the chair.

Using a Stretcher

The procedure to move the helpless patient from a bed to a stretcher may require three or four people, and two people are necessary when transferring the patient by stretcher down the hall. Transport the patient feet first and be careful turning corners in the hallway. Never leave a patient alone on a stretcher. You are responsible for the patient's safety until someone else takes over. Reverse the procedure to transfer the patient from the stretcher to a bed.

Guidelines for Repositioning the Patient in a Wheelchair

- Get help if necessary. Two people may be required with one lifting from each side.
- Lock the brakes and move the footrests aside.
- Stand behind the chair and place your arms around the patient's body, under the arms.
- On the count of three, lift and reposition the patient.
- Do not pull the patient up by the arms.
- Reposition the footrests and make sure the patient is in good body alignment.

Procedure for Moving the Patient from the Bed to a Stretcher

Beginning Steps

- Identify the patient and explain the procedure.
- Collect necessary equipment and supplies.
- Wash your hands and use standard precautions.
- Protect the patient's privacy.
- Use correct body mechanics.

1. Arrange for two or three co-workers to help.
2. Raise the bed to a comfortable working height and lock the wheels.
3. Remove the top linen while covering the patient with a bath blanket. Loosen the draw sheet.
4. Lower the side rail on your side.
5. Using the draw sheet, move the patient toward you.
6. Two co-workers will go to the other side of the bed, lower the rail, and steady the patient to prevent a fall.
7. Position the stretcher against the near side of the bed and lock the wheels. Adjust the height of the bed even with the stretcher (Figure 18–21A).
8. Two co-workers will stand at the side of the bed, one near the patient's shoulders and the other near the thighs. You and the other co-worker stand at the side of the stretcher.
9. Roll the draw sheet close to the sides of the patient's body.
10. On the count of three, move the patient from the bed to the stretcher.
11. Center the patient on the stretcher and place a pillow under the head and shoulders, if allowed.

12. Fasten the safety straps and raise the side rails (Figure 18–21B).
13. Unlock the wheels and transport the patient feet-first with the help of one co-worker.
14. Stay with the patient until someone else takes over.

Ending Steps

- Wash your hands.
- Report and record your observations.

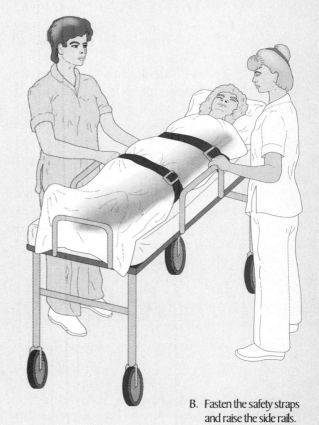

B. Fasten the safety straps and raise the side rails.

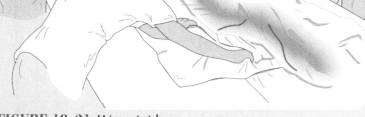

A. Adjust the height of the bed even with the stretcher.

FIGURE 18–21 Using a stretcher.

Review

Read each sentence and fill in the blank with the vocabulary term that best completes the sentence.

1. A wasting and decrease in the size of muscle tissue is called _____.
2. A _____ is a large amount of hard, dry stool overloading the bowel.
3. The patient in a _____ position is lying on his side.
4. The patient in a _____ position is lying on his abdomen.
5. _____ refers to sitting on the side of the bed with the feet hanging down.

Remember

1. Exercise and activity are necessary for a healthy mind and body.
2. Encourage the patient to move independently as much as possible.
3. Using correct body mechanics when assisting patients in moving helps protect you and the patient from injury.
4. A patient who is not in correct body alignment is at increased risk of complications.
5. Restorative equipment is available to help the patient maintain body alignment.
6. A bedbound patient needs to be turned at least every two hours.
7. It is safer and easier to move and position the patient with a lift sheet.
8. You will need to logroll the patient who has had spinal surgery or has a back or neck disorder.
9. Dangling on the side of the bed helps the patient to regain balance.
10. The patient should always transfer toward the strong side.
11. A gait/transfer belt helps prevent falls and injuries.
12. The wheels should be locked on the wheelchair any time it is stopped.
13. The patient in a wheelchair should be repositioned at least every 2 hours.
14. You will need to learn how to operate the mechanical lifts in your facility.
15. Never leave a patient alone on a stretcher.

Reflect

Read the following case study and answer the questions.

Case Study

Jim Worth is a 19-year-old patient recovering from an auto accident. He has several broken bones and bruised ribs. Jim has a lot of pain and avoids moving around. He is 6 feet tall and weighs 250 pounds. You have orders to get him up in a wheelchair today.

1. What kind of complications could occur because of Jim's inactivity?
2. What can you do to help prevent those complications?
3. What piece of equipment would be most helpful in getting Jim out of bed?
4. What can you do to make the procedure less painful for Jim?

Respond

Choose the best answer for each question.

1. A breakdown in skin tissue that occurs when blood flow to an area is interrupted is called a/an
   A. Contracture
   B. Atrophy
   C. Pressure ulcer
   D. Fecal impaction

2. A wasting and shortening of a muscle due to lack of use is called a/an
   A. Contracture
   B. Atrophy
   C. Pressure ulcer
   D. Fecal impaction

3. Which of the following is NOT correct body mechanics to use when lifting a patient?
   A. Keep your back straight.
   B. Bend your knees.
   C. Use the large muscles in your legs.
   D. Stand with your feet together.

4. Placing the patient in correct anatomical position is called
   A. Body alignment
   B. Body mechanics
   C. Atrophy
   D. Contracture

' 5. A patient who is sitting up in bed is in what position?
   A. Prone position
   B. Fowler's position
   C. Sims' position
   D. Lateral position

6. A procedure that keeps the patient's back straight while turning patients with spinal injuries is called
   A. Logrolling
   B. Dangling
   C. Pooling
   D. Flexing

7. The patient who is dangling complains of feeling faint. What should you do?
   A. Go get the nurse immediately.
   B. Return the patient to a supine position.
   C. Tell him to try to sit for a few minutes longer.
   D. Get the patient into a wheelchair.

8. Which of these statements about transferring patients is correct?
   A. Weight bearing should be on the strong side first.
   B. The weak side leads.
   C. Always use a gait belt when transferring patients.
   D. Unlock the brakes before getting a patient out of a wheelchair.

9. Which of the following statements about gait/transfer belts is FALSE?
   A. The gait belt helps patients feel secure.
   B. The gait belt is not appropriate for all patients.
   C. Apply the gait belt snugly around the patient's waist.
   D. Fasten the buckle exactly in the center of the patient's body.

10. What is the correct way to take a patient down a ramp in a wheelchair?
   A. Turn the wheelchair around and back down the ramp.
   B. Push the wheelchair forward down the ramp.
   C. Lift the footrests out of the way before starting down the ramp.
   D. Lock the brakes before starting down the ramp.

Chapter Nineteen

Ambulation *and* Exercise

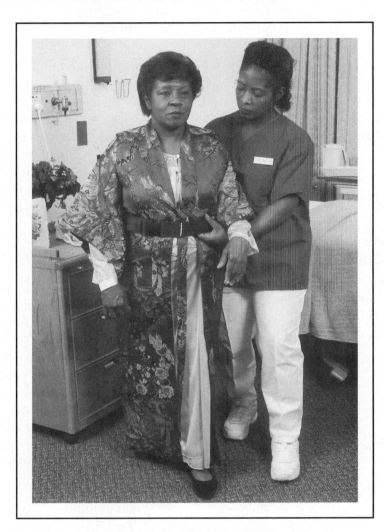

O B J E C T I V E S

1. Identify four benefits of ambulation.

2. Briefly describe the restorative ambulation program.

3. List four guidelines for protecting a falling patient.

4. Identify five guidelines for using assistive ambulation devices.

After studying this chapter, you will be able to _____

5. Describe two types of restorative exercises.

6. Identify three safety measures to follow for performing range-of-motion exercises.

7. Demonstrate the procedures described in this chapter.

ambulate   To walk.

empowerment   To give power to a person; to enable a person to make decisions independently.

range-of-motion exercises   Movements of joints through the normal area of movement.

The Benefits of Ambulation

The ability to *ambulate* (walk) provides mobility, independence, and the opportunity to experience the environment. Ambulation also makes life more interesting and enjoyable. It helps relieve stress and anxiety and it contributes to mental and emotional well-being. Walking is a form of exercise that is available to almost everyone. It costs no money and requires no special equipment. Muscle strength and stamina are increased by walking. Appetite, digestion, and elimination are improved. A brisk walk stimulates the cardiovascular system and increases blood flow to the cells. But even a leisurely stroll through the park is beneficial.

When patients lose the ability to walk, their self-esteem may be damaged because their independence is threatened. Socializing and participating in activities require greater effort when patients cannot walk. Feelings of frustration, anger, or sadness may lead to withdrawal or depression. Treatment must focus on the patient's feelings as well as on the physical needs.

Restorative Ambulation Program

A restorative ambulation program helps the patient learn to walk again. It focuses on building muscle strength and regaining stamina. Special equipment is available in physical therapy to strengthen the patient and assist in ambulation. For example, parallel bars support the patient while practicing walking. Physical therapists and aides instruct and assist as necessary. As a nursing assistant, you may have the opportunity to work in physical therapy. It can be very rewarding to observe the satisfaction the patient experiences from relearning to walk. (See Figure 19–1.)

A restorative ambulation program must meet the needs of the whole person. Although walking is primarily a physical activity, it is affected by many psychosocial factors. Fear, anxiety, and joy are some of the feelings that may arise during rehabilitation. Motivation and personal goals must also be taken into consideration. Hence, the program is designed for the individual patient. The patient is encouraged

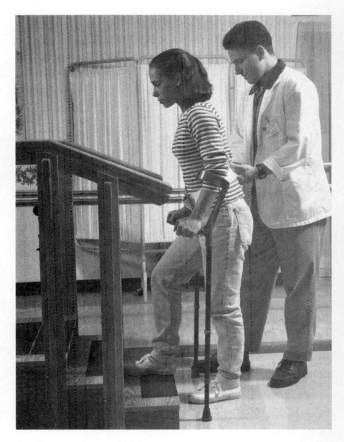

FIGURE 19–1
The patient may need special equipment to assist her in ambulation.

to be involved in planning the program. This can be a great motivator because it provides patient empowerment. *Empowerment* means to give power to or to enable a person to take charge of his or her life. It then becomes the patient's plan and focuses on the patient's goals.

Assisting the Patient to Walk

A patient who cannot walk or is relearning to walk will need both physical and emotional support. The same technique will not work for every patient, so check the care plan and become familiar with the patient's individualized plan. Know the distance the patient is supposed to walk. Usually, the patient starts out walking only a few steps and gradually increases the distance as strength returns. When assisting the patient to ambulate, walk at the patient's side and slightly behind. If the patient should feel faint or lose balance, you can quickly pull the patient close to your body. Do not support the patient by holding to his clothing or belt. The safest way to protect both of you is by using a gait/transfer belt.

Using a Gait/Transfer Belt

It is easier and safer if a gait/transfer belt is used for assisting the patient to ambulate. The gait/transfer belt gives you better control over the patient during ambulation. If the patient begins to fall, you can ease him down to the floor with more control, using the belt. Not only do you feel safer with the gait/transfer belt, but so does the patient.

There are times when you will not be able to use the gait/transfer belt to assist the patient with ambulation. For example, it would not be appropriate to use the gait/transfer belt if a patient has broken ribs, has had recent abdominal surgery, or has respiratory difficulties. In any of those situations, you would need to place one arm around the patient's waist and support the patient's arm with your other hand. If the patient is very weak or unsteady, it would be better to have two people assisting with ambulation, one on either side of the patient.

Procedure for Using a Gait/Transfer Belt to Assist the Patient to Ambulate

Beginning Steps

◼ Identify the patient and explain the procedure.

◼ Collect necessary equipment and supplies.

◼ Wash your hands and use standard precautions.

◼ Protect the patient's privacy.

◼ Use correct body mechanics.

1. Apply the gait/transfer belt around the patient's waist.

   a. Apply the belt snugly around the waist, over the clothing.

   b. Fasten the safety buckle in the front, slightly off-center.

2. Bring the patient to a standing position, using the correct procedure (Figure 19–2A).

3. Stand at the patient's side until balance is regained. Keep your hands on the gait/transfer belt.

4. While holding onto the gait/transfer belt, change the position of your hands. One hand should be holding the belt at the side, and the other hand holding the belt in the back (Figure 19–2B).

5. Assist the patient to walk. Walk at the patient's side, and slightly behind, while holding the belt with both hands (Figure 19–2C).

6. Encourage the patient to stand straight and walk as normally as possible.

7. Return the patient to the chair or bed.

Ending Steps

◼ Check to see that the patient is comfortable.

◼ Lower the bed to the floor and raise the side rails, if appropriate.

◼ Place the call signal within the patient's reach.

◼ Wash your hands.

◼ Report and record your observations.

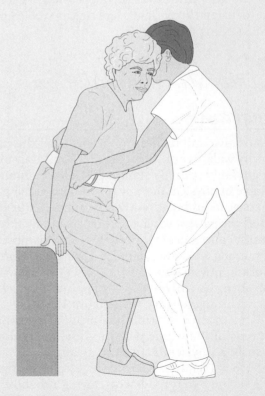

FIGURE 19–2 Using a gait/transfer belt to assist the patient in ambulation.

A. Bring the patient to a standing position.

Procedure for Using a Gait/Transfer Belt to Assist the Patient to Ambulate (cont.)

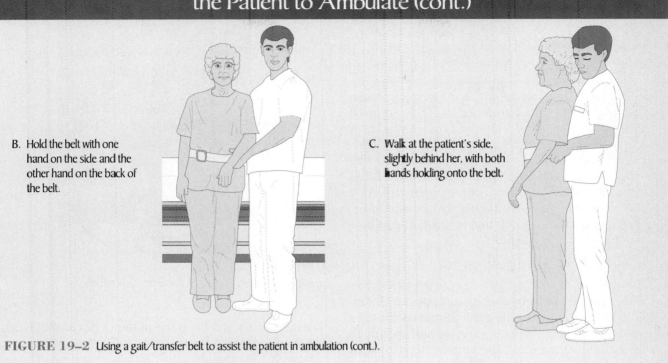

B. Hold the belt with one hand on the side and the other hand on the back of the belt.

C. Walk at the patient's side, slightly behind her, with both hands holding onto the belt.

FIGURE 19–2 Using a gait/transfer belt to assist the patient in ambulation (cont.).

Protecting a Falling Patient

If the patient begins to fall when standing or ambulating, do not attempt to prevent the fall. You could lose your balance and hurt the patient as well as yourself. Lower the patient to the floor while protecting the head from injury. Anytime a patient falls, call for assistance immediately. Do not leave or attempt to move the patient until the nurse tells you to do so. An incident report is written when a patient falls, even if there is no apparent injury. Incident reports are explained in Chapter 6.

Guidelines for Protecting the Falling Patient

- Walk at the patient's side and slightly behind.
- If the patient starts to fall, move your feet apart to increase stability.
- Pull the falling patient close to your body with the gait/transfer belt or place your arms under the patient's arms (Figure 19–3A).
- Position your leg so the patient's body can rest on it.
- Let the patient slide slowly down your leg to the floor (Figure 19–3B).
- Bend your knees as you lower the patient to the floor.
- Protect the patient's head from injury.
- Call for assistance and stay with the patient.
- Do not move the patient until the nurse tells you to do so.
- Report the details to the charge nurse and write an incident report.

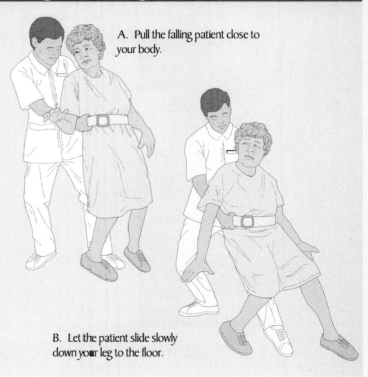

A. Pull the falling patient close to your body.

B. Let the patient slide slowly down your leg to the floor.

FIGURE 19–3 Protecting a falling patient.

Assistive Ambulation Devices: Canes, Walkers, and Crutches

Canes, walkers, and crutches are examples of devices used to assist patients in ambulation. They are used by patients who have been injured or have weakness or poor balance. These devices can make the difference between immobility and independence. The physical therapist or occupational therapist teaches patients how to use the equipment properly. As a nursing assistant, you will frequently be helping patients to use assistive ambulation devices. The following guidelines will be helpful.

Canes

A cane is usually held by the hand opposite the affected leg. To ambulate, the cane is moved forward and placed just ahead of the strong leg and slightly to the side of the strong foot. The patient steps forward with the affected leg and brings the foot even with the cane. The strong leg is then moved forward beyond the weak leg and the cane. To assist, you should stand at the patient's side opposite the cane. Steady or support the patient with your arm or a gait/transfer belt, if necessary. (See Figure 19–4.)

Walkers

There is a variety of walkers available to meet the patient's individual needs. (See Figure 19–5.) Some walkers have wheels, and some do not. The walker

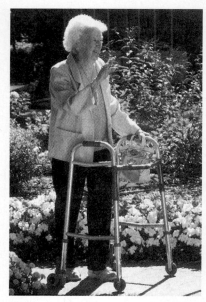

FIGURE 19–5
A walker can help a patient to ambulate independently.

handgrips should be at the patient's hip level. The patient should use both hands to lift the walker and move it forward about six inches at a time. The patient steps forward toward the walker with the affected foot first and then brings the strong foot forward, up to the affected foot.

Crutches

Crutch length must be fitted correctly, according to the patient's height. It is important that handgrips and underarm braces also fit (see Figure 19–6). A patient who uses crutches will be taught a specific step

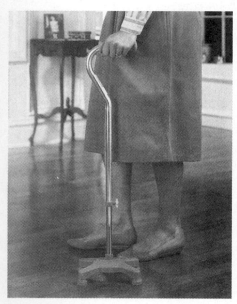

FIGURE 19–4
A cane may help the weak patient maintain independence.

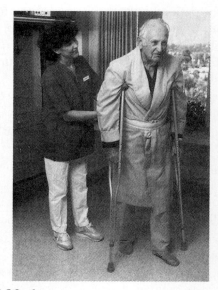

FIGURE 19–6
Remind the patient using crutches to place his or her weight on the handgrips.

and gait pattern. Remind the patient to place his or her weight on the handgrips, not under the arms. The top of the crutches should rest against the patient's upper side torso area—not against the axilla.

Guidelines for Using Assistive Ambulation Devices

■ Check the patient's care plan.

■ Check the ends of canes, walkers, and crutches to see that the rubber tips are intact.

■ Make sure all screws and bolts are in place and that the device is in good condition.

■ Instruct the patient not to use the walker or cane to pull up to a standing position.

■ Ensure that the hand piece of each device is level with the hips so there is a slight bend in the elbow when standing.

■ Encourage the patient to follow the therapist's instructions.

■ Repeat and reinforce the instructions as necessary.

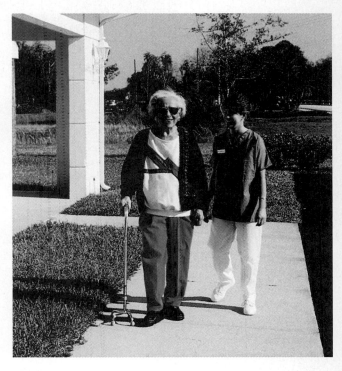

FIGURE 19–7
Walking is an excellent form of exercise.

Restorative Exercises

Restorative Exercise Programs

Restorative exercise programs help to prevent the complications of inactivity. They help patients to feel better physically and emotionally. Exercise improves circulation and helps to relieve anxiety, stress, and depression. Restorative exercise programs include aerobics, walking, and range of motion. Dangling and rocking are also forms of exercise.

A restorative exercise program is individually designed to meet each patient's needs. The patient will begin with light exercises and progress as tolerated. The exercise program should be challenging, but not exhausting. The program becomes a part of the patient's plan of care and is evaluated and changed as needed.

Walking

Walking is an excellent form of exercise that requires no special knowledge or equipment. Many people who are reluctant to do other exercises will enjoy walking. It is easily adapted to meet individual needs and preferences. A patient might enjoy a walk in the garden, a stroll through the gift shop, or just taking a few steps in the hallway. Walking allows the patient to make different choices from day to day. (See Figure 19–7.)

Dangling

For the patient who is unable to walk, dangling might be the exercise choice. Sitting on the edge of the bed places the patient in an upright position. It improves circulation and other bodily functions. Dangling increases strength and helps the patient regain balance. If able, the patient can swing the legs and move the feet and toes while dangling. Otherwise, the feet should be supported by a footstool. Remain nearby while a patient is dangling. The patient who complains of feeling faint should be returned to bed immediately.

Rocking

Rocking is a form of exercise that is often overlooked. It is an old-fashioned remedy that works just as well today. The back and forth motion of the rocking chair provides gentle exercise. It helps calm, soothe, and reduce stress. Confused patients, particularly those with Alzheimer's disease, may benefit from this type of exercise.

Range-of-Motion Exercises

Range-of-motion exercises are exercises that are performed to move each joint through its normal range of movement. They are a form of exercise for people who are weak or unable to move about on their own. Range-of-motion exercises help the patient to regain mobility after an illness and help to prevent complications, such as contractures (shortening of muscles due to lack of use).

Range-of-motion exercises may be active, assisted, or passive. The patient performs active range-of-motion exercises without assistance. Assisted range-of-motion exercises are performed with patients who cannot do the exercises by themselves. Your assistance would be to offer hands-on help, while encouraging the patient to do as much as possible independently. Passive range-of-motion exercises are done by someone else without assistance from the patient.

Range-of-motion exercises can be a part of self-care or activities of daily living. Brushing the hair, taking a bath, and feeding oneself provide opportunities for range of motion. Report any increase or decrease in range of motion to the charge nurse. Complaints of pain should also be reported.

Safety Factors for Range-of-Motion Exercises

Check the care plan or consult the charge nurse to find out which joints should be exercised and how much the patient can do independently. Use both hands to support the joint you are exercising. The exercise should be done with a slow, easy rhythm. Stop at the point of resistance or if the patient complains of pain. Watch the patient's face for signs of pain or discomfort. The exercises should be pleasant and relaxing, never painful. The number of times you repeat each exercise will depend on the patient's condition and tolerance. If range-of-motion is limited, exercise within those limitations and do not be discouraged. A small amount of mobility is better than none.

Many facilities do not allow nursing assistants to perform range-of-motion exercises on the patient's neck. These exercises are usually done by physical therapists. Follow the policy of the facility where you work. The terms used to describe movement and direction when performing range-of-motion exercises are described in the table in Figure 19–8.

Directions and Body Movements

- Abduction: Moving the arm or leg away from the body
- Adduction: Moving the arm or leg toward the body
- Extension: Straightening a body part
- Flexion: Bending a body part
- Rotation: Moving the joint in a circular motion
- Supination: Turning the palm upward
- Pronation: Turning the palm downward

- Radial deviation: Bending the wrist toward the thumb
- Ulnar deviation: Bending the wrist away from the thumb
- Dorsal flexion: Bending the foot backward toward the body
- Plantar flexion: Bending the foot toward the sole of the foot

FIGURE 19–8
Directions and body movements for range-of-motion exercises.

Procedure for Performing Range-of-Motion Exercises

Beginning Steps

- Identify the patient and explain the procedure.
- Collect necessary equipment and supplies.
- Wash your hands and use standard precautions.
- Protect the patient's privacy.
- Use correct body mechanics.

1. Raise the side rails and raise the bed to a comfortable working height. Lock the wheels and lower the side rail on your working side.
2. Place the patient in a supine position with the head supported on a pillow.
3. Exercise the shoulder as shown in Figure 19–9A and B.

4. Exercise the elbow and the forearm as shown in Figure 19–10.
5. Exercise the wrist as shown in Figure 19–11A, B, C, and D.
6. Exercise the fingers as shown in Figure 19–12A, B, and C.
7. Exercise the hip as shown in Figure 19–13A, B, and C.
8. Exercise the knee as shown in Figure 19–14.
9. Exercise the ankle as shown in Figure 19–15A and B.
10. Exercise toes as shown in Figure 19–16A and B.

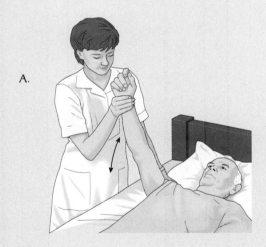

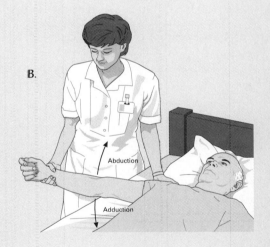

FIGURE 19–9
Range-of-motion exercises.

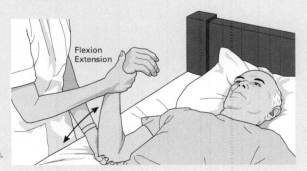

FIGURE 19–10
Exercise the elbow and the forearm.

Procedure for Performing Range-of-Motion Exercises (cont.)

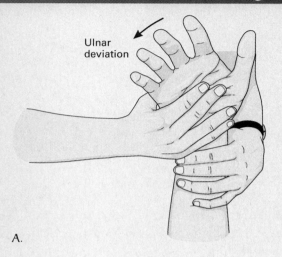

Ulnar deviation

A.

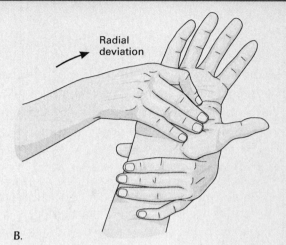

Radial deviation

B.

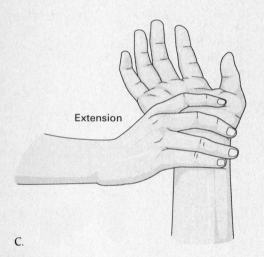

Extension

C.

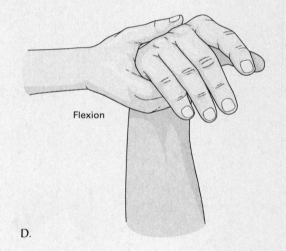

Flexion

D.

FIGURE 19–11
Exercise the wrist.

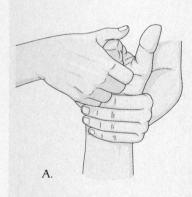

A.

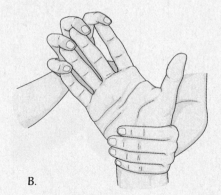

B.

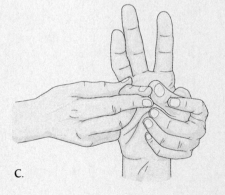

C.

FIGURE 19–12
Exercise the fingers.

Procedure for Performing Range-of-Motion Exercises (cont.)

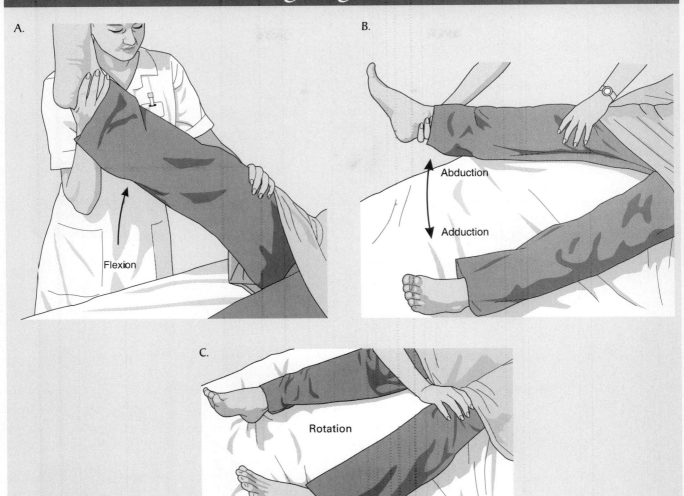

A.

Flexion

B.

Abduction

Adduction

C.

Rotation

FIGURE 19-13
Exercise the hip.

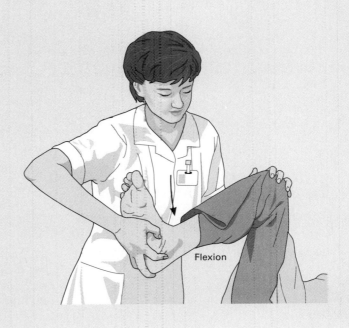

Flexion

FIGURE 19-14
Exercise the knee.

Procedure for Performing Range-of-Motion Exercises (cont.)

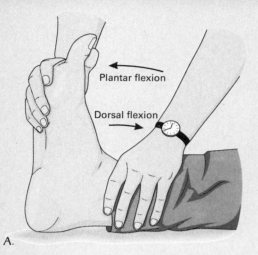

Plantar flexion

Dorsal flexion

A.

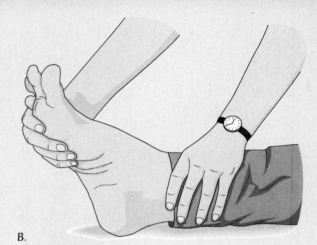

B.

FIGURE 19–15
Exercise the ankle.

A.

Extension

B.

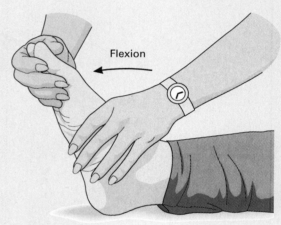

Flexion

FIGURE 19–16
Exercise the toes.

Review

Read each sentence and fill in the blank with the vocabulary term that best completes the sentence.

1. To _____ is to walk.
2. Giving power to enable a person to take charge of his or her own life is called _____.

3. _____ is the ability to move.
4. Bending a body part is called _____.
5. _____ are exercises that are performed to move each joint through its normal range of motion.

Remember

1. A restorative ambulation program must be designed for the individual patient.
2. Use correct body mechanics when you are assisting the patient with ambulation.
3. Using a gait/transfer belt reduces the risk of injury while you are assisting the patient with ambulation.
4. Canes provide balance and support when one side of the body is weak.
5. The walker handgrips should be at hip level.

6. Remind the patient using crutches to place his or her weight on the handgrips, not under the arms.
7. Restorative programs help to prevent the complications of limited activity.
8. Walking is an excellent form of exercise that requires no special knowledge or equipment.
9. Range-of-motion exercises help to prevent contractures.
10. Plan range-of-motion exercises as a part of the patient's daily care routines.

Reflect

Read the following case study and answer the questions.

Case Study

Melissa, a home health aide, is assigned to visit Mrs. Washington, who is recovering from a stroke that left her with weakness of the left side. Mrs. Washington has been taught to perform active range-of-motion exercises by the physical therapist. Melissa visits twice a week to assist her with activities of daily living. Part of her assignment is to assist Mrs. Washington with her exercises. Mrs. Washington begins the exercises of her left arm but gets mixed up and starts over several times. Melissa becomes impatient and says, "Don't worry about it.

I'll do the exercises for you." She moves each joint rapidly through the motions. While exercising the shoulder, Mrs. Washington complains of pain. Melissa continues the exercise and responds, "That's to be expected. Remember—no pain, no gain."

1. List four benefits of range-of-motion exercises?
2. What type of exercises did Melissa perform on Mrs. Washington? Was that the correct type?
3. What should Melissa have done when Mrs. Washington got mixed up in performing her exercises?
4. Identify two mistakes Melissa made while performing range-of-motion exercises.

Respond

Choose the best answer for each question.

1. Which of the following are benefits of ambulation?
   A. Increased muscle strength
   B. Stress reduction
   C. Increased appetite
   D. All of the above
2. Which of the following statements about using a gait belt to assist in ambulation is FALSE?
   A. Apply the gait belt around the patient's waist.
   B. Fasten the buckle slightly off-center.
   C. Walk directly behind the patient to keep him or her from falling.
   D. Keep both hands on the gait belt during ambulation.

3. The patient begins to fall while you are ambulating him. Which action is correct?
   A. Let him slide slowly down your leg to the floor.
   B. Place your feet together to increase stability.
   C. Grab him around the waist and try to hold him upright.
   D. Get out of the way so you don't get hurt.
4. The hand piece of the walker or cane should be at what level of the patient's body?
   A. Waist level
   B. Hip level
   C. Knee level
   D. Fingertip level

5. The patient using crutches should place his or her weight on the handgrips.
   A. True
   B. False
6. Which of the following are restorative exercises?
   A. Walking
   B. Dangling
   C. Rocking
   D. All of the above
7. Range-of-motion exercises the patient performs without assistance are called
   A. Active exercises
   B. Assisted exercises
   C. Passive exercises
   D. Aerobic exercises
8. A patient complains of pain while you are exercising his shoulder. Which response is correct?
   A. Tell him to take deep breaths and the pain will go away.
   B. Stop the exercises and notify the nurse.
   C. Continue the exercises and record his response.
   D. Stop exercising that joint and go to another.
9. Moving the arm or leg away from the body is called
   A. Abduction
   B. Adduction
   C. Extension
   D. Flexion
10. Moving a joint in a circular motion is called
   A. Abduction
   B. Flexion
   C. Rotation
   D. Pronation

Chapter Twenty

Personal Care *and* Hygiene

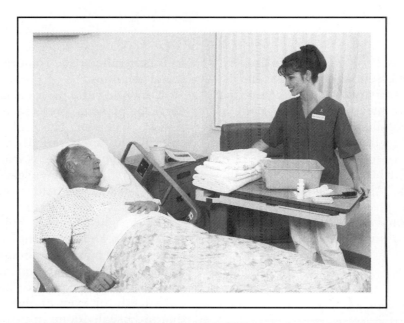

axilla   The armpit.
dentures   A partial or complete set of artificial teeth.
oral hygiene   Cleaning and care of the mouth, teeth, and gums.

perineal care (peri-care)   Cleansing the genital and anal areas.

A ssisting patients with personal care and hygiene can provide essential services for the patient and bring satisfaction to the nursing assistant. Personal care measures include many of the patient's activities of daily living (ADLs) such as bathing, brushing the teeth, combing the hair, and dressing. Hygiene refers to cleanliness and health. These procedures contribute to the patient's comfort and quality of life. Always encourage the patient to do as much as possible independently. The ability to provide personal care and hygiene for oneself is a true measure of independence. (See Figure 20–1.)

*H*olistic Personal Care

The concept of treating the whole person as an individual especially applies to personal care and hygiene. While these procedures provide for physical needs, such as cleanliness and infection control, they meet psychosocial needs as well. For example, shampooing and combing the patient's hair not only keeps it clean and manageable, but it also improves appearance and self-esteem. Because the patient

feels better, he or she is more likely to participate in social activities.

Grooming and personal care practices are influenced by personal preference and vary greatly from person to person. The preferences are affected by culture and family practices. For example, patients from areas where water is scarce or the climate is extremely cold may view cleanliness differently than others. Most people hold strong opinions about how, when, and where to perform personal care. Patients have the right to make choices according to their preferences, and those choices should be respected and followed whenever possible.

Personal care and hygiene practices are private activities for most people. Taking a bath, brushing one's teeth, or even applying deodorant are tasks that are usually done in private. A patient may become embarrassed if these intimate activities are performed in the presence of others. It is important that you do all that you can to protect the patient's privacy. Do not unnecessarily expose the patient's body during personal care procedures. Close the door, the window drapes, and the privacy curtain when you are assisting with patient care. If the door is closed, knock and wait for a response before entering.

Communicate with the patient while assisting with personal care and hygiene. Encourage the patient to talk, and listen attentively. Use your skills of observation. Look at the patient's skin as you help with the bath, listen to breath sounds, notice any unusual smells. Pay close attention to the patient's complaints. These observations will make reporting and recording more meaningful.

Special restorative equipment is available to help patients with personal care and hygiene. This type of equipment helps patients perform procedures independently. Check the care plan to see what equipment has been ordered for the patient. (See Figure 20–2.)

Infection Control

Use aseptic practices and standard precautions with all patients. Be aware of the policies of your facility regarding the use of protective equipment such as gloves and gowns. For example, some facilities require that gloves be worn during the entire bath pro-

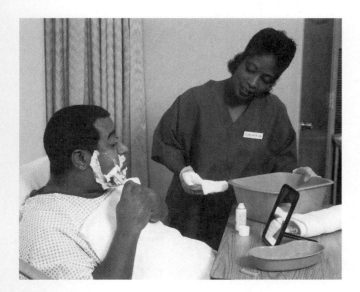

FIGURE 20–1
Encourage the patient to do as much as possible independently.

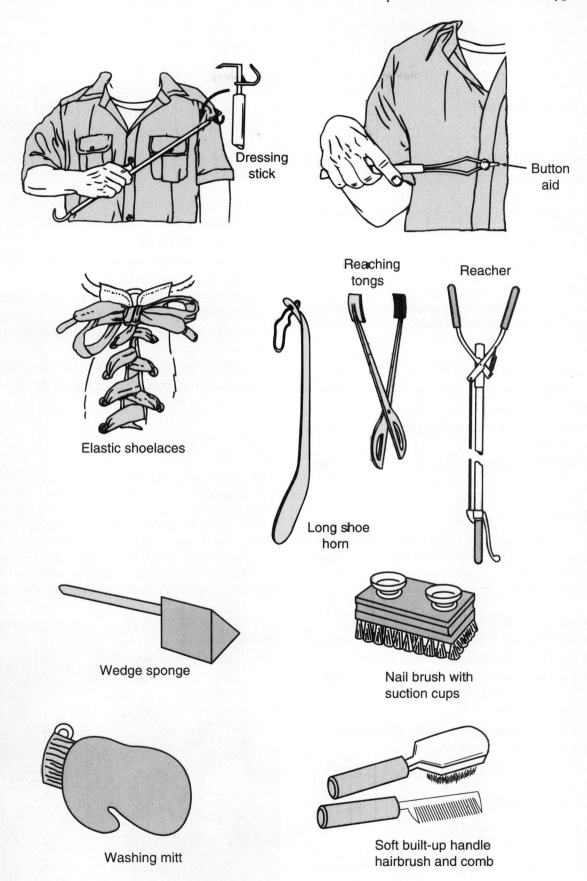

Dressing stick

Button aid

Elastic shoelaces

Reaching tongs

Reacher

Long shoe horn

Wedge sponge

Nail brush with suction cups

Washing mitt

Soft built-up handle hairbrush and comb

FIGURE 20–2
Examples of restorative equipment used for personal care and hygiene.

cedure, while others do not. Always wear gloves when there is a possibility of contact with blood, body fluids, or nonintact skin. Wear gloves if you have a rash or open wound on your hands. Handle soiled linen carefully. Handwashing may be necessary several times during a procedure.

Daily Care Routines

Health care facilities follow daily routines or schedules in order to ensure that patients receive personal care and hygiene. These routines should be flexible enough to allow for patient choice and personal preference.

Early A.M. Care

Early A.M., or early morning, care is given before breakfast to help the patient wake up and get ready for breakfast. Early A.M. care tasks include:

- Assisting with toileting
- Assisting the patient to wash the face and hands
- Providing *oral hygiene* (mouth care)
- Seeing that eyeglasses and hearing aide are available, if needed
- Positioning the patient for breakfast or assisting to the dining area

A.M. Care

A.M. care or morning care is provided after breakfast. Check the patient's care plan to determine if the patient is to have a complete bath, partial bath, tub bath, or shower. A.M. care tasks include:

- Assisting with toileting
- Assisting with oral hygiene
- Assisting with bathing and giving a backrub
- Assisting with *perineal care (peri-care)* (cleansing the genital and anal areas)
- Assisting the patient to dress.
- Assisting the patient with grooming (hair care, shaving, and applying makeup)
- Assisting the patient to the chair or wheelchair
- Making the bed
- Tidying the patient's unit

Afternoon Care

Afternoon care is given after lunch and includes the following tasks:

- Assisting with toileting
- Assisting the patient to wash the face and hands

- Assisting with oral hygiene
- Straightening the bed linens and tidying the unit

H.S. Care

The abbreviation H.S. stands for hour of sleep or bedtime. It is given when the patient is preparing for sleep and may be called evening care or P.M. care. The purpose of H.S. care is to help the patient relax and prepare for sleep. H.S. care tasks include:

- Assisting with toileting
- Providing peri-care when necessary
- Assisting with oral hygiene
- Assisting the patient to wash the face and hands
- Giving a relaxing backrub
- Changing the patient's gown or assisting into nightclothes
- Straightening bed linens and providing an extra blanket, if needed
- Assisting the patient to a comfortable position
- Straightening the unit (See Figure 20–3.)

Oral Hygiene

Oral care is important to patient health and comfort. Illness, treatment, or medication may cause an unpleasant taste in the mouth or an odor to the breath. Oral hygiene involves brushing the teeth, gums, and tongue. Flossing the teeth and rinsing the mouth with mouthwash can also be included. Cleaning *dentures* (false teeth) is also part of oral hygiene. Oral hygiene is provided in the morning,

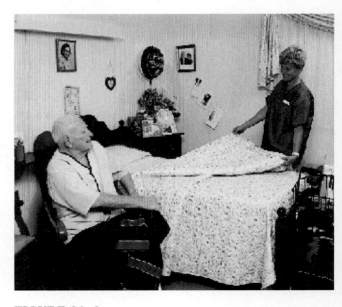

FIGURE 20–3
H.S. care helps the patient relax and prepare for sleep.

Procedure for Assisting the Patient to Brush the Teeth

Beginning Steps

■ Identify the patient and explain the procedure.
■ Collect necessary equipment and supplies.
■ Wash your hands and use standard precautions.
■ Protect the patient's privacy.
■ Use correct body mechanics.

1. Place equipment and supplies on the overbed table.
2. Raise the side rails, raise the bed to a comfortable working height, and lock the wheels.
3. Raise the head of the bed and lower the side rail on your working side.
4. Place a bath towel across the patient's chest.
5. Place the overbed table across the bed in front of the patient.
6. Put on gloves if you will be assisting the patient in brushing the teeth.
7. Place toothpaste on a wet toothbrush and encourage the patient to do the brushing. All surfaces of the teeth, gums, and the tongue should be brushed.
8. Allow the patient to rinse the mouth with water or diluted mouthwash. You may need to hold the emesis basin to the chin for expectoration (Figure 20–4).
9. Assist with flossing the teeth, if necessary.
10. Assist the patient to rinse the mouth and expectorate into the emesis basin. Wipe the patient's mouth, if necessary.

11. Clean and put away equipment. Discard disposables in the proper container.
12. Wipe off the overbed table.
13. Remove the gloves and dispose of them in the proper container. Wash your hands.

Ending Steps

■ Check to see that the patient is comfortable.
■ Lower the bed and raise the side rails, if appropriate.
■ Place the call signal within the patient's reach.
■ Wash your hands.
■ Report and record your observations.

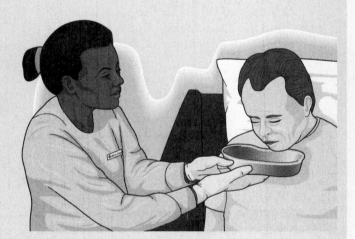

FIGURE 20–4
Hold the emesis basin under the patient's chin for expectoration.

after meals, and at bedtime. It is necessary at least every two hours for the comatose (unconscious or unresponsive) patient. A patient with a tube in the nose or a patient receiving oxygen will require oral care more frequently.

Assisting the patient with oral hygiene allows an excellent time for observation. Remember that listening is a part of observation because there are some things that you cannot know unless the patient tells you. For example, you cannot observe that the patient has a toothache or a bad taste in the mouth. Observations of the mouth that should be reported include:

■ Loose, broken, decayed teeth, or cavities (holes in the teeth)
■ Spongy, pale, swollen, or bleeding gums
■ White, gray, or black patches or coating on the tongue

■ Swelling, redness, sores, bleeding, or white patches on the mucous membranes of the mouth
■ Chapped, blistered, cracked, or swollen lips
■ Unpleasant mouth odor
■ Loose, chipped, or broken dentures
■ Patient complaints

Some patients will be able to perform oral hygiene independently, while others will need you to assist or provide the care for them. Confused or forgetful patients may be able to provide their own oral care if reminded and assisted to do so. The procedure for assisting the patient to brush the teeth is shown above.

Flossing the Teeth

The teeth are flossed to remove food particles from between the teeth. It also helps to remove sub-

Procedure for Giving Oral Care to the Comatose Patient

Beginning Steps

- Identify the patient and explain the procedure.
- Collect necessary equipment and supplies.
- Wash your hands and use standard precautions.
- Protect the patient's privacy.
- Use correct body mechanics.

1. Place equipment and supplies on the overbed table.
2. Raise the side rails, raise the bed to a comfortable working height, and lock the wheels.
3. Put on gloves and lower the side rail nearest you.
4. Position the patient with the head to one side.
5. Place a bath towel under the patient's head and face and the emesis basin under the side of the chin to catch secretions or fluid coming from the mouth.
6. Use a padded tongue blade to separate the teeth and open the mouth (Figure 20–5).
7. Clean the mouth using toothettes, commercially prepared swabs, or a padded tongue blade with diluted mouth wash. Clean inner surfaces of the mouth including the gums, teeth, and tongue. Wipe secretions from the lips and corners of the mouth.
8. Apply lubricant to the lips, if needed.
9. Reposition the patient and raise the side rail.
10. Clean and put away equipment and discard disposables.
11. Wipe off the overbed table.

12. Remove your gloves and wash your hands. Dispose of gloves in the proper container.

Ending Steps

- Check to see that the patient is comfortable.
- Lower the bed to the floor and raise the side rails, if appropriate.
- Place the call signal within the patient's reach.
- Wash your hands.
- Report and record your observations.

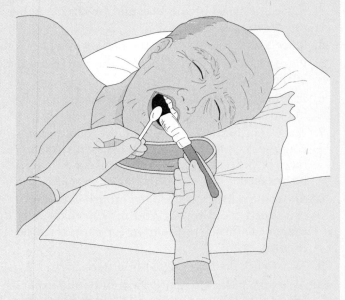

FIGURE 20–5
Use a padded tongue blade to separate the teeth and open the mouth of the comatose patient.

stances from tooth surfaces. A special string called dental floss is pulled between the teeth and to the gumline next to each tooth. Some patients are unable to floss their own teeth, and you will need to perform the procedure for them.

Providing Oral Care for the Comatose Patient

Mouth care on an unconscious patient must be performed more frequently to prevent infection, odor, and discomfort. When a person becomes unconscious, muscles relax. As the jaw muscles relax, the mouth hangs open, causing the mouth, tongue, and lips to become dry. Oral secretions may accumulate due to the inability to cough or clear the throat. These conditions create discomfort and provide an environment for the growth of pathogens. Oral hygiene should be performed at least every two hours for the comatose patient.

Most comatose patients are unable to swallow. Position the comatose patient on his or her side for oral care to prevent aspiration (choking). Commercially prepared swabs or toothettes may be used in place of a toothbrush. A tongue blade wrapped in gauze and moistened with diluted mouthwash may be used if commercial products are not available.

Always assume that the comatose patient can hear you. Explain the procedure and talk to the patient. Carefully explain what you are going to do and what equipment you are going to use. You might say something like, "Do not be frightened. I am going to clean your mouth using a special swab. It is moist and has a lemony taste."

Procedure for Care of Dentures

Beginning Steps

- Identify the patient and explain the procedure.
- Collect necessary equipment and supplies.
- Wash your hands and use standard precautions.
- Protect the patient's privacy.
- Use correct body mechanics.

1. Place the necessary equipment at the sink.
2. Take the emesis basin, mouth wash, glass of water, and gloves to the bedside. Line the basin with a paper towel.
3. Place the towel over the patient's chest.
4. Put on the gloves.
5. Ask the patient to remove the dentures, and place them in the emesis basin.
6. If the patient cannot remove the dentures, you may do so as follows:
   a. Move the upper denture up and down slightly by grasping it with your thumb and index finger at the front. This breaks the seal.
   b. Remove the denture and place it into the emesis basin.
   c. Grasp the lower denture at the front with your thumb and index finger.
   d. Remove it gently, turning it to bring the end of one side out before the other. Place the lower denture into the emesis basin.
7. Take the dentures in the lined emesis basin to the sink (Figure 20–6A).

8. Place a paper towel or clean washcloth in the sink and fill the sink with water to cushion the dentures in case they slip from your hands.
9. Place toothpaste or denture cleaner on each denture.
10. Holding one denture in your palm, brush all surfaces thoroughly. Return it to the emesis basin while you brush the other denture (Figure 20–6B).
11. Rinse each denture thoroughly, one at a time, under cool running water.
12. Place the dentures in the denture cup labeled with the patient's name and fill with fresh cool water.
13. Rinse the emesis basin.
14. Bring the emesis basin and dentures to the patient.
15. Brush the patient's tongue and gums and assist the patient to rinse out the mouth. You may hold the emesis basin to one side of the patient's chin for expectoration.
16. Have the patient replace the dentures.
17. If the patient is unable to replace dentures, proceed as follows:
   a. With your thumb and finger at the front of the upper denture, insert it into the patient's mouth. Lift the upper lip with your other hand.
   b. If necessary, turn the denture slightly to the side to insert one side, and then turn it gently against the inner cheek to insert the other side.

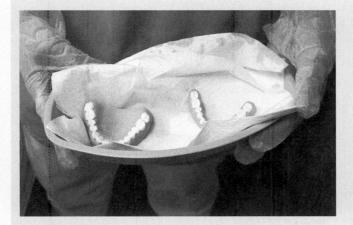

A. Take the dentures in a lined emesis basin to the sink.

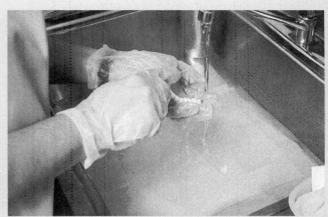

B. Holding the dentures in your palm, brush all surfaces thoroughly.

FIGURE 20–6 Performing denture care.

Procedure for Care of Dentures (cont.)

c. Secure it by pressing it into place lightly.

d. With your thumb and index finger at the front of the lower denture, insert it. Lower the bottom lip and if necessary, turn the denture to insert it. Gently press downward to secure it.

18. Cover the labeled denture cup, which has been filled with clean water, and leave it at the patient's bedside. If dentures are not to be replaced in the patient's mouth, place them in the denture cup. Put the cup in the top drawer of the bedside table.

19. Return equipment and supplies to proper storage.

20. Remove the gloves and discard them in the proper container. Wash your hands.

Ending Steps

■ Check to see that the patient is comfortable.

■ Lower the bed and raise the side rails, if appropriate.

■ Place the call signal within the patient's reach.

■ Wash your hands.

■ Report and record your observations.

Denture Care

Dentures should be cleaned as often as natural teeth. A patient may have an upper plate (denture), a lower plate, or both.

The patient may have a special brush and cleanser for cleaning dentures. However, a regular toothbrush and toothpaste will work just as well. If denture tablets are used for cleaning and soaking, the dentures should be brushed and rinsed first. The mouth should be cleaned and rinsed while the dentures are out. Do not forget to wash and rinse the denture cup after using it.

People who wear dentures are sometimes embarrassed about their use. Always provide privacy and encourage self-care when possible. However, it will be necessary for you to clean some patients' dentures yourself. Examine the dentures carefully for cracks and missing teeth. Observe the inside of the mouth, gums, and tongue. Report to the nurse if dentures are damaged or do not fit properly.

Handle the dentures carefully while removing, cleaning, and returning them to the patient's mouth. Carry them to the bathroom in an emesis basin lined with tissues or filled with water. Use cool water for cleaning the dentures because hot water may cause them to warp. You may be guilty of negligence if dentures are damaged because you failed to use proper precautions. These precautions are included in the procedure for care of dentures located on page 259.

Encourage the patient to place the dentures in cool water in the denture cup when not wearing them. Label the container or cup with the patient's name and room number. When stripping the bed, look for dentures mixed up with the linen. Also check the meal tray before returning it to the food cart because some patients remove their dentures while they eat.

Restorative Skin Care

Personal care procedures provide excellent opportunities for observation of the skin. While giving a complete bath, you can examine the patient's entire body. Pay special attention to the bony prominences (areas where the bone is close to the skin, and there is little padding) such as the hips, coccyx (tailbone), and ankles. Check skin folds and creases under the arms and behind the knees. Observe and report skin that is

■ Pale, dark, or reddened in color.

■ Rough or chapped in texture.

■ Dry or flaking, lacking in moisture.

■ Injured (blisters, bruises, or lacerations).

■ Sore (pressure sores or infection).

One of the best ways to prevent pressure sores is to keep the skin clean, dry, and healthy. Skin is healthier when it receives adequate circulation of blood. Washing, rinsing, and drying the skin stimulates circulation and increases blood flow. Giving a backrub and massaging the skin with lotion also increases circulation and helps keep the skin moist. If the patient is incontinent (unable to control urine or feces), the skin must be cleaned and dried immediately after each incontinent episode to prevent skin breakdown or infection.

Giving a Backrub and Applying Lotion

A backrub or massage is enjoyed and appreciated by most patients. It relaxes muscles and relieves ten-

Procedure for Giving a Backrub

Beginning Steps

- Identify the patient and explain the procedure.
- Collect necessary equipment and supplies.
- Wash your hands and use standard precautions.
- Protect the patient's privacy.
- Use correct body mechanics.

1. Raise the side rails, raise the head of the bed to a comfortable working height, and lock the wheels.
2. Lower the side rail on the side nearest you.
3. Assist the patient onto the abdomen or the side, with the patient's back toward you.
4. Expose the patient's back and drape the rest of the body with a bath blanket or sheet.
5. Pour lotion onto your hands and warm it by rubbing your hands together briskly.
6. Warn the patient that the lotion may feel cool and moist.
7. Apply lotion by using long, firm strokes with both hands. Do not lift your hands from the skin.

8. Stroke upward from the buttocks toward the shoulders. Circle with your hands at the shoulders and stroke down the upper arm. Stroke back up the arms, across the shoulders, and down the back. (See Figure 20–7.)
9. Repeat step 8 for approximately three minutes.
10. Using a circular motion, massage the bony areas of the back.
11. Let the patient know when you are finished.
12. Remove the bath blanket and assist the patient to dress. Straighten the linen.

Ending Steps

- Check to see that the patient is comfortable.
- Lower the bed and raise the side rails, if appropriate.
- Place the call signal within the patient's reach.
- Wash your hands.
- Report and record your observations.

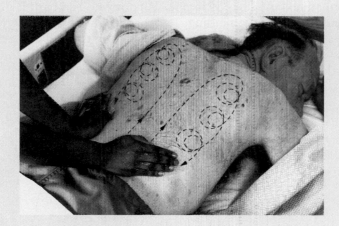

FIGURE 20–7
When giving a backrub, use circular motions to promote circulation over bony prominences.

sion. Massaging backrubs help prevent skin breakdown by stimulating and increasing circulation to the area. Backrubs are routinely given with A.M. care, H.S. care, and after repositioning a bedbound patient.

Warm the lotion before using it by holding the bottle under warm, running water or by rubbing the lotion between your hands. The feel of cold lotion or cold hands is neither pleasant nor relaxing. There are some patients who do not like a backrub or who are not allowed to have one. Check the patient's care plan or ask the nurse if you are not sure

what to do. The procedure for giving a backrub is shown above.

Applying Lotion to Dry Skin

Certain areas of the skin, such as the elbows and heels, tend to be very dry. Applying lotion to these areas helps keep the skin soft and prevent cracking. Massaging and rubbing the lotion into the skin is relaxing and also increases blood circulation. If there is a reddened area on the skin, massage around it. Massaging over a reddened area can cause further skin breakdown.

Bathing

Bathing is one of the most appreciated procedures that you may assist the patient to perform. It cleanses the body by removing dirt and dead skin cells while promoting comfort, controlling odor, and helping to prevent infection. Bathing also provides exercise, increases circulation, and helps prevent skin breakdown.

Methods of bathing include the complete bed bath, partial bath, tub bath, specialty bath, and shower. The patient's personal preference, physical condition, and level of independence will determine the method of bathing required. In long-term care facilities, showers or specialty baths are most frequently used because of their restorative value. The type of bath the patient is to have will be indicated on the care plan.

Encourage patients to do as much of the bath as possible for themselves. Place bath equipment and supplies within the patient's reach to promote patient independence. Praise all efforts, regardless of success. For example, if a patient wants to wash the perineal area himself, but does not thoroughly clean the area, you will need to finish the procedure. Avoid negative comments like, "You didn't get the area clean. I'll have to do it for you." That kind of statement can embarrass and discourage the patient. Try saying something like, "You did great! Let me make sure that all the soap is rinsed off." Then you can clean the area correctly without making the patient feel inadequate.

Offer toileting before beginning the bath because water stimulates the urge to urinate. Make sure that the room temperature is comfortable and that the bath water temperature is between 105° and 115° Fahrenheit. Change the water as often as needed if it cools or becomes soapy or dirty. Uncover, wash, rinse, and dry only one body part at a time. The rest of the patient's body should be covered by a bath blanket for warmth and privacy. Make a mitt of the washcloth to prevent loose ends from splashing water (Figure 20–8). Rinse soap thoroughly from the patient's body and thoroughly pat the skin dry. If the patient is incontinent during the bath, the skin must be cleansed and the linen changed immediately. Wash, rinse, and dry the soiled areas before obtaining a clean towel, washcloth, and water and continuing the bath.

Giving the patient a good bath can be a lengthy procedure. Use the time wisely for communication and observation. Observe the patient's skin while giving the bath and report your observations to the nurse. Bathing is a nurturing process that should be pleasant for both you and the patient.

The Complete Bed Bath

A complete bed bath is given to patients who are not able to bathe themselves. Patients who need this type of bath may be seriously ill, completely helpless, or comatose. Encourage the patient to participate if allowed.

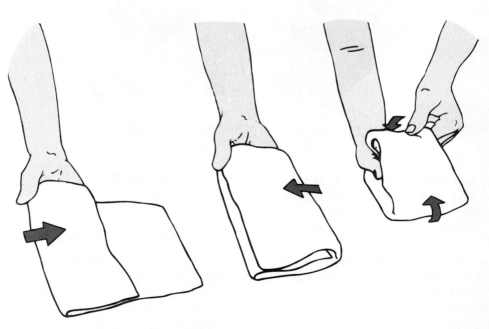

FIGURE 20–8
Make a mitt of the washcloth.

Procedure for Giving a Complete Bed Bath

Beginning Steps

■ Identify the patient and explain the procedure.
■ Collect necessary equipment and supplies.
■ Wash your hands and use standard precautions.
■ Protect the patient's privacy.
■ Use correct body mechanics.

1. Raise the side rails, raise the bed to a comfortable working height, and lock the wheels.
2. Offer the bedpan to the patient.
3. Adjust the bed to as flat a position as possible.
4. Check for drafts and proper room temperature.
5. Arrange the equipment on the overbed table.
6. Remove the bedspread and blanket from the bed. Fold them over the back of the chair.
7. Lower the side rail nearest you and position the patient on that side of the bed.
8. Place the bath blanket over the top sheet. Remove the top sheet from under the bath blanket without uncovering the patient (see Figure 20–9).
9. Remove the patient's clothes. Raise the side rail.
10. Fill the bath basin two-thirds full with water that is a comfortable temperature (approximately 105° F to 115° F).

11. Lower the side rail on the side of the bed nearest you while leaving the rail on the opposite side raised.
12. Place the towel over the patient's chest.
13. Make a mitt with the washcloth.
14. Wash the eyes from the nose (inner part) toward the ear (outer part), using a different corner of the mitt for each eye. Do not use soap. Wash and rinse the face, ears, and neck. Pat dry.
15. Place a towel lengthwise under the arm farthest from you. Support the arm with your palm under the elbow while using long firm strokes to wash the arm, the *axilla* (underarm), and the shoulder. Observe these areas carefully. The hand may be soaked in the basin of water when possible (Figure 20–10). Rinse, pat dry, and cover the arm.
16. While the fingernails are damp, clean under them with an orange stick and push back the cuticle (extra skin at the base of the fingernail), if needed.
17. Repeat steps 15 and 16 for the arm nearest you.
18. Place the bath towel across the patient's chest. Reach under the towel and fold the bath blanket to the waist. Lifting the towel partially, wash, rinse, and dry the chest. Observe the skin under the female patient's breasts carefully for reddened areas.

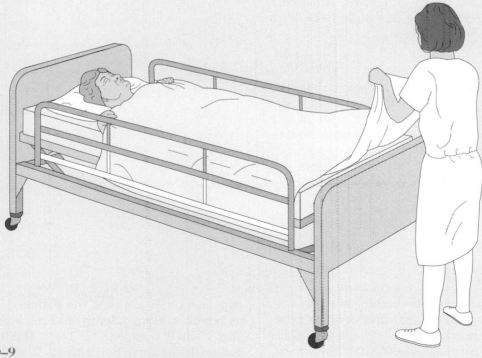

FIGURE 20–9
Remove the top sheet from under the bath blanket without uncovering the patient.

Procedure for Giving a Complete Bed Bath (cont.)

19. With the towel covering the chest, fold the bath blanket to the pubic area. Wash the abdomen and navel. Observe any abdominal skin folds for irritation. Rinse and pat dry. Cover the chest and abdomen with the bath blanket and remove the towel.

20. Uncover the leg farther from you and place a towel under it lengthwise. Have the patient flex the knee if possible, or place your palm under the knee to support the leg. Wash the leg and foot, carefully observing for skin problems at the knee, ankle, and heel, and between the toes. Wash thoroughly between the toes. The foot may be soaked in a basin of water if possible. Pat dry, taking special care to dry thoroughly between the toes.

21. Observe the toenails and perform nail care according to facility policy (see Nail Care on page 270). Cover the leg and foot with the bath blanket.

22. Repeat steps 20 and 21 for the leg nearest you.

23. Change the bath water and rinse the basin. Raise the side rail whenever you leave the bedside.

24. Lower the side rail and assist the patient to turn onto the side facing away from you.

25. Place the towel lengthwise on the bed along the patient's back. Wash the back, the back of the neck, and the buttocks with firm, long, and circular strokes. Carefully observe bony prominences at the shoulder blades, sacrum, coccyx, and hips. Dry the area and remove the towel. A backrub may be given at this time (see Backrub on page 261). Assist the patient to return to the back.

26. Change the bath water and rinse the basin. Raise the side rail when you leave the bedside.

27. Lower the side rail and place a towel under the thighs and buttocks. Put on gloves and use a clean washcloth to wash the perineal area (see Perineal Care on page 269). Wash from front to back on the female patient. For male patients, wash the penis and scrotum. Rinse and dry thoroughly. Observe the perineal area carefully.

Patients who are able to do so may prefer to do this part of the bath themselves.

28. Remove the gloves and discard them in the proper container. Wash your hands.

29. Assist the patient to dress and complete grooming.

30. Raise the side rail.

31. Empty, rinse, and dry the bath basin and return equipment and supplies to their proper place. Place soiled linen in the hamper.

32. Wipe off the overbed table with a paper towel.

33. Assist the patient out of bed, when possible, and make the bed.

34. If the patient is to remain in bed, make an occupied bed.

Ending Steps

■ Check to see that the patient is comfortable.
■ Lower the bed and raise the side rails, if appropriate.
■ Place the call signal within the patient's reach.
■ Wash your hands.
■ Report and record your observations.

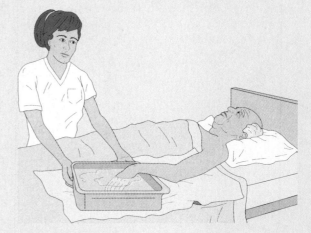

FIGURE 20–10
Soak the patient's hands in a basin of warm water when possible.

The Partial Bath

A partial bath usually involves bathing the areas of the body that cause discomfort and odor or need daily cleaning. These areas include the face, hands, axillae, back, and perineal area. Collect the necessary equipment and supplies and place them within the patient's reach to help promote the patient's independence. Encourage the patient to do as much as possible independently and reassure him or her that you will complete the bath. The following procedure is for a partial bath for a self-care patient. The procedure for assisting a self-care patient with a partial bath is shown on the facing page.

Procedure for Assisting a Self-Care Patient with a Partial Bath

Beginning Steps

■ Identify the patient and explain the procedure.
■ Collect necessary equipment and supplies.
■ Wash your hands and use standard precautions.
■ Protect the patient's privacy.
■ Use correct body mechanics.

1. Raise the side rails, raise the bed to a comfortable working height, and lock the wheels.
2. Raise the head of the bed so that the patient is in a sitting position.
3. Lower the side rail on your near side and position the overbed table in front of the patient.
4. Place a paper towel on the overbed table and arrange the bathing supplies within the patient's reach. (See Figure 20–11.)
5. Fill the bath basin two-thirds full with water that is a comfortable temperature (between 105° F and 115° F).
6. Place the basin of water on the paper towels on the overbed table.
7. Instruct the patient to wash as much of his or her body as possible. Provide assurance that you will wash areas that the patient is unable to reach.
8. Place the call signal within the patient's reach and instruct him to call when finished or if help is needed.
9. Wash your hands and leave the room, closing the door behind you.
10. Return to the room when the patient signals. Check on the patient at regular intervals if it seems to be taking a long time. However, do not take over until it is necessary.
11. Wash your hands and put on gloves.
12. Wash the areas of the body that the patient could not reach.

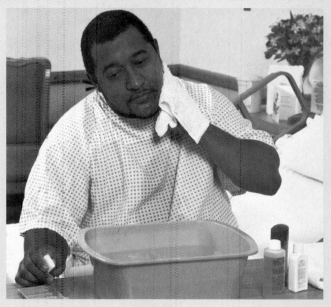

FIGURE 20–11
Place the bath basin of water and other supplies within the patient's reach and allow him to do as much of his bath as possible.

13. Apply lotion and give the patient a backrub. Lotion may also be applied to dry skin areas, such as the heels.
14. Apply deodorant or antiperspirant if the patient has not already done so.
15. Assist the patient to dress.
16. Remove your gloves and discard them in the proper container. Wash your hands.

Ending Steps

■ Check to see that the patient is comfortable.
■ Lower the bed and raise the side rails if appropriate.
■ Place the call signal within the patient's reach.
■ Wash your hands.
■ Report and record your observations.

Assisting the Patient to Shower

Using a shower to bathe provides many advantages. A continuous flow of clean water does a thorough job of rinsing off dirt and soap. It is easier to get in and out of a shower stall than it is a bathtub. A patient may stand in the shower or sit in a shower chair (a wheeled chair, usually made of plastic, that can remain in the shower during the procedure). Because a shower chair is lightweight and easily turned over, the patient should never be left alone in it. A lightweight shower stretcher that the patient can lie on while receiving a shower may also be available. Water runs through the mesh material of the stretcher. For some very weak patients, it is preferable to a shower chair.

Safety in the Shower or Tub

The safety rules listed on page 267 will help protect the patient from injury, infection, and chilling during a shower or a tub bath:

Procedure for Assisting the Patient to Shower

Beginning Steps

- Identify the patient and explain the procedure.
- Collect necessary equipment and supplies.
- Wash your hands and use standard precautions.
- Protect the patient's privacy.
- Use correct body mechanics.

1. Arrange supplies and equipment on a chair near the shower.
2. Assist the patient to the shower room. Transfer to a shower chair if necessary, once the patient is in the shower area. (See Figure 20–12.)
3. Turn the water on and adjust the temperature and pressure.
4. Assist the patient to undress.
5. Assist the patient into the shower. If a shower chair is used, lock the wheels.
6. Provide the patient with soap and a washcloth. Encourage self-care and stand by to assist as needed.
7. After the patient has finished bathing and rinsing, turn off the water.
8. Provide towels for drying. Assist as necessary to be sure the patient is completely dry.
9. If gloves were used, remove the gloves and discard them in the proper container. Wash your hands.
10. Assist the patient to dress and leave the shower area.
11. Return equipment and supplies to their proper place.
12. Put on gloves to clean the shower. Place soiled linen in the hamper.
13. Remove gloves and discard them in the proper container. Wash your hands.
14. Assist the patient with complete grooming.

Ending Steps

- Check to see that the patient is comfortable.
- Lower the bed and raise the side rails if appropriate.
- Place the call signal within the patient's reach.
- Wash your hands.
- Report and record your observations.

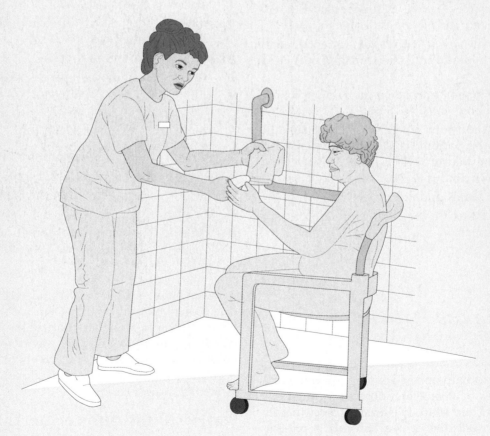

FIGURE 20–12
The patient may sit in a shower chair while taking a shower.

- Never leave a patient alone in the shower or tub.
- Adjust the water temperature and pressure before the patient enters the shower.
- Assist the patient in and out of the shower or tub to prevent falling on slippery floors.

- Provide a large towel for cover and adjust the room temperature to avoid chilling.
- Clean the shower or tub before and after use.
- Wear gloves for the entire procedure if required by facility policy.

Procedure for Assisting the Patient with a Tub Bath

Beginning Steps

- Identify the patient and explain the procedure.
- Collect necessary equipment and supplies.
- Wash your hands and use standard precautions.
- Protect the patient's privacy.
- Use correct body mechanics.

1. Arrange supplies and equipment on a chair near the tub.
2. Assist the patient to the bathroom (see Figure 20–13).
3. Put on gloves and clean the tub.
4. Remove gloves and discard them in the proper container. Wash your hands.
5. Fill the tub half-full of water that is a comfortable temperature (approximately 105° F).
6. Place a towel or bath mat on the floor beside the tub.
7. Assist the patient to undress.
8. Assist the patient into the tub.
9. Provide the patient with soap and a washcloth. Encourage self-care but be prepared to assist. Wear gloves if necessary.

10. Place a towel on the chair and drain the tub.
11. Put a towel around the patient's shoulders to prevent chilling.
12. Provide towels for drying and assist as necessary.
13. If gloves were used, remove the gloves and dispose of them in the proper container. Wash your hands.
14. Assist the patient to dress and leave the bathroom.
15. Return supplies and equipment to their proper place.
16. Put on gloves and wash the tub. Place soiled linen in the hamper.
17. Remove gloves and discard them in the proper container. Wash your hands.
18. Assist the patient with grooming.

Ending Steps

- Check to see that the patient is comfortable.
- Lower the bed and raise the side rails if appropriate.
- Place the call signal within the patient's reach.
- Wash your hands.
- Report and record your observations.

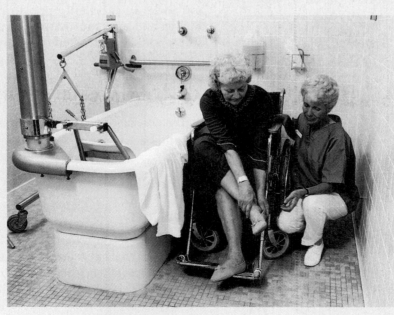

FIGURE 20–13
Assisting the patient with a tub bath.

Assisting with a Tub Bath

Patients who usually take a tub bath at home may wish to follow the same routine in the health care facility. Bathing in a warm tub of water can be relaxing and satisfying, as well as a way to get clean.

The Specialty Bath

Most specialty tubs combine bathing with whirlpool action to stimulate circulation and relax muscles. The tubs usually have some form of hydraulic lift to move patients in and out of the tub safely. The procedure is not the same for all types of tubs. You will need to know the correct procedure for each tub that you use.

Guidelines for Assisting with a Specialty Bath

- Follow the safety rules for assisting with a tub bath.
- Follow procedural steps for the tub that you are using.
- Fill the tub and check the water temperature before the patient enters the tub.
- Fasten safety belts when available.
- Activate whirlpool action after patient is in the tub. (See Figure 20–14.)
- Wear gloves for the entire procedure if they are required by the facility.
- Prevent chilling and protect privacy.
- Clean the tub before and after use.
- Report your observations to the nurse.

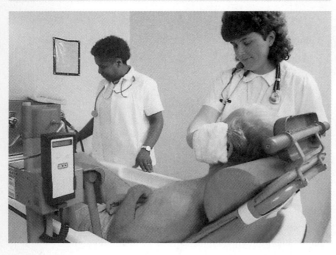

FIGURE 20–14
Most specialty tubs combine bathing with whirlpool action.

Perineal Care

Perineal care (peri-care) is the cleansing of the genital and anal areas of the body. The purposes of this procedure are to cleanse the area, provide comfort, control odor, and prevent skin breakdown or infection. Because the perineal area is warm, dark, and moist, it provides an ideal environment for the growth of pathogens. Peri-care is a part of the daily bath routine for all patients. It may also be ordered for patients after surgery or childbirth. Peri-care should be provided after each incontinent episode, because a buildup of ammonia and other body substances can cause skin breakdown. The procedure for perineal care is located on the facing page

Infection Control

When performing peri-care, always cleanse from the urinary meatus toward the anus. This helps to keep pathogens from the rectal area away from the entrance to the urinary system. The facility may provide a peri-kit or spray solution for peri-care. However, the most common method of performing peri-care is washing with soap and water. Check with the nurse if you are not sure what to use and follow facility policy.

Care of the Nails and Feet

You have an excellent opportunity for observation during nail and foot care. The following observations should be reported to the nurse:

- Ingrown nails
- Hangnails
- Broken or torn nails
- Blisters, rash, or reddened area
- Calluses and corns
- Skin breaks and other injuries
- Complaints of pain or itching

Nail Care

Nail care is frequently done with the bath routine, because damp nails are softer and easier to clean and trim. Soaking the hands or feet in a pan of warm water 105° F to 115° F is also helpful. Trim the fingernails to a reasonable length using a nail clipper and an emery board. Scissors could injure skin tissue and should not be used. In many facilities, nursing assistants are not allowed to trim toe-

Procedure for Perineal Care

Beginning Steps

- Identify the patient and explain the procedure.
- Collect necessary equipment and supplies.
- Wash your hands and use standard precautions.
- Protect the patient's privacy.
- Use correct body mechanics.

1. Raise the side rails, raise the bed to a comfortable working height, and lock the wheels.
2. Lower the side rail on the side nearest you.
3. Assist the patient to a supine position (lying on the back). Separate the legs and bend the knees if possible.
4. Place a protective pad or towel under the buttocks.
5. Cover the patient with a bath blanket. Fold the top linens to the foot of the bed. Raise the side rail when you leave the bedside.
6. Fill a wash basin with water at a comfortable temperature (approximately 105° F) and place it on the overbed table.
7. Put on gloves and uncover the perineal area.
8. Provide peri-care for the female or male patient using the following steps.

For the female:

a. Separate the labia and wash from front to back (from the urinary meatus toward the anus) with the soapy washcloth. Use a different area of the cloth for each stroke.
b. With a clean washcloth, rinse in the same manner. Dry thoroughly (Figure 20–15A).

c. Turn the patient to the side facing away from you.
d. Cleanse with soapy washcloth from the vagina to the anus. Wash the rectal area well. Use a different area of the cloth for each stroke.
e. Rinse in the same manner. Dry thoroughly.

For the male:

a. Cleanse the penis with the soapy washcloth, using circular motions away from the urinary meatus.
b. Using a clean washcloth, rinse in the same manner. Dry thoroughly (Figure 20–15B).
c. If the patient is uncircumcised, the foreskin must be retracted to cleanse around the head of the penis. After rinsing and drying, the foreskin must be returned to its natural position.
d. Turn the patient to the side facing away from you.
e. Cleanse with soapy washcloth from the scrotum to the anus. Wash the rectal area well. Use a different area of the cloth for each stroke. Rinse in the same manner. Dry thoroughly.

9. Remove and discard the protective pad. Cover the patient and raise the side rail.
10. Empty, rinse, and dry the basin.
11. Remove the gloves and discard them in the proper container. Wash your hands.
12. Return equipment and supplies to their proper location.

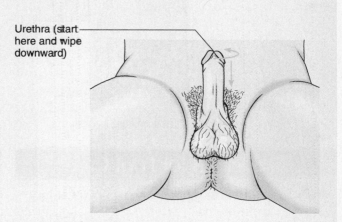

A. Cleanse the perineal area from the urinary meatus toward the anus and rinse in the same manner.

B. Use circular motions away from the urinary meatus when performing male perineal care.

FIGURE 20–15
The cleansing motion for peri-care should be away from the urinary meatus.

Procedure for Perineal Care (cont.)

Ending Steps

- Check to see that the patient is comfortable.
- Lower the bed and raise the side rails, if appropriate.

- Place the call signal within the patient's reach.
- Wash your hands.
- Report and record your observations.

Guidelines for Nail Care

- Soak the hands in water before nail care.
- Use an orange stick to gently clean under the nails and push back the cuticle. Wipe the orange stick on a paper towel after each nail.
- Use a nail clipper—not scissors—to trim nails.
- Smooth the nails with an emery board or nail file, if allowed. (Figure 20–16.)
- Apply lotion to the hands and feet.
- Do not trim toenails unless you know it is allowed in your facility.
- Check with the nurse about nail care for diabetic patients.
- Follow facility policy regarding nail care.

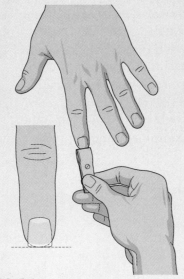

FIGURE 20–16
The fingernails should be clipped and shaped straight across.

Guidelines for Foot Care

- Examine the feet at least once daily for injury or other problems.
- Wash, rinse, and dry the feet thoroughly, especially between the toes.
- Massage the feet with lotion to soften the skin, moisturize the skin, and stimulate circulation.

- Encourage the patient to ambulate and exercise the feet.
- Check to see that shoes and socks fit well.
- Report any injury, no matter how slight.

nails. They do not usually trim fingernails or toenais for diabetic patients. Let the nurse know if the patient's nails need trimming, and follow facility policies.

Foot Care

The patient's feet need special attention. This is particularly true for patients who have diabetes or some other disease that causes poor circulation in the extremities. Closely examine all areas of the foot. Soaking the feet in a pan of warm water softens the skin and is also very relaxing. Massaging the feet with lotion stimulates circulation and increases blood flow to the area. Many elderly patients have problems with their feet. Also, their toenails may get hard and difficult to trim. Most long-term care facilities arrange for a podiatrist (a doctor who specializes in problems of the feet) to visit on a regular basis.

Care of the Hair

Hair care affects appearance, mood, and self-esteem. Generally, we feel better about ourselves when our hair looks attractive. This is true whether we are well or sick, male or female. Hair care, styling, and brushing involve personal choice and habit. Patients who are not able to do their own hair should be consulted as to personal preference. Family members may want to participate in this procedure. For example, brushing her sick child's hair can relieve some of the mother's feelings of helplessness. (See Figure 20–17.)

The hair is brushed and combed as a part of A.M. care and as often as necessary throughout the day. Try not to pull or tangle the hair. A small amount of alcohol or a commercial detangler ap-

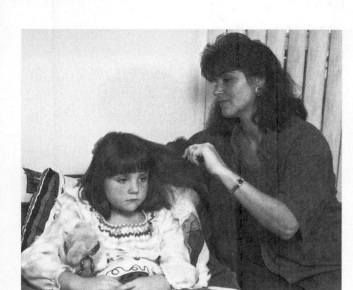

FIGURE 20–17
Brushing her child's hair may relieve some of the mother's feelings of help-lessness.

plied to the hair helps to remove tangles. Do not change a patient's hairstyle without permission. Nursing assistants never cut patients' hair. Let the patient and family know if a professional beautician is available in your facility. Help patients set and keep their hair appointments.

Shampooing the Hair

The hair is usually shampooed while the patient is in the shower or tub, if it is not done in the beauty salon. However, the bedbound patient may receive a shampoo without getting out of bed. The hair should be dried as quickly as possible to avoid chilling. Shampooing is generally done once or twice a week.

Guidelines for Combing and Brushing the Patient's Hair

- Place a towel over the pillow or around the shoulders if the patient can sit up.
- If the patient is wearing glasses, remove them, wash them if necessary, and place them in an eyeglass case.
- Part the hair into sections and comb or brush from the roots to the ends.
- Tangles should be removed by combing or brushing from the ends and working your way to the roots.
- Arrange the hair in the style the patient prefers.
- Allow the patient to use a hand mirror if one is available.
- Make any changes the patient suggests.

Your assignment sheet will indicate which patients are to be shampooed. The procedure for shampooing a patient in bed is located on page 269.

Shaving the Patient

Most men shave daily, usually in the morning or at bath time. Patients decide the shape and length of a beard, mustache, or sideburns and choose when and if they want to shave. Some female patients may want to shave their legs, underarms, or excess facial hair. Shaving can be done with an electric razor, a safety razor, or a disposable razor. Patients may use their own shaving equipment or the facility may provide it.

Always wear gloves when shaving a patient. If you accidentally cut or nick the patient, apply pressure with a tissue or washcloth to stop the bleeding. Report the incident to the nurse immediately. The procedure for shaving a male patient is located on page 273.

Assisting with Dressing

In the acute care hospital, patients usually wear hospital gowns or their own nightclothes. Most patients in nursing homes, rehabilitation centers, and mental hospitals wear street clothes during the day. Patients should be encouraged to choose the clothing that they want to wear.

Make it easier for patients to dress themselves whenever possible by organizing the clothing and placing it within reach. The clothing should be placed in the order in which it will be put on, with the undergarments on top. Dressing will be easier if patients are able to sit on the side of the bed or in a chair. Check the care plan to see if any special equipment has been ordered.

Allow the patient to move at his or her own speed. A patient who has had a stroke or a brain injury may be relearning to dress and undress. Your patience and understanding will encourage self-care. Praise the patient's small accomplishments as well as the major ones. You will need to dress and undress patients who are unable to care for themselves. It is easier and safer to dress these patients in bed. (See Figure 20–20 on page 274.) Put the patient's socks and shoes on before getting the patient out of bed. Support weak or paralyzed limbs while changing the clothing.

Remove clothing from the unaffected limb first and place clothing on the affected limb first. The term "affected" means there is something wrong with the arm or leg. It might be weak, paralyzed, or contracted (locked in one position because of a shortened muscle). The extremity might also have a cast or an IV in

Procedure for Giving a Bed Shampoo

Beginning Steps

- Identify the patient and explain the procedure.
- Collect necessary equipment and supplies.
- Wash your hands and use standard precautions.
- Protect the patient's privacy.
- Use correct body mechanics.

1. Raise the side rails, raise the bed to a comfortable working height, and lock the brakes.
2. Place a chair at the side of the bed near the patient's head. Put a towel on the chair and place a large basin or bucket on the towel to catch the rinse water.
3. Fill a large container or several pitchers with warm water (approximately 105° F), and arrange the supplies on the overbed table.
4. Lower the side rail on the side nearest you.
5. Place a disposable bed protector under the patient's head and shoulders. Use towels to keep the patient dry during the procedure.
6. Position a shampoo trough under the patient's head. The trough can be made from plastic bags if a commercial trough is not available. The trough should drain into the large container on the chair.
7. Brush and comb the patient's hair to remove snarls and tangles.
8. Place cotton in the patient's ears and apply a damp washcloth over the eyes (see Figure 20–18).
9. Wet the hair completely with water from the pitcher. Let the waste water run from the trough into the container on the chair.
10. Apply a small amount of shampoo and gently work up a lather with both hands.
11. Wash the hair and massage the scalp with the fingertips.
12. Rinse the hair by pouring water from the pitcher over it until the hair is free of shampoo.
13. Use conditioner as directed.
14. Remove the cotton from the ears and the washcloth from the eyes.
15. Raise the patient's head and wrap it in a towel.
16. Dry the patient's face and neck with a towel.
17. Rub the patient's hair and scalp to dry it as much as possible.
18. Comb the hair to remove snarls and tangles.
19. Dry the hair as quickly as possible. If using a hair dryer, select the low or warm setting to avoid burning.
20. Style the hair as the patient desires.
21. Remove the supplies and change any wet linens.
22. Place a dry gown on the patient.

Ending Steps

- Check to see that the patient is comfortable.
- Lower the bed and raise the side rails if appropriate.
- Place the call signal within the patient's reach.
- Wash your hands.
- Report and record your observations.

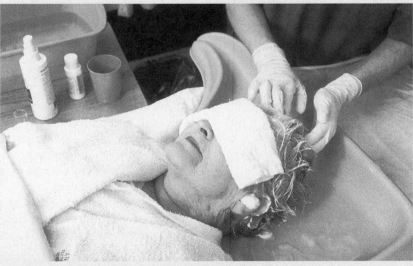

FIGURE 20–18
When giving a bed shampoo, place a shampoo tray under the patient's head to catch the water.

Procedure for Shaving the Male Patient

Beginning Steps

■ Identify the patient and explain the procedure.
■ Collect necessary equipment and supplies.
■ Wash your hands and use standard precautions.
■ Protect the patient's privacy.
■ Use correct body mechanics.

1. Raise the side rails, raise the bed to a comfortable working height, and lock the wheels.
2. Arrange supplies on the overbed table and place the table within your reach.
3. Lower the side rail on the side nearest you.
4. Place the patient in a semi-Fowler's position, if possible.
5. Place a towel over the patient's chest. Put on gloves.
6. Follow these steps, depending on the type of razor used:

If you are using a disposable or safety razor:
   a. Wet the washcloth in the basin of warm water (approximately 105° F) and gently wring it out. Apply the washcloth to the patient's face for a few minutes to soften the beard.
   b. Apply shaving cream or gel to the beard.
   c. Shave in the direction of hair growth while holding the skin taut with your other hand. Shave downward under the sideburns and over the cheek. Shave upward on the neck under the chin. Be careful around the sensitive areas of the nose and lips (Figure 20–19).

   d. Rinse the razor frequently in the basin of water.
   e. When shaving is completed, remove the remaining shaving cream with a damp washcloth.
   f. Pat the skin dry and apply shaving lotion, if desired.

If using an electric or rechargeable razor:
   a. Check to be sure the razor is clean. Clean with a small brush if necessary.
   b. Turn on the razor and shave in the direction of hair growth. Hold the skin taut with the fingers of the other hand.
   c. Apply shaving lotion if the patient desires.
7. Allow the patient to check the shave in a mirror.
8. Clean and return equipment and supplies to the proper location. Clean the electric razor according to the manufacturer's directions. Clean the safety razor carefully. Discard razor blades or the disposable razor in a sharps container. Place linen in the soiled linen hamper.
9. Remove your gloves and discard them in the proper container.

Ending Steps

■ Check to see that the patient is comfortable.
■ Lower the bed to the floor and raise the side rails if appropriate.
■ Place the call signal within the patient's reach.
■ Wash your hands.
■ Report and record your observations.

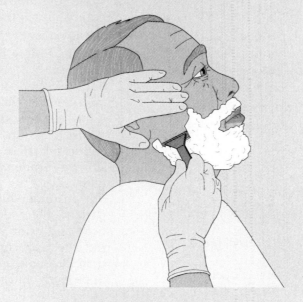

FIGURE 20–19
Shave in the direction of hair growth.

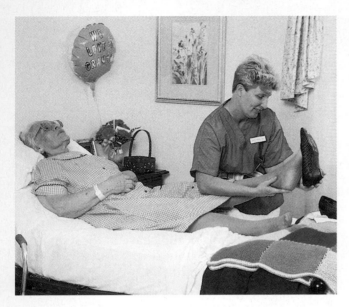

FIGURE 20–20
If the patient is unable to help herself, it is easier and safer to dress her in bed.

place. That limb is called the affected limb, and the "good" arm or leg is referred to as unaffected. See the procedure for assisting the patient to dress below.

The Hospital Gown

Hospital gowns are frequently used in health care facilities. They are loose and comfortable, as well as easy to get on and off the patient. Most hospital gowns open down the back and close with ties or snaps. Some have snaps on the shoulder that make it easier to change the gown on patients who have IVs. Hospital gowns come in pediatric, adult, and extra large sizes. Pajama bottoms are also available.

There are advantages and disadvantages to using hospital gowns. Sizes are limited, so they do not fit well if the patient is very tall, short, or heavy. The opening down the back does not provide much privacy, and they are not very attractive or stylish. However, hospital gowns are ideal for patients who require frequent clothing changes or treatments. The patient who has vomiting, diarrhea, or wound drainage is more comfortable and easier to care for when wearing a hospital gown. Gowns are changed at bath time, bedtime, and as needed during the day or night. A gown is changed immediately if it becomes wet or soiled. Guidelines for dressing the patient with an IV are located in Chapter 31.

Procedure for Assisting the Patient to Dress

Beginning Steps

■ Identify the patient and explain the procedure.
■ Collect necessary equipment and supplies.
■ Wash your hands and use standard precautions.
■ Protect the patient's privacy.
■ Use correct body mechanics.

1. Raise the side rails, raise the bed to a comfortable working height, and lock the wheels.
2. Arrange clothing on the overbed table and place the table within your reach.
3. Lower the side rail on the side nearest you.
4. Assist the patient to a supine position and cover with a bath blanket.
5. Remove the patient's nightclothes.
   a. Remove garments from the unaffected side first, then remove garments from the affected side. Encourage the patient to assist as much as possible.
6. With the upper part of the body covered, put on the underpants.
   a. Place the feet through the correct openings in the pants. Bring the pants up over the

legs and buttocks, rolling the patient from side-to-side, if necessary. Adjust the waistband at the waist and fasten snaps or buttons. Straighten the elastic band.
7. Apply slacks or pantyhose following step 6.
8. Put on socks or hose one at a time. Align the socks over the toes and heels. Leave toe room and do not stretch the socks too tightly.
9. Put on the patient's shoes and fasten them.
10. Uncover the patient's upper body and apply undergarments.
    a. Put a brassiere on a female patient by guiding the arms through the shoulder straps. Adjust the brassiere cups over the breasts. Adjust the straps on the shoulders and fasten the brassiere hooks so the brassiere fits snugly. (Some women prefer to wear an undershirt.)
    b. Put an undershirt or T-shirt on the male patient. Place the shirt over the patient's head and bring it down to the neck. Place the affected arm through the sleeve hole, then the unaffected arm. Adjust the shirt to fit properly and smooth out wrinkles.

Procedure for Assisting the Patient to Dress (cont.)

11. Put on the outer garment.
    a. A knit shirt is put on as indicated in step 10b.
    b. If the shirt opens in the front or back, place the affected arm in the armhole first, then bring the shirt around and insert the unaffected arm. Straighten the shirt and fasten it.
    c. If the female patient is wearing a dress that does not open all the way down, pull it on over the head as indicated in step 10b.
12. Straighten and adjust the clothing. This is easier to do if the patient is sitting up or standing. Otherwise, it may be necessary to roll the patient from side-to-side in order to straighten the clothing (Figure 20–21).

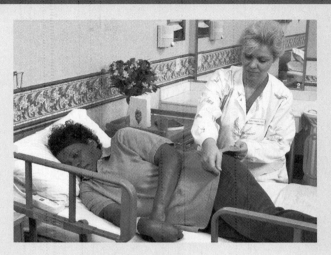

FIGURE 20–21
It may be necessary to roll the patient from side to side to straighten the clothing.

*R*eview

Read each sentence and fill in the blank with the vocabulary term that best completes the sentence.

1. The medical term for mouth care is _____.
2. The nursing care to help patients relax and prepare for sleep is called _____.
3. _____ are false teeth.
4. The medical term for armpit is _____
5. _____ is the medical term for cleansing the genital and anal areas of the body.

*R*emember

1. The ability to perform personal care and hygiene procedures for oneself is a true measure of independence.
2. It is important to protect the patient's privacy during personal care.
3. Daily care routines should be flexible to allow for patient preference.
4. Oral care should be performed at least every two hours for the comatose patient.
5. You may be guilty of negligence if dentures are broken because you failed to use proper precautions.
6. Personal care procedures help to keep the skin healthy and free from tissue breakdown.
7. An incontinent patient must be cleaned and dried immediately to prevent skin breakdown or infection.
8. Backrubs help relax muscles, relieve tension, and stimulate circulation.
9. Bathing is a nurturing process that should be pleasant for you and the patient.
10. Never leave a patient unattended in the tub or shower.
11. When performing peri-care, always cleanse from the urinary meatus toward the anus.
12. Wash, rinse, and dry the feet thoroughly, especially the area between the toes.
13. Hair care affects appearance, mood, and self-esteem.
14. Encourage patients to choose the clothing they want to wear.
15. Remove clothing from the unaffected limb first. Place it on the affected limb first.

Reflect

Read the following case study and answer the questions.

Case Study

You are assigned to care for Mrs. Oliver this morning. Mrs. Oliver has emphysema and diabetes. She wears dentures. Your assignment includes providing A.M. care with a partial bath and getting her up in a wheelchair. She is scheduled for physical therapy at 10:00. Mrs. Oliver asks you to do her bath for her so she will be ready on time.

1. Where should you place Mrs. Oliver's morning care on your priority list? Explain your answer.
2. List four tasks that are included in A.M. care.
3. How should you respond to Mrs. Oliver's request for bathing?
4. How will you protect Mrs. Oliver's dentures while cleaning them?

Respond

Choose the best answer for each question.

1. You are assigned to give Mr. Allen a bed bath, but he says he wants to shower. What should you do?
   A. Tell him he has to have a bed bath because that's what's ordered.
   B. Tell him you will ask the nurse to talk to him about his request.
   C. Help him take a shower.
   D. Skip his bath today.

2. Which of the following will NOT protect the patient's privacy during personal care?
   A. Knock before entering.
   B. Close the drapes and curtains.
   C. Cover the patient with a bath blanket.
   D. Open the door for ventilation.

3. You have a cut on your hand that has not healed. What is the best action to protect the patient and yourself while providing personal care?
   A. Wear gloves during procedures.
   B. Get someone else to do the personal care.
   C. Get a shot to prevent infection.
   D. Stay home until the cut has healed.

4. How often should oral care be provided for the unconscious patient?
   A. Every hour
   B. Every 2 hours
   C. Every 4 hours
   D. Every shift

5. While carrying the patient's dentures to the bathroom, they slip out of your fingers, fall to the floor, and break. This is an example of what legal issue?
   A. Assault
   B. Battery

C. Negligence
D. Slander

6. To protect the patient from infection while performing peri-care, which direction should you cleanse?
   A. From side to side
   B. Away from the urinary meatus
   C. Away from the anus
   D. All of the above

7. You observe that the patient's toenails are long and yellow-colored. What should you do?
   A. Cut the toenails immediately.
   B. Report it to the nurse.
   C. Ignore the long toenails.
   D. Call a podiatrist.

8. The patient's hair is tangled. What should you do?
   A. Apply a small amount of alcohol and comb carefully.
   B. Get scissors and cut out the tangles.
   C. Report it to the nurse immediately.
   D. Call a beautician to help.

9. Which of the following is correct procedure for shaving a patient?
   A. Shave upward over the cheek.
   B. Shave downward on the neck.
   C. Shave upward toward the sideburns.
   D. Shave in the direction of hair growth.

10. Which of the following is NOT correct procedure for assisting a patient to dress?
    A. Remove clothing from the unaffected arm first.
    B. Remove clothing from the affected arm first.
    C. Organize clothing in the order it will be used.
    D. Support weak limbs when changing the clothing.

Chapter Twenty-One

Measuring Vital Signs

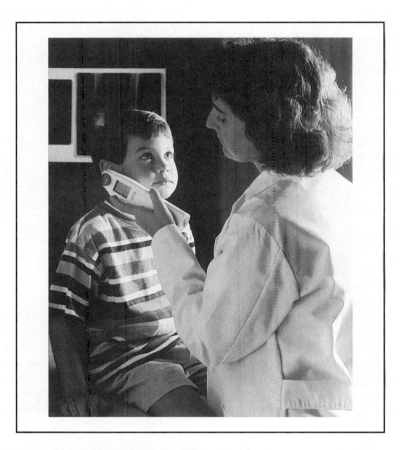

O B J E C T I V E S

After studying this chapter, you will be able to

1. Identify four factors that affect vital signs.

2. Record and report vital signs accurately.

3. Identify the normal adult temperature values.

4. Describe three guidelines for reading a glass thermometer.

5. Identify and locate the radial and apical pulse sites.

6. List three guidelines for using a stethoscope.

7. Identify the normal adult rates for pulses and respirations.

8. Describe the proper method for applying a blood pressure cuff.

9. Identify the normal pediatric rates for pulse and respirations.

10. Perform the procedures described in this chapter.

apical pulse The number of heartbeats per minute as heard over the apex of the heart.

blood pressure A measurement of the amount of force the blood exerts against the artery walls.

body temperature A measurement of the amount of heat in the body.

diastolic pressure A measurement of blood pressure against the artery wall when the heart is relaxing between beats (diastole).

dyspnea Labored or difficult breathing.

fever A body temperature that is above normal.

hypertension An abnormally high blood pressure reading.

hypotension An abnormally low blood pressure reading.

sphygmomanometer An instrument for measuring blood pressure.

stethoscope An instrument that amplifies body sounds.

systolic pressure A measurement of blood pressure against the artery wall when the heart is contracting (systole).

tympanic membrane Thin layer of tissue separating the outer ear from the middle ear; eardrum.

The key to understanding vital signs is the word "vital." When taking vital signs, you are measuring body functions that are vital to life: heart function, breathing, and body heat. Vital signs include temperature, pulse, respirations, and blood pressure. It is essential that vital signs are measured, reported, and recorded accurately. Medications and treatments are frequently based on vital sign measurements. Accurate measurement and prompt reporting of vital signs could save a patient's life.

If you are not sure of a measurement you have taken, repeat the procedure. You may not have performed the procedure correctly the first time, or perhaps you were not concentrating. If you are still not certain after taking the measurement the second time, report the problem to the nurse. **Never** guess or estimate a vital signs measurement. Other members of the team should be able to rely on the accuracy of your measurements.

Factors
That Affect Vital Signs

A person's pulse, respirations, blood pressure, and body temperature may vary slightly from time to time. Factors that may affect vital signs include:

- Illness
- Emotions
- Exercise and activity
- Age
- Sex
- Environment
- Climate and weather
- Food and fluid intake
- Medications
- Time of day

Heart function, breathing, and body heat are closely related. Therefore, a change in one of the vital signs will frequently cause a change in the others. For example, when body temperature goes up, the pulse and respiratory rate usually increase as well.

Recording
and Reporting Vital Signs

Record vital signs measurements as soon as possible after taking them. (See Figure 21–1.) The longer you wait, the more likely you are to forget or make a mistake. Carry a small notepad in your pocket so you can jot down vital signs measurements as soon as you have taken them. The vital signs are abbreviated as follows:

- Temperature (T)
- Pulse (P)

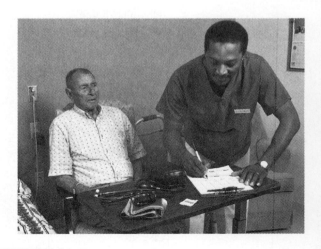

FIGURE 21–1
Record vital signs measurements as soon as possible after taking them.

■ Respirations (R)
■ Blood pressure (BP)

Check to be sure that the right measurement is charted in the right place for the right patient. Record vital signs measurements according to facility policy. Some facilities provide a vital signs board or sheet. Others will expect you to chart directly on the patient's flow sheet. It is your responsibility to know the policy of the facility in which you are working.

Immediately report to the nurse any measurements that are not within normal range. Include in your report other observations that you made while taking the patient's vital signs. Respond to patient and visitor questions about vital signs measurements according to facility policy. Although patients have the right to know about their condition, you may not be the appropriate person to give out this information. It is best to refer their questions to the nurse.

Body Temperature

Body temperature is a measurement of the amount of heat in the body. The temperature is measured to determine the difference between the amount of heat produced by the body and the amount that is lost. Body heat is produced by the contraction of muscles during exercise, the breakdown of food during digestion, and the environmental temperature. Body heat is lost through urine, feces, respirations, and perspiration. Body temperature must remain fairly constant in order to maintain health. Although temperature is controlled by the brain, other body systems assist in regulation.

It is best to take a patient's temperature at the same time every day because body temperature is usually slightly lower in the morning and slightly higher in the evening. An above-normal body temperature is called a *fever*.

Temperature Measurement Sites

Body temperature is usually measured in one of four areas of the body:

■ The mouth—oral
■ The rectum—rectal
■ The axilla (underarm)—axillary
■ The ear—tympanic or aural

The site for measurement is determined by the patient's age and condition. Most temperatures are taken orally because the mouth is a convenient, acceptable area. Patients do not usually object to a thermometer being placed in the mouth. A rectal

temperature is the most accurate measurement, and an axillary temperature is the least accurate. A tympanic measurement is also very accurate and can be taken very quickly.

Normal Body Temperature Values

Normal body temperature depends on the site of measurement. Normal adult body temperatures are as follows:

Oral:	98.6° F (37° C)
Rectal:	99.6° F (37.5° C)
Axillary:	97.6° F (36.5° C)
Tympanic:	98.6° F (37° C)

A patient may have a body temperature that is higher or lower than these figures and still be considered normal if the temperature falls within a certain range. Normal adult temperature ranges include:

Oral:	97.6° F to 99.6° F (36.5° C to 37.5° C)
Rectal:	98.6° F to 100.6° F (37° C to 38.1° C)
Axillary:	96.6° F to 98.6° F (36° C to 37° C)
Tympanic:	98.6° F (37° C)

Types of Thermometers

There are many types of thermometers available to measure body temperature, including glass and electronic thermometers, disposable oral thermometers, temperature-sensitive tape, and tympanic (ear) thermometers. Although the most commonly used type of thermometer in a health care facility is electronic, using a glass thermometer is a basic nursing skill that you will need to learn.

The use of glass thermometers has been discontinued in many health care facilities because they contain mercury, a toxic substance. Exposure to mercury can cause severe poisoning. If you break a glass thermometer, do not attempt to pick up the mercury with your bare hands. It must be treated as toxic waste.

Glass Thermometers

The glass thermometer is a small glass tube that contains mercury in a bulb at one end. Body heat causes the mercury to expand and rise inside the tube. The outside of the thermometer is calibrated (marked with lines and numbers) for measurement. The temperature is read at whatever point the mercury stops rising.

There are three common types of glass thermometers that may be identified by shape and color markings (see Figure 21–2).

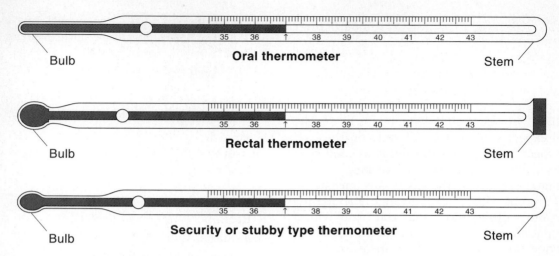

FIGURE 21–2 Types of glass thermometers.

- **Oral:** A glass oral thermometer has a long, slender bulb of mercury. The stem end is usually blue. It is used to take an oral or axillary temperature.
- **Rectal:** A glass rectal thermometer has a round bulb and the stem end is red. It is used to take a rectal temperature.
- **Security or universal:** A security thermometer has a pear-shaped bulb. The stem end is usually blue. It is used for an oral or axillary temperature. A security thermometer is also used for taking the temperature of an infant.

A glass thermometer must be shaken down before and after use until the mercury is below 96° F. Hold the thermometer stem firmly with your thumb and index finger and snap your wrist. The thermometer is usually covered by a disposable plastic shield before it's put in the patient's mouth to prevent the spread of pathogens. If a cover is not used, wipe the thermometer with a tissue, cleansing from the stem end to the bulb. Always check the thermometer for chips or breaks before using it.

Glass thermometers should be washed in cool, soapy water before disinfection. Clean and store the thermometers according to facility policy. Remember to rinse the thermometer with cool water when removing it from the disinfectant solution.

Reading a Glass Thermometer   Temperature measurements may be expressed by the Fahrenheit scale, indicated by an "F," or the Celsius (centigrade) scale, indicated by a "C" (see Figure 21–3). The Fahrenheit scale is more commonly used in the United States.

Fahrenheit Scale

- The scale is marked from 94° F to 108° F.
- The long lines represent one degree.
- The short lines represent two tenths of a degree.

Centigrade Scale

- The scale is marked from 34° C to 42° C.
- The long lines represent one degree.
- The short lines represent one- tenth of a degree.

Electronic Thermometers

Although there are a variety of electronic thermometers, most are battery-operated, handheld units. Electronic thermometers like the one shown in Figure 21–4, are equipped with an oral probe (color-coded blue) and a rectal probe (color-coded red). A probe cover is placed on the probe before use and discarded after each use. A box or supply of probe covers is usually attached to the unit for ready availability. The temperature reading is digitally displayed on the unit.

Tympanic or Aural (Ear) Thermometers

The ear thermometer is a relatively new type of electronic thermometer (see Figure 21–5). It measures the temperature from blood vessels in the *tympanic*

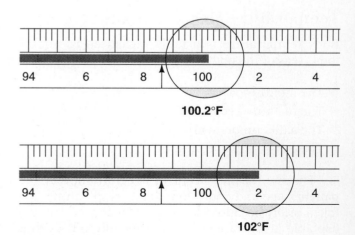

FIGURE 21–3 A Fahrenheit thermometer.

Guidelines for Reading a Glass Thermometer

■ Hold the thermometer at the stem end, in a horizontal position at eye level.

■ Rotate the thermometer until you can see both the numbers and the lines.

■ Slowly roll the thermometer back and forth between the thumb and forefinger until you can see the line of mercury.

■ Read the temperature to the nearest degree (long line) and then to the nearest tenth of a degree (short line).

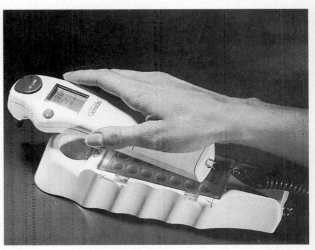

FIGURE 21–5 A tympanic thermometer.

membrane (eardrum). A disposable probe is gently inserted into the ear canal, and within a few seconds the temperature is digitally displayed in the window on the unit. Some tympanic thermometers have a built-in converter that provides equivalent oral or rectal values in either Fahrenheit or centigrade. Like other electronic thermometers, the unit works quickly and accurately. Because of its speed of operation the ear thermometer is useful for children and confused patients. The procedure for taking a tympanic temperature is located on page 287.

Reporting and Recording Temperatures

Any temperature that is outside the normal range should be reported to the nurse immediately.

Remember that the normal range depends on the site of the measurement. It is important that you record temperatures accurately. Temperatures are usually recorded in decimals. For example, an oral temperature might be recorded 98.2. A rectal temperature of the same reading would be recorded 98.2 R, and an axillary temperature would be recorded 98.2 A. A tympanic temperature may be recorded 98.2 TY. No letter is placed after an oral temperature when you are recording. It is assumed that all temperatures are oral unless otherwise indicated. It is usually not necessary to designate Fahrenheit or centigrade because a facility will use one system or the other.

*M*easuring Body *Temperature*

Taking an Oral Temperature

The patient should be in bed or sitting in a chair when the oral temperature is being taken. Place the bulb end of the thermometer under the patient's tongue, on one side of the mouth. Ask the patient to lower the tongue and close the lips around the thermometer. If the patient is paralyzed or weak on one side, place the thermometer on the unaffected side of the mouth. Instruct the patient not to talk and to keep the mouth closed firmly while the thermometer is in place. The glass thermometer is held in place for 3 to 5 minutes or as indicated by facility policy. The electronic thermometer measures the temperature within 2 to 60 seconds and beeps or flashes when measurement is completed.

Although it is the most common method of measurement, you would not take an oral temperature on patients who have tubes in the nose or mouth, are receiving oxygen, are unconscious, breathe through the mouth, have seizures, or are confused or disoriented. Another method would

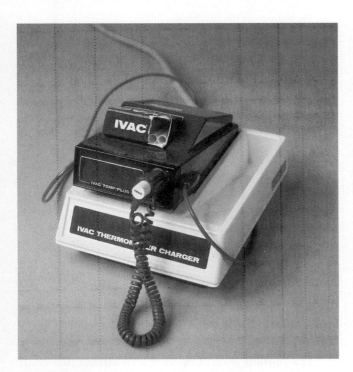

FIGURE 21–4 An Electronic thermometer.

Procedure for Taking an Oral Temperature Using a Glass Thermometer

Beginning Steps

■ Identify the patient and explain the procedure.
■ Collect necessary equipment and supplies.
■ Wash your hands and use standard precautions.
■ Protect the patient's privacy.
■ Use correct body mechanics.

1. After rinsing and drying the glass thermometer, check it for cracks, shake it down, and place a cover on it.
2. Ask the patient to wet the lips so that the thermometer does not stick to them.
3. Place the bulb under the patient's tongue, on one side of the mouth (see Figure 21–6).
4. Ask the patient to lower the tongue and close the lips around the thermometer.
5. Leave the glass thermometer in place three to five minutes or as required by facility policy.
6. Remove the thermometer from the patient's mouth.
7. Remove the cover from the glass thermometer or wipe an uncovered thermometer from stem to bulb with a tissue.
8. Read the temperature at eye level.
9. Make a note of the patient's name and temperature measurement.

10. Ensure the patient's comfort and safety.
11. Shake down and prepare the glass thermometer for disinfection and storage, according to facility policy.

Ending Steps

■ Check to see that the patient is comfortable.
■ Place the call signal within the patient's reach.
■ Wash your hands.
■ Report and record your observations.

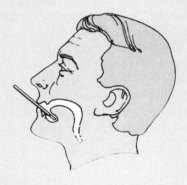

FIGURE 21–6
Place the bulb of the oral thermometer under the patient's tongue on one side of the mouth.

---

also be used for patients who have had recent surgery of the mouth, nose, or face. Oral temperatures are not taken on infants or small children.

If the patient has just finished eating, drinking, smoking, or chewing gum, you will need to wait 15 minutes before taking the oral temperature. These activities can raise or lower the oral temperature, and you will not get an accurate measurement.

Taking a Rectal Temperature

A rectal temperature is taken if an oral temperature cannot be taken. Although this is the most accurate method of temperature measurement, it is not the most commonly used. A rectal temperature is not taken if there has been rectal injury or surgery or if the patient has heart disease. It is often used for measuring the temperature of infants and children.

The mucous membranes of the rectum are delicate and easily damaged. That is why the rectal thermometer has a round bulb and must be lubricated. A small amount of water-soluble lubricant is placed on the bulb end of the thermometer, probe, or cover before inserting it into the anus (the opening to the rectum).

Place the patient in a side-lying position to take a rectal temperature. The thermometer is left in place for 3 to 5 minutes. Hold both the thermometer and the patient's hip throughout the procedure to prevent the thermometer from injuring the rectum or falling out onto the bed. The temperature is recorded with an "R" after the measurement to indicate that it was taken rectally. The procedure for taking a rectal temperature begins on page 284.

Taking an Axillary Temperature

An axillary temperature is taken only when no other temperature site can be used, because axillary temperatures are the least accurate. The axillary temperature can be measured with an oral glass thermometer or oral probe from the electronic thermometer.

The patient should be in bed or sitting in a chair while the axillary temperature is being measured.

Procedure for Taking an Oral Temperature Using an Electronic Thermometer

Beginning Steps

- Identify the patient and explain the procedure.
- Collect necessary equipment and supplies.
- Wash your hands and use standard precautions.
- Protect the patient's privacy.
- Use correct body mechanics.

1. Make sure the oral probe is attached to the electronic thermometer.
2. Insert the electronic probe firmly into the probe cover (see Figure 21–7A).
3. Ask the patient to wet the lips, lower the tongue, and close the lips around the thermometer.
4. Place the probe under the patient's tongue, on one side of the mouth.
5. Leave the probe in place until the thermometer signals.

6. Remove the probe and read the temperature on the digital display.
7. Discard the cover (see Figure 21–7B), and return the probe to its holder (see Figure 21–7C).
8. Make a note of the patient's name and temperature measurement.
9. Return the electronic thermometer to the charging or storage unit.

Ending Steps

- Check to see that the patient is comfortable.
- Place the call signal within the patient's reach.
- Wash your hands.
- Report and record your observations.

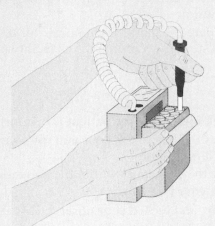

A. Insert the electronic probe into the probe cover.

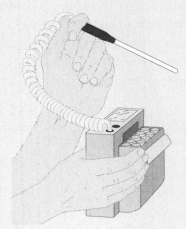

B. After reading the temperature on the digital display, discard the probe cover.

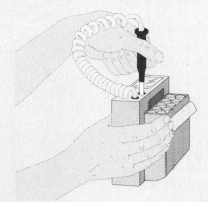

C. Return the probe to its holder.

FIGURE 21–7 Using an electronic thermometer.

Make sure that the axilla is clean and dry. The patient's arm is held close to the body to create a warm pocket of air. The glass thermometer must be left in place for 10 minutes. You may need to hold the thermometer or hold the patient's arm in place during the procedure. Place an "A" after the measurement when you are recording to indicate that the axillary method was used. The procedure for taking an axillary temperature begins on the facing page.

The Pulse

When you measure the pulse, you are counting the patient's heartbeats per minute. A wave of blood is pumped through the arteries into circulation each time the heart contracts. The pulse is counted at pulse sites where an artery is near the surface of the skin. The most commonly used pulse site is the radial artery on the wrist.

When measuring the pulse rate, you must also note the rhythm or regularity of the pulse. The heart normally beats in a steady, regular rhythm, with the same amount of time between each beat. An irregular pulse has unequal amounts of time between beats.

You also need to observe the force or strength of the heartbeat. The terms "weak," "thready," "full," and "bounding" are frequently used to describe the pulse. A weak, thready pulse tends to disappear from under your fingers, even with the

Procedure for Taking a Rectal Temperature Using a Glass Thermometer

Beginning Steps

■ Identify the patient and explain the procedure.
■ Collect necessary equipment and supplies.
■ Wash your hands and use standard precautions.
■ Protect the patient's privacy.
■ Use correct body mechanics.

1. After rinsing and drying the glass rectal thermometer, check it for damage, shake it down, and place a cover on it.
2. Flatten the bed and place the patient in a left side-lying position.
3. Put on disposable gloves.
4. Apply lubricant to the bulb end of the thermometer.
5. Fold the top linens back to expose the rectal area.
6. Raise the upper buttock with one hand so you can see the anus.
7. Gently insert the lubricated end of the glass thermometer one inch into the rectum (see Figure 21–8). Remove your hand from the upper buttock.
8. Hold the glass thermometer and the patient's hip in place for three to five minutes.
9. Remove the thermometer and place it on a clean paper towel.
10. Wipe the anal area with toilet tissue to remove excess lubricant and feces. Discard the tissue into the toilet.
11. Remove the cover from the glass thermometer or wipe it from stem to bulb with a tissue. Read the temperature.

12. Remove the gloves and wash your hands.
13. Make a note of the patient's name and temperature.
14. Prepare the glass thermometer for disinfection and storage according to the facility policy.

Ending Steps

■ Check to see that the patient is comfortable.
■ Lower the bed to the floor and raise the side rails if appropriate.
■ Place the call signal within the patient's reach.
■ Wash your hands.
■ Report and record your observations.

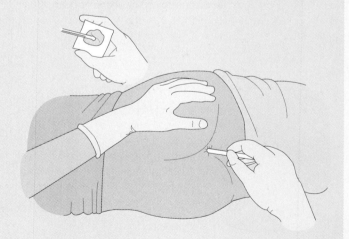

FIGURE 21–8
Gently insert the lubricated end of the rectal thermometer one inch into the patient's rectum.

Procedure for Taking a Rectal Temperature Using an Electronic Thermometer

Beginning Steps

- Identify the patient and explain the procedure.
- Collect necessary equipment and supplies.
- Wash your hands and use standard precautions.
- Protect the patient's privacy.
- Use correct body mechanics.

1. Make sure the rectal probe is connected to the electronic thermometer.
2. Insert the rectal probe firmly into a probe cover (see Figure 21–7A on page 283).
3. Flatten the bed and place the patient in a left side-lying position.
4. Put on disposable gloves.
5. Apply lubricant to the tip of the probe cover.
6. Fold the top linens back to expose the rectal area.
7. Raise the upper buttock with one hand so you can see the anus.
8. Gently insert the tip of the electronic probe one-half inch into the rectum. Remove your hand from the upper buttock.
9. Hold the electronic probe and the patient's hip in place until the thermometer signals.
10. Remove the probe from the patient's rectum and read the temperature on the digital display of the electronic thermometer.
11. Dispose of the probe cover (see Figure 21–7B on page 283) and return the probe to its holder (see Figure 21–7C on page 283).
12. Make a note of the patient's name and temperature.
13. Wipe the anal area with toilet tissue to remove excess lubricant and feces. Discard the tissue into the toilet.
14. Remove the gloves and wash your hands.
15. Return the electronic thermometer to the charging or storage unit.

Ending Steps

- Check to see that the patient is comfortable.
- Lower the bed and raise the side rails, if appropriate.
- Place the call signal within the patient's reach.
- Wash your hands.
- Report and record your observations.

Procedure for Taking an Axillary Temperature Using an Electronic Thermometer

Beginning Steps

- Identify the patient and explain the procedure.
- Collect necessary equipment and supplies.
- Wash your hands and use standard precautions.
- Protect the patient's privacy.
- Use correct body mechanics.

1. Make sure the oral probe is attached to the electronic thermometer.
2. Insert the electronic probe firmly into the probe cover (see Figure 21–7A on page 283).
3. Expose the axilla (underarm).
4. Place the bulb of the thermometer into the center of the axilla. Place the patient's arm over the chest.
5. Hold the patient's arm in place over the probe until the thermometer signals.
6. Remove the thermometer from under the arm and straighten the patient's clothing.
7. Read the temperature on the digital display.
8. Discard the cover (see Figure 21–7B on page 283) and return the probe to its holder (see Figure 21–7C on page 283).
9. Make a note of the patient's name and temperature measurement.
10. Return the electronic thermometer to the charging or storage unit.

Ending Steps

- Check to see that the patient is comfortable.
- Lower the bed and raise the side rails, if appropriate.
- Place the call signal within the patient's reach.
- Wash your hands.
- Report and record your observations.

Procedure for Taking an Axillary Temperature Using a Glass Thermometer

Beginning Steps

■ Identify the patient and explain the procedure.
■ Collect necessary equipment and supplies.
■ Wash your hands and use standard precautions.
■ Protect the patient's privacy.
■ Use correct body mechanics.

1. After rinsing and drying the glass thermometer, check it for cracks, shake it down, and place a cover on it.
2. Expose the axilla (underarm).
3. Place the bulb of the thermometer into the center of the axilla. Place the patient's arm over the chest (see Figure 21–9).
4. Hold the patient's arm and the glass thermometer in place for 10 minutes.

5. Remove the thermometer from under the arm and straighten the patient's clothing.
6. Remove the plastic cover from the glass thermometer or wipe it from stem to bulb with a tissue. Read the temperature.
7. Make a note of the patient's name and temperature.
8. Shake down and prepare the glass thermometer for disinfection and storage according to facility policy.

Ending Steps

■ Check to see that the patient is comfortable.
■ Place the call signal within the patient's reach.
■ Wash your hands.
■ Report and record your observations.

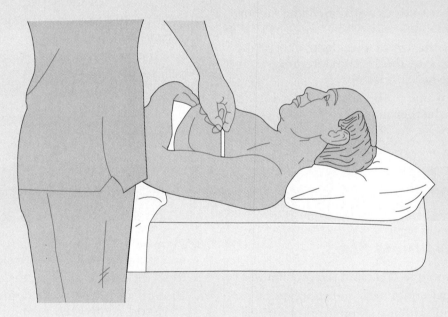

FIGURE 21–9
Place the bulb of the thermometer into the center of the axilla and position the patient's arm over the chest.

gentlest of pressure. A full, bounding pulse is so strong that you may be able to see the pulse movement at the wrist. It may be strong enough to move your fingers as it beats. The normal adult pulse should have a steady and regular rate, rhythm, and force.

The normal pulse rate changes with age. A newborn baby has a very rapid rate. The pulse rate gradually slows as the infant matures. The normal adult pulse rate ranges between 60 and 100 beats per minute. Report any pulse rate above or below the

normal range and include your observations concerning rhythm and force. An irregular pulse must be reported immediately.

The Radial Pulse

The radial pulse is located on the thumb side of the wrist. To locate the radial pulse, apply gentle pressure at the base of the thumb. If you do not feel the pulse, turn the patient's wrist slightly. The artery may have rolled under a bone. Practice locating the

Procedure for Taking a Tympanic, or Aural (Ear), Temperature

Beginning Steps

■ Identify the patient and explain the procedure.
■ Collect necessary equipment and supplies.
■ Wash your hands and use standard precautions.
■ Protect the patient's privacy.
■ Use correct body mechanics.

1. Make sure the probe is connected to the unit.
2. Insert the cone-shaped end of the thermometer into a probe cover.
3. Position the patient's head so that it is directly in front of you.
4. For adults, pull the outer ear up and back to open the ear canal. Pull the ear straight back for infants (see Figure 21–10).
5. Gently insert the probe into the ear canal. If necessary, use a slight rocking motion to insert the probe as far as possible and seal the ear canal.

6. Watch and listen for a signal such as a flashing light or beep that indicates measurement is complete.
7. Remove the probe from the patient's ear and read the digital display.
8. Eject the probe cover into the wastebasket.
9. Make a note of the patient's name and temperature.
10. Assure the patient's comfort and safety.
11. Return the tympanic thermometer to the battery charger or storage unit.

Ending Steps

■ Check to see that the patient is comfortable.
■ Place the call signal within the patient's reach.
■ Wash your hands.
■ Report and record your observations.

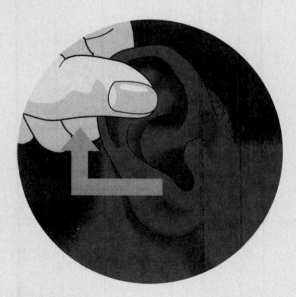

A. For adults and children over the age of one year, grasp the outer ear and pull up and back.

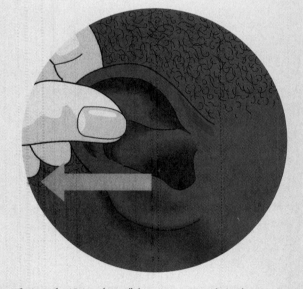

B. For infants under 12 months, pull the outer ear straight back.

FIGURE 21–10 Using a tympanic thermometer.

radial pulse on yourself to gain confidence. Always feel the pulse with the first three fingers, never the thumb. The thumb has a pulse, and you may be counting your own pulse rather than the patient's. Use gentle pressure, particularly if the patient's pulse is weak.

Usually, you will count the pulse for 30 seconds and multiply by two to obtain the rate per minute. For example, let's say that you have measured the radial pulse for 30 seconds and counted 38 heartbeats. By multiplying 38 by two you find that the patient's pulse is 76 per minute. You would record the patient's pulse as 76. The most accurate way to measure the radial pulse is to count it for one full minute. This allows more time to observe for irregularities and eliminates the possibility of a mathematics error. A pulse that is abnormal in any way is always counted for one full minute.

Procedure for Taking a Radial Pulse

Beginning Steps

- Identify the patient and explain the procedure.
- Collect necessary equipment and supplies.
- Wash your hands and use standard precautions.
- Protect the patient's privacy.
- Use correct body mechanics.

1. Place the patient in a comfortable position, either lying down or sitting. The arm should be resting on a table or across the patient's chest.
2. Locate the radial pulse with the first three fingers of one hand and apply gentle pressure (see Figure 21–11).

3. Using the second hand of your watch, count for 30 seconds, or one full minute.
4. Note the rhythm and strength of the pulse.
5. Remove your fingers from the pulse site and make a note of the patient's name and the pulse rate. If you counted for 30 seconds, multiply the count by two.

Ending Steps

- Check to see that the patient is comfortable.
- Place the call signal within the patient's reach.
- Wash your hands.
- Report and record your observations.

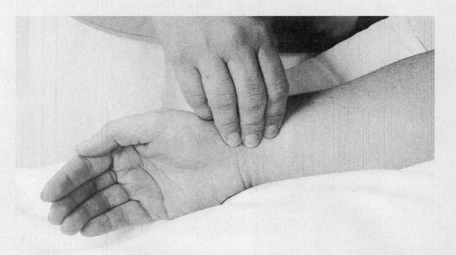

FIGURE 21–11
Locate the radial pulse with the first three fingers of one hand and apply gentle pressure.

Using a Stethoscope

A *stethoscope* amplifies body sounds and is used to listen to sounds produced by the heart, lungs, stomach, and other organs. (See Figure 21–12.) You will use a stethoscope when taking an apical pulse or measuring blood pressure. Because the stethoscope is placed directly on the skin of many patients, infection control is a concern. The following guidelines will help you use a stethoscope correctly and safely.

The Apical Pulse

The *apical pulse* is a measurement of the heart beats per minute over the apex or bottom point of the heart. Since the apical pulse is a more accurate measurement of heart rate, it is often used for cardiac patients or anyone with an irregular heart rate.

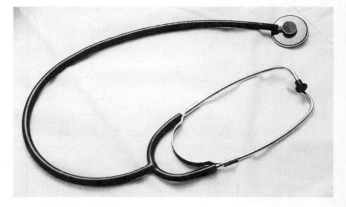

FIGURE 21–12
You may use a stethoscope to take an apical pulse or measure a blood pressure.

Guidelines for Using a Stethoscope

- Clean the earpieces and diaphragm (flat part) with alcohol before and after each use.
- Position the earpieces slightly forward to fit correctly in the ears.
- Warm the diaphragm in the palm of your hand before placing it on the patient's skin.
- Use two fingers to hold the diaphragm in place. Never use your thumb.
- Avoid noise. Ask the patient not to talk during the procedure, and do not let anything touch the tubing.
- Report and record measurements and observations promptly.

It is the preferred method for infants and small children. The apical pulse is located on the left chest, slightly below the nipple. It is measured by listening through a stethoscope (an instrument that amplifies body sounds). (See Figure 21–13 below.)

The Apical–Radial Pulse

The procedure for taking an apical–radial pulse requires two people, with one person counting the apical pulse and the other counting the radial pulse. The pulse is taken for one full minute by both persons, starting and ending at the same time and using one watch. The purpose of taking an apical–radial pulse is to determine the pulse deficit (the difference between the two pulses). Chart the apical pulse first, then the radial pulse and indicate that an apical–radial pulse was taken with an "A-R." In some facilities, this procedure is only performed by nurses.

Procedure for Measuring an Apical Pulse

Beginning Steps

- Identify the patient and explain the procedure.
- Collect necessary equipment and supplies.
- Wash your hands and use standard precautions.
- Protect the patient's privacy.
- Use correct body mechanics.

1. Clean the earpieces and diaphragm of the stethoscope with alcohol.
2. Position the patient lying down or sitting in a chair.
3. Warm the diaphragm in the palm of your hand and place the earpieces in your ears.
4. Locate the apical pulse. Place the diaphragm 2 to 3 inches to the left of the sternum (breastbone) and below the left nipple. (See Figure 21–13.)
5. Count the pulse for one full minute. Note its volume and regularity. The heartbeat will be heard as two sounds "lub-dub." Each pair of sounds count as one pulse beat.
6. Remove the earpieces and diaphragm and straighten the patient's clothing.
7. Note the patient's name, apical pulse measurement, and regularity of the pulse. When recording the reading, place "AP" after the measurement to indicate an apical pulse.

Ending Steps

- Check to see that the patient is comfortable.
- Lower the bed and raise the side rails if appropriate.
- Place the call signal within the patient's reach.
- Wash your hands.
- Report and record your observations.

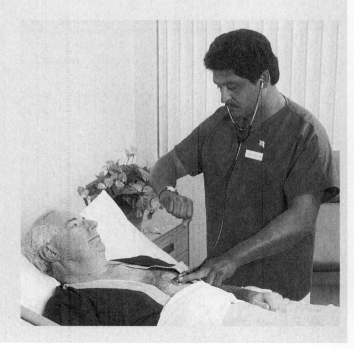

FIGURE 21–13
The apical pulse is measured over the apex or bottom point of the heart.

Counting Respirations

Respiration is the process of breathing air in and out of the lungs. One respiration consists of one inspiration (breathing in) and one expiration (breathing out). The chest rises during inspiration and falls during expiration. When counting respirations (see Figure 21–14 below), you will count one each time the chest rises to determine the number of breaths per minute. Count for one full minute, or for 30 seconds and multiply by two, as you did when counting the pulse.

Because there is some voluntary control of breathing, it is important to count respirations without the patient's awareness of what you are doing. Otherwise, the patient may change the pattern of breathing. One way to measure respirations accurately is to take the pulse first. When you've finished counting the pulse, keep your hand in place at the wrist while continuing to exert slight pressure with your fingers. Raise your eyes to observe the chest and count the respirations. The patient will assume you are still taking the pulse (see Figure 21–14 below).

While you are counting respirations, there are observations to make other than rate or speed. You will need to observe depth, regularity, and sounds. Let the nurse know if the patient has *dyspnea* (difficult breathing). Normal breathing is regular, even, quiet, and painless.

The normal range of respirations for adults is 12 to 20 respirations per minute. Infants and children breathe faster than adults. Report any abnormalities to the nurse immediately.

Blood Pressure

The function of the heart is to circulate blood throughout the body. It uses pressure to pump blood and force it to circulate. Measurement of this pressure helps determine heart function. *Blood pressure* is the amount of force the blood exerts against the artery walls. Blood pressure is affected by internal factors, such as the strength of the heart contractions, the amount of blood flowing, and the elasticity of the blood vessels. Blood pressure that is abnormally high is called *hypertension*, and abnormally low blood pressure is called *hypotension*.

Procedure for Counting Respirations

Beginning Steps

■ Identify the patient and explain the procedure.
■ Collect necessary equipment and supplies.
■ Wash your hands and use standard precautions.
■ Protect the patient's privacy.
■ Use correct body mechanics.

1. Place the patient in a comfortable position, either lying down or sitting. Count the radial pulse first.
2. Keep your fingers in place at the patient's wrist and continue to exert a slight pressure. Look at the patient's chest (see Figure 21–14).
3. Using the second hand of your watch, count one respiration each time the chest rises. Count for 30 seconds or one full minute.
4. Observe for depth, rhythm, and breath sounds.
5. Remove your fingers from the pulse site and make a note of the patient's name and the respiratory rate. If you counted for 30 seconds, multiply the count by two.

Ending Steps

■ Check to see that the patient is comfortable.
■ Place the call signal within the patient's reach.
■ Wash your hands.
■ Report and record your observations.

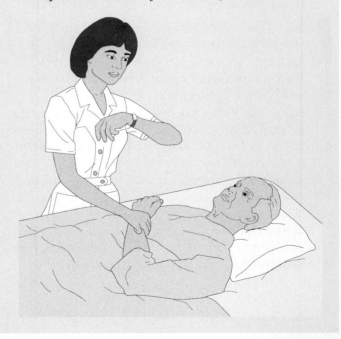

FIGURE 21–14
After counting the pulse, keep your hand in place at the wrist, raise your eyes to observe the chest, and count the respirations.

Systolic and Diastolic Pressures

When you are taking a blood pressure, both the systolic and the diastolic pressure are measured. The *systolic pressure* is the pressure exerted when the heart is contracting during systole. The *diastolic pressure* is the pressure of the blood during diastole, when the heart is relaxing between beats. The blood pressure is recorded as a fraction, with the systolic pressure (the higher number) on the top and the diastolic (the lower number) on the bottom (130/80). The abbreviation for blood pressure is BP.

The adult average systolic pressure range is 100 to 140 and the average adult diastolic pressure ranges from 60 to 90. A systolic measurement below 100 or above 140, and a diastolic measurement below 60 or above 90 should be reported to the nurse immediately.

Using Blood Pressure Equipment

A stethoscope and a sphygmomanometer are used to measure the blood pressure. Guidelines for using a stethoscope are located on page 289. The *sphygmomanometer* consists of a cuff, bladder, bulb, valve, tubing, and measuring device (manometer or gauge). One type of manometer has a column of mercury inside a calibrated (marked with measurements) tube. The mercury manometer may be portable or attached to the wall. The aneroid manometer has a circular dial and a needle that points to the calibrations. Electronic sphygmomanometers are attached to a unit that digitally displays the blood pressure reading. (See Figure 21–15.)

The blood pressure cuff is wrapped around the upper arm and fastened securely. A bladder inside

the cuff is connected to a valve and bulb by a soft tube. When the valve is closed (clockwise), the bulb can be squeezed by hand to inflate the cuff. This inflates the bladder with air and causes pressure over the brachial artery. To deflate the cuff, turn the valve counterclockwise and allow the air to escape from the bladder. A tube connects the bladder to the manometer, which indicates the pressure.

The blood pressure cuff must fit the patient's arm snugly and must stay fastened when inflated. A cuff that is too big or too small can result in an inaccurate blood pressure measurement. Do not take the blood pressure on an arm that is paralyzed or has a wound, a cast, a surgical site, or an IV.

Measuring Blood Pressure

The blood pressure is measured over the brachial artery, which is located on the inner part of the arm at the bend of the elbow. Position the lower edge of the cuff approximately one inch above the elbow. Apply the cuff snugly and fasten it securely on bare skin, not over clothing. Inflate the cuff to 160 mm Hg or 30 mm Hg above the patient's usual systolic pressure. Slowly open the valve and allow the air to escape. The first clear sound you hear is the systolic pressure, and the last clear sound is the diastolic pressure.

If you immediately hear a sound as you open the valve, it means the systolic blood pressure is 160 mm Hg or greater. Deflate the cuff and wait one minute. Then reinflate the cuff to 200 mm Hg and complete the procedure. It is not wise to routinely inflate the cuff to 200 mm Hg. Too much air in the cuff can cause the patient pain and discomfort.

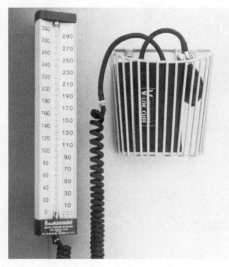

A. A mercury sphygmomanometer.

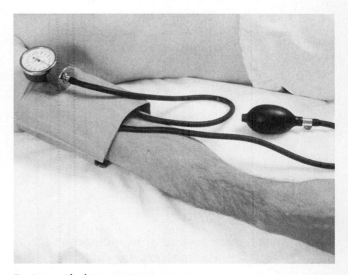

B. A aneroid sphygmomanometer.

FIGURE 21–15
A sphygmomanometer is an instrument used to measure blood pressure.

Procedure for Measuring the Blood Pressure

Beginning Steps

- Identify the patient and explain the procedure.
- Collect necessary equipment and supplies.
- Wash your hands and use standard precautions.
- Protect the patient's privacy.
- Use correct body mechanics.

1. Clean the stethoscope earpieces and diaphragm with alcohol wipes.
2. Have the patient sitting or lying down with the arm extended at heart level. The palm of the hand should be turned up.
3. Remove clothing over the area of the arm where the cuff will be placed.
4. With the valve open, squeeze the cuff to be sure it is completely deflated.
5. Locate the brachial pulse with your fingertips (see Figure 21–16).
6. Wrap the cuff around the arm approximately one inch above the elbow with the arrow pointing to the brachial artery. Fasten the cuff so that it fits snugly.
7. The gauge should be clearly visible.
8. Place the bell or diaphragm of the stethoscope flat on the pulse site, holding it firmly in place with the index and middle fingers of one hand.
9. Close the valve by turning it to the right (clockwise) until it stops.
10. Place the stethoscope earpieces (turned slightly forward) snugly into your ears.
11. Inflate the cuff to 160 mm Hg (or 30 mm Hg above the patient's usual systolic pressure). You will no longer hear a pulse.
12. Deflate the cuff slowly by opening the valve slightly and turning it counterclockwise (to the left) with your thumb and index finger. Allow the air to escape slowly while listening for a pulse sound.

13. Note the reading at which you hear the first clear, regular pulse sound. This number is the systolic pressure.
14. Continue listening until the sound disappears. The diastolic pressure is the reading when the sound disappears. Note this reading.
15. Open the valve completely to deflate the cuff. Remove the cuff from the patient's arm.
16. Record your reading.
17. Wipe the stethoscope earpieces and diaphragm with alcohol.
18. Return the stethoscope and sphygmomanometer to storage.

Ending Steps

- Check to see that the patient is comfortable.
- Place the call signal within the patient's reach.
- Wash your hands.
- Report and record your observations.

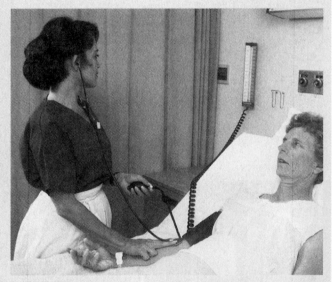

FIGURE 21–16
The blood pressure is measured over the brachial pulse.

Reading the Manometer (Gauge)

Blood pressures are measured in millimeters (mm) of mercury (Hg). Manometers are calibrated with long lines, which represent 10 mm Hg, and short lines, which represent 2 mm Hg. The systolic, or upper, pressure is read first, and the diastolic, or lower, pressure is read last.

Measuring Vital Signs of Pediatric Patients

Measuring vital signs of infants and children requires special care. It is important that you explain the procedure and the equipment you are using before you begin. Gather your supplies and perform the procedure quickly and confidently. Children become impatient and are easily distracted. Crying can cause an increase in heart and respiratory rate, so vital signs should be taken when the child is quiet or asleep. Follow infection control practices to prevent cross-contamination between the children.

Take Pediatric Temperatures

Most facilities prefer that the rectal temperature is measured with infants and small children. A tympanic thermometer may also be used. An oral thermometer is used only on children who are able to understand the procedure. Normal temperature rates for children are the same as for adults: oral 98.6° F or 37.0° C; rectal 99.6° F or 37.5° C; axillary 97.6° F or 36.4° C.

Taking Pediatric Pulses

The infant or young child's pulse is usually measured apically. A radial pulse may be measured if the child is over 6 years old. Normal pediatric pulse rates differ from adults and depend on the age of the child. The older the child gets, the closer the heart rate gets to a normal adult rate. Normal pediatric pulse rates (per minute) for different age groups:

- Birth to 4 weeks: 120 to 160
- 4 weeks to 1 year: 80 to 160
- Above 1 year: 80 to 115

Taking Pediatric Respirations

Children normally breathe faster than adults. Infants frequently use the stomach muscles to breathe and you will need to count the rise and fall of the stomach as one respiration. You cannot count respirations accurately if the child is upset or crying, so wait until the child is quiet. It is especially important that the child not be aware you are counting respirations. Adolescent respiratory rates are similar to normal adult rates. Normal pediatric respiratory rates (per minute):

- Infants: 30 to 60
- Toddlers: 24 to 40
- Preschoolers: 22 to 34
- School age: 18 to 30

Measuring Pediatric Blood Pressures

When measuring the blood pressure of a pediatric patient, make sure you use a cuff that is small enough to fit snugly around the patient's arm (see Figure 21–17). Normal pediatric blood pressure rates depend on the age of the child. Adolescent blood pressure rates are similar to adult rates. Normal pediatric blood pressure rates:

Systolic Pressure	Diastolic Pressure
Infants: 74 to 100	50 to 70
Toddlers: 80 to 112	50 to 80
Preschoolers: 82 to 110	50 to 78
School age: 84 to 120	54 to 80

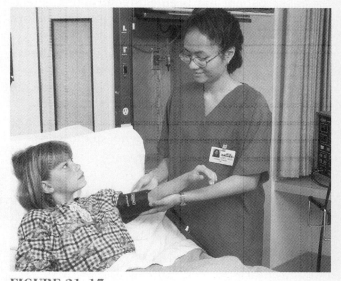

FIGURE 21–17
When measuring the blood pressure of a child, be sure the cuff is small enough to fit snugly around the patient's arm.

Review

Read each sentence and fill in the blank with the vocabulary term that best completes the sentence.

1. The medical term for eardrum is _____.
2. A/an _____ is an above normal body temperature.
3. An abnormally high blood pressure is called _____.
4. The _____ is the blood pressure measurement when the heart is contracting.
5. The _____ is the pulse rate measured by listening through a stethoscope over the apex of the heart.

Remember

1. It is essential that vital signs be measured, reported, and recorded accurately.
2. A change in one of the vital signs will frequently cause a change in the others.
3. If you are unsure of the vital signs that you have just measured, report your problem to the nurse.
4. Report any measurements that are not within the normal range.
5. If the patient has been eating, drinking, smoking, or chewing gum, wait 15 minutes before taking an oral temperature.
6. Hold the rectal thermometer and the patient's hip in place throughout the procedure.
7. The most commonly used pulse site is over the radial artery on the thumb side of the wrist.
8. The apical pulse is measured over the apex of the heart by listening through a stethoscope.
9. It is important to count respirations without the patient's awareness.
10. The first clear sound you hear when taking a blood pressure is the systolic pressure. The point at which the sound disappears is the diastolic pressure.
11. Clean the earpieces and the diaphragm of the stethoscope between use.
12. The blood pressure cuff must be deflated slowly for accurate measurement.
13. Do not take a blood pressure on an arm that is paralyzed or has a cast, surgical site, or IV.
14. Crying can cause an increase in heart and respiratory rates, so take the child's vital signs when he or she is quiet.

Reflect

Read the following case study and answer the questions.

Case Study

Bob needs to take the vital signs on two of his assigned nursing home patients. Mr. Green is comatose and has an IV in his left arm. Bob takes his temperature orally by holding Mr. Green's mouth closed around the thermometer. Bob measures the blood pressure in Mr. Green's right arm. Mr Green's vital signs are T 98.2, P 80, R 14, BP 164/92. Bob also takes Mr. Long's vital signs, which are T 102, P 104, R 26, BP 120/60.

1. Was Bob correct in taking Mr. Green's temperature orally? Explain your answer.
2. Was Bob correct in taking Mr Green's blood pressure in the right arm? Explain your answer.
3. Were Mr. Green's vital signs within normal range? If not, which were abnormal?
4. Were Mr. Long's vital signs within normal range? If not, which were abnormal?

Respond

Choose the best answer for each question.

1. You are not sure of the pulse rate you have just counted. What should you do?
    A. Record what you think it was. You are probably right.
    B. Check the chart and record what the pulse was the last time it was recorded.
    C. Retake the pulse. Let the nurse know if you are not certain.
    D. Get someone else to take the vital signs for you.

2. The vital signs you have just taken are: T 98, P 72, R 12, and BP 120/70. What should you do?
    A. Record the vital signs promptly. They are within normal range.
    B. Notify the nurse immediately.
    C. Retake the vital signs then record them promptly.
    D. Ask a co-worker to retake the vital signs.

3. Glass thermometers are not being used in many facilities because they contain a toxic substance called
    A. Oxygen
    B. Iron
    C. Mercury
    D. Emesis

4. A tympanic thermometer measures the temperature in the
    A. Mouth
    B. Ear
    C. Rectum
    D. Axilla

5. A glass rectal thermometer should be left in place for
    A. 1 to 3 minutes
    B. 3 to 5 minutes
    C. 6 to 8 minutes
    D. 10 to 12 minutes

6. Where is the radial pulse located?
    A. Over the apex of the heart
    B. On the side of the neck
    C. In the groin area
    D. On the thumb side of the wrist

7. Which pulse is measured by listening to it over the heart through a stethoscope?
    A. A radial pulse
    B. A carotid pulse
    C. An apical pulse
    D. A pedal pulse

8. What is the most accurate way to count respirations?
    A. Ask the patient to breathe nromally.
    B. Ask the patient to take deep breaths.
    C. Keep the patient unaware that you are counting respirations.
    D. Watch the chest for a few minutes and estimate respirations.

9. The blood pressure reading you just took was 190/80. Which part of the pressure is abnormal?
    A. Systolic pressure
    B. Diastolic pressure
    C. Average pressure
    D. All of the above

10. What type of thermometer is preferred when taking an infant's temperature?
    A. Oral thermometer
    B. Axillary thermometer
    C. Rectal thermometer
    D. Temperature-sensitive tape

Chapter Twenty-Two

Nutrition *and* Fluids

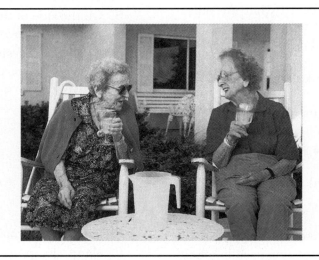

OBJECTIVES

After studying this chapter, you will be able to

1. Explain what is meant by proper nutrition.

2. List two guidelines for using the food guide pyramid.

3. Describe two therapeutic diets.

4. Identify three factors that affect nutrition.

5. Describe four guidelines to follow when you are feeding a patient.

6. List four guidelines for caring for the patient with a feeding tube.

7. Identify five guidelines for caring for a patient with an IV.

8. Explain how fluid balance is maintained.

9. Describe four guidelines for providing patients with drinking water.

10. Calculate fluid intake and output correctly.

calorie A unit of heat produced as the body oxidizes food.
dehydration Lack of adequate fluid in the body.
dysphagia Difficulty chewing and swallowing.
graduate A calibrated container for measuring fluids.
hydration The amount of fluid in the body.
intake and output (I&O) A record of all fluids taken into the body and all fluids eliminated from the body.

NPO Abbreviation for the Latin phrase, *"non per os,"* which means "nothing by mouth."
nutrients Substances contained in foods that are necessary for metabolism.
nutrition The intake and metabolism of food by the body.
PO Abbreviation for the Latin phrase *"per os,"* which means "by mouth."

Food helps meet the needs of the whole person and contributes to the quality of life. Because food provides energy for all the body processes, it is essential to life. However, food does more than meet physical needs. Eating together allows social interactions that help meet emotional and spiritual needs. Sharing food with the sick, the bereaved, and the less fortunate conveys love and caring. Think about what food means to you and how you use it to meet your needs and the needs of your loved ones (see Figure 22–1).

Proper Nutrition

Nutrition is the intake and metabolism of food by the body. Food is oxidized (burned) by the body to create energy needed for all body functions. The amount of heat produced as the body oxidizes food for its use is measured in *calories*. Proper nutrition involves well-balanced meals and the appropriate number of calories.

Nutrients

Foods and fluids contain *nutrients*, substances that are necessary for metabolism. The proper combination of nutrients is necessary for physical and mental health. Most foods contain more than one type of nutrient, but no one food contains all the essential nutrients.

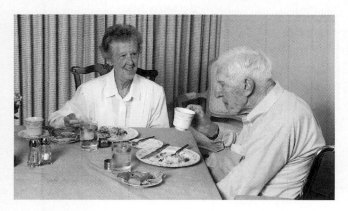

FIGURE 22–1
Food meets physical, emotional, social, and spiritual needs.

Carbohydrates

Carbohydrates (sugars and starches) are the body's major source of energy and also provide fiber or bulk that aids elimination. Carbohydrates are found in breads, cereals, grains, pasta, fruits, and vegetables.

Fats

Fats provide energy, carry vitamins, conserve body heat, and protect internal organs from injury. Fats are found in meat, mayonnaise, butter, margarine, oil, milk, cheese, and nuts. They are higher in calories than any other nutrient.

Proteins

Protein is necessary for tissue growth and repair. It is basic to the structure of all cells and builds muscle, blood, and other tissue. Protein is found in meat, poultry, fish, eggs, milk, cheese, nuts, peanut butter, dry beans, and whole-grain cereals.

Minerals

Minerals needed by the body include calcium, sodium, potassium, iron, phosphorous, iodine, and zinc. Although they are important to health, some minerals are used in very small amounts.

- **Calcium** is used for building bones and teeth, blood clotting, muscle contraction, and nerve function. Milk, cheese, sardines, and green leafy vegetables contain calcium.
- **Sodium** helps with nerve and muscle function and helps the body maintain fluid balance. Foods high in sodium include lunch meat, hot dogs, catsup, mustard, pickles, commercially prepared foods, and all salty foods.
- **Potassium** is necessary for healthy nerves, muscles, and heart function. Foods high in potassium include bananas, oranges, prunes, and cranberries.
- **Iron** is necessary for hemoglobin, which carries oxygen in the blood. Foods high in iron include meat, eggs, dry beans, whole-grain cereals, and green, leafy vegetables.

Vitamins

Vitamins that are needed by the body include vitamin A, B-complex vitamins, vitamin C, vitamin D, vitamin E, and vitamin K.

- **Vitamin A** is needed for vision, healthy hair, skin, and mucous membranes and to help fight infection. Foods containing vitamin A include yellow fruits and vegetables, milk, cheese, liver, and green leafy vegetables.
- **B-complex vitamins** are used for digestion, muscle tone, growth, nerve function, and metabolism. Foods that contain the B-complex vitamins include meat, fish, milk, eggs, cereals, bread, and green leafy vegetables.
- **Vitamin C** is necessary for tissue formation, mineral absorption, healthy skin and mucous membranes, and resistance to infection. Oranges, lemons, tomatoes, strawberries, melon, and cabbage contain vitamin C.
- **Vitamin D** is needed by the body to build healthy bones and teeth. Foods containing vitamin D include milk, butter, eggs, and liver. Many foods, such as bread and milk, have vitamin D added.
- **Vitamin E** is used for the formation of red blood cells and for healthy muscle function. Vitamin E is found in green leafy vegetables, liver, eggs, and vegetable oils.
- **Vitamin K** is necessary for blood clotting. Vitamin K is found in liver, eggs, and green leafy vegetables.

Water

Although water is not a nutrient, it is an essential ingredient of a well-balanced diet. Adequate *hydration* (amount of fluid) is necessary for good health. Water and other fluids are addressed later in this chapter.

The Food Guide Pyramid

In 1992 the United States Department of Agriculture developed the Food Guide Pyramid to replace the Basic Four Food Groups to use as a guide for good nutrition (see Figure 22–2). The Food Guide Pyramid dramatically changed the recommended amounts of food within each group. Remember that the most important part of a pyramid is the base. Therefore, you should eat more foods located at the base and decrease amounts located higher on the pyramid. The emphasis is on bread, cereals, and pasta, with vegetables and fruits next in importance. The key is to avoid the simple carbohydrates, such as candy and desserts that digest quickly, while increasing the amount of complex carbohydrates, such as cereal and other grain foods that take longer to digest. Complex carbohydrates satisfy hunger because they remain in the body longer and make you feel full.

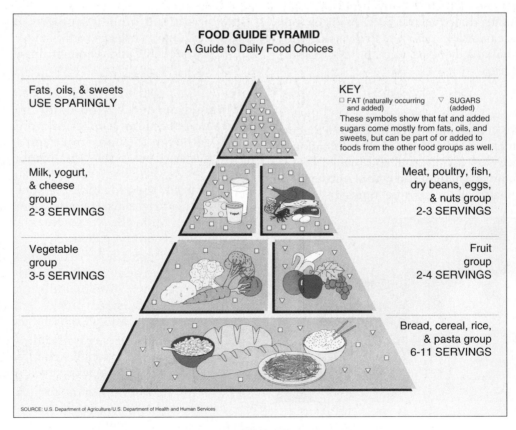

FOOD GUIDE PYRAMID
A Guide to Daily Food Choices

Fats, oils, & sweets
USE SPARINGLY

KEY
▫ FAT (naturally occurring and added)   ▽ SUGARS (added)
These symbols show that fat and added sugars come mostly from fats, oils, and sweets, but can be part of or added to foods from the other food groups as well.

Milk, yogurt, & cheese group
2-3 SERVINGS

Meat, poultry, fish, dry beans, eggs, & nuts group
2-3 SERVINGS

Vegetable group
3-5 SERVINGS

Fruit group
2-4 SERVINGS

Bread, cereal, rice, & pasta group
6-11 SERVINGS

SOURCE: U.S. Department of Agriculture/U.S. Department of Health and Human Services

FIGURE 22–2 The Food Guide Pyramid developed by the U.S. Department of Agriculture.

Guidelines for Using the Food Guide Pyramid

- Eat a variety of foods.
- Eat 6 to 11 servings of complex carbohydrates daily.
- Select fresh fruits and vegetables when available.
- Eat fats, oils, and sweets sparingly.

The Food Guide Pyramid can easily be adapted for patients with special needs. For example, it is unrealistic to expect a frail, elderly person to eat the recommended amounts of each food group.

However, the elderly diet can still follow the principles of using more carbohydrates and less fats.

Types of Diets

Patients in health care facilities may receive either a regular diet or a therapeutic diet. (See Figure 22–3.) A regular or general diet is a well-balanced diet in which there are no restrictions or limits. Therapeutic or special diets are ordered for patients who have special nutritional needs. A therapeutic diet may be ordered to treat disease, correct nutritional problems, or to promote weight loss. Two of the most commonly used therapeutic diets are mechanical diets and diabetic diets.

TYPE OF DIET	DESCRIPTION	COMMON PURPOSE
Regular	Provides a well-balanced variety of complete nutrition. This diet must be tailored for age.	To maintain or attain optimal nutrition status in patients who do not require a special diet.
Clear liquid	Clear broth and juices, ginger ale, gelatin, popsicles, clear coffee, and tea.	To provide calories and fluid in a form that requires minimal digestion. Commonly ordered after surgery.
Full liquid	Strained soups/cereals, coffee, fruit and vegetable juices, ginger ale, gelatin, custard, ice cream, sherbet, pudding, tea.	For those unable to chew or swallow solid food. Used as a transitional diet between clear liquids and solid foods.
Soft	Foods soft in consistency; no strongly flavored foods that could cause distress.	Used for patients who are unable to chew or swallow hard or coarse foods.
Mechanical soft	Same food included in a soft diet except food is ground or strained.	For patients with difficulty chewing or swallowing soft food.
Bland	Foods mild in flavor; omits spicy food, caffeine, and alcohol.	Omits food that may cause excessive gastric acid secretion (ulcers).
Low residue	Food low in fiber and bulk, also omits all foods that contain seeds.	Used for patients with acute colitis, enteritis, and diverticulitis.
High residue/fiber	Food high in fiber such as whole grains, cereals, fruit, vegetables, and legumes.	Used for bowel regulation, high cholesterol, and high glucose; protects against colon cancer and diverticulosis.
Low calorie	Low in calorically dense food such as fat.	For patients who need to lose weight.
Diabetic	Precise balance of carbohydrates, protein, and fats, devised according to the needs of the individual patient.	For diabetic patients; matches food intake with the insulin requirements.
High protein	Meals supplemented with high-protein foods such as meat, fish, cheese, milk, and eggs and oral supplements.	Assists in the repair of tissues wasted by disease. Used for increased protein needs (wound healing).
Low fat; low cholesterol	Limited amounts of butter, cream, oil, and margarine. Limit fried food, high fat meat, and dairy.	For patients who have difficulty digesting fat. Examples include pancreatitis, cholestasis, heart and hepatic disease.
Lactose free or low lactose	Excludes or limits food that contains lactose (milk products).	Used to prevent cramping and diarrhea in patients with a lactose deficiency.
Low sodium (low salt)	Limited amounts of foods containing sodium; no salt packet on tray. This diet may be restricted in protein, sodium, phosphorus, fluid, and potassium.	May be needed for patients with liver, cardiac, and renal disease. Used for patients with acute or chronic renal failure.
Gluten restricted	Restricts gluten-containing foods such as wheat, rye, barley, and oats.	Used for patients with gluten-sensitive enteropathy.

FIGURE 22–3 Examples of patient's diets.

The Mechanical Diet

A mechanical diet may be ordered for the patient who has difficulty chewing or swallowing. The consistency of the food is changed by chopping, pureeing, or blending the food. The mechanical diet may include foods offered on a regular or therapeutic diet.

The Diabetic Diet

A diabetic diet is ordered for patients who have diabetes mellitus. Carbohydrates, protein, and fats are strictly controlled. Patients are discouraged from eating candy and desserts and from drinking soft drinks. The diet emphasizes complex carbohydrates, which the body digests slowly. Patients are provided with exchange lists that indicate the nutritional and caloric values of common foods. Using the list allows the patient to choose the desired foods that are within the diet restrictions.

Factors

That Affect Nutrition

The patient's eating habits may interfere with nutrition. Factors that influence eating habits include age, health, finances, culture, religion, and personal preference.

Age

Infants up to the age of six months usually eat when they are hungry and are offered food, regardless of where they are or who is feeding them. Older infants and small children may be "picky" eaters, especially in a strange environment. While teenagers have higher nutritional needs, many of them have poor eating habits. Older adults may have a decreased appetite or difficulty chewing or swallowing.

Health

Illness may affect appetite and choice of foods. Pain, nausea, and other symptoms interfere with the desire to eat. Medications may reduce hunger or leave an unpleasant taste in the mouth. Confused patients may not recognize the signs of hunger or may be afraid to eat. Sometimes food is restricted or even forbidden for a time.

Finances

Finances affect nutrition in many ways. Some people do not have enough money to buy the food needed for a well-balanced diet. Many elderly people on fixed incomes cannot afford to eat properly. Others can afford to buy whatever they want, but do not choose wisely.

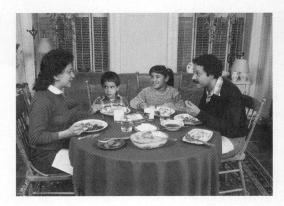

FIGURE 22–4
Many people have specific ethnic food preferences.

Culture

Culture influences food choices and eating habits. When we think of the influence of culture on foods, we often think internationally. We associate rice with the Far East and pasta with Italy. However, there are various cultures within the United States. These differences are reflected in the names of some foods. Think about southern fried chicken, New England clam chowder, or Tex-Mex tacos. Providing food that meets each patient's cultural needs is not easy in a health care facility. It is important to know if patients have specific ethnic food preferences (see Figure 22-4).

Religion

Many religions have rules regarding cooking, serving, and eating certain foods. Pork is forbidden to Muslims, and some Adventists do not eat meat. According to the Jewish faith, foods must be kosher (prepared in special ways according to Jewish laws). Many religions forbid the use of alcohol, coffee, and tea.

Personal Preference

Personal preference is influenced by family practices. For example, if mother or father do not like vegetables, the children may decide that they do not like vegetables either. People usually like foods that bring back pleasant memories and tend to avoid foods that caused an unpleasant reaction. Personal preference is very individual and should be respected.

Nutritional Assessment

The initial nutritional assessment is completed on the patient at admission, and a care plan is established. The care plan will address how well the patient eats; any chewing, swallowing, or digestive problems; and the need for weight loss or gain. The doctor, the dietitian, and the nurses are responsible for regular evaluations of the dietary care plan. Since nursing assistants assist the patients with dining, you may be the one who identifies a problem. You contribute to the care plan by reporting your observations to the nurse.

Resident's Rights as Related to Nutrition

The Residents' Bill of Rights specifically addresses nutrition and food in long-term care facilities. Residents have the right to

- Be served food according to ethnic, cultural, or religious beliefs.
- Be served food according to personal preference.
- Be served attractive, tasty food at correct temperatures.
- Participate in traditional holiday meals.

*A*ssisting the Patient to Eat

You may be assisting the patient to eat in the dining room or in the patient's room. Patients in long-term care facilities are encouraged to go to the dining room if possible because it is a more normal setting and provides opportunities for socialization. Assist the patient who is eating in his room to sit up in a chair whenever possible. If the patient cannot get out of bed, assist him or her to sit up as straight as possible in the bed to improve digestion and prevent choking. Although it is important to encourage independence, some patients will need to be fed.

Provide assistance as needed with oral care, washing the face and hands, and toileting before meals. Make sure the patient is neat and well-groomed. Patients eat better when they are clean and refreshed, even if they are eating alone in their rooms.

Serving Trays

Serving food trays involves much more than just setting a tray in front of the patient. Remember that the goal is self-care, so do not do more for the patient than is necessary. However, you can aid independence by preparing the tray correctly.

Picking Up Food Trays

Make sure the patient is through eating before you remove the tray. Observe and record the amount of food that the patient has eaten. Let the nurse know

Guidelines for Serving Food Trays

- Match the name tag on the tray with the patient's identification bracelet.
- Note if there are any allergies identified.
- Check the food on the tray with the diet that is ordered.
- Offer to replace any food the patient does not like.
- Remove food covers and unwrap the silverware.
- Open cartons and small packages.
- Butter the bread and cut up the meat, if necessary.
- Provide adaptive equipment as needed (see Figure 22–5).

if the patient has not eaten well or has eaten only certain foods. Calculate and record the fluid intake if necessary.

Assisting the Vision-Impaired Patient with Meals

Use the clock method to help the vision-impaired patient with eating. The location of the food is compared to the face of a clock (see Figure 22–6). Remember, the vision-impaired patient cannot see what is on the plate and has no idea what to expect. Ask vision-impaired patients if they want assistance. Most vision-impaired patients guard their independence carefully.

Feeding the Patient

A patient who is very sick, weak, or confused may need to be fed. You may be feeding patients who are in the dining room, in their rooms, or in the bed. Make sure the patient is positioned correctly, sitting up as straight as possible. If the patient is in a geri-chair, bring the recliner forward to an upright position. Do not attempt to feed the patient while the head is tilted back or the patient may aspirate (choke).

Assisting Patients with Dysphagia

Patients who have *dysphagia*, difficulty chewing and swallowing, may need assistance with their food. They must eat slowly and carefully to avoid choking. The doctor may order a mechanical diet using foods that have been chopped or pureed. Thickener may be ordered to use with fluids. A speech therapist is usually involved in the care of these patients. You may be the one who observes that the patient has trouble swallowing. Notify the nurse immediately if you notice that a

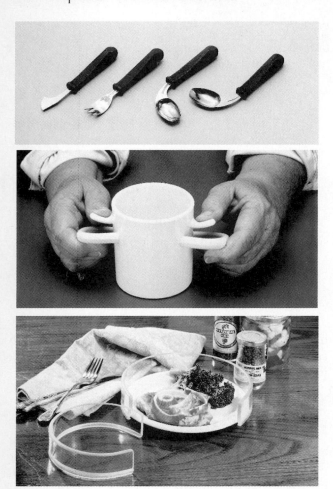
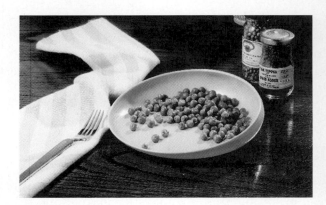
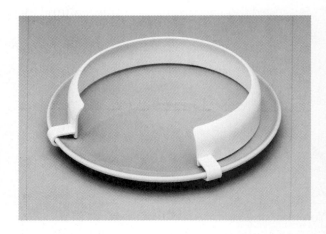
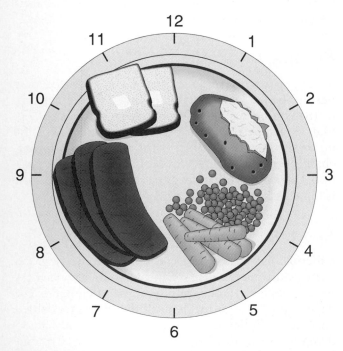

FIGURE 22–5 Examples of adaptive equipment available to help the patient feed himself.

FIGURE 22–6
When assisting the blind patient, compare the location of food to the face of the clock.

Guidelines for Feeding a Patient

- Introduce yourself and tell the patient what you are going to do.
- Provide a clothing protector if needed.
- Sit down facing the patient and make eye contact. (See Figure 22–7.)
- Communicate with the patient, even if there is no response.
- Season the food as the patient desires.
- Make sure that liquids are not too hot.
- Encourage the patient to help as much as possible.
- Identify each food as it is offered.
- Alternate foods and fluids.
- Fill the spoon about one-half full and feed with the tip of the spoon.
- Feed on the unaffected side of the patient's mouth if the patient is paralyzed on one side.
- Allow time for chewing and swallowing and do not rush.

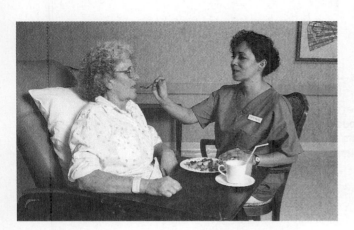

FIGURE 22–7
Sit down facing the patient and make eye contact.

■ Make sure the patient swallows after each bite.
■ Gently stroke the patient's throat if necessary and remind him to swallow.
■ Use a different straw for each liquid.

patient coughs, drools, or pockets food in the cheek while eating. These are symptoms of dysphagia. (*Note:* Do not confuse the medical term "dysphagia" with "dysphasia," which means difficulty speaking.)

Guidelines for Assisting Patients with Dysphagia

■ Check the patient's care plan for special orders.
■ Assist the patient to as upright a position as possible.
■ Add butter or syrup to dry foods, such as bread.
■ Allow the patient time to chew and swallow.
■ Encourage the patient to swallow twice after each bite.
■ Make sure swallowing is complete before offering more food.
■ Special ices may be used between bites.
■ Use thickener with fluids as ordered.
■ Encourage the patient to remain sitting up for 30 minutes after eating.
■ Report any problems to the nurse immediately.

Supplemental Nutrition

Between-Meal Nourishments

This type of food and drink is provided for extra nourishment or to create an enjoyable break in rou-

tine. Snacks are usually offered midmorning, midafternoon, and late evening before bedtime. Jell-O™, ice cream, milkshakes, cookies, cheese, crackers, or fruit may be offered, along with appropriate fluids. For patients on special diets, these snacks are included in their daily dietary allowances.

Some patients receive between-meal snacks because they need extra nourishment. It is important that you serve the snacks to the patients and that you encourage them to eat. Never just leave the snacks at the bedside. Let the nurse know if the patient refuses extra nourishment.

Liquid Oral Supplements

Liquid oral supplements may be ordered for some patients to provide extra calories. These supplements provide necessary nutrients and calories in a small amount of fluid. Liquid supplements may be mixed with ice cream, bananas, or other fruit for variety.

Alternative Methods of Feeding and Hydration

Tube Feedings

Patients who are unable to take food or fluids by mouth or are unable to swallow may be fed through a tube. If the situation is considered to be temporary or short-term, a nasogastric tube will probably be used. A nasogastric (NG) tube is a tube that is inserted through the nose into the stomach (see Figure 22–8).

If the tube feeding is expected to be necessary for a long period of time, a gastrostomy tube will be used. A gastrostomy (G) tube is a tube that is

Guidelines for Care of the Patient with a Feeding Tube

■ Observe the patient frequently.
■ Call the nurse if the feeding pump alarm sounds.
■ Make sure the tubing is not kinked, tangled, or under the patient's body.
■ Avoid pulling on the tube.
■ Keep the head of the bed elevated as ordered.
■ Provide frequent oral care.
■ Observe the area for skin damage where the NG tube is taped.
■ Check with the nurse before giving food or fluids.

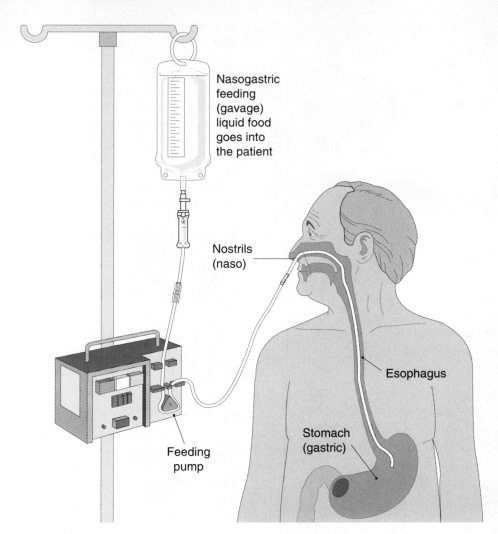

Nasogastric
feeding
(gavage)
liquid food
goes into
the patient

Nostrils
(naso)

Esophagus

Stomach
(gastric)

Feeding
pump

FIGURE 22–8
A nasogastric tube is inserted through the nose into the stomach.

placed through a small surgical opening through the abdominal wall into the stomach. (See Figure 22–9.) The tube is sutured (surgically stitched) to hold it in place.

Most feeding tubes are attached to electronic feeding pumps that control the flow of fluid. An alarm on the pump sounds if the flow rate is disturbed or interrupted. Notify the nurse immediately if the alarm sounds. Although you are not allowed to adjust the flow rate of the feeding, it is important to let the nurse know if it stops or seems to be going too fast or too slow. Do not give the patient who has a feeding tube anything to eat or drink without checking with the nurse, because the patient may be *NPO* (the abbreviation for "nothing by mouth"). The abbreviation used for "by mouth" is *PO*.

The patient who has a feeding tube requires special care. The NG tube can irritate the nose and throat, so oral care is needed more frequently. The skin may become irritated at the site of insertion of the G-tube. Observe the skin carefully and report

any redness or signs of skin breakdown to the nurse immediately. It is important to use aseptic practices to prevent infection. The head of the bed should be slightly elevated for patients who have feeding tubes.

Intravenous (IV) Therapy

Intravenous (IV) means "within a vein." A needle or special catheter is inserted into the vein to deliver water, nutrients, or medications into the bloodstream. A sterile dressing covers the insertion site. Tubing connects the needle or catheter to a bag of fluids, which hangs from an IV pole (see Figure 22–10 on page 306). Usually there is a pump attached to control the flow rate of the fluid. A nursing assistant may NOT start, stop, adjust the rate of, or change the dressing of an IV. These tasks are the responsibility of licensed nurses. Observe the patient frequently and report any problems to the nurse immediately.

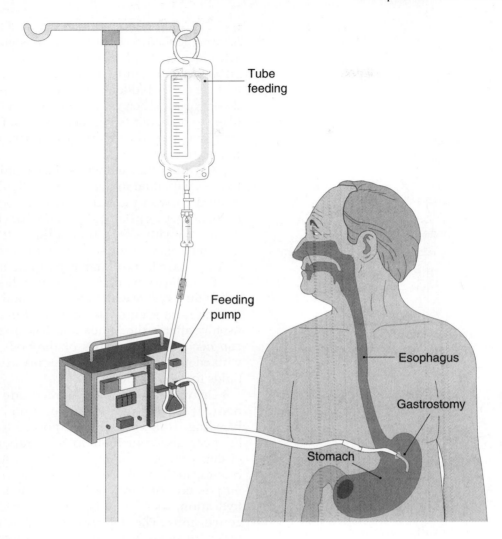

Tube feeding

Feeding pump

Esophagus

Gastrostomy

Stomach

FIGURE 22–9
A gastrostomy tube is placed through a small surgical opening into the stomach.

Guidelines for Care of the Patient with an IV

■ Keep the fluid bag above the level of the insertion site.

■ Avoid pulling on the tubing when assisting the patient to turn or reposition.

■ Make sure that the tubing is not kinked, tangled, under the patient's body, or caught in the side rails.

■ Change the patient's clothing carefully to avoid pulling on the tubing.

■ Do not take a blood pressure in the arm that has an IV.

■ Avoid getting the insertion site wet.

■ Ask the nurse to check the IV after you have completed the patient's care.

■ Report to the nurse immediately if you observe
  a. Swelling, redness, bleeding, leaking at the insertion site.
  b. Complaints of pain, burning, or shortness of breath.
  c. Elevated temperature.
  d. Low fluid level in the container.
  e. A change in the flow rate
  f. The tubing becomes disconnected.

Hyperalimentation

Hyperalimentation is a type of intravenous feeding that contains concentrated amounts of nutrients and flows through a tube directly into a major vein on the upper chest. It may also be called total parenteral nutrition (TPN), or Hyper-Al. This type of feeding contains a patient's total nutritional needs,

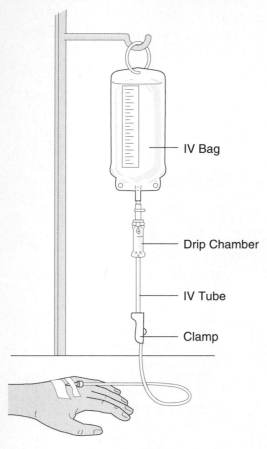

IV Bag

Drip Chamber

IV Tube

Clamp

FIGURE 22–10
Intravenous (IV) equipment.

while a regular IV generally provides only fluid, medication, or up to 900 calories of nutrition. Nursing assistants are not allowed to administer or regulate hyperalimentation. However, it is important to follow the same guidelines as you observe for a regular IV.

The Importance of Water

Water is as essential to life as oxygen and food. Water is the major component of blood, which transports oxygen and nutrients to the cells and carries waste products away from the cells. Water helps regulate body temperature, chemical balance, and fluid balance. It also provides moisture and lubrication.

Maintaining Fluid Balance

In order to maintain fluid balance, the amount of fluid taken into the body must equal the amount that is eliminated or used by the body. Adequate hydration for the adult is between two and three

quarts (2,000 cc to 3,000 cc) daily. Fluid intake is also influenced by culture and personal preference. The choice of fluid or the amount consumed may be affected. For example, caffeine drinks such as coffee and tea are forbidden in many religions. People who do not drink much water when they are well are not likely to do better when they are sick. Find out what fluids the patient prefers, and report this information to the nurse.

Anything that increases fluid elimination or interferes with fluid intake can affect fluid balance. For example, if you mow the lawn in August, you will probably get very hot and perspire heavily. Your body warns you with a sensation of thirst. It is telling you that you need to drink some water to replace the fluid that you have lost through perspiration.

Complications that can occur when the body is not in fluid balance include edema and dehydration. Edema is an accumulation of fluid in the tissues. It usually affects the hands and feet first, although it can occur in other parts of the body. The patient with edema may be on a sodium-restricted diet and fluids may be limited.

Dehydration is lack of adequate fluid in the body. It can be caused by vomiting, diarrhea, or bleeding. Hot weather or exposure to strong sunlight can also contribute to dehydration. Symptoms of dehydration include dry skin and mucous membranes, sunken eyes, weight loss, decreased urinary output, constipation, or fever. In cases of severe dehydration, there may be irritability, confusion, or convulsions. The dehydrated patient may have an order for increased fluids. Fluids should be offered frequently, and the amount taken must be measured and recorded.

Providing Patients with Drinking Water

One of the nursing assistant's responsibilities is to provide patients with fresh drinking water. This usually involves filling a disposable water pitcher that is kept at the patient's bedside. Water pitchers are collected every day, cleaned, refilled, and returned to the patient's room. Be aware that some patients may be restricted to specific amounts of fluids and some may not be allowed any fluids for a period of time. Check your assignment carefully before distributing water pitchers. Cleaning the pitchers may also be the responsibility of the nursing assistant. In long-term care facilities where dehydration is a major concern, a hydration cart may be used. The cart contains ice, spring water, juice, and a variety of other fluids. Each patient is offered a choice of fluids at regular intervals. Failure to provide adequate fluids is considered negligence, so be sure you know what your responsibilities are.

Guidelines for Providing Patients with Drinking Water

■ Identify patients who are NPO. Remove the water pitcher from the room or follow facility policy.

■ Identify patients who are on diets with restricted fluids.

■ Identify patients who are not to have ice in their water.

■ Empty, clean, and refill the water pitcher according to facility policy.

■ Make sure that a clean cup is available.

■ Place the water pitcher and the cup within the patient's reach.

■ Check and refill the pitcher with fresh water at regular intervals.

■ Offer fluids at least every 2 hours and assist as needed.

■ Measure fluid intake and record if necessary.

■ Report to the nurse immediately if the patient is not taking adequate fluids.

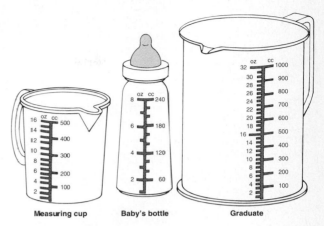

FIGURE 22–11 Examples of graduates.

*M*easuring Fluid Intake and Output

Intake and Output

An order to record a patient's *intake and output (I&O)* means that a record must be kept of all fluids that are taken into the body and all fluids that are eliminated. It is very important to measure and record all fluids accurately, because this information is used in evaluating a patient's fluid balance and in planning care and treatment. Fluids are measured in a container called a *graduate*. The graduate may be a measuring cup, bottle, or pitcher with measuring marks (see Figure 22–11).

Measuring Fluid Intake

Fluid intake includes all the water and other liquids that are taken into the body. Popsicles, ice cream, sherbet, pudding, and custard are examples of solid or semisolid foods that are counted as liquids. Usually, any food that will melt at room temperature is included. Tell the patient and the family that the patient's fluid intake is being measured. If I&O is to be accurate, their cooperation will be necessary. Encourage them to help you keep track of the amount of fluid the patient drinks.

Measuring Urinary Output

Urinary output is measured after each voiding. Empty the bedpan into the graduate for measuring. If the urinal has measurements on the side, you will not have to use a graduate to measure the urine. If the patient is able to be out of bed for toileting, a specimen pan can be placed under the seat of the toilet or bedside commode to collect and measure the urine (see Figure 22–12). Ask the patient not to put toilet tissue in the bedpan, urinal, or specimen pan. Instruct the patient to call you when he or she has finished urinating, so that you can measure and discard the urine. Measuring urine from a urinary catheter is discussed in Chapter 23.

When I&O is ordered, it will also be necessary to measure and record emesis (vomitus) and liquid stool. If the patient has bleeding, drainage, or excessive perspiration, the nurse will help you estimate the amount of these fluids.

Recording Intake and Output

The amount of fluid the patient takes in and the amount eliminated are recorded on the I&O form (see Figure 22–13 on page 309). Check with the nurse if you are not sure if a certain food is counted as fluid. Record fluid intake as soon as the patient is finished eating or drinking. Mark the I&O form before the tray is removed at mealtimes. Do not forget to record between-meal nourishments. You are responsible for recording all oral fluid intake. Tube feedings and IV solutions are recorded by the nurse.

*F*luid Calculations

In health care facilities, fluids are generally measured in cubic centimeters (cc) or milliliters (ml). One milliliter equals 1 cubic centimeter and 30 cubic centimeters or 30 milliliters equals 1 ounce (oz). You will use this formula of 30 cc = 1 oz to cal-

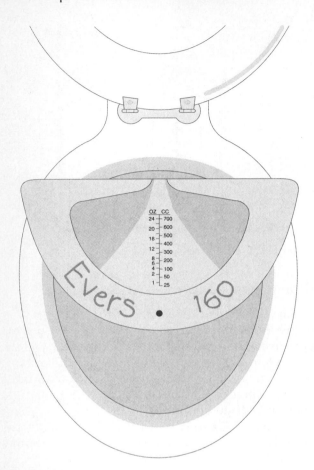

OZ | CC
24 — 700
20 — 600
18 — 500
— 400
12 — 300
8 — 200
6
4 — 100
2 — 50
1 — 25

Evers • 160

FIGURE 22–12 A specimen pan.

culate intake and output. Graduates are usually marked in both ounces and cubic centimeters (see Figure 22–11 on page 307). If you know only the number of ounces in a container, you will need to multiply the number of ounces by 30 to determine cubic centimeters. For example, to figure the number of cubic centimeters in an 8-ounce cup, you would multiply by 30 (8 oz × 30 = 240 cc). A table of common measurements is usually included on each I&O form (see Figure 22–13 on facing page). This table indicates the capacity of various containers used in the facility.

The following example may help you to understand fluid calculation. A milk carton contained 240 cc. You measured 80 cc left in the carton. Subtract 80 from 240 to determine that the patient drank 160 cc of milk. She also drank a full cup of coffee that held 180 cc. Add 160 and 180 for a total intake of 340 cc.

Procedure for Intake and Output

Beginning Steps

■ Identify the patient and explain the procedure.
■ Collect necessary equipment and supplies.
■ Wash your hands and use standard precautions.

1. Measure fluid intake, using the following steps:
   a. Determine the amount of fluid that was originally in the container. Check the I&O form, if necessary.
   b. Pour the remaining fluid into a graduate and measure it.
   c. Subtract the amount remaining from the amount originally in the container.
   d. Repeat steps a–c for each liquid.
   e. Total the amounts and record in cubic centimeters on the I&O form.

2. Measure fluid output, using the following steps:
   a. Pour the urine or other fluid output into a graduate.
   b. Read the measurement at eye level.
   c. Record the amount in cubic centimeters on the I&O form.

Ending Steps

■ Empty the contents of the graduate into the toilet. Rinse the graduate and replace it.
■ Wash your hands.
■ Report and record your observations.

CITY MEMORIAL HOSPITAL

DAILY INTAKE AND OUTPUT RECORD

Name _____

Solutions	Rate (cc/hr)	Solutions	Rate (cc/hr)
A		D	
B		E	
C		F	

Date: _____   Yesterday's Weight: _____   Today's Weight: _____

		INTAKE								OUTPUT				
HOUR	ORAL	Feeding Tube		IV		IV		IVPB		Other	Other	Urine	Emesis	Stool	Other
		Amt. Up	Amt. Abs.	Amt. Up	Amt. Abs.	Amt. Up	Amt. Abs.	Amt. Up	Amt. Abs.						
11 p.m.															
12 p.m.															
1 a.m.															
2 a.m.															
3 a.m.															
4 a.m.															
5 a.m.															
6 a.m.															
8 hr. total															
7 a.m.															
8 a.m.															
9 a.m.															
10 a.m.															
11 a.m.															
12 noon															
1 p.m.															
2 p.m.															
8 hr. total															
3 p.m.															
4 p.m.															
5 p.m.															
6 p.m.															
7 p.m.															
8 p.m.															
9 p.m.															
10 p.m.															
8 hr. total															
24 hr. total															

Combined 24 hour total   INTAKE   OUTPUT

GUIDE FOR RECORDING I & O:

Juice Glass...................120 cc	Insulated Hot Mug........210 cc	Cereal Bowl...................180 cc	Ice Cream.....................120 cc
Coffee Cup...................210 cc	Cold Cup (small)...... ....120 cc	Milkshake Container......210 cc	Jello Container...... ....120 cc
	Jumbo Paper Cup.........300 cc	Water Pitcher................900 cc	Milk Container...............240 cc

FIGURE 22–13 A sample I&O sheet with a table of common measurements at the bottom.

Review

Read each sentence and fill in the blank with the vocabulary term that best completes the sentence.

1. _____ is the intake and metabolism of food by the body.
2. The amount of heat produced as the body oxidizes food for its use is measured in _____.
3. Patients who have _____, difficulty chewing and swallowing, may need assistance with their food.
4. _____ is lack of adequate fluid in the body.
5. Fluids are measured in a container called a _____.

Remember

1. Food helps meet the needs of the whole person and contributes to the quality of life.
2. Proper nutrition involves well-balanced meals and the appropriate number of calories.
3. The Food Guide Pyramid stresses the importance of complex carbohydrates.
4. A mechanical diet may be ordered for patients who have difficulty chewing or swallowing.
5. Eating habits are influenced by age, health, finances, culture, religion, and personal preference.
6. The location of food can be described to the vision-impaired patient by using the clock method.
7. Allow time for eating and socialization. Do not rush the patient.
8. Provide adaptive equipment and help the patient maintain proper positioning while eating.
9. Patients with dysphagia must eat slowly and carefully.
10. Observe, report, and record the amount of food the patient has eaten.
11. Check with the nurse before giving the patient with a feeding tube anything to eat or drink.
12. Nursing assistants do not start, stop, or adjust the flow rate of an IV.
13. To maintain fluid balance, the amount of fluid taken into the body must equal the amount that is eliminated or used by the body.
14. It is important to measure and record intake and output accurately.
15. Offer fluids to patients at least every 2 hours and assist them as needed.
16. Fluids are usually calculated in cubic centimeters in the health care setting.

Reflect

Read the following case study and answer the questions.

Case Study

Mrs. Gonzalez is an 85-year-old woman who immigrated to Florida from Cuba many years ago. She was admitted to the hospital with a diagnosis of dehydration and weight loss. Although Mrs. Gonzalez is legally blind, she lived alone in her own home until her recent hospitalization. Her fluid balance has been restored and the IV therapy discontinued. Mrs. Gonzalez is still eating poorly and continues to lose weight. Efforts to get her to eat more only make her angry. Discharge goals are to maintain her independence, increase food intake, and stop the weight loss. She is then to be discharged to live with her daughter in New York. You have been assigned to care for her.

1. How can you help Mrs. Gonzalez maintain her independence?
2. What effect might culture have on her eating habits?
3. What emotional factors might be causing Mrs. Gonzalez's behavior?
4. How can you respond appropriately to her angry behavior?

Respond

Choose the best answer for each question.

1. The nutrient found in meat that is necessary for tissue growth and repair is
   A. Carbohydrate
   B. Fat
   C. Protein
   D. Calcium

2. Which of the following foods is the best example of a complex carbohydrate?
   A. Cereal
   B. Dessert
   C. Meat
   D. Milk

3. The diet most often ordered for people who have difficulty chewing and swallowing is a
   A. Regular diet
   B. Clear liquid diet
   C. Low-calorie diet
   D. Mechanical diet

4. Which of the following foods would NOT likely be found on a diabetic diet?
   A. Chocolate cake
   B. Rye bread
   C. Green beans
   D. Cabbage salad

5. Eating habits and choices may be affected by
   A. Health
   B. Religion
   C. Culture
   D. All of the above

6. What is the safest way to be sure a patient gets the right food tray?
   A. Ask the patient what his or her name is.
   B. Match the name tag on the tray with the patient's identification bracelet.
   C. Match the name tag on the tray with the room number on the door.
   D. Ask another nursing assistant to help.

7. The medical term for difficulty chewing and swallowing is
   A. Dysphasia
   B. Dysphagia
   C. Dysphnea
   D. Dysuria

8. A patient tells you she likes fresh lemon in her drinking water. What is the appropriate response?
   A. "We don't have any fresh lemons."
   B. "Plain water is better for you."
   C. "I'll go to the kitchen and get you a fresh lemon."
   D. "I'll check with the nurse and see if you can have lemon."

9. Which of the following is a guideline for caring for a patient with an IV?
   A. Slow the rate if the IV is running too fast.
   B. Discontinue the IV when the bag is empty.
   C. Keep the fluid bag above the level of the insertion site.
   D. All of the above.

10. How many cubic centimeters are in an 8-ounce cup of milk?
    A. 120 cc
    B. 240 cc
    C. 360 cc
    D. 480 cc

Chapter Twenty-Three

Elimination

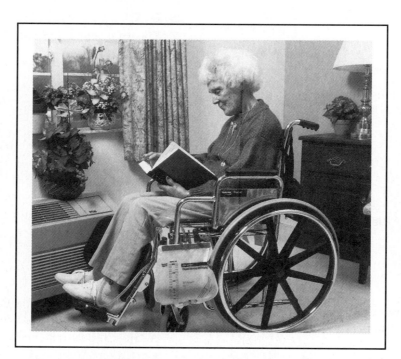

OBJECTIVES

After studying this chapter, you will be able to

1. Identify three factors that affect elimination.

2. Identify three guidelines for assisting a patient with a bedside commode.

3. Describe three common urinary problems

4. List two nursing measures to stimulate urination.

5. List three methods to prevent incontinence.

6. List four guidelines for care of a urinary drainage system.

7. Identify four guidelines for restorative bowel and bladder retraining.

8. List four guidelines for inserting a rectal suppository.

9. List four guidelines for providing ostomy care.

10. Perform the procedures described in this chapter.

Glossary

colostomy   A surgically created opening through the abdominal wall into the colon.

dysuria   Painful urination or difficulty urinating.

enema   Procedure to introduce fluid into the lower colon and rectum for the purpose of removing feces.

flatus   Air or gas expelled from the digestive tract.

incontinence   The inability to control urine or feces.

nocturia   Excessive urination during the night.

ostomy   A surgical procedure to form an artificial opening from an organ to an exit site.

stoma   The artificially created opening of an ostomy on the outside of the body.

suppository   A cone-shaped, semisolid substance inserted in the rectum where it dissolves.

void   To expel urine.

The process of elimination removes waste products from the body and is essential to a healthy life. The elimination of liquid waste or urine is called urination and the elimination of solid waste or feces is called defecation. Feces may be called stool, bowel movement, or B.M. Most adults are able to control elimination until the time and place are appropriate. The inability to control urine or feces is called *incontinence*.

Factors
That Affect Elimination

Elimination may be affected by nutrition, fluid intake, privacy, exercise, and medications. Eating a well-balanced diet and drinking plenty of fluids helps to promote elimination. Water increases urination and helps keep stool soft-formed for defecation. Foods high in fiber, such as whole-grain cereals, create bulk that assists in elimination. Some foods, such as beans and cabbage, may produce *flatus* (air or gas expelled from the colon).

It is important to protect the patients' privacy during elimination. Since most people prefer to perform these functions alone and independently, they may have difficulty urinating or defecating if another person is present. Close the door, pull the curtain, and close the window drapes or blinds. Always knock on the door and wait for a response before entering. (See Figure 23–1.)

Exercise, such as walking or range-of-motion, aids digestion and helps keep bowel elimination regular. Whenever possible, patients should be sitting upright for defecation. The normal position for a woman when urinating is sitting, while the man normally stands. Patients should be assisted to a position as nearly normal as possible.

Certain medications can increase or decrease urination and may cause the urine to turn red or purple. Medication can be given to soften stool and stimulate defecation. Constipation is a side effect of some medications.

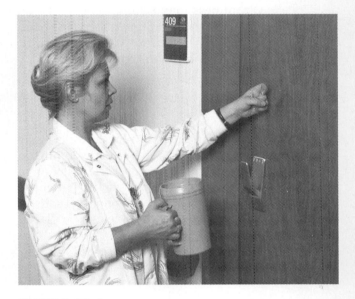

FIGURE 23–1
Knock on the door and wait for a response before entering.

Assisting the Patient
with Elimination

Infection Control

Gloves should be worn when you are assisting a patient with elimination because of the possibility of contact with body fluids, body substances, or mucous membranes. Remember to wash your hands after removing the gloves and assist the patient to wash his or her hands.

Restorative Measures

Assist the patient to meet elimination needs as independently as possible. Provide adaptive equipment as needed. A cane, walker, or wheelchair may allow the patient to go to the bathroom for elimination. A raised toilet seat can bring the seat to a height that is easier for the patient to use (see Figure

23–2). Check the patient's care plan to see if any equipment is recommended.

Whenever it is possible, the patient should be encouraged to go to the bathroom for elimination. Going to the bathroom is a restorative measure because it provides a more normal environment and helps confused patients to be aware of the need for elimination. Make sure that the patient knows the location of the bathroom call signal that is to be used for emergencies.

Be aware of cultural influences when assisting patients with elimination. Culture and personal habits can affect how, where, and when elimination takes place. Cleanliness may be an important issue. For example, in some Arab cultures, the right hand is considered unclean, because it is the hand most often used to perform elimination procedures.

Using a Bedside Commode

A bedside commode (a portable chair with a toilet seat that fits over a container or regular toilet) may be helpful (see Figure 23–3). The bedside commode may be placed in the bathroom over the toilet or in the patient's room beside the bed. If the patient is able to get to the bathroom but does not feel safe on the toilet, then the bedside commode can be placed in the bathroom.

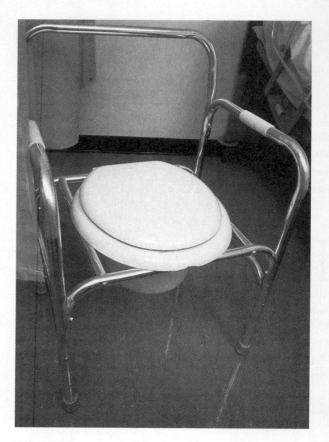

FIGURE 23–3 A bedside commode.

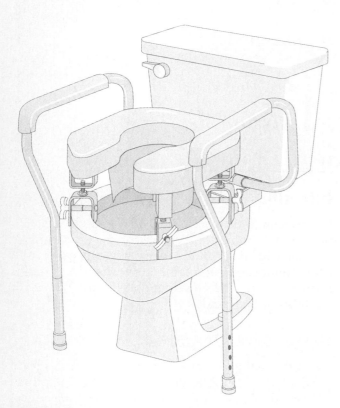

FIGURE 23–2
A raised toilet seat brings the toilet seat to a height that is easier for the patient to use.

Using the Bedpan

A patient who is unable to get out of bed will need to use a bedpan for elimination. A regular bedpan or a fracture pan is the most commonly used (see Figure 23–4). A fracture pan is a bedpan that usu-

Guidelines for Assisting a Patient with a Bedside Commode

- Lock the brakes to prevent the bedside commode from moving.
- Wear gloves and follow standard precautions.
- Allow the patient as much privacy as possible.
- Remain nearby while the patient is on the bedside commode.
- Place toilet tissue and the call signal within reach.
- Never restrain a patient to a bedside commode.
- Assist the patient to wash his or her hands after elimination.
- Clean the bedside commode after each use.
- Place water in the bottom of the commode to make cleaning easier.
- Report and record elimination results.

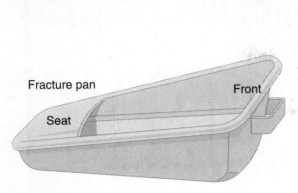

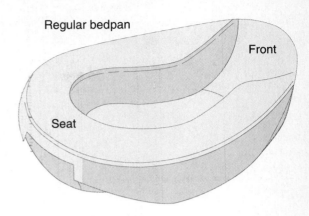

FIGURE 23-4 Types of bedpans.

Procedure for Assisting the Patient with a Bedpan

Beginning Steps

■ Identify the patient and explain the procedure.
■ Collect necessary equipment and supplies.
■ Wash your hands and use standard precautions.
■ Protect the patient's privacy.
■ Use correct body mechanics.

1. Raise the side rails, raise the bed to a correct working height, and lock the brakes. Adjust bed to as flat a position as possible.
2. Lower the side rail on the side nearest you.

3. Assist the patient to a supine position (on the back). Move the top linens aside.
4. Put on gloves.
5. Position the patient on the bedpan, using Method 1 or Method 2.

Method 1
  a. Ask the patient to raise the hips. Bending the knees and pushing with the feet may make this easier.
  b. Slide the bedpan under the patient's buttocks (see Figure 23-5A).

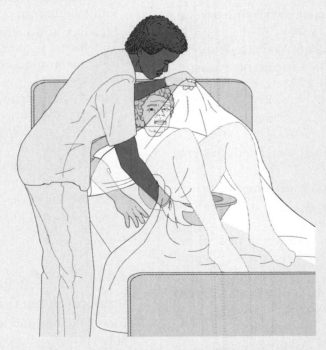

A. Method I: Ask the patient to raise her hips, while you slide the bedpan under her buttocks.

FIGURE 23-5 Assisting the patient onto a bedpan.

Procedure for Assisting the Patient with a Bedpan (cont.)

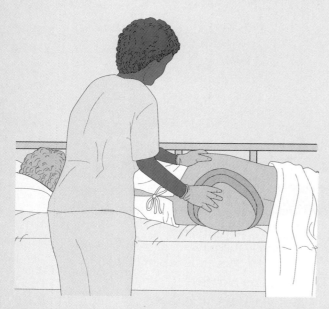

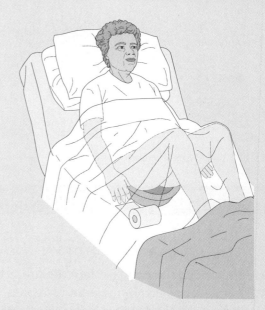

B. Method 2: With the patient on her side, place the bedpan against her buttocks, and roll her onto the bedpan.

C. Adjust the head of the bed so that the patient is in a sitting position on the bedpan.

FIGURE 23–5 Assisting the patient onto a bedpan (cont.).

Method 2

    a. Turn the patient onto the side facing away from you.

    b. Place the bedpan against the patient's buttocks (see Figure 23–5B).

    c. Roll the patient back onto the bedpan.

6. Adjust the head of the bed so that the patient is in a sitting position (see Figure 23–5C). Cover the patient to provide privacy.

7. Place toilet tissue and the call signal within the patient's reach.

8. Raise the side rail and tell the patient to signal when finished.

9. Remove your gloves and wash your hands.

10. Leave the room only if the patient can be left alone on the bedpan.

11. If you leave the room, lower the bed, check back frequently, and answer the call signal promptly.

12. To remove the patient from the bedpan, lower the side rail and the head of the bed.

13. Put on gloves.

14. Remove the bedpan by asking the patient to raise the hips or by turning the patient onto the side facing away from you. Cover the bedpan immediately.

15. Assist the patient as needed to clean the perineal area.

16. Raise the side rail and take the covered bedpan to the bathroom or soiled utility room.

17. Measure the urine if I&O has been ordered and collect a specimen if needed. Observe the color, amount, and character of the urine or feces.

18. Empty the bedpan into the toilet. Rinse, clean, and dry the pan with disinfectant or follow facility policy. Place the used linen in the dirty linen hamper.

19. Return the bedpan and other equipment to their proper places.

20. Remove the gloves and wash your hands.

21. Assist the patient in handwashing.

Ending Steps

■ Check to see that the patient is comfortable.

■ Lower the bed and raise the side rails, if appropriate.

■ Place the call signal within the patient's reach.

■ Wash your hands.

■ Report and record your observations.

ally has a handle on the front and a flat end that is placed under the patient. Although the fracture pan is more comfortable for the patient, it holds less urine and is easy to spill.

There are basically two methods for assisting a patient with the bedpan. The simplest way is to ask the patient to raise the hips while you slide the bedpan under the buttocks. If the patient is not able to raise the hips, you will need to turn the patient onto the side, place the bedpan against the buttocks, and roll the patient back onto the bedpan. To prevent discomfort and skin breakdown, do not leave the patient on the pan for a prolonged period. When rolling the patient off the bedpan, hold the pan to prevent spilling. Place a bedpan cover over the pan as soon as you remove it. Assist the patient to clean the perineal area.

Using the Urinal

The urinal used by the male patient when urinating usually has a handle to hold on to and a lid to cover the top. Because it is calibrated (marked with measurements) on the side, the urinal does not need to be emptied into a graduate for measuring the urine. Some male patients will want to keep the urinal within reach when they are in bed. This helps to protect independence by allowing them to use the urinal without calling for help. Check frequently to see if the urinal has been used. If so, empty and rinse it immediately. (See Figure 23–6.)

The patient may stand to use the urinal, or he may use it while in bed. If the patient is unable to stand, raise the head of the bed to a sitting position, if possible.

Urine is normally pale yellow (straw-colored) and contains no visible substances. Changes in

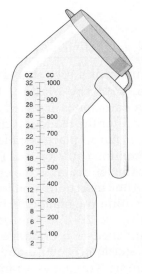

FIGURE 23–6 A urinal.

Guidelines for Using a Urinal

- Wear gloves and use aseptic technique.
- Do not put the urinal on the overbed table or on the floor.
- Empty and clean the urinal promptly after it has been used.
- Help the patient position the urinal, if necessary.
- Assist the patient to remove the urinal, if necessary.
- Measure the urine if I&O is being measured.
- Collect a specimen if one is needed.
- Observe the urine carefully for abnormalities.
- Empty the urinal into the toilet.
- Clean the urinal, replace the lid, and return it to its proper place.

urine color, clearness, or odor may be caused by a disease condition or medication. Notify the nurse if you observe any of the following conditions:

- Blood or mucus, stones, gravel, or sediment in the urine
- Dark- or pale-colored urine
- Concentration (thickening of urine)
- Unusual urine odor
- Complaints of pain, burning, or itching in the perineal area
- *Dysuria* (difficult or painful urination)
- Inability to *void* (urinate)

Common Urinary Problems

Some of the most common problems that affect urinary elimination are:

- Urinary tract infection
- Urinary frequency and urgency
- Urinary hesitancy
- *Nocturia* (excessive urination during the night)
- Urinary incontinence

Urinary Tract Infection

Urinary tract infections (UTIs) are caused by pathogens that enter the urinary system and multiply. A UTI may occur because of improper cleansing of the perineal area. Always cleanse from the urinary meatus toward the anus when performing perineal care and use the same technique when using toilet tissue. Practice aseptic technique at all times and change the incontinent patient immediately.

Urinary Frequency and Urgency

The need to urinate often is called urinary frequency. Urgency is a sudden, strong urge to urinate. Normally the urge to void occurs when the bladder contains about 350 cc of urine. In urinary frequency, the urge may occur when there is only a small amount of urine in the bladder. The patient may need to urinate every hour and pass only 50 to 100 cc each time. Urinary frequency and urgency often occur together and are more common in elderly women. These problems can result from a disease condition, an injury, or the changes of aging. Answering call signals promptly helps to reduce incontinent episodes for these patients.

Urinary Hesitancy

The patient with urinary hesitancy has trouble starting to urinate. This condition is more common in older men, when the prostate gland enlarges, causing a narrowing of the urethra. Swelling in the perineal area can also interfere with urination. It helps to assist the patient to as near normal positioning as possible. Measures to stimulate urination include:

- Turn on the faucet and let the water run.
- Place the patient's fingers in warm water.
- Pour warm water over the patient's genitals.

Nocturia

Nocturia is a common problem in older patients. The patient may need to get up several times at night and go to the bathroom or use the bedpan or urinal. Nocturia can contribute to urinary incontinence and interfere with sound sleep.

Urinary Incontinence

Urinary incontinence is the inability to control urinary elimination. Although any patient may have this problem, it is more common in elderly patients, confused patients, and children. Although incontinence is **not** a normal change of aging, some changes do contribute to incontinence because they make it more difficult to control elimination. Other causes of incontinence include disease, confusion, medications, decreased mobility, and failure to toilet frequently.

Incontinence can affect the patient physically, emotionally, and socially. Urine provides a warm, moist environment for pathogens that may cause either skin breakdown or a UTI. Falls and fractures may result from a patient's attempt to reach the bathroom in time. Incontinent patients may feel embarrassed, ashamed, or angry. Families may have difficulty dealing with their loved one's incontinence. Self-esteem may be damaged and depression may result. The patient may withdraw and avoid social activities.

Preventing Incontinence

Incontinence may be prevented by using the following measures:

- Offer toileting at regular intervals.
- Answer call signals promptly.
- Remind confused patients to use the bathroom on a regular basis.
- Observe for signs of the need for toileting such as restlessness, crying, or holding the genitals.

Caring for the Incontinent Patient

The patient who has an incontinent episode requires immediate care. Wash, rinse, and dry the soiled areas of the patient's body after each episode. Clean the wet area of the skin with soap and water, then rinse and dry the area well. Wiping the urine with a dry towel, without using soap and water, leaves germs and chemicals on the skin that can cause skin breakdown or infection. Change the patient's clothes and bed linen as necessary. Be pleasant, understanding, empathetic, and never shame or scold the patient. Clean the patient in a professional, matter-of-fact manner.

Urinary Catheters

A urinary catheter is a tube that is inserted through the urethra, into the bladder to drain urine. Sometimes a catheter is inserted temporarily and then removed after the bladder is drained. A urinary catheter that is left in place is called an in-dwelling catheter, a retention catheter, or a Foley catheter. An in-dwelling catheter drains urine continuously from the bladder. After insertion, a balloon on the end of the catheter within the bladder is inflated with sterile water (Figure 23–7). The other end of the catheter is attached to a drainage bag. Inserting a catheter is a sterile procedure and requires special skill and training. Nursing assistants do not usually perform catheterizations.

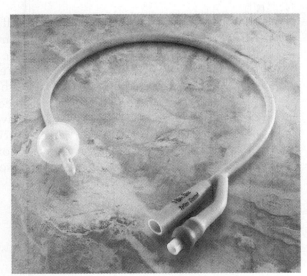

FIGURE 23-7
A balloon, inflated with sterile water, holds the catheter in place in the bladder.

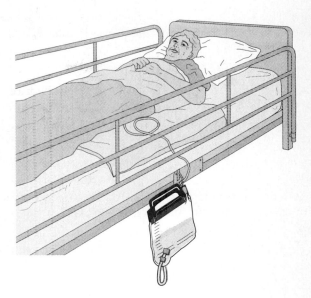

FIGURE 23-8
The urinary drainage bag is attached to the bedframe.

Guidelines for Care of a Urinary Drainage System

- Keep the system closed and connected to prevent contamination.
- Report any leaks in the system immediately.
- Keep the drainage bag below the level of the bladder.
- Keep the catheter and drainage tubing free of kinks.
- Avoid pulling on the catheter when moving the patient.
- Attach the drainage bag to the bed frame when the patient is in bed (see Figure 23-8).
- Never attach the drainage bag to the side rail or any moving part of the bed.

provide a catheter care kit containing antiseptic, swabs, cotton balls, and disposable gloves. Although catheter care procedures vary among facilities, the principles remain the same: Wear gloves and follow standard precautions; wash away from the urinary meatus; and use a different part of the washcloth or a separate wipe for each stroke. The procedure for providing catheter care is located on page 320.

Urinary Leg Bags

Some patients prefer a small drainage bag that is worn on the upper leg. It may be held in place by a Velcro band. The leg bag holds a small amount of urine and must be emptied frequently. Each time it is emptied, the urinary tract is exposed to infection, so be careful not to contaminate the inside of the catheter or the tubing. (See Figure 23-9.)

Providing Catheter Care

The catheter site will need regular cleaning to help prevent infection. Perform peri-care before you touch the catheter. The most common method for performing catheter care is washing the area and the catheter with soap and water. Some facilities

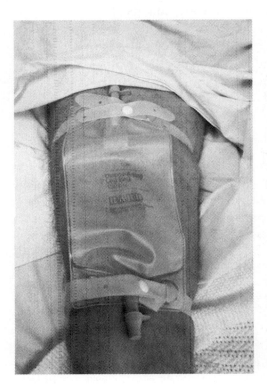

FIGURE 23-9
A urinary drainage leg bag.

Procedure for Providing Catheter Care

Beginning Steps

- Identify the patient and explain the procedure.
- Collect necessary equipment and supplies.
- Wash your hands and use standard precautions.
- Protect the patient's privacy.
- Use correct body mechanics.

1. Raise the side rails, raise the bed to a correct working height, and lock the brakes.
2. Lower the rail on the side nearest you.
3. Assist the patient to a supine position with the legs separated and the knees bent, if possible.
4. Place a protective pad or towel under the patient's buttocks and drape as you would for perineal care.
5. Put on disposable gloves.
6. Perform perineal care, following the procedure explained in Chapter 20.
7. Check carefully for dried secretions, sores, bleeding, or leakage.
8. Using a clean washcloth, wash 3 or 4 inches of the catheter. Begin at the urinary meatus and wash away from the body, using a different part of the washcloth for each stroke (see Figure 23–10). Avoid pulling on the catheter.
9. Rinse and dry thoroughly.
10. Make sure there are no kinks in the catheter or the tubing.
11. Remove the bed protector and raise the side rail.
12. Empty, rinse, and dry the basin.
13. Remove the gloves and discard them in the proper container. Wash your hands.
14. Remove the bath blanket after covering the patient with the top linen.
15. Return equipment and supplies to the proper location.

Ending Steps

- Check to see that the patient is comfortable.
- Lower the bed and raise the side rails, if appropriate.
- Place the call signal within the patient's reach.
- Wash your hands.
- Report and record your observations.

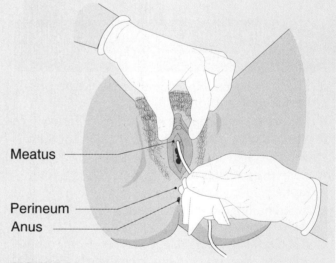

FIGURE 23–10
Wash the catheter from the urinary meatus down the catheter about 3 or 4 inches.

External Catheter

An external catheter (also called a condom catheter or a Texas catheter) may be ordered for the incontinent male patient. The catheter consists of a soft rubber condom sheath that is applied over the penis (see Figure 23–11). A tube leading from the sheath connects to a urinary drainage bag. The external catheter can irritate the skin or interfere with circulation if not applied correctly.

Emptying the Urinary Drainage Bag and Measuring Urine

The urinary drainage bag is emptied at the end of every shift, and the amount of urine is measured

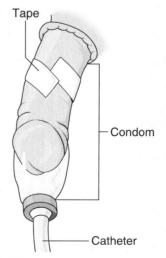

FIGURE 23–11
An external urinary catheter.

Guidelines for Applying an External Catheter

- Wear gloves and follow standard precautions.
- Provide peri-care.
- Remove the protective backing from the adhesive surface.
- Roll the catheter onto the penis, rolling from the end of the penis toward the body.
- Leave one inch of space between the penis and the end of the catheter.
- Apply tape spirally to secure the catheter. Do not completely encircle the penis.
- Connect the catheter to the drainage bag.
- Fasten the drainage bag to the bedframe.

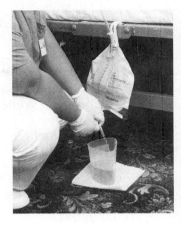

FIGURE 23–12
Empty the urinary drainage bag into a graduate.

and recorded on the intake and output record. The amount of urine from all shifts is totaled every 24 hours. If the bag fills before the end of your shift, empty it and record the amount. Use a graduate (a container used to measure fluids) and do not use the measurements on the side of the drainage bag, as they may not be accurate. (See Figure 23–12.)

Check the amount of urine in the drainage bag frequently. Although this check does not give you an accurate measurement, it allows you to observe if urinary output has decreased or increased. When you make rounds to check on your patients at the beginning of your shift, carefully observe those with catheters. Make sure that the bag has been emptied and the tubing is free of kinks. Refer to Chapter 22

for a thorough description of the procedure for intake and output.

Restorative Bladder Retraining

Some incontinent patients may be in a restorative bladder retraining program. The goal is to restore control of urinary elimination to as nearly normal as possible. An individual plan of retraining is developed for each patient in the program. Close observation and participation by the staff will be necessary during the retraining period. Restorative bladder retraining involves determining normal voiding habits, establishing a regular routine of toileting, evaluating results, and adjusting the routine as necessary.

The nursing assistant plays an important role in restorative bladder retraining. When you are assigned a patient who is on bladder retraining, his or her schedule must be a priority as you organize your work. You will help to prevent incontinence by toileting the patient according to the established schedule.

Guidelines for Emptying a Urinary Drainage Bag

- Follow standard precautions and wear disposable gloves.
- Do not raise the drainage bag above the level of the bladder.
- Place a paper towel on the floor under the graduate.
- Empty the drainage bag into a graduate.
- Do not allow the drain to touch the inside of the graduate.
- Do not allow the drainage bag to touch the floor.
- Replace the closed clamp in the holder.
- Read the amount on the graduate at eye level.
- Record output on the I&O record.

Guidelines for Restorative Bladder Retraining

- Observe and record the patient's normal voiding pattern—24 hours a day for at least three days.
- Offer fluids and encourage voiding at scheduled times.
- Use methods to stimulate urination, as needed.
- Be consistent on all shifts.
- Maintain a positive attitude. Never shame or scold the patient.
- Maintain accurate records.

Bowel Elimination

Normal feces is soft-formed and brown. Let the nurse know if the stool is too soft, too hard, contains blood, or is abnormal in any way. While defecation usually takes place every day or two, remember that elimination patterns are individualized. Some people defecate only once or twice a week.

Common Problems of Bowel Elimination

Constipation

The most common problem of bowel elimination is constipation, which is hard, dry stool that collects in the rectum because it cannot pass easily through the anus. Constipation can be caused by poor fluid intake, eating the wrong foods, medication, disease, lack of exercise, or ignoring the urge to defecate. Constipation can often be prevented by adequate fluid intake, increasing exercise, and eating foods that are high in fiber and bulk.

Constipation that is not relieved can result in a fecal impaction, a large amount of very hard, dry stool that cannot be expelled normally from the rectum. The patient may complain of pain or nausea, the abdomen may appear swollen and hard, and smears of stool may be noticed on clothing or linen. An impaction may affect urinary elimination because of pressure exerted on the bladder by the mass of stool. Report these signs and symptoms to the nurse immediately because the fecal impaction may completely block the bowel and prevent elimination of wastes. Enemas may need to be given, or the fecal impaction may have to be manually removed.

Diarrhea

Diarrhea is loose, watery stool that occurs when peristalsis pushes food too rapidly through the intestines. Diarrhea can be caused by food, medication, infection, or other diseases and can be very serious for infants, small children, and elderly patients. The patient with diarrhea will need to defecate frequently and urgently, and fecal incontinence may occur. Answer call lights promptly and provide toileting as often as needed. Thorough cleansing of the rectal and perineal area is important to prevent skin damage. Report each occurrence of diarrhea to the nurse, noting the time, amount, and frequency of the diarrhea.

Fecal Incontinence

Fecal incontinence is the inability to control bowel movements. It can be caused by poor muscle tone, a change in peristalsis, nervous system damage, or confusion. An illness such as infectious diarrhea may cause temporary incontinence. Fecal incontinence can cause skin breakdown and urinary tract infection. Feelings of embarrassment, guilt, loss of control, and depression may result. Act promptly and professionally when assisting the patient after an incontinent episode.

Restorative Bowel Retraining

A bowel retraining program is developed specifically for each patient. The goal of restorative bowel retraining is to restore the patient's control of fecal elimination. The retraining program usually includes increased activity, adequate fluid intake, and a high-fiber diet. The steps are similar to those in bladder retraining. The usual pattern of bowel elimination is determined, a regular schedule is established, and the program is evaluated and altered as necessary.

Enemas

An *enema* is the introduction of fluid into the rectum and colon in order to remove feces and cleanse the lower bowel. Some x-ray tests require a cleansing enema, or the doctor may order an enema to relieve constipation or an impaction. Many health care facilities do not allow nursing assistants to give enemas. It is your responsibility to know the policy where you work.

Guidelines for Restorative Bowel Retraining

- Check the patient's care plan.
- Offer fluids frequently.
- Encourage the patient to eat foods that create bulk.
- Assist with regular exercises.
- Be alert for signs that indicate a need for defecation (perspiration, goose pimples, restlessness, or rubbing the abdomen).
- Offer toileting promptly.
- Never scold or embarrass the patient.

Procedure for Giving a Cleansing Enema

Beginning Steps

- Identify the patient and explain the procedure.
- Collect necessary equipment and supplies.
- Wash your hands and use standard precautions.
- Protect the patient's privacy.
- Use correct body mechanics.

1. Raise the side rails, raise the bed to a comfortable working height, and lock the wheels.
2. Lower the side rail on the side nearest you.
3. Assist the patient onto the left side (see Figure 23–13A) and cover with a bath blanket.
4. Place an IV pole beside the bed and raise the side rail.
5. Clamp the tubing on the enema tube and prepare the solution that is ordered to 105° F or 40.5° C.
6. Allow a small amount of solution to run through the tubing to expel the air. Clamp the tubing again.
7. Hang the enema bag on the IV pole with the tubing at the bottom. Make sure that the enema bag is no more than 18 inches above the bed or 12 inches above the anus (see Figure 23–13B).
8. Wash your hands and put on disposable gloves.

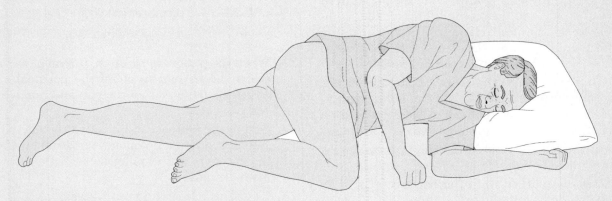

A. Position the patient on the left side.

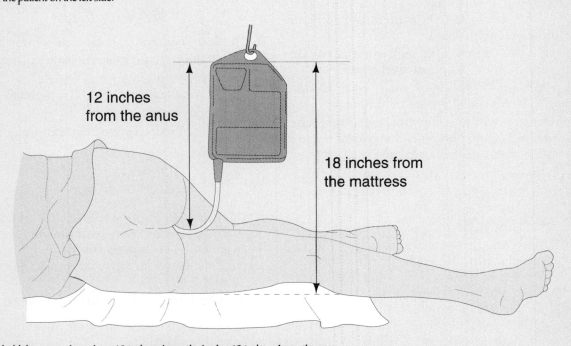

12 inches from the anus

18 inches from the mattress

B. Hang or hold the enema bag about 18 inches above the bed or 12 inches above the anus.

FIGURE 23–13
A cleansing enema.

Procedure for Giving a Cleansing Enema (cont.)

9. Lower the side rail and uncover the patient enough to expose the anus.

10. Place the disposable bed protector under the patient's buttocks. Place the bedpan close to the patient's body.

11. Lubricate 4 inches of the tip of the enema tubing.

12. Ask the patient to breathe deeply during the procedure to help relieve cramps.

13. With one hand, lift the upper buttock to expose the anus. With the other hand, insert the tip of the tubing into the rectum (see Figure 23–13C).

14. Rotate the tubing 2 to 4 inches into the rectum. Stop if you feel resistance or if the patient complains of pain. Call the nurse if this happens.

15. Unclamp the tubing and allow the solution to flow slowly into the rectum. If the patient complains of cramping, clamp the tubing and stop for a minute or so. Encourage the patient to take as much of the solution as possible.

16. When the solution is almost gone, clamp the tubing and remove the tip from the rectum. Place the tip of the tubing into the empty enema bag. Do not let it contaminate you or the linens.

17. Ask the patient to hold the solution as long as possible.

18. Assist the patient onto the bedpan or bedside commode or into the bathroom.

19. Make sure that toilet paper and the call signal are within reach. Ask the patient not to flush the toilet when finished.

20. Discard the disposable equipment in the proper container and clean up the area.

21. Remove your gloves and wash your hands. Discard gloves in the proper container.

22. Leave the room for a few minutes, if possible. Lower the bed and remind the patient to use the call signal. Check back frequently.

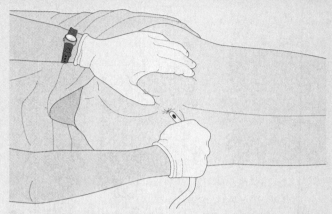

C. Lift the upper buttock to expose the anus and insert the top of the tubing into the rectum.

FIGURE 23–13 A cleansing enema (cont.).

23. When the patient is through, put on gloves and assist the patient to clean the perineal area. Assist the patient from the pan and remove the bed protector.

24. Empty the bedpan and observe the enema results for amount, color, and consistency. Check the contents of the toilet if the patient was in the bathroom.

25. Clean the bedpan and put it away.

Ending Steps

■ Check to see that the patient is comfortable.

■ Lower the bed and raise the side rails, if appropriate.

■ Place the call signal within the patient's reach.

■ Wash your hands.

■ Report and record your observations.

Cleansing Enemas

A cleansing enema involves introducing 750 to 1,000 cc of a solution ordered by the doctor into the patient's rectum and colon. (See Figure 23–13.) The water temperature for the enema solution should be 105° F or 40.5° C. Wear gloves and use aseptic technique when giving an enema. Hold the tubing during the procedure as the force of the water may dislodge it. If the patient complains of cramps, close the clamp and wait a few minutes before resuming the enema. Encourage the patient to breathe through the mouth. Report to the nurse if the patient is unable to hold the solution or does not release all the solution that has been given. (The procedure for giving a cleansing enema is located on pages 323 and 324.)

Commercially Prepared Enemas

The commercially prepared enema comes prepackaged and ready to use. The most common type is a disposable plastic container filled with solution. Sometimes an oil retention solution is used to soften and lubricate the stool. Some facilities do not allow nursing assistants to give commercially

Procedure for Giving a Commercially Prepared Enema

Beginning Steps

■ Identify the patient and explain the procedure.
■ Collect necessary equipment and supplies.
■ Wash your hands and use standard precautions.
■ Protect the patient's privacy.
■ Use correct body mechanics.

1. Raise the side rails, raise the bed to a comfortable working height, and lock the brakes.
2. Lower the side rail nearest you.
3. Assist the patient onto the left side and cover with a bath blanket.
4. Put on disposable gloves.
5. Uncover the patient enough to expose the anus. Place a bed protector under the buttocks.
6. Remove the cap of the commercially prepared enema and expose the tip of the container (see Figure 23–14A).
7. Separate the buttocks and ask the patient to take a deep breath.
8. Insert the lubricated tip of the container into the rectum (see Figure 23–14B).
9. Squeeze the container gently until all the solution has been given.
10. Remove the tip of the container from the anus.

11. Place the tip of the used container into the original container (see Figure 23–14C).
12. Encourage the patient to lie quietly and hold the solution as long as possible.
13. Assist the patient onto the bedpan or into the bathroom.
14. Place toilet tissue and the call signal within reach.
15. Discard the disposable equipment in the proper container.
16. Remove your gloves and wash your hands. Discard the gloves in the proper container.
17. Leave the room for a few minutes if possible. Check back frequently.
18. When the patient is through, put on gloves and assist the patient to clean the perineal area.
19. Observe the enema results and empty the bedpan or flush the commode.
20. Clean and put away equipment and supplies.

Ending Steps

■ Check to see that the patient is comfortable.
■ Lower the bed and raise the side rails if appropriate.
■ Place the call signal within the patient's reach.
■ Wash your hands.
■ Report and record your observations.

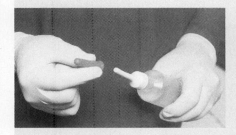

A. Remove the cap and expose the tip of the enema container.

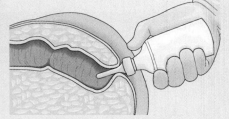

B. Insert the lubricated tip of the enema container into the rectum.

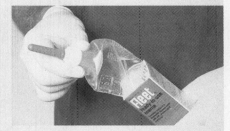

C. The tip of the used container is placed into the original container to prevent contamination.

FIGURE 23–14
Giving a commercially prepared enema.

prepared enemas. It is your responsibility to know the policy of the facility where you work.

Rectal Tubes

A rectal tube may be ordered to help eliminate flatus from the patient's colon. In some facilities, nursing

assistants are not allowed to insert rectal tubes. Be sure that you know the policy of your facility.

Inserting a Suppository

A *suppository* is a cone-shaped, semisolid substance that is inserted into the rectum. It may be used to

Procedure for Inserting a Rectal Tube

Beginning Steps

- Identify the patient and explain the procedure.
- Collect necessary equipment and supplies.
- Wash your hands and use standard precautions.
- Protect the patient's privacy.
- Use correct body mechanics.

1. Raise the side rails, raise the bed to a comfortable working height, and lock the wheels.
2. Lower the rail on the side nearest you.
3. Assist the patient onto the left side and place a disposable bed protector under the patient's buttocks. Cover with a bath blanket.
4. Put on gloves.
5. Lubricate 2 to 4 inches of the tip of the rectal tube.
6. Fold the blanket back. Raise the upper buttock so you can see the anus.
7. Gently insert the rectal tube 2 to 4 inches through the anus into the rectum (see Figure 23–15).
8. Apply a small piece of adhesive tape to secure the tube to the buttocks, or follow facility policy if tape is not allowed.
9. Place the flatus bag on the bed protector. If there is no flatus bag available, place the open end of the flatus tube into a paper cup filled with cotton balls.

10. Cover the patient and leave the tube in place for 20 minutes, or as ordered. Ask the patient to remain lying on the side until the procedure is complete.
11. Remove gloves and wash your hands. Discard gloves in the proper container.
12. Lower the bed and raise the side rails, if appropriate. Make sure the call signal is within reach.
13. Leave the room and check on the patient frequently.
14. Return to the room when the time specified is up.
15. Put on gloves and remove the rectal tube.
16. Wipe the rectal area with toilet tissue and place the tissue on a paper towel.
17. Remove the bed protector and the bath blanket after covering the patient with linen.
18. Clean and put away equipment and discard disposables in the proper container.
19. Ask the patient about the amount of gas expelled and if he or she is more comfortable.

Ending Steps

- Check to see that the patient is comfortable.
- Lower the bed and raise the side rails, if appropriate.
- Place the call signal within the patient's reach.
- Wash your hands.
- Report and record your observations.

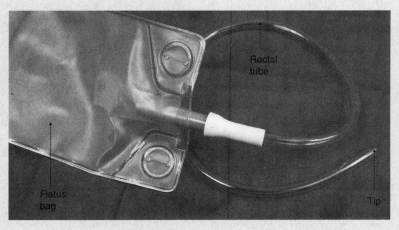

FIGURE 23–15
A rectal tube may be used to relieve flatus from the colon.

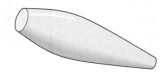

FIGURE 23–16   A rectal suppository.

soften the stool and stimulate defecation. Many facilities do not allow nursing assistants to insert suppositories. Some suppositories are medicated, and nursing assistants are not allowed to give medication of any kind. (See Figure 23–16.)

Guidelines for Inserting a Suppository

- Wear gloves and use aseptic technique.
- Remove any foil cover from the suppository.
- Lubricate the suppository before inserting it.
- Insert the narrow end into the anus (opening to the rectum).
- Gently push the suppository 2 to 3 inches into the rectum.
- Ask the patient to try to retain the suppository for as long as possible.
- Record and report the results.

Ostomies

An *ostomy* is a procedure in which a surgical opening is made into the body. The artificial opening of the ostomy is called a *stoma*. An ostomy bag or appliance is usually placed over the stoma to collect the waste material that is expelled. Some ostomies do not require an appliance. A gauze or large Band-Aid may be placed over the stoma.

The patient with an ostomy may have feelings of anxiety, embarrassment, and anger. Having an artificial opening in the body can affect body image and lead to depression and social withdrawal. The loss of control can lower self-esteem. Most people eventually adjust and learn to care for their own ostomy and continue to live normal lives. As a nursing assistant, you can help the patient adjust to the ostomy. Allow the patient to do as much of the ostomy care as possible. This helps build confidence and promote independence. (See Figure 23–17.)

Colostomy

A *colostomy* is a surgical opening through the abdominal wall into the colon. A colostomy may

Guidelines for Performing Ostomy Care

- Wear gloves and use standard precautions.
- Gently remove appliances that are applied to the skin.
- Clean the skin around the stoma with soap and water.
- Observe the skin around the stoma for redness and irritation.
- Use skin cream or protector around the stoma, as ordered.
- Empty the bag and observe the contents.
- Clean the reusable bag with soap and water.
- Attach the appliance and fasten the clamp securely to prevent leakage.
- Report and record your observations.

be necessary when disease or injury prevents elimination of stool from the anus. A section of the colon is brought to the surface of the abdomen and a stoma is created. Feces and flatus pass through the stoma to the outside of the body.

The colostomy site depends on the location of the injury or disease. The consistency of the feces expelled through the stoma depends on the location of the colostomy. Water is removed from the feces as it moves through the colon, so the nearer the colostomy is to the rectum, the more normal the feces will appear. See Figure 23–18 for examples of colostomy locations.

Be aware of your feelings while providing care for the patient with a colostomy and avoid facial

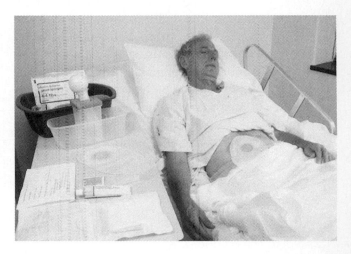

FIGURE 23–17
Allow the patient to do as much of his own ostomy care as possible.

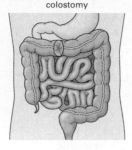

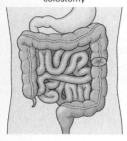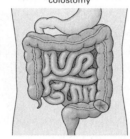

FIGURE 23–18
Colostomy site locations.

expressions that indicate distaste for the procedure. Caring for the ostomy in an accepting, professional manner may help the patient be more accepting as well.

Providing Colostomy Care

Colostomy care should be provided every time the patient has a bowel movement. This might involve emptying and cleaning the bag, or it might include changing the entire appliance. Keep the patient's skin clean and dry and observe for redness, rash, or skin breakdown. An adhesive may be used to secure the appliance to the skin and prevent leaking around the stoma. However, these adhesives may also irritate the skin. Proper cleaning and emptying of the ostomy appliance helps to prevent odor and infection. Empty the bag every time soiling occurs, and clean or replace it immediately. Deodorants are available to prevent odor in the bag.

 Review

Read each sentence and fill in the blank with the vocabulary term that best completes the sentence.
1. The inability to control urine or feces is called _____.
2. _____ is air or gas expelled from the rectum.
3. Excessive urination during the night is called _____.
4. A/an _____ is a cone-shaped semisolid substance that is inserted into the rectum.
5. The artificial opening of an ostomy is called the _____.

 Remember

1. Eating a well-balanced diet and drinking plenty of fluids help promote elimination.
2. Be aware of cultural influences when assisting patients with elimination.
3. Follow standard precautions and wear gloves when you are assisting patients with elimination.
4. Assist patients to meet elimination needs as independently as possible.
5. The patient who has an incontinent episode requires immediate care.
6. The urinary drainage system should be left closed and connected as much as possible to prevent infection.
7. Always keep the urinary drainage bag below the level of the bladder.
8. When assisting with peri-care, clean from the urinary meatus toward the anus.
9. Empty the urinary drainage bag into a graduate. Do not use the measurements on the side of the drainage bag.
10. The goal of bowel and bladder retraining is to restore elimination to as nearly normal as possible.
11. Constipation can often be prevented by increasing fluids and exercise.
12. Encourage patients to hold enema fluid for as long as possible.
13. Follow facility policy regarding administration of enemas, rectal tubes, and suppositories.
14. Colostomy care should be provided every time the patient has a bowel movement.

Reflect

Read the following case study and answer the questions.

Case Study

While making rounds, Patty discovers that Mrs. Mayberry's bed is wet. Mrs. Mayberry is weak, frail, and confused. She tells Patty that "someone else" has wet her bed. Patty answers, "Mrs. Mayberry, you know better than that. No one else has been in your room. You wet your bed." Patty observes that the liquid in the bed is dark in color. There are smears of stool on the gown and on the sheet. Mrs. Mayberry is not usually incontinent. Patty tells Mrs. Mayberry that she will clean her up when she does her bath later. Patty reports and records the incontinent episode.

1. Was Patty's comment to Mrs. Mayberry appropriate? Explain your answer.
2. What might the dark-colored liquid and smears of stool indicate?
3. When should Patty plan to cleanse and change Mrs. Mayberry?
4. How should Patty chart this information and what should she report to the nurse?

Respond

Choose the best answer for each question.

1. You observe that the patient has red-colored urine that looks like blood. What should you do?
   A. Ignore it. The color probably is a result of medication.
   B. Report to the nurse that the patient has red-colored urine.
   C. Report to the nurse that the patient has blood in the urine.
   D. None of the above.
2. The patient on a bedside commode is slightly confused. Which action is best?
   A. Stay with the patient to prevent an accident.
   B. Leave the room to allow patient privacy.
   C. Restrain the patient to the bedside commode and leave the room.
   D. Put the patient on a bedpan instead of the bedside commode.
3. Urinary incontinence is a normal change of aging.
   A. True
   B. False
4. Which of the following is NOT a guideline for caring for a urinary drainage system?
   A. Keep the system closed and connected.
   B. Report any leaks immediately.
   C. Keep the tubing free of kinks.
   D. Keep the drainage bag above the level of the bladder.
5. A catheter that is placed into the bladder and left in place to drain urine is often called
   A. A French catheter
   B. A straight catheter
   C. A Foley catheter
   D. A curved catheter
6. A large amount of hard, dry stool that cannot be expelled normally from the rectum is called a fecal
   A. Diarrhea
   B. Stoma
   C. Impaction
   D. Colostomy
7. Loose, watery stool that is caused when peristalsis pushes food too rapidly through the intestines is
   A. Diarrhea
   B. Constipation
   C. Impaction
   D. Colostomy
8. How deep into the rectum should a suppository be inserted?
   A. 1/2 to 1 inch
   B. 2 to 3 inches
   C. 4 to 5 inches
   D. 6 to 8 inches
9. A surgical opening through the abdominal wall into the colon is a/an
   A. Tracheostomy
   B. Colostomy
   C. Hysterectomy
   D. Impaction
10. How often should colostomy care be provided?
    A. Every 2 hours
    B. Once a shift
    C. As often as soiling occurs
    D. As often as time allows

Chapter Twenty-Four

Special Care *and* Procedures

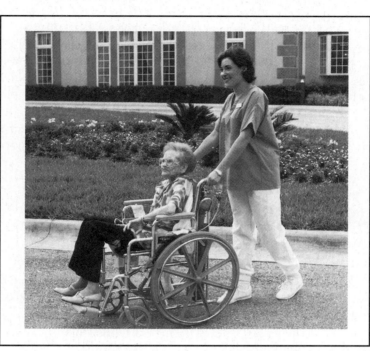

OBJECTIVES

After studying this chapter, you will be able to _____

1. Identify four guidelines for care of the patient receiving oxygen.

2. List four guidelines for care of the patient in traction.

3. Describe four guidelines for cast care.

4. Explain the method for measuring the height of a patient in bed.

5. List four guidelines each for collecting a fresh-fractional urine specimen and a 24-hour urine specimen.

6. Identify two methods for diabetic testing for sugar and acetone.

7. Describe four guidelines for administration of a vaginal irrigation.

8. List four guidelines for applying elastic support hose.

9. Describe six guidelines for heat and cold applications.

10. Perform the procedures described in this chapter that are appropriate in your facility.

Glossary

oxygen   A colorless, odorless gas, that is essential to life.

fracture   A break in a bone.

immobilize   To position a limb or body part to prevent movement.

This chapter includes a variety of tasks that are not done on a routine basis. The tasks are grouped into a category called special procedures. Included are procedures or guidelines for care of patients with oxygen, fractures, traction, and casts; measuring height and weight; collecting specimens; straining urine; diabetic testing for sugar and acetone; applying support hose and elastic bandages; giving vaginal irrigations; and applying heat and cold applications. Nursing assistant responsibilities regarding these procedures vary from state to state and even from facility to facility. Your instructor will decide which of these procedures is appropriate for you to learn. Remember, however, that you are responsible for knowing what your duties are in the facility in which you are working.

Care of the Patient Receiving Oxygen

Oxygen, a colorless, odorless gas, is essential to life. Oxygen (O_2) is found naturally in the air, and we bring it into our bodies through respiration (breathing). An illness or injury may interfere with the respiratory process and decrease the amount of oxygen in the body. When this happens, the doctor may order additional oxygen. The doctor's order includes the method, rate, and length of time for oxygen administration.

In most facilities, nursing assistants may not start, adjust, or discontinue the flow rate of oxygen. However, because you will care for patients receiving oxygen, you need to have a clear understanding of how it is administered and how it effects the body. You play an important role in helping meet the needs of patients who are receiving oxygen.

Oxygen may be supplied by piped-in wall outlets, freestanding tanks, or concentrators. The flow rate of oxygen from wall outlets is regulated by a flow gauge. An oxygen tank has a flow gauge and a pressure gauge that indicates the amount of oxygen remaining in the tank. Oxygen concentrators concentrate the O_2 from the air in the room. Because oxygen is very drying, it goes through distilled water in a humidifier before reaching the patient. The water container must be kept at the proper level indicated on the side of the humidifier.

As a nursing assistant, you need to understand how the oxygen equipment works. If a tank is used, check the pressure gauge and let the nurse know when the amount of oxygen remaining in the tank is low. Be aware of the flow gauge, and report any changes to the nurse. Special safety precautions must be taken when oxygen is being used. Because oxygen supports combustion, fire prevention methods are very important. Follow the guidelines for oxygen safety given in Chapter 6.

Oxygen is usually administered by face mask or nasal cannula (see Figure 24–1). Face masks are used in an emergency situation when oxygen is needed quickly. The mask covers the mouth and nose and is a fast, efficient way of providing oxygen. However, with the mask in place it is difficult for the patient to communicate, and some people feel smothered by the mask.

The nasal cannula is the most comfortable method of oxygen administration. Oxygen flows through two prongs inserted into the nostrils. The tubing loops up over the ears and under the chin to keep it in place. The top of the ears may need to be padded to prevent irritation from the tubing.

The patient receiving oxygen has special needs. Dyspnea (difficult breathing) may cause the patient to feel tired or uncomfortable and can be very frightening. When oxygen does not ease breathing, the patient may become even more upset. Check the patient frequently and offer reassurance. Listen to the patient's concerns and report any problems to the nurse. Providing emotional support is as important as meeting physical needs.

The mouth and nose may become dry and irritated from the oxygen or the equipment, so frequent mouth care is necessary. Lubrication of the lips and the area around the nostrils will help prevent skin breakdown. Because the patient may perspire heavily, frequent linen changes and proper skin care will be required.

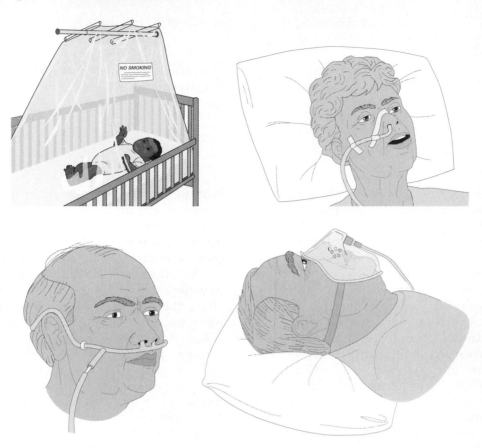

FIGURE 24–1 Methods of oxygen administration.

The patient with respiratory problems may cough or sneeze frequently. Do not handle contaminated tissues without gloves. Provide the patient with a convenient container or bag for disposing of tissues. Follow standard precautions any time you are in contact with mucus or other body fluids.

Guidelines for Assisting the Patient Who Is Receiving Oxygen

- Follow safety precautions when oxygen is in use.
- Follow standard precautions and wear gloves when necessary.
- Check the patient frequently to identify needs and anxieties.
- Help the patient conserve energy and strength.
- Provide periods of rest after activities.
- Provide frequent mouth care.
- Prevent pressure or discomfort caused by oxygen devices.
- Provide bathing, skin care, linen changes, and clothing changes as necessary.
- Assist the patient to a comfortable position. An upright position often makes breathing easier. (See Figure 24–2.)
- Check for and report changes in gauges and humidifiers.

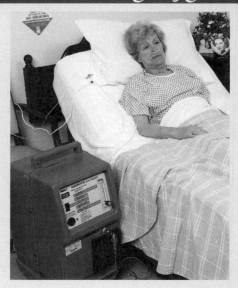

FIGURE 24–2
Remember that the patient receiving oxygen has special needs.

Care of the Patient with a Fracture

A *fracture* (broken bone) may be classified as an open fracture if the skin is broken, or a closed fracture if the skin remains intact. A fracture may be treated with a cast, splint, pins, nails, or traction to *immobilize* (prevent movement of) the bone while it is healing.

Immobilized patients require special care because they are at increased risk for skin breakdown, constipation, blood clots, and pneumonia. Exercise of unaffected limbs is important. Keep the skin clean and dry and observe carefully for skin irritation.

Care of the patient with a fracture depends on the patient's age and general physical condition, other injuries, and the type of fracture. For example, care of an elderly patient with a hip fracture would not be the same as the care of a 10-year-old with a fractured arm. Check the care plan daily. Patient care routines and treatments will change as the fracture begins to heal.

A fractured hip may be repaired with a pin, a plate, or a prosthesis. The affected leg is to be kept abducted (away from the mid-line of the body) to prevent strain on the operative site. The patient should not cross the legs or rotate or twist the affected leg outward. Check with the nurse regarding movement and positioning of the patient with a hip fracture (see Figure 24–3).

Traction

Traction is the use of a pulling force to immobilize a fracture or realign broken bones. Traction can be applied to the skin or to the bone. Although many types of traction are available, most types involve weights, ropes, and pulleys. Some traction can be removed at intervals, while other types of traction must be kept in place continuously. Nursing assistants are not allowed to remove or adjust traction equipment. Check with the nurse if you are not sure how to care for the patient in traction.

Guidelines for Care of the Patient in Traction

- Keep the patient pulled up in bed in order for the traction to pull properly.
- Never lift, remove, or adjust the weights or allow the weights to touch the floor.
- Observe for skin pressure that may result from the equipment or from immobilization.
- Exercise unaffected limbs if permitted.
- Observe for circulation in the affected area. Check for swelling, odor, change in skin color, or a change in skin temperature.
- Report patient complaints of pain, numbness, tingling, or discomfort. (See Figure 24–4.)

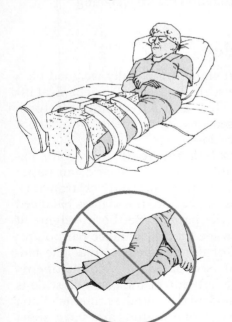

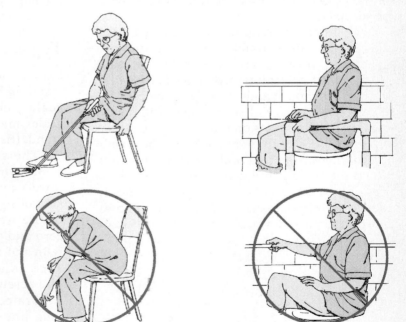

FIGURE 24–3
Some precautions for patients with hip fractures include:
  Use an abduction device to keep the fracture in the proper position.
  Do not allow the patient to lie on his or her side with legs together.
  Do not rotate or turn the operated leg outward.
  Have patient use a device for reaching objects on the floor or shelves.

Do not allow the patient to bend forward from the waist more than 90 degrees—to pull up blankets or socks, for example, or to tie shoes. Provide adaptive devices for these purposes.
Have the patient sit in a high chair.
Do not allow the patient to cross his or her legs or raise the knee on the affected side higher than the hip.

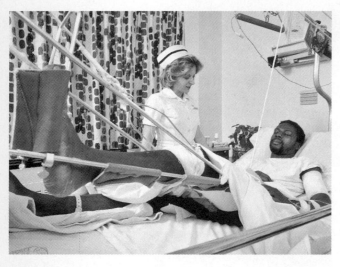

FIGURE 24-4
A patient in traction requires special nursing care.

Guidelines for Cast Care

- Observe and report changes in skin color, swelling, or temperature.
- Check the skin area around a cast for pressure or irritation. Report any problems to the nurse.
- Keep the cast dry.
- Report patient complaints of numbness, pain, or tingling to the nurse.
- Report stains or color changes in the cast material that may indicate bleeding or drainage inside the cast.
- Report any odor coming from the cast that could indicate infection.
- Discourage the patient from inserting anything into the cast to relieve itching.

Cast Care

A cast may be made of plaster or fiberglass. Fiberglass is often used because it is lightweight, easily removed or adjusted, and more comfortable than plaster. The patient with a cast must be observed frequently for signs of complications. Skin must be assessed carefully for pressure or irritation that may result from the appliance, swelling, or immobilization. Toes and fingers are left exposed for this purpose. The skin should be warm to the touch and of normal color.

A new plaster cast requires special care until it dries. Fiberglass dries quickly, but a plaster cast may take a day or two to dry completely. The shape of the cast must be maintained while it is drying. Use the palms of your hands to support the cast, because even the pressure of your fingers will dent it and create pressure points on the underlying skin. A bed cradle over lower extremities keeps the weight of the bedding off the cast and allows air to circulate. Turn the patient frequently to expose all the surfaces of the cast and allow the cast to dry evenly. A casted extremity is usually elevated on pillows. Check with the nurse if you are not sure how to care for the cast.

Measuring the Patient's Weight

Patients are usually weighed on admission to a health care facility. The doctor may order a one-time weight measurement or that the patient be weighed on a regular schedule. A change in weight may indicate a change in the patient's condition. Doses of medication, treatments, and diet may be based on the patient's weight.

To ensure accuracy in weight measurements, weigh the patient on the same scale, in the same type of clothing, and at the same time of day. Assist the patient with toileting before weighing.

Types of Scales

Patients who can stand are usually weighed on a standing balance scale. Bed scales, mechanical lift scales, chair scales, and wheelchair platform scales may be used to weigh patients who cannot stand. (See Figure 24-5.)

The **standing balance scale** is used for patients who are able to stand. Place clean paper towels on the platform to prevent the transmission of pathogens. Make sure the scale is balanced before weighing the patient. Set both weights at zero and check to see that the balance bar pointer is in the middle of the designated area. The balance adjustment is usually set by adjustments of a screw on the left side of the bar. The scale is calibrated in one-fourth pound segments. Each long line designates one pound, and each short line designates one-fourth of a pound. Instructions for weighing a patient using a standing balance scale are included in the procedure for measuring height and weight located on page 336.

A bed scale is used to weigh patients who are bedbound. The patient is rolled onto a plat-

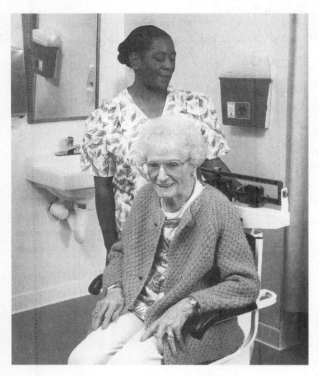

FIGURE 24-5
A chair scale may be used to weigh patients.

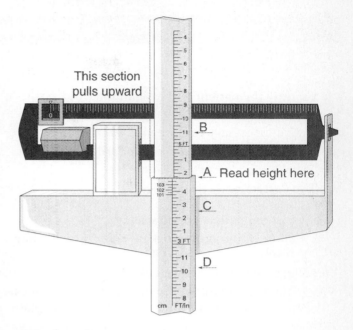

FIGURE 24-6
Reading the height measurement rod on a standing balance scale.

form that is placed on the bed. The scale is then raised above the bed, and the weight is measured. The mechanical lift scale is a hydraulic lift that raises the patient off the bed to be measured. A chair scale is an armchair balanced on a weight mechanism with a foot rest to support the patient's feet. A wheelchair platform scale weighs the patient and the wheelchair together. The weight of the empty wheelchair is subtracted from the total weight of the patient and the chair.

Measuring the Patient's Height

The height of the patient who can stand can be measured with the height measurement rod that is attached to the standing balance scale. The rod measures the height in inches and fractions of inches. It is calibrated in 1/4 inch segments (see Figure 24-6). To measure the height of a patient in bed, place a mark at the top of the patient's head and another at the bottom of the feet, and measure the distance between the marks with a tape measure. If the patient has contractures and cannot lie in a straight position, use the tape measure and follow the curves of the spine and legs. Instructions for measuring the height of a patient who can stand are included in the procedure for measuring height and weight located on page 336.

Collecting Specimens

The doctor may order that a specimen of tissue or fluid from the patient's body be collected. Wear gloves and use aseptic practices to avoid contaminating yourself or the specimen. Label the specimen container accurately before you collect the specimen. (See Figure 24-7.)

Collecting a Urine Specimen

Urine specimens may be collected and sent to the lab, or they may be tested in the work area. Urine specimens that you will most commonly collect in-

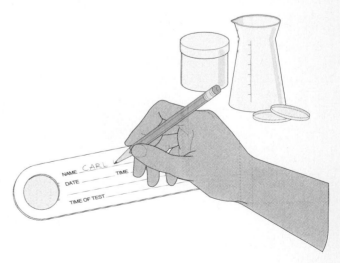

FIGURE 24-7
Label the specimen container accurately.

Procedure for Using a Standing Balance Scale

Beginning Steps

- Identify the patient and explain the procedure.
- Collect necessary equipment and supplies.
- Wash your hands and use standard precautions.
- Protect the patient's privacy.
- Use correct body mechanics.

1. Assist the patient to the scale.
2. Balance the scale so that the balance bar is level.
3. Place clean paper towels on the platform.
4. Assist the patient to step out of his or her shoes and robe and onto the center of the scale platform.
5. Slide the bottom weight (marked in 50-pound segments) to the approximate patient weight (see Figure 24–8).
6. Slide the top weight until the pointer is balanced in the middle.

7. Add the bottom and top numbers together. For example, if the bottom number is 150 and the top number is 15, the patient's weight is 165 pounds. Make a note of the weight.
8. Ask the patient to stand up straight with the arms at the side.
9. Lower the height rod until it rests on the patient's head
10. Note the height and record it.
11. Assist the patient off the scale and into his or her shoes.
12. Dispose of paper towels.

Ending Steps

- Check to see that the patient is comfortable.
- Place the call signal within the patient's reach.
- Wash your hands.
- Report and record your observations.

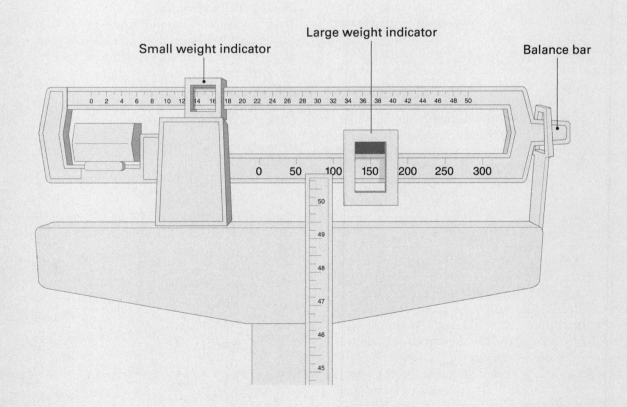

FIGURE 24–8
This scale indicates a weight of 165 pounds. (Add the bottom measurement of 150 and the top measurement of 15.)

Procedure for Collecting a Routine Urine Specimen

Beginning Steps

- Identify the patient and explain the procedure.
- Collect necessary equipment and supplies.
- Wash your hands and use standard precautions.
- Protect the patient's privacy.
- Use correct body mechanics.

1. Select and label the specimen container with the patient's name and any other information required by the facility.
2. Put on disposable gloves.
3. Ask the patient to urinate into a clean bedpan or urinal. Assist as necessary.
4. Pour the urine from the bedpan or urinal into the specimen container.

5. Place the lid on the container, being careful not to touch the inside of either the lid or the container.
6. Clean and replace the equipment.
7. Remove the gloves and discard them in the proper container. Wash your hands.
8. Take the labeled container to the designated area.

Ending Steps

- Check to see that the patient is comfortable.
- Place the call signal within the patient's reach.
- Wash your hands.
- Report and record your observations.

---

clude routine urine specimens, clean-catch urine specimens, fresh-fractional urine specimens, and 24-hour urine specimens. Make sure the urinal or bedpan is clean and dry before you collect the urine specimen. Ask the patient not to have a bowel movement or place toilet tissue in the pan to avoid contaminating the specimen.

A **routine urine specimen** requires no special preparation. It is routinely collected on admission. The nurse will tell you when to collect the specimen.

A **clean-catch urine specimen** is collected to obtain a clean specimen that is as free from contamination as possible. It may also be called a

Procedure for Collecting a Clean-Catch Urine Specimen

Beginning Steps

- Identify the patient and explain the procedure.
- Collect necessary equipment and supplies.
- Wash your hands and use standard precautions.
- Protect the patient's privacy.
- Use correct body mechanics.

1. Select and label the specimen container.
2. Put on disposable gloves.
3. Provide perineal care.
4. Place the patient on a clean, dry bedpan, provide a urinal, or assist to the bathroom.
5. Ask the patient to begin voiding and then stop.
6. Hold the specimen container under the patient and ask him or her to resume voiding.

7. Ask the patient to stop voiding when the urine has been collected.
8. Allow the patient to finish voiding.
9. Place the lid on the container, being careful not to touch the inside.
10. Clean and replace the equipment.
11. Remove the gloves and discard them in the proper container. Wash your hands.
12. Assist the patient with handwashing.
13. Take the labeled container to the designated area.

Ending Steps

- Check to see that the patient is comfortable.
- Place the call signal within the patient's reach.
- Wash your hands.
- Report and record your observations.

midstream or a clean-voided urine specimen. Perform perineal care first to help prevent contamination.

A **fresh-fractional urine specimen**, or a double-voided specimen, is collected to obtain a freshly voided urine specimen. A fresh-fractional urine specimen may be obtained to test for the presence of sugar or acetone in the urine.

A **24-hour urine specimen** requires collecting all the urine that is voided during a 24-hour period. The collection begins after the patient empties the bladder. The urine from the first void-

Guidelines for Collecting a 24-Hour Urine Specimen

■ Wear gloves and use aseptic technique.
■ Follow the general guidelines for collecting a urine specimen.
■ Ask the patient to void. Discard that first urine and start the test collection.
■ Keep ice in the bucket or pan that holds the collection container.
■ Explain to the patient and family that all urine must be saved for the next 24 hours.
■ Place all the urine collected in the large container. (See Figure 24–9.)
■ Save the last voided urine during the 24-hour period. It is part of the test.
■ Let the nurse know immediately if incontinence occurs or urine is accidentally discarded.

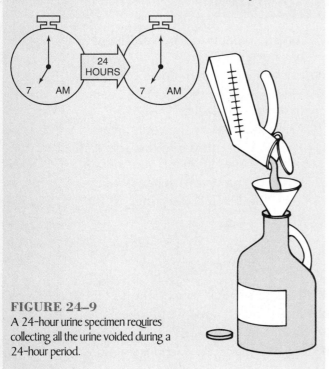

FIGURE 24–9
A 24-hour urine specimen requires collecting all the urine voided during a 24-hour period.

Guidelines for Collecting a Fresh-Fractional Urine Specimen

■ Wear gloves and use aseptic technique.
■ Follow the general guidelines for collecting a urine specimen.
■ Ask the patient to void at the specified time.
■ Collect a specimen. (This specimen will not be used unless a second specimen cannot be obtained.)
■ Return in 30 minutes and ask the patient to void again. Collect a specimen.
■ If the specimen is collected for diabetic urine testing, test the second specimen.
■ Let the nurse know if you were unable to collect a second specimen.

ing is discarded and is not considered a part of the collection. All the urine that is collected must be kept chilled to prevent the growth of microorganisms.

Collecting a Urine Specimen from an Infant

A special procedure is used to collect a urine specimen from an infant or small child who is not yet toilet trained. A collective device is applied over the genital area and the urinary meatus (outer opening to the urethra). The device is usually a plastic bag with an adhesive that is applied to the child's skin.

Straining Urine

The doctor may order that the patient's urine be strained for stones or other material that may be present in the urinary system. Inform the patient and the family that all the urine must be saved for this purpose. Guidelines for straining urine are located on page 340.

Collecting a Stool Specimen

Stool specimens are collected to test for blood, fat, microorganisms, parasites (worms), or other conditions. Make sure the bedpan is clean and dry and ask the patient not to urinate or place toilet tissue in the pan. A stool specimen from an infant may be collected from the diaper. If a warm stool specimen is required, the specimen must go to the laboratory promptly. The procedure for collecting a stool specimen is located on page 340.

Procedure for Collecting a Urine Specimen from an Infant

Beginning Steps

- Identify the patient and explain the procedure.
- Collect necessary equipment and supplies.
- Wash your hands and use standard precautions.
- Protect the patient's privacy.
- Use correct body mechanics.

1. Select and label the specimen container.
2. Put on disposable gloves.
3. Remove the diaper from the infant.
4. Clean the perineal area.
5. Remove the protective backing from the collection device, exposing the adhesive.
6. Apply the collection device to the perineum. Do not cover the anus (see Figure 24–10).
7. Diaper the infant.
8. Remove your gloves and wash your hands. Discard gloves in the proper container.

9. Check back frequently to see if the infant has urinated.
10. After the infant urinates, put on gloves and carefully remove the collection device.
11. Clean the perineal area and replace the diaper.
12. Put the specimen into a labeled specimen container and cover it.
13. Make sure the baby is clean, dry, and comfortable.
14. Clean and replace equipment.
15. Remove the gloves and discard them in the proper container. Wash your hands.
16. Take the labeled container to the designated area.

Ending Steps

- Wash your hands.
- Report and record your observations.

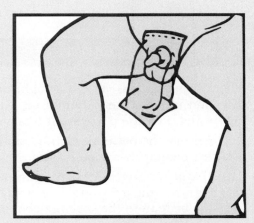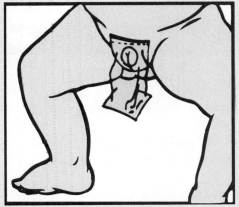

FIGURE 24–10 A urine specimen collection device for an infant.

Collecting a Sputum Specimen

A sputum specimen is collected to test for infection or disease. Sputum is a thick, sticky mucus from the lungs and indicates respiratory problems. In some facilities, nursing assistants are not allowed to collect sputum specimens. Guidelines for collecting a sputum specimen are located on page 341.

Diabetic Testing for Sugar and Acetone

Either urine or blood from the diabetic patient may be tested for sugar and acetone. Urine testing for glucose (sugar) is a procedure that is rarely used today because studies have shown that blood testing is more accurate. However, since some facilities may still do urine testing, information regarding the procedure has been included. Follow the policy and procedures of the facility where you work.

The urine test for sugar and acetone is called an S&A test, and there are many types of tests. Some test only for sugar in the urine, and others test only for acetone, while some test for both sugar and acetone. The procedure is different for performing each of these tests. Directions for testing the urine and reading the results are on each container. Follow the directions carefully to ensure accuracy, and re-

Guidelines for Straining Urine

- Wear gloves and follow standard precautions.
- Collect the urine in a urinal, bedpan, or specimen pan.
- Ask the patient not to have a bowel movement or put toilet paper in the pan.
- Pour the urine through a disposable strainer into a graduate (see Figure 24–11).
- If any particles are observed, place the strainer in a plastic bag or specimen container.
- Label the specimen carefully.
- Measure and record the urine for I&O if necessary.
- Report and record your observations and results.

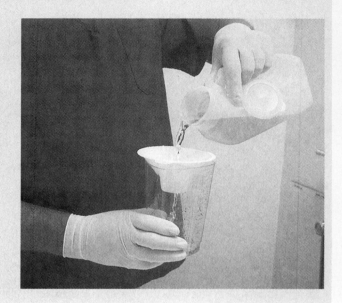

FIGURE 24–11
When straining urine, pour the urine through a disposable strainer into a graduate.

Procedure for Collecting a Stool Specimen

Beginning Steps

- Identify the patient and explain the procedure.
- Collect necessary equipment and supplies.
- Wash your hands and use standard precautions.
- Protect the patient's privacy.
- Use correct body mechanics.

1. Select and label the specimen container.
2. Put on disposable gloves.
3. Assist the patient to urinate, if necessary.
4. Place the patient on a clean, dry bedpan or place a specimen pan under the toilet seat.
5. Instruct the patient not to put toilet tissue into the bedpan or specimen pan. Provide a disposable bag for used toilet tissue.
6. Place the toilet tissue and call signal within the patient's reach.
7. Remove your gloves and discard them in the proper container. Wash your hands. Leave the room if the patient can be left alone.

8. When the patient is through, put on gloves and remove the patient from the bedpan or toilet. Provide peri-care if it is needed.
9. Ensure the patient's comfort and safety. Take the bedpan to the bathroom.
10. Use a tongue blade (tongue depressor) to transfer one or two tablespoons of stool from the bedpan to the specimen container (Figure 24–12).
11. Place the lid on the specimen container without contaminating it. Wrap the specimen container according to facility policy.
12. Empty, clean, and dry the bedpan or specimen pan.
13. Wrap the tongue blade in a paper towel and discard it in the disposable bag.
14. Clean and replace equipment. Place the disposable plastic bag in a biohazardous waste container.
15. Remove the gloves and discard them in the proper container. Wash your hands.
16. Take the labeled specimen container to the designated area.

Procedure for Collecting a Stool Specimen (cont.)

Ending Steps

■ Check to see that the patient is comfortable.

■ Place the call signal within the patient's reach.

■ Wash your hands.

■ Report and record your observations.

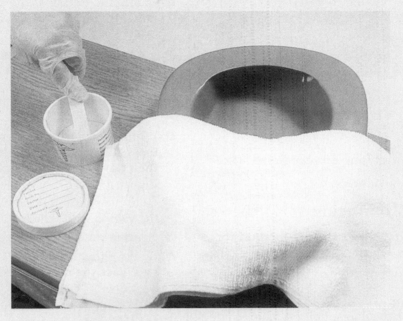

FIGURE 24–12
Use a tongue blade to transfer one or two tablespoons of stool from the bedpan to the specimen container.

Guidelines for Collecting a Sputum Specimen

■ Wear gloves and use aseptic technique. A mask and gown may be necessary.

■ Label a sputum specimen container.

■ Allow the patient to rinse the mouth with plain water. Do not use mouthwash.

■ Instruct the patient to take a few deep breaths and cough.

■ The patient should expectorate directly into the specimen container (see Figure 24–13).

■ Cover the container immediately. Do not contaminate yourself or the specimen.

■ Remove your gloves and wash your hands.

■ Take the contents to the designated area.

■ Record the procedure and report your observations.

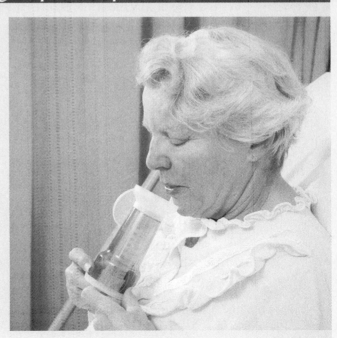

FIGURE 24–13
The patient should expectorate directly into the sputum specimen container.

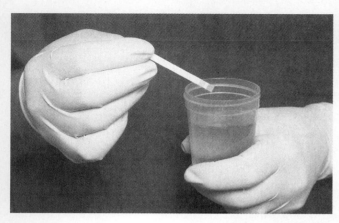

FIGURE 24–14
Test strips may be used to check for sugar or acetone in the urine.

port the test results to the nurse immediately. (See Figure 24–14.)

Blood Glucose Monitoring

Blood glucose testing is the preferred method for monitoring blood sugar level in the diabetic patient. It gives a more accurate current assessment than urine testing and is less subject to human error. In most areas, nursing assistants are not allowed to perform blood tests. Be aware of the policies and procedures of your facility.

Vaginal Irrigations

A vaginal irrigation (douche) is the introduction of fluid into the vagina for cleansing or medical treatment. It may be used to apply heat or cold or to medicate vaginal tissues. In some areas, nursing assistants are not allowed to give vaginal irrigations. Follow the policy of the facility where you are working.

Elastic Support Hose and Elastic Bandages

Elastic support hose and elastic bandages may be used to prevent and treat blood clots, provide comfort and support, or reduce swelling in the legs. They are often ordered for patients with heart disease and other circulatory problems. They improve circulation by exerting pressure on the veins, which promotes blood return to the heart. Always apply elastic support hose and elastic bandages properly to prevent discomfort and injury.

Guidelines for Administering a Vaginal Irrigation

- Assist the patient to empty the bladder.
- Provide peri-care.
- Place the patient on a clean bedpan.
- Clamp the tubing of the douche kit and fill the douche container with warm solution (105° F or 40.5° C).
- Expel air from the tubing by releasing the clamp and allowing the solution to flow through the nozzle and over the genitals, without allowing the nozzle to touch the vulva.
- While the solution flows, insert the nozzle 2 to 3 inches into the vagina, in an upward, then downward and backward motion (see Figure 24–15).
- Hold the solution container 12 inches above the vagina while the solution flows.
- Gently rotate the nozzle.
- Remove the nozzle after clamping the tubing and place the nozzle inside the solution container.
- Ask the patient to sit upright on the bedpan to allow the solution to drain from the vagina.
- Record and report your observations.

Elastic Support Hose

Elastic support hose are also called anti-embolism stockings or TED hose. The hose may be knee high or full length, and various sizes are available (see Figure 24–16). The nurse measures the patient to determine the correct size.

Elastic Bandages

Elastic bandages are strips of elasticized material of varying lengths and widths. Begin applying the bandage at the smallest part of the extremity, farthest from the heart, leaving the fingers or toes exposed. Use as many bandages as you need to cover the area. Reapply bandages if they become loose or wrinkled. Check frequently for edema, skin discoloration, or changes in skin temperature. Also check for complaints of pain, numbness, or tingling.

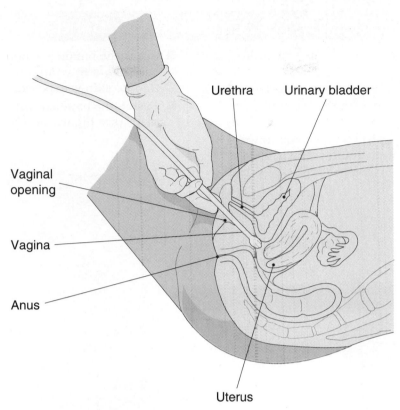

Urethra

Urinary bladder

Vaginal opening

Vagina

Anus

Uterus

FIGURE 24–15
While the solution flows, insert the nozzle 2 to 3 inches into the vagina.

Guidelines for Applying Elastic Support Hose

- Apply the hose **before** the patient gets out of bed.
- Hold the heel of the stocking and gather the rest of the stocking in your hand.
- Support the patient's foot at the heel.
- Slip the front of the stocking over the toes, foot, and heel.
- Pull the stocking snugly and evenly up over the leg.
- Check frequently to see that the hose are not twisted or wrinkled.
- Remove the hose at least twice a day.
- Remove the hose completely during the bath.
- Check for edema or discolored areas.

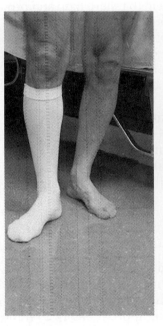
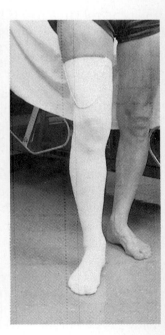

FIGURE 24–16
Elastic support hose may be knee-high or full-length size.

Guidelines for Applying Elastic Bandages

- Hold the bandage with the loose end at the bottom of the roll.
- Make two circular turns to anchor the bandage around the smallest part of the extremity (see Figure 24–17A).
- Make overlapping spiral wraps in an upward direction. Each wrap should overlap about one-half the width of the bandage (see Figure 24–17B).

- Apply the bandage smoothly and firmly, being careful not to wrap it too tightly. Make sure that no skin is exposed.
- Fasten the bandage with clips to hold it in place (see Figure 24–17C).

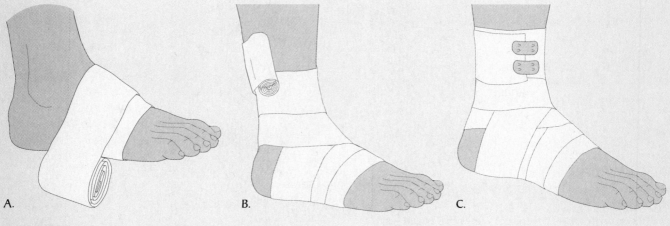

A. B. C.

FIGURE 24–17 Applying an elastic bandage on the foot.

Heat and Cold Applications

Heat and cold treatments help to relieve pain and promote healing. Heat dilates (expands) blood vessels and increases circulation, providing more oxygen and nutrients necessary for tissue repair. Heat may also reduce inflammation and relieve pain. Cold constricts (narrows) blood vessels and helps to prevent or reduce bleeding and swelling. Cold may also be used to reduce fever and pain. Heat or cold may be applied dry or moist. (See Figure 24–18.)

Dry heat application includes warm water bottles, heat lamps, and aquamatic pads. Warm compresses, soaks, and sitz baths are examples of moist heat treatments.

The Sitz Bath

A sitz bath may be ordered to relieve pain, improve circulation, or cleanse wounds in the perineal area. During the procedure, the patient sits in warm water (105° F or 40.5° C) for approximately 20 minutes. A sitz bath may be given using a disposable plastic sitz bath that fits under the toilet seat or in the bathtub. Some facilities use portable sitz bath chairs or have built-in models. Stay with the patient during the sitz bath because fatigue, weakness, or faintness may occur.

Dry, cold applications include ice bags, cold packs, and ice collars. Cold compresses, soaks, and sponge baths are examples of moist cold applications.

A Cooling Sponge Bath

A cooling sponge bath using water or alcohol may be ordered by the doctor to reduce a patient's fever. Alcohol or cool water is sponged onto the patient's skin and is left to evaporate. One area of the body is uncovered and sponged at a time. Evaporation of moisture from the skin has a cooling effect. Alcohol evaporates very quickly and usually cools more effectively than plain water. Do not apply alcohol near the face or the perineal area. Stop the procedure and notify the nurse if the patient's body temperature returns to normal or near normal, if the patient starts shivering or shows other signs of chilling, or if the patient's skin becomes cyanotic (bluish color).

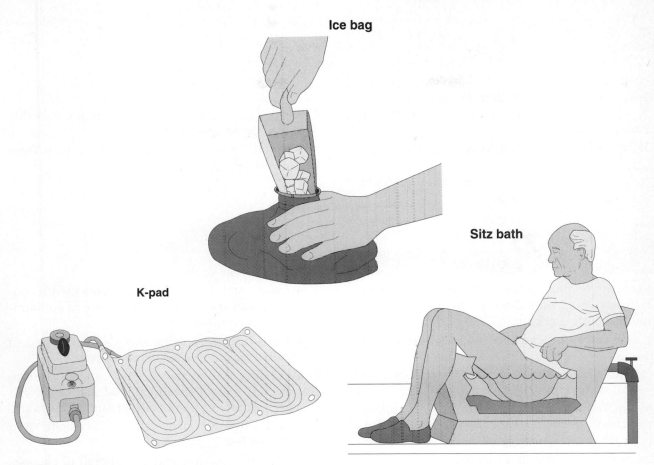

FIGURE 24-18
Examples of heat and cold applications.

Safety Factors When Using Heat and Cold

Heat or cold applications can cause serious injury if not applied and monitored properly. In many facili-

ties nursing assistants are not allowed to apply heat or cold applications because of safety concerns. The following guidelines will help you to perform these procedures safely.

Guidelines for Safe Application of Heat and Cold

- Follow facility policies and procedures regarding the application of heat and cold.
- Maintain a temperature of heat applications between 100° F and 115° F (37.8° C and 46.5° C, respectively).
- Check the water temperature of solutions with a bath thermometer.
- Keep electrical equipment away from water.
- Place a waterproof pad under moist heat to keep the bed dry.
- Add ice to cold applications as necessary to maintain constant temperature.
- Check for leaks in ice bags, collars, packs, and water bottles.
- Be sure ice bags are dry before applying.

- Cover ice bags, hot water bottles, or vinyl containers with cloth before applying to the skin.
- Be sure that caps or firm parts of bags are away from the skin.
- Do not fill ice bags or water bottles more than half full.
- Check the skin frequently under the application and report pale, cyanotic, red, white, or dark coloring.
- Report patient complaints of discomfort to the nurse promptly.
- Apply the treatment for the length of time ordered.

Review

Read each sentence and fill in the blank with the vocabulary term that best completes the sentence.

1. _____ is a colorless, odorless gas that is essential to life.

2. The medical term for a broken bone is a/an _____.

3. To _____ is to position a limb or body part to prevent movement.

4. A _____ is collected to obtain a freshly voided urine specimen.

5. The medical term for thick, sticky mucus from the lungs is _____.

Remember

1. It is your responsibility to know what procedures you can and cannot do in the facility in which you are working.

2. Follow safety precautions when oxygen is in use.

3. Immobilized patients require special care to prevent complications of limited activity.

4. Do not remove traction from patients unless specifically instructed to do so by the nurse. Never lift or remove weights.

5. Check the skin around a cast for pressure or irritation.

6. To ensure accuracy, weigh the patient on the same scale, in the same type of clothing, and at the same time of day.

7. Label the specimen container accurately before you collect the specimen.

8. A clean-catch urine sample is collected to obtain a clean specimen that is as free of contamination as possible.

9. A fresh-fractional urine sample is collected to obtain a freshly voided urine specimen.

10. Make sure the bedpan is clean and dry before collecting a stool specimen, and ask the patient not to urinate or place toilet tissue in the pan.

11. Blood glucose testing is more accurate than urine testing.

12. A vaginal irrigation may be ordered to cleanse, apply heat or cold, or medicate vaginal tissues.

13. Elastic support hose and bandages may be used to prevent or treat blood clots or to provide comfort and support.

14. Heat or cold applications can cause injury if not applied and monitored properly.

Reflect

Read the following case study and answer the questions.

Case Study

Mr. Winslow is a hospital patient who has oxygen ordered to relieve dyspnea. The oxygen is being delivered through a concentrator and nasal cannula. Mr. Winslow complains that he has a bad taste in his mouth and his nose is sore from the prongs. He seems anxious and irritable this morning. You have been assigned to give him a complete bed bath and to collect a fresh-fractional urine specimen.

1. What can you do to relieve Mr. Winslow's sore nose and the bad taste in his mouth?

2. What may be causing Mr. Winslow's anxiety, and how can you help?

3. How will you collect the fresh-fractional urine specimen?

4. What is the purpose of collecting the fresh-fractional urine specimen?

Respond

Choose the best answer for each question.

1. The medical term for difficult breathing is
   A. Fracture
   B. Dyspnea
   C. Dysuria
   D. Emesis

2. Which of the following is a guideline or precaution for caring for a patient with a hip fracture?
   A. Encourage the patient to lie on his or her side with the legs together.
   B. Allow the patient to cross the legs.
   C. Do not rotate the operated leg outward.
   D. Do not allow the patient to use an abduction device.

3. How can you measure the height of a patient who cannot stand?
   A. Estimate the height.
   B. Get someone to help you hold the patient upright on the standing balance scale.
   C. Use a tape measure and measure from head to toe.
   D. Use a yardstick and measure from head to toe.

4. You have weighed the patient on a standing balance scale. The bottom weight reads 150 and the top weight reads 35. How much does the patient weigh?
   A. 150 pounds
   B. 160 pounds
   C. 175 pounds
   D. 185 pounds

5. What special preparation is necessary when collecting a routine urine specimen?
   A. Ask the patient to void twice and test the second voiding.
   B. Ask the patient to eat nothing for 24 hours before the test.
   C. Ask the patient to interrupt voiding and begin again.
   D. None of the above.

6. What is the purpose of straining urine?
   A. To obtain a clean-catch urine specimen
   B. To look for stones or other particles in the urine
   C. To test for sugar and acetone
   D. None of the above.

7. The preferred method for diabetic testing for sugar is an S&A test?
   A. True
   B. False

8. The correct temperature for the solution used in a vaginal irrigation is
   A. 80° F
   B. 90° F
   C. 105° F
   D. 125° F

9. Which of the following is NOT a guideline for applying elastic support hose?
   A. Apply the hose after the patient gets out of bed.
   B. Adjust the stocking evenly over the leg.
   C. Remove the hose at least twice a day.
   D. Check for edema or discoloration.

10. Which of the following is NOT a guideline for heat and cold applications?
    A. Maintain a temperature of 125° F on heat applications.
    B. Keep electrical equipment away from water.
    C. Be sure caps of ice bags are away from the patient.
    D. Be sure ice bags are dry before applying.

Chapter Twenty-Five

The Geriatric Patient

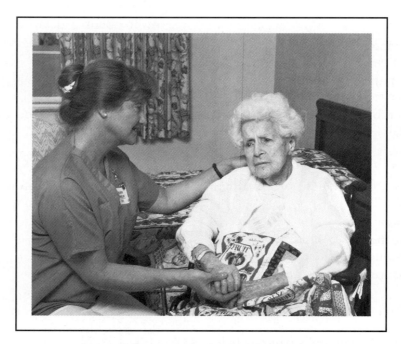

After studying this chapter, you will be able to

1. Describe three factors that affect aging.

2. List four false beliefs about aging.

3. Identify three losses and role changes of the elderly.

4. Describe the attitude toward aging in the American culture.

5. Briefly explain two theories of aging.

6. List four guidelines for assisting the elderly patient to meet basic needs.

environment The surroundings, conditions, and influences that affect an organism.
geriatric Refers to the aging person.
gerontology The branch of science that studies aging.

heredity Characteristics passed down from one's ancestors.
pollution Contamination of the environment.

Americans are living longer and healthier lives than ever before in history. There are more than 35 million people over the age of 65 with an increasing number over 85 years of age. The "baby boomers," the large number of people born at the end of World War II, will soon increase the number of elderly citizens. Unfortunately, living longer increases the risk of chronic disease.

There are many elderly patients in hospitals, in long-term care facilities, and in their homes. The majority of the elderly live alone or with their families in the community, and many of them have health care needs. This is particularly true of the frail elderly over the age of 85. Individuals in this age group are frequently admitted to health care facilities. A large percentage of residents of long-term care facilities are over the age of 85. (See Figure 25–1.)

Health care workers must be prepared to meet the needs of the elderly. They must be able to provide care that takes into consideration the changes that take place with aging and the unique needs of the elderly individual. Much of that care will be provided by nursing assistants. You will play an important role in the health and well-being of the elderly.

The goals of health care of the elderly are to delay illness, prevent illness from becoming a disability, assist the disabled to function, and prevent further disability. Rehabilitation and restorative care are the keys to meeting these goals and helping elderly patients maintain or improve their level of function and independence.

This chapter identifies the needs of the elderly patient and offers suggestions and guidelines for meeting those needs. This information will help you to become more aware of the special needs of the *geriatric* (relating to the elderly) patient. Your journey into *gerontology* (study or science of aging) will help you to care for elderly patients, friends, and family members. It will help you to understand your own aging as well.

The Aging Process

Aging is not a sudden event that begins at 65. We are aging from the moment we are born. When aging stops, death occurs. The process of aging is individualized, and no two people age at exactly the same rate. Aging is influenced by heredity, lifestyle, health, and environment. *Heredity* refers to characteristics that one inherits from one's ancestors, such as life span or length of life. If the older members of your family seem to age well and live long lives, your chances of aging well are increased.

Living a healthy lifestyle will slow the aging process and help you live longer. Eating a well-balanced diet, getting adequate rest, and exercising regularly contribute to a healthy lifestyle. Smoking and the abuse of alcohol or drugs lead to an unhealthy lifestyle and may hasten the aging process. A negative attitude or inability to handle stress may lead to depression and an overall decline in health, in turn leading to an earlier death (see Figure 25–2).

People who are in good health usually do not age as quickly because they are able to be more active and involved. Due to improvements in health care, elderly people today are in much better health than those of a generation ago. The discovery of new medicines and treatments has reduced and prevented many diseases.

Environment (all the conditions and influences around us) affects aging. Environmental factors include air and water quality, temperature, humidity, and noise levels. People who live in the city are more exposed to *pollution* (contamination of the environment). Automobile emissions, tobacco smoke, insecticides, and hazardous garbage contribute to

FIGURE 25–1
Frail patients over the age of 85 have many health care needs.

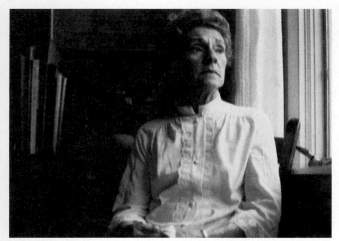

FIGURE 25–2
The inability to handle stress may lead to depression.

pollution. People live longer in an environment that is clean, quiet, and not polluted.

False Beliefs About Aging

There are several old-fashioned beliefs about aging that are no longer true, but can interfere with the care of geriatric patients. These false beliefs include:

- Age 65 is old.
- Most old people are sick and helpless.
- All old people are confused.
- Most of the elderly live in nursing homes.

In truth, age 65 is only a statistic used by government agencies and insurance companies. Most old people are healthy, mentally competent, and live in their own homes or with family members. These ideas might have once been true but certainly do not represent today's elderly.

Losses and Role Changes of Aging

Elderly patients may have experienced many losses. Since the majority of the elderly are widows or widowers, they have already lost their spouses. There is often a loss of financial resources because many retired elderly persons are on a fixed income. Some of the losses of aging include

- Health
- Independence
- Socialization
- Spouse

- Work role
- Finances
- Mobility

Elderly patients who enter long-term care facilities may also lose their homes, possessions, privacy, neighbors, friends, and pets. These patients may be greatly affected by the losses in their lives, particularly if the loss is recent. They need our understanding and empathy.

Grief is one of the primary reactions to loss. A person may feel angry, frustrated, or depressed when a loss occurs. There may be tears and suffering that interfere with normal activities. A great loss, such as that of a loved one, can affect an individual's well-being for a long time. (See Figure 25–3.)

Role Changes

We all play a role in life, and many of us occupy multiple roles. The longer we live, the more roles we assume. Roles of the elderly may include that of spouse, parent, grandparent, retiree, homemaker, and widow or widower. When an elderly person becomes ill, he or she must exchange the role of a healthy, independent person for the role of a patient.

Role changes can be very stressful, and most people have very little preparation for the major role changes in life. The change from spouse to widow or widower may require learning new skills at a difficult time in life. Changing from an inde-

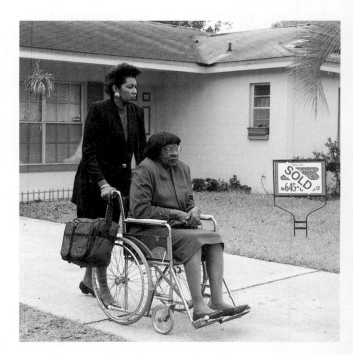

FIGURE 25–3
Elderly patients may suffer many losses.

pendent role to one of dependency can be devastating. Loss of a role without a satisfactory replacement is damaging to self-esteem. This may frequently be observed in the person who retires and has nothing to do.

Role Reversal

Many elderly persons experience role reversal, with adult children now caring for the parent. It is important to remember that the parent does **not** become a child again and should not be treated as a child. Patients can be helped to deal with role reversal by including them in discussions that involve their care. Assist them to remain independent and encourage decision making. Each person should be allowed to function at maximum capacity.

Cultural Diversity

Different cultures have different expectations for their elderly. For example, in some Hispanic families a widow is expected to lean heavily on her children. She is treated with much kindness and respect. She has an important role in the family structure and may continue to function as the leader. The children and other family members assume responsibility for her when she is no longer healthy or independent.

The American culture emphasizes youth and beauty. In many families, there is no role for the elderly individual. This is particularly true for the older male. Grandmother can help with the babies or the housework, but of what use is an old man? This attitude has not always been present. In earlier, simpler times, there was a place for everyone, and families respected and took care of their own.

Much of today's attitude came about as a result of the shift from farms to cities in America. On the farm there was a role and a need for every member of the family. The head of the family was generally the father, who controlled whatever money the family had acquired. The city had no place for the elderly farmer or his wife. Urban culture focused on young, healthy people.

It will be interesting to see if this attitude changes as the elderly population continues to grow larger and become more visible. Older people are banding together in support groups that are active in politics, industry, and social issues. Legislation now prevents discrimination based on age, and many retired people are reentering the workforce. Employers are discovering that older workers are often more knowledgeable and dependable than younger workers. What is emerging is a new picture and definition of the "older American."

Theories of Aging

The aging process is very complex. Although studies have been ongoing for years to find out why we age, no single theory explains what happens. However, two major groups of theories are generally recognized. One group includes the "programmed" theories, and the other consists of "error" theories.

Programmed Theories of Aging

Programmed theories believe that aging follows some kind of internal timetable, much like that of growth during childhood. One programmed theory is that each of us has a "biological clock" that eventually stops running. Death is "programmed" into the system from birth and, barring accident or disease, death occurs at the end of the program.

Error Theories of Aging

According to the error theory, an accumulation of errors in cell development, as well as cell changes caused over time by radiation or chemicals, produces faulty cells that interfere with normal function. Included in this group is the "wear and tear" theory, which holds that cells and tissues have vital parts that wear out with age.

All the theories provide clues to aging, but there is no single theory accepted by medical science. In the past, most of the studies of the elderly concentrated on the sick individual who had already entered the health care system. We really know very little about the majority of the elderly population that is well and productive.

The Elderly Patient

The majority of geriatric patients are women, most of whom are widowed. The personalities of geriatric patients are as varied as those of any other age group. We cannot classify people by groups. Individual elderly patients are no more alike than are the individual members of your class. (See Figure 25–4.)

The basic personality that a person has developed over the years does not change with age. However, certain characteristics often get stronger and more noticeable. Older people are more likely to speak their mind, rather than say what they think other people want to hear. A pleasant, happy, young person usually becomes a pleasant, happy older person, and the older person who is hard to get along with now probably was disagreeable earlier in life.

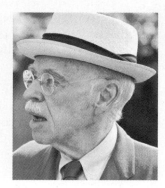
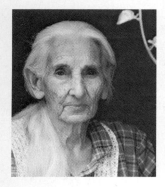
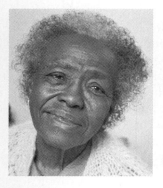
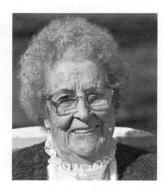

FIGURE 25–4
Older adults are concerned with their own individuality.

Guidelines for Meeting the Needs of the Geriatric Patient

- Provide assistance as needed with activities of daily living (ADLs).
- Focus on safety because accidents happen more frequently to older people and often result in more serious injuries.
- Remember that the elderly patient may be miles away from family and may turn to you for assistance in meeting the need for love and belonging.
- Encourage elderly patients to do as much as possible for themselves. Independence raises self-esteem.
- Listen to their stories of the "olden days" because remembering helps remind them of who they are now.
- Encourage patients to set realistic goals and assist them to meet those goals.
- Reassure patients who become discouraged and remind them that recovery takes time.
- Provide comfort and privacy for spiritual advisors and other visitors (see Figure 25–5).

Geriatric patients may have many health problems. Some are caused by body changes that take place as one ages. All the body systems slow down as a person gets older. Response and coordination decrease. Stiff joints and weak muscles may make mobility difficult. Bones become brittle and break more easily. Vision and hearing loss may occur. These changes place the elderly person at greater risk of injury from falls and other accidents. The body does not heal as quickly as a person ages, and rehabilitation may take a longer time. Some geriatric patients who are confused or disoriented have communication problems because they cannot always follow directions or understand what is being said to them. They have difficulty keeping facts straight. Remember, however, that most geriatric patients are neither confused nor disoriented.

It is important that you develop an understanding of geriatric patients and their problems. Protection of their health and safety is your main concern. Use empathy and care for the geriatric patients as though they were elderly members of your own family.

End-of-Life Issues

End-of-life issues are important to the elderly person. Decisions regarding advance directives must be made while a person is alert and competent. Most elderly patients have given a lot of thought to the issues and many have taken the necessary steps to ensure autonomy for the remainder of their lives. They have discussed the matter with members of their family as well as the medical team. The ethical and legal aspects of end-of-life issues are addressed in Chapter 3, and caring for patients at the end of life is discussed in Chapter 26.

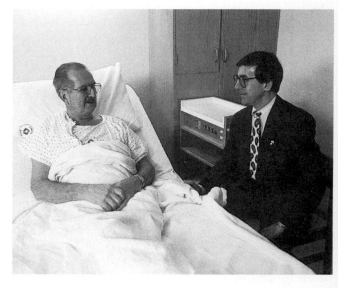

FIGURE 25–5
Provide comfort and privacy for spiritual advisors and other visitors.

Meeting the Needs of the Geriatric Patient

In Chapter 13, you learned that all human beings have basic needs. Elderly patients may need assistance with any of the basic needs. It is important to remember that each patient is a unique individual whose personal beliefs and values need to be honored and respected. Do not expect certain behaviors just because the patient is elderly.

Review

Read each sentence and fill in the blank with a vocabulary term that best completes the sentence.

1. _____ is the term used to refer to the aging person.
2. _____ is the branch of science that studies aging.
3. All the conditions and influences around us are part of our _____.
4. Contamination of the environment is called _____.
5. _____ are characteristics passed down from one's ancestors.

Remember

1. The process of aging is individualized, and no two people age at exactly the same rate.
2. The aging process is affected by heredity, lifestyle, health, and environment.
3. Belief in false ideas about aging can interfere with the care of geriatric patients.
4. Role changes can be damaging to self-esteem.
5. Different cultures have different expectations for their elderly.
6. At present, there is no single theory of aging that is accepted by medical science.
7. Elderly patients are at greater risk of injuries from falls and other accidents.
8. You may be the person the patient turns to for assistance in meeting the need for love and belonging.
9. Reassure patients who become discouraged that recovery takes time.

Reflect

Read the following case study and answer the questions.

Case Study
You are a home health aide assigned to Mr. Williams, a geriatric patient who had a stroke two months ago. He is depressed and moody and refuses to let you help him with range-of-motion exercises. He says he is "of no use to anyone anymore." His daughter says he cries a lot when he thinks no one is watching. Mr. Williams has been a farmer all his life. Since his stroke and his wife's recent death, he has had to move into the city with his daughter.

1. What cultural attitude might be contributing to Mr. Williams's depression?
2. What factors might be causing his grief?
3. What role changes have taken place in his life?
4. How can you help raise Mr. Williams's self-esteem?

Respond

Choose the best answer for each question.

1. The term "baby boomers" refers to the large number of people born
   A. During the 1970s and 1980s
   B. At the beginning of the last century
   C. At the end of World War II
   D. At the end of the war in Vietnam

2. Which of the following contribute to a healthy lifestyle?
   A. Eating a high-fat diet
   B. Smoking cigarettes
   C. Drinking alcohol
   D. Learning to handle stress

3. Which of the following contribute to pollution?
   A. Automobile emissions
   B. Tobacco smoke
   C. Hazardous garbage
   D. All of the above

4. The elderly woman living with her daughter is depressed. The depression is most likely a result of
   A. Role reversal
   B. Old age
   C. Poor health
   D. Pollution

5. In many Hispanic cultures an elderly widow is expected to
   A. Become independent and take care of herself
   B. Lean heavily on her children
   C. Remarry as soon as possible
   D. Get a job and support herself

6. What theory of aging contains the belief that each of us has a "biological clock" that eventually stops running?
   A. Programmed theory of aging
   B. Error theory of aging
   C. "Wear and tear" theory of aging
   D. Faulty cell theory of aging

7. Most of the elderly live in nursing homes.
   A. True
   B. False

8. Which of the following is NOT true about end-of-life issues?
   A. Decisions regarding advance directives must be made while a person is competent.
   B. Most elderly people have given a lot of thought to end-of-life issues.
   C. Advanced directives ensure autonomy for the elderly person.
   D. Decisions regarding end-of-life issues are not necessary until death is near.

9. Which of the following help meet the needs of geriatric patients?
   A. Provide assistance as needed with ADLs.
   B. Encourage independence.
   C. Focus on safety.
   D. All of the above.

10. Which statement would be most helpful to the patient who is doing range-of-motion exercises and recovering from a stroke?
    A. "Exercise harder. Remember—no pain, no gain."
    B. "Be patient. Remember that recovery takes time."
    C. "Quit worrying. This is as good as you're going to get."
    D. "Slow down. You're not a kid anymore."

Chapter Twenty-Six

The Dying Patient

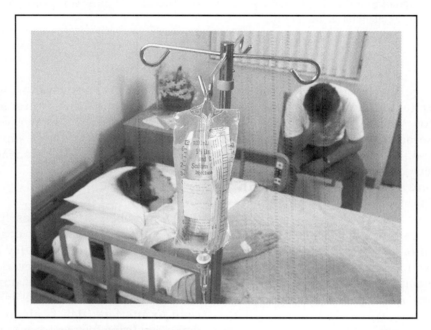

OBJECTIVES

After studying this chapter, you will be able to

1. Explain how your attitude toward death affects the way you respond to dying patients.

2. List four services provided by hospice.

3. Describe the five stages of grief according to Kübler-Ross.

4. Explain how you can help provide end-of-life care.

5. Briefly describe ways to help meet the needs of the patient's family.

6. List two ways to help other patients deal with their grief.

7. Identify five signs of approaching death.

8. Perform the procedure for postmortem care.

acceptance stage   The last stage of grief, during which the grieving person is calm and peaceful.

anger stage   The second stage of grief, during which the grieving person becomes hostile.

bargaining stage   The third stage of grief, during which the grieving person attempts to gain more time.

denial stage   The first stage of grief, during which the grieving person refuses to believe what is happening.

depression stage   The fourth stage of grief, during which the grieving person becomes saddened and quiet.

hospice   A type of health care agency that treats patients who are terminally ill, and offers support services to their families.

postmortem care   Care of the body after death.

respite care   A program to provide relief for the caregiver.

Today's health care focuses on quality of life. When planning techniques and procedures, we first ask, "How will this affect the quality of the patient's life?" Because we're living longer and better, death and end-of-life care has not been given enough emphasis. Perhaps we also need to question the effect of health care on the quality of death.

This chapter explores attitudes toward death and dying. It explains the grief process and how grief affects patients, families, and staff. Most importantly, it offers information about end-of-life care that will allow you to become a more compassionate and effective caregiver. Caring for dying patients can be the most rewarding nursing you will ever do.

Attitudes Toward Death and Dying

Most of us have no clear-cut concept of death. We are uncomfortable talking about it and attempt to distance ourselves from the reality of death. We shun reality out of fear, and this fear of death affects our attitude. Attitude toward death and dying may be influenced by culture, religion, experience, and age.

Culture

Culture influences the way people grieve and deal with death. For example, Buddhists believe that a person's state of mind at the time of death influences events after death. Therefore, it is important to maintain calmness and serenity around the dying person. On the other hand, some Native Americans will chant loudly and sing mourning songs as death occurs. Muslim culture requires that dying persons should never be left alone, so a family member must remain at the patient's bedside. People from many cultures expect to be able to bathe, position, and dress the dead body.

As a nursing assistant, you will need to be aware of the cultural diversity, beliefs, and practices within your community. You will also need to be sensitive to your own cultural attitudes and beliefs and how they may influence your care. Dying patients have a right to expect support and respect for their cultural beliefs and practices.

Religion

Religious beliefs are very closely tied to culture and affect one's attitude about death. Some religions emphasize that people must pay for the wrong things they do in life. Believers may be convinced that illness and death are punishment for sins. Others believe in "God's will" and that man has no right to interfere. Beliefs about what happens after death can bring fear or acceptance.

Age

Age can affect our attitude toward death. Younger people are usually more afraid of dying than older people. They are also more concerned about having death extended by artificial means. Some elderly people actually see death as a welcome relief from pain and disability. Children and the very old usually have less fear of death (see Figure 26–1).

Your attitude toward death affects the way you respond to dying patients. If you feel frightened and uncomfortable talking about death, you will not be able to comfort dying patients or their families. On the other hand, if you can accept death as a natural part of the life cycle, you may be able to help patients become more accepting.

Advance Directives

An advance directive is a document that gives instructions as to the patient's desires about health care treatment. The directive becomes effective when the terminally ill patient is not able to make decisions about his or her care. Examples of advance directives include a living will, power of attorney for health care, and health care surrogate.

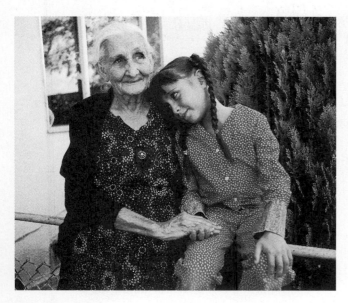

FIGURE 26–1
Children and the elderly have less fear of death.

The goal is to help return control to the patient and dignity to the dying process.

The issue of death with dignity has been a controversial subject for the past 20 or 30 years. It is a relatively new issue, because only in recent years have we been interfering with death. Once death was accorded dignity and respect as a natural event that occurred at the end of life. However, medical and technical advances now allow us to postpone death by means of artificial support of the circulatory and the respiratory system.

Legislation at the state and federal level has addressed the issue of returning control to the dying patient. A federal law called the Patient Self-Determination Act gives patients the right to refuse medical or surgical treatment and the right to prepare legally binding advance directives. Advance directives are discussed in more detail in Chapter 3 of this text.

Hospice

Hospice is an organization that treats patients who are terminally ill and at the same time offers supportive services to their families. (See Figure 26–2.) St. Christophers, founded in England in the 1960s by Dame Cicely Saunders, was the beginning of the modern hospice movement. The first hospice in the United States was founded in New Haven, Connecticut, in 1974.

Hospice care may be provided in a hospice facility, a hospital, a long-term care facility, or at home. It is a family-oriented program that treats the patient and family as a unit. Quality of life and effective pain control are emphasized.

Hospice care is managed by a team of professionals and trained volunteers. Physicians, nurses, nurse aides, social workers, chaplains, and volunteers all work together to meet the needs of the patient and the family. Hospice volunteers assist the family, run errands, offer friendship, and provide respite care. *Respite care* (providing relief for the caregiver) is one of hospice's most appreciated services. Other services provided by hospice may include the following:

- Symptom and pain control, comfort measures, and continuity of care
- A holistic approach to physical and psychosocial care
- Skilled nursing care
- Personal care and assistance, as needed, with activities of daily living (ADLs)
- Training and support to encourage family participation
- Open communication among staff, volunteers, patients, and families
- Crisis intervention to help families deal with emergencies
- Legal and financial counseling
- Assistance with advance directives and living wills
- Family bereavement counseling after the patient dies

As a nursing assistant, you may want to become a part of the hospice team. You will need to complete home health as well as nursing assistant training. Most hospices require at least one year of experience. They look for individuals who have effective communication skills and a genuine concern for people. It takes a lot of skill, competence, and compassion to care for dying patients and their families.

The Stages of Grief

Dr. Elisabeth Kübler-Ross, who devoted much of her life to working with terminally ill patients, divided grief into five stages. According to Dr. Kübler-Ross, the five stages of grief are denial, anger, bargaining, depression, and acceptance. (See Figure 26–3.)

Denial Stage

In the first stage of grief, the *denial stage*, the grieving person is refusing to believe what is happening. Denial is like a shock absorber, giving the person

National Hospice Standards

The following are the National Hospice Organization Standards of a Hospice Program of Care, published by the National Hospice Association.

- Appropriate therapy is the goal of hospice care.

- Palliative care is the most appropriate form of care when cure is no longer possible.

- The goal of palliative care is the prevention of distress from chronic signs and symptoms.

- Admission to a hospice program of care depends on patient and family needs.

- Hospice care consists of a blending of professional and nonprofessional services.

- Hospice care considers all aspects of the lives of patients and their families as valid areas of therapeutic concern.

- Hospice care is respectful of all patient and family belief systems and will employ resources to meet the personal philosophic, moral, and religious needs of patients and their families.

- Hospice care provides continuity of care.

- A hospice care program considers the patient and the family together as the unit of care.

- The patient's family is considered to be a central part of the hospice care team.

- Hospice care programs seek to identify, coordinate, and supervise persons who can give care to patients who do not have a family member available to take on the responsibility of giving care.

- Hospice care for the family continues into the bereavement period.

- Care is available 24 hours a day, 7 days a week.

- Hospice care is provided by an interdisciplinary team.

- Hospice programs will have structured and informal means of providing support to staff.

- Hospice programs will be in compliance with the standards of the National Hospice Organization and the applicable laws and regulations governing the organization and delivery of care to patients and families.

- The services of the hospice program are coordinated under a central administration.

- The optimal control of distressful symptoms is an essential part of a hospice care program requiring medical, nursing, and other services of the interdisciplinary team.

- The hospice care team will have a medical director on staff, physicians on staff, and a working relationship with the physicians.

- On the basis of patient's needs and preferences as determining factors in the setting and location for care, a hospice program provides inpatient care and care in the home setting.

- Education, training, and evaluation of hospice services is an ongoing activity of a hospice care program.

- Accurate and current records are kept on all patients.

FIGURE 26–2
Hospice care is delivered by a team of professionals and trained volunteers.

time to adjust. It delays the shock until the person has more emotional control. Sometimes people need denial because they are not ready for the truth. This can be frustrating to others because the truth seems obvious. Your best response to this stage is to allow the grieving person as much denial as he or she appears to need.

Anger Stage

During the second stage of grief, the *anger stage*, the grieving person becomes very hostile. Although anger may be directed at anyone, the most common target is the caregiver. At home, that is usually a family member, while in the health care facility, it might be you. Remember, the anger is not about you, it is about dying. (See Figure 26–4.)

Bargaining Stage

The third stage of grief, the *bargaining stage*, is an attempt to gain more time by promising something in return. Bargaining is often between the grieving person and God or a Higher Power and may be expressed in the form of prayer. During this stage a dying patient might say something like, "If I could just live until Christmas, I'd be ready to die." Encourage the patient to express feelings, and be an empathetic listener.

Depression Stage

The fourth stage of grief, the *depression stage*, is experienced with sadness and quiet. Denial and anger are gone in this stage, replaced by a deep sadness with

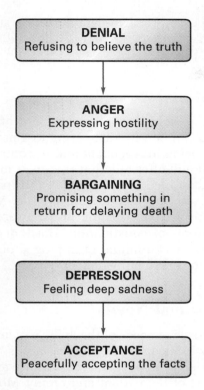

FIGURE 26–3   The stages of grief.

thoughts of loss of health, loss of independence, and eventually, loss of life. Your help may be refused as the grieving person withdraws. Your concern is comforting, so continue to offer your assistance.

Acceptance Stage

In the *acceptance stage*, the fifth and last stage of grief, the grieving person is calm and peaceful. It is

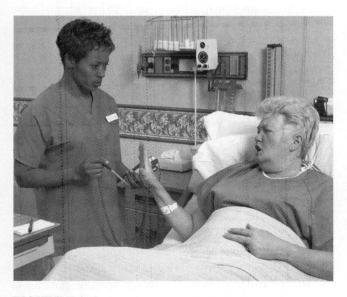

FIGURE 26–4
Acting out in anger toward those who provide care may be the only way the grieving person can express hostility.

an easier time for everyone, as anger fades and depression lifts. You may hear the grieving patient say something like, "I'm ready to die now." This doesn't always mean that death is really desired. It simply means that the patient has accepted that there is limited time left to live. You can help by trying to understand and accept the situation. At this time, you might use some of your energy to assist family members or other patients with their grief.

Grief does not always progress evenly or in a certain order. The stages are not clearly defined and may overlap or be repeated. Loved ones may not be in the same stage as the patient. Do not try to place a person in a certain stage or anticipate the next one. Simply remember that the stages are normal reactions to the dying process.

End-of-Life Care

End-of-life care focuses on meeting the needs of the whole person—both the physical needs and the psychosocial needs. Dying patients are entitled to the same rights as other patients. That includes the right to be treated in a holistic and humanistic manner. While the physical needs are most important, do not become so involved in meeting those needs that you may overlook the psychosocial needs.

Physical Needs

The physical needs of the dying patient include comfort, personal care, nutrition, fluids, elimination, and mobility. As a nursing assistant, you will assist with many of the physical needs of the dying patient.

Comfort and Pain Control

Quality end-of-life care depends on keeping the patient as comfortable and pain free as possible. Patients are often more afraid of experiencing pain than they are of dying. With modern medicines, no patient has to die in pain. The nursing assistant plays a very important role in keeping patients comfortable. The best assessment of pain is the patient's own report. Listen carefully to the patient's complaints and watch for restlessness or facial expressions that may indicate pain. Sometimes all that is needed is to help the patient into a more comfortable position. Accurate observations and prompt reporting help to assure prompt relief from pain.

If dyspnea (difficult breathing) is present, assist the patient to either an upright or side-lying position. When breathing is difficult, the patient may become anxious and upset. Promptly report episodes of dyspnea to the nurse. Stay with the patient until the nurse arrives. It may comfort the patient to know that someone who can help is nearby.

Personal Care

The dying patient may need assistance with bathing and personal care. A bath stimulates circulation and helps the patient feel refreshed and more comfortable. It can also be comforting to family members to see that their loved one is being cared for. Encourage family participation to help meet the patient's personal care needs.

Oral care should be provided at least every two hours. A decreased cough reflex makes it more difficult for the patient to handle oral secretions. As fluid intake decreases, the lips and mucous membranes in the mouth tend to dry. Small sips of fluid or ice chips help keep oral tissues moist. The lips may need to be lubricated to prevent cracking.

A decrease in physical activity and slowed circulation, as well as poor nutrition and fluid intake, increases the risk of skin breakdown. Frequent turning and positioning help to prevent pressure on bony areas. Use foam pads, heel protectors, and elbow protectors when necessary. Keep the skin clean and dry and massage with lotion each time the person is repositioned. Change linens as often as necessary to keep the patient dry and comfortable. (See Figure 26–5.)

Nutrition and Fluids

Dying patients gradually lose interest in food and fluids. Medications and treatments may affect appetite and the taste of food. The patient may be too weak to eat, and swallowing problems may occur. Frequent, small amounts of soft feedings may be

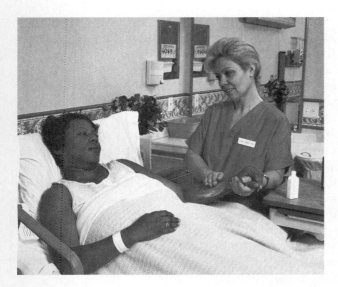

FIGURE 26–5
Lotion and the touch of your hand may be comforting.

helpful. The dying patient will eventually stop eating and drinking. Family members will need your support when this occurs.

Elimination

The dying patient may be incontinent of urine or stool. This can be very distressing to a patient who is used to being independent and in control. Check the patient and offer toileting at regular intervals to prevent incontinence. Clean and dry the patient immediately after an incontinent episode. Most pain medications are constipating, so be aware of signs and symptoms of constipation. Hard, dry stool or complaints of abdominal cramping should be reported to the nurse immediately.

Psychosocial Needs

The psychosocial needs of the dying patient may not be as easy to meet as the physical needs. However, your emotional support and reassurance are vital to the comfort of the patient and family. Most people who are dying are comforted by company. There is often a fear of dying alone. Encourage family members to visit and participate in the patient's care, and allow privacy so that the patient can be alone with family and friends.

Independence is lost as patients require more and more care. Dying patients may feel as if they are not as important as other patients who have a chance to get well. Sometimes staff members reinforce these feelings because they are uncomfortable with death and avoid contact with dying patients. You can help by making regular visits to dying patients and answering call lights promptly. Be caring, gentle, and empathetic, and think about how you would want a loved one of your own to be treated.

Communication

It is important to maintain open communication among the dying patient, the family, and staff members. Sometimes people avoid talking about dying because they want to protect their loved ones from sadness. However, open communication encourages people to express their feelings more honestly.

If the patient chooses to talk to you about dying, try to respond with honesty and compassion. There are no right or wrong words to comfort the patient. It is your presence that is comforting, not what you say. While the dying patient may express many questions and concerns, answers are not really expected. Listen carefully, as speech may be difficult. Remember that touch and listening are valuable forms of communication so, if you are not sure what to do, a pat on the hand or touch on the shoulder often speaks louder than words.

Spiritual Needs

Spiritual needs may be increased when a patient is dying. There may be unfinished business to take care of, such as settling family differences. Provide comfort and privacy for visitors. While most spiritual advisors will bring with them the supplies and equipment needed, be prepared to help if necessary. Be respectful and supportive of religious beliefs and practices. Let the nurse know if the patient expresses a need for spiritual advice.

The Dying Patient's Family

It is important that the dying patient and his or her family members be together. (See Figure 26–6.) This provides an opportunity to share memories, make apologies, and discuss the future. Facility visiting hours are usually extended to allow friends and family members to visit whenever possible. Anything that you do for the family also helps the patient. Help them to locate bathrooms, telephones, the waiting room, and the cafeteria. Let them know if guest trays are available. A cup of hot coffee or tea may be welcome, especially during the long hours of the night. Encourage them to share their feelings and provide opportunities for private conversations.

The Other Patients

When a patient is dying, other patients, especially the roommate, may be frightened and upset. They hear and see the distress of the dying patient and family members. The roommate may actually witness the death of the patient. Thoughts such as "I may be next" are not uncommon.

Residents of long-term care facilities often form close relationships and depend on each other for companionship. Because of this closeness, the loss of one of the residents is like a death in the family. Grieving may go on for a long time. If you notice behavior changes, such as pouting, crying, or frequent complaining, these may be clues that the residents need to talk about the loss. Take time to listen and help them to work through their grief. (See Figure 26–7.)

Signs That Death Is Near

All the systems of the body gradually slow as death approaches. Although the dying process varies from one person to another, some common signs are often observed.

Cardiovascular System

- A slowing of circulation
- Cyanosis of the lips, nose, nails, hands, and feet
- Pale or ashen skin color
- Skin feels cold to the touch
- An increased pulse and decreased blood pressure

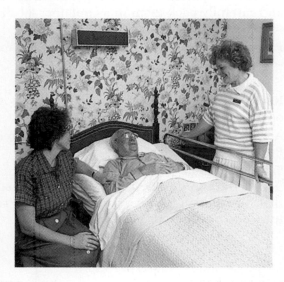

FIGURE 26–6
It is important that the dying patient and his family members have time together.

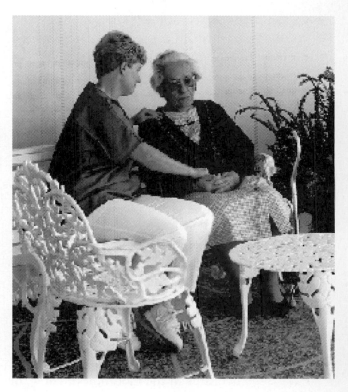

FIGURE 26–7
You can help other patients by showing concern and understanding.

Respiratory System

- Dyspnea with shallow, noisy respirations
- A decreased cough reflex, making it difficult to expel secretions
- Cheyne-Stokes respirations, a cycle of rapid breathing, followed by slow breathing and periods of no breathing

Digestive System

- Loss of appetite and thirst
- Difficulty swallowing
- Peristalsis slows
- The abdomen may become swollen
- Nausea and vomiting
- Bowel incontinence

Urinary System

- Impaired kidney function
- Urinary incontinence
- Decreased urinary output

Muscular System

- Decreased body movement
- Decreased muscle tone
- Muscles relax and become flaccid (limp)
- The jaw drops and the mouth remains partially opened

Sensory System

- Decreased awareness
- Dilated pupils and staring eyes
- Decreased pain sensation
- Unconsciousness or coma

Psychosocial Changes

The patient may be unresponsive and withdrawn. This indicates preparation for "letting go" or detaching oneself from surroundings and relationships. The patient may speak to or claim to have seen people who have already died. Reassure the patient that these are common experiences.

Signs of Death

Death occurs when there is no pulse, respirations, or blood pressure.

Procedure for Providing Postmortem Care

Beginning Steps

- Collect necessary equipment and supplies.
- Wash your hands and use standard precautions.
- Protect the privacy of the body.
- Use correct body mechanics.

1. Raise the bed to a comfortable working height, lock the wheels, and lower the side rails on the side nearest you.
2. Lower the head of the bed and place the body in a supine position. Place a pillow under the head and shoulders.
3. Put on gloves and remove tubes and drainage bags, if allowed. Turn off oxygen, suction, or other equipment, if instructed to do so by the nurse.
4. Wash the body and comb the hair. Protect privacy with a bath blanket.
5. Place a clean gown on the body and position a bed protector under the body.
6. Close the eyes gently, without applying pressure.
7. Place the dentures in the mouth, if possible, or place them in a labeled container.
8. Leave identification on the body. You may need to apply additional identification according to facility policy.
9. Handle jewelry according to facility policy.
10. Remove the bath blanket, straighten the body, and cover with clean linen. Do not cover the face.
11. Collect the patient's belongings, make a list, and carefully pack them in a container labeled with the patient's name. (See Figure 26–8.)
12. Remove all equipment, used supplies, and soiled linen from the room.
13. Straighten the room and dim the light.
14. Remove gloves and wash your hands. Dispose of gloves in the proper container.
15. Allow the family to view the body, if desired. Provide privacy and assist as needed.
16. Take the patient's belongings to the nurse's station or the appropriate area. The nurse will see that all belongings are accounted for and returned to the appropriate family member.

Ending Steps

- Wash your hands.
- Report and record your observations.

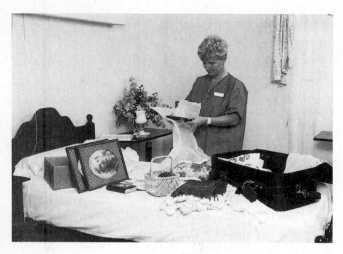

FIGURE 26–8
Carefully pack the patient's belongings in a container labeled with the patient's name.

Postmortem Care

When death occurs, family members may want to sit at the bedside and say their goodbyes. The need to see the body varies and is the individual's decision. Allow time and provide privacy for family members to express their grief. Tears are a normal part of the grief process, so reassure them that it is okay to cry. The nurse will tell you when to begin *postmortem care* (care of the body after death). Postmortem care includes caring for the body, straightening the room, and collecting the patient's personal belongings. Wear gloves and follow standard precautions as you may be in contact with body fluids. The body must be treated with respect, dignity, and privacy at all times. The procedure for postmortem care is not the same in all facilities. In some facilities, a shroud (a cover for wrapping the dead body) may be used. If you feel uneasy the first time you perform postmortem care, talk about your feelings with the nurse.

Review

Read each sentence and fill in the blank with the vocabulary term that best completes the sentence.

1. _____ is care of the body after death.
2. A program to provide relief for the caregiver is called _____.
3. The first stage of grief is the _____.
4. The _____ is the last stage of grief.
5. The _____ is the stage of grief during which the grieving person attempts to gain more time.

Remember

1. Your attitude toward death affects the way you respond to dying patients.
2. Culture influences the way people grieve and deal with death.
3. Patients have the right to prepare legally binding advance directives.
4. Hospice treats patients who are terminally ill and offers support services to the families.
5. Grief does not always progress evenly or in a certain order.
6. Quality end-of-life care depends on keeping the patient as comfortable and pain free as possible.
7. You can help the family members by being a supportive listener and allowing them to express their grief.
8. When a patient is dying, other patients may need your comfort and support.
9. All the body systems gradually slow as death approaches.
10. Death occurs when there is no pulse, respirations, and blood pressure.
11. The body must be treated with respect, dignity, and privacy at all times.
12. Provide time and privacy for the family members if they wish to sit at the bedside and say their goodbyes.
13. Follow facility policy when you are performing postmortem care.

Reflect

Read the following case study and answer the questions.

Case Study

Mr. Duncan is a lung cancer patient who is near death. He has a productive cough with thick sputum and sometimes expectorates blood. He is being medicated for pain on a regular basis. His wife stays at his bedside most of the time. She keeps urging him to eat more and he tries to please her, although it usually makes him sick. She tells you that she knows he is getting better and will soon be able to go home.

1. What measures can you take to make Mr. Duncan more comfortable?
2. What infection control practices will be necessary when caring for Mr. Duncan?
3. What stage of grief does Mrs. Duncan seem to be experiencing?
4. How can you assist Mrs. Duncan in dealing with her grief?

Respond

Choose the best answer for each question.

1. Your attitude toward death and dying is influenced by
   A. Culture
   B. Religion
   C. Age
   D. All of the above
2. A document that gives instructions as to the patient's desires about health care treatment is a/an
   A. Hospice care
   B. Advance directive
   C. Respite care
   D. Acceptance directive
3. The modern hospice movement began in what country?
   A. England
   B. United States
   C. Germany
   D. Spain
4. What is the second stage of grief in which the person may show hostility?
   A. Acceptance stage
   B. Bargaining stage
   C. Anger stage
   D. Denial stage
5. The stage of grief that is experienced with sadness and withdrawal is the
   A. Denial stage
   B. Anger stage
   C. Depression stage
   D. Acceptance stage
6. The medical term for difficult breathing is
   A. Dysuria
   B. Dyspnea
   C. Respite
   D. Depression
7. How often should oral care be provided for the dying patient?
   A. Every two hours
   B. Every four hours
   C. Every shift
   D. Every day
8. The patient tells you that he thinks he is dying. What is your best response?
   A. "Don't be so gloomy."
   B. "You'll be better tomorrow."
   C. "Let me call your pastor."
   D. "Would you like to talk about it?"
9. All body systems slow as death approaches.
   A. True
   B. False
10. Which of the following are nursing assistant responsibilities in providing postmortem care?
    A. Remove the IV.
    B. Notify the family.
    C. Discard the patient's medications.
    D. Collect the patient's belongings.

Chapter Twenty-Seven

Dementia
and Alzheimer's Disease

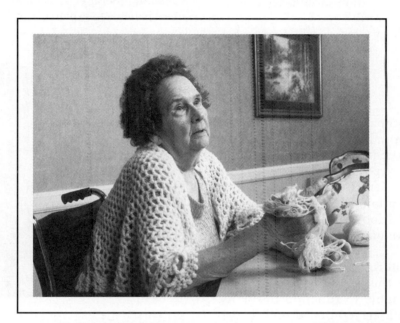

OBJECTIVES

After studying this chapter, you will be able to

1. Briefly explain how dementia affects patients.

2. Describe the stages of Alzheimer's disease.

3. List four guidelines for caring for the patient with Alzheimer's disease.

4. Identify three causes of confusion.

5. List six guidelines for care of the confused patient.

6. Briefly describe reality orientation and validation therapy.

7. List four guidelines for care of the aggressive/combative patient.

8. List three symptoms of depression.

9. List four guidelines for care of the depressed patient.

delusions   False ideas or beliefs.

dementia   A general impairment of brain function that interferes with normal social and occupational activities.

hallucinations   False perception unrelated to reality; may be seeing, hearing, or smelling nonexistent things.

paranoia   Suspicious thinking that one is being treated wrongly, harassed, or persecuted.

reality orientation   A technique used with confused patients involving repeated verbal and nonverbal information to remind them of time, place, and person.

sundowner's syndrome   A condition in which confusion and agitation increase as the evening progresses.

validation therapy   A technique used to encourage confused patients to explore their thoughts.

Dementia

Dementia is a general impairment of brain function that interferes with normal social and occupational activities. Half of all patients in long-term care facilities suffer from some type of dementia. Although many older people have dementia, it is not a normal change of aging. Dementia interferes with independence and quality of life. It interrupts rational thinking and sound judgment and threatens personal safety.

Dementia is difficult for families and friends to understand, because their loved one may look healthy and yet be unable to function normally. Patients with dementia are confused and disoriented (confused as to person, place, or time). They are often irritable and angry as they try to adapt to a changing world. As their focus narrows, they may appear demanding and thoughtless. It is frightening to lose control of both self and environment.

Dementia may be reversible (curable) or irreversible (not curable). Reversible dementia may be caused by vitamin deficiency, metal poisoning, or depression. This type of dementia can be reversed by correcting the problem that caused it. While irreversible dementia can sometimes be controlled by treatments and medications, no cure is available. The two most common types of irreversible dementias are multi-infarct dementia and Alzheimer's disease. (See Figure 27–1.)

Multi-Infarct Dementia

The term "multi-infarct dementia" means impairment of mental function that results from many small strokes that each destroy small areas of the brain. These strokes may be so slight that the patient is unaware of them. However, collectively they destroy enough brain cells to affect memory and mental function. Approximately 20 percent of all dementias are of this type.

Symptoms of multi-infarct dementia usually begin suddenly. There may be numbness or weakness

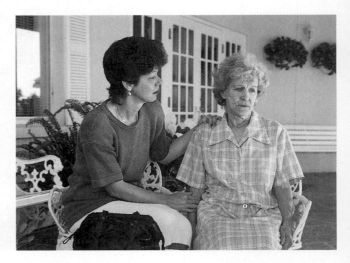

FIGURE 27–1
Dementia is difficult for the family to understand. The patient may look healthy but not be able to function independently.

of one side of the body. Vision or speech may be affected. Patients with multi-infarct dementia may seem to improve or remain stable for a period of time; then, suddenly, new symptoms will appear. The effects of multi-infarct dementia depend upon the amount of brain cell damage and the area of the brain that is involved. Symptoms vary widely among patients.

Alzheimer's Disease

Alzheimer's disease (AD) is a progressive nervous disorder that eventually destroys all mental and physical function. It is the most common form of dementia, affecting over 4 million Americans. Alzheimer's disease has no economic, social, racial, or national boundaries and affects both men and women. Although it can affect people in their forties or fifties, most patients with Alzheimer's disease are over age 65. The disease causes problems in thinking, communication, and behavior. There is no "typical" Alzheimer's patient. Some patients are angry and agitated, while others are sweet and gentle. Some endlessly pace the floor, while others may sit in one spot for hours. Personality and behavior can change quickly. As the disease progresses, physical symptoms appear that eventually lead to death.

Cause

The cause of Alzheimer's disease is not yet known, although a great deal of research is taking place. What is known is that changes occur in the outer layer of the brain, and nerve endings weaken, disrupting brain signals. Patches of material called plaque appear on neurons (basic cells of the nervous system), and nerve endings that transmit messages become tangled (see Figure 27–2). An accurate diagnosis can be obtained only by an autopsy after death.

Stages of Alzheimer's Disease

Alzheimer's disease can be divided into stages, each of which gets progressively worse. Although there are several different theories, one of the most commonly used scales of measuring disease progression is the Three-Stage theory.

Early Stage

The disease at this stage is mild, and patients are often unaware of their problems. Symptoms include mild memory loss, disorientation, difficulty learning and concentrating, personality changes, disinterest in grooming, overreaction to stress, and inability to use familiar items correctly.

Middle Stage

In the middle stage, symptoms are intensified and losses become too severe to ignore. Symptoms include short-term memory loss, increased disorientation, difficulty in performing activities of daily living (ADLs), language difficulties, inappropriate behavior, *delusions* (false ideas and beliefs), anxiety and *paranoia* (overly suspicious), *hallucinations* (seeing or hearing things that aren't there), withdrawal and depression, increased irritability, chronic wandering, and decreased interest in food. (See Figure 27–3.)

Late Stage

During the late stage, patients may become totally dependent. Eventually, the patient lapses into a coma and dies. Symptoms of this stage include little or no ability to remember, loss of ability to communicate, helplessness and confusion, inability to recognize family or friends, loss of bowel and bladder control, unsteady gait and balance, loss of gag and swallowing reflexes, inability to walk, inability to perform ADLs, unresponsiveness, and coma.

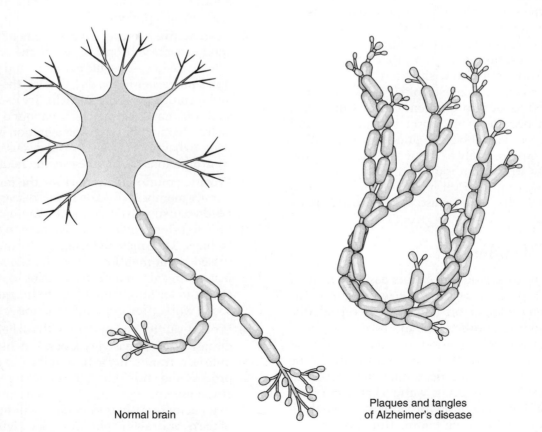

Normal brain

Plaques and tangles of Alzheimer's disease

FIGURE 27–2
Plaques and tangles in the brain are associated with Alzheimer's disease.

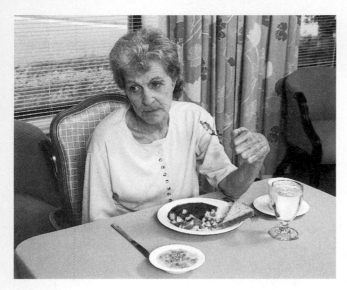

FIGURE 27–3
Patients with Alzheimer's disease frequently lose interest in food.

Symptoms of Alzheimer's Disease

The first noticeable symptom of Alzheimer's disease is a loss of memory. It is unlike the normal memory loss that comes with aging. As people get older, they often have difficulty remembering names and telephone numbers. The person with Alzheimer's disease may frequently get lost because he cannot remember the way to the office or where home is.

Another early symptom of Alzheimer's disease is the occurrence of catastrophic reactions. Catastrophic reaction is the term that is used to describe an overreaction to a situation. For example, the patient may have a catastrophic reaction because he was asked to sit in a different chair at the table. The patient becomes very upset and may cry and scream or become stubborn, agitated, or combative. These reactions are likely to occur when there are too many things to think about at once or there is a change in the routine. Even pleasant surprises such as a birthday party may cause a catastrophic reaction.

Chronic Wandering

One of the most serious problems associated with Alzheimer's disease is chronic wandering. Individuals may wander off and get lost repeatedly. They may go into another patient's room, into staff areas, or outside. When a door opens, they may be outside like a flash, with no regard for traffic or other dangers. Protecting personal safety becomes a real challenge. Sometimes wandering occurs because the patient is looking for something, such as the bathroom or his own room. But most of the time it seems to happen without reason or purpose.

Guidelines for Care of Patients with Alzheimer's Disease

■ **Provide a calm, quiet environment:** Too much stimulation such as noise, lights, and groups of people can cause anxiety or a catastrophic reaction. Turn down or turn off the radio or television if the patient begins to get agitated. Avoid placing the patient among large numbers of people. Keep the environment simple, orderly, and uncluttered.

■ **Provide a consistent routine:** Keep the patient on a regular daily schedule. Try to offer bathing, toileting, and other ADLs at approximately the same time each day. Avoid changes in routine or environment. Transferring the patient to a different room or changing the seating arrangement at dinner may have disastrous results.

■ **Reassure and explain frequently:** Speak in short, simple sentences, and move calmly and slowly. Do not force the patient to make decisions or perform tasks that cause frustration. Explain tasks one step at a time. Give the patient time to complete each step. Reassure patients who are suspicious and paranoid. Do not argue, but try to distract them with another activity. Touch is often effective in reassuring a patient.

■ **Restructure evening events:** Remember that sundowner's syndrome occurs in the evenings. When possible, schedule activities and procedures for earlier in the day. Closing the drapes and turning on lights may help. Try using soft, soothing music. Music has been found to be especially effective in decreasing agitation in patients with Alzheimer's disease. Avoid discussions and confrontations during the evening hours.

■ **Provide emotional support for the family:** Family members of Alzheimer's disease patients need your support and understanding. Take time to listen, and encourage them to express feelings. They may be feeling guilty or embarrassed about their loved one's behavior. Often, just talking about a problem helps to relieve stress. Refer family members to the nurse or the social worker for more information.

■ **Protect safety:** The patient with Alzheimer's disease is at increased risk of accidents and injuries. Wandering is part of the disease process and should be allowed within a safe environment. Try to get the patient involved in an activity such as sweeping, winding a ball of yarn, or drawing pictures. (See Figure 27–4.)

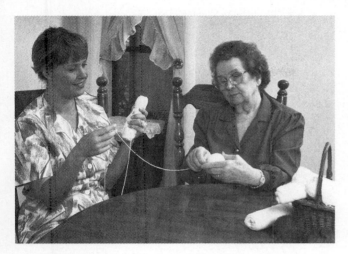

FIGURE 27–4
Getting the patient involved in a simple activity may distract her from wandering.

Sundowner's Syndrome

Patients who suffer from *sundowner's syndrome* have an increase in problems, confusion, and agitation as the sun sets in the evening. For some reason, this is a very common problem in patients who have Alzheimer's disease. It may occur because patients are tired at the end of the day. By evening, there is less ability to cope with the frustrations and stimulation that are taking place.

Many people who have Alzheimer's disease are in long-term care facilities because the care they require is so time-consuming that caring for them at home is extremely difficult. Confusion, mood swings, depression, wandering, and poor judgment require special care that must be provided for these patients. Many facilities maintain an area or unit specifically for patients with Alzheimer's disease. Special training is usually required to work in an Alzheimer's unit. Speak to your employer if you are interested in working with patients who have Alzheimer's disease.

In the final stage of disease, the patient with Alzheimer's disease will become totally dependent on the staff. The patient may need to be bathed, dressed, and fed. Remember that each patient is an individual, and no two patients will react in the same way. It takes patience and compassion to care for patients with Alzheimer's disease.

The Confused Patient

Patients who are confused have difficulty thinking in an orderly manner. Decision-making skills are impaired, and the confused patient may also be disoriented. Alzheimer's patients are confused, especially during the later stages. However, most confused patients do not have dementia. Their con-

fusion is temporary and goes away when the cause of the confusion is identified and treated.

Causes of Confusion

The cause of confusion may be physical or psychological. Some causes of confusion include the following:

- Disease or injury—dementia, diabetes, kidney disease, heart disease, pneumonia, cancer, tumor, stroke, or brain injury.
- Physical condition—infection, dehydration, immobilization (inability to move), pain, sleep disturbance, chemical imbalance, vitamin deficiency, or metal poisoning.
- Medication—drug interactions, side effects, or drug buildup.
- Sensory changes—hearing, vision, speech, or touch impairment that causes the patient to misunderstand.
- Stress, anxiety, and grief—relocating, hospitalization, surgery, or the death of a loved one.
- Change in routine or environment—unfamiliarity.
- Language and cultural differences—misunderstanding.

Common Problems of Confusion

Confused patients tend to live in the past because it is easier and more pleasant to remember earlier times. They tell the same stories over and over in an attempt to recall who they were and what they did. A

Guidelines for Care of the Confused Patient

- Provide activities to distract the patient from inappropriate behavior.
- Build rapport (a trusting relationship).
- Observe for causes of confusion.
- Maintain a regular routine.
- Use patience and understanding.
- Maintain a calm, quiet environment.
- Use simple, clear words and sentences.
- Give step-by-step directions.
- Give frequent praise and reassurance.
- Use touch and other forms of nonverbal communication.
- Be sure the patient understands.
- Use reality orientation or validation therapy, as appropriate.

fear of failure may cause them to resist activities that once were easy. Writing a letter or even taking a bath may be a challenge they do not wish to attempt. Purposeless activity such as pacing or wandering may occur. Patients may spend hours buttoning and unbuttoning clothing or folding and pleating bed linens. Inappropriate activity such as hiding things or getting into other patient's belongings may cause problems with the staff or with other patients.

Most confused patients have difficulty expressing feelings appropriately. Frequent crying may occur, and patients may easily become anxious, impatient, and agitated. They may become paranoid and suspicious. They suspect caregivers of trying to harm them or keep them from going home. Delusions of being a young child again are common. There may be a fear of being alone that causes patients to cling to a caregiver or hover around the nurses's station. Confused patients often place themselves in unsafe situations.

Caring for Confused Patients

Listen carefully to what the confused patients tells you. Do not assume that all complaints and questions are related to confusion. Very few patients are confused all the time. Before you dismiss the patient's complaint that she has not had her breakfast, check to see if it is true or not. Maybe she did not get her breakfast, or perhaps she is hungry again. Confused patients experience discomfort, cold, and hunger in the same way as other patients do. (See Figure 27–5.)

Many of the patients you care for use English as a second language, and some do not speak English at all.

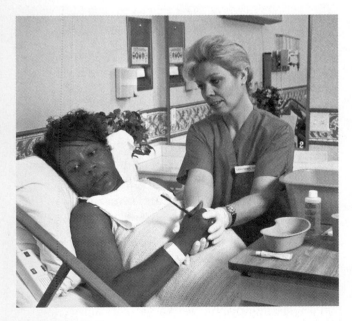

FIGURE 27–5
You may need to assist the patient with ADLs.

They may act or answer inappropriately at times. These people often get labeled as "confused" when, in fact, their confusion comes from not understanding. Individuals from some Latin cultures consider it rude and ignorant to admit they don't understand. They will smile and nod their heads and pretend to understand when they have no idea what has been said. Always verify understanding when working with these patients. Ask them to repeat what you said in their own words or rephrase your message to be more clear.

Reality Orientation and Validation Therapy

Reality orientation and validation therapy are two restorative techniques that may be used with confused patients. *Reality orientation* is a technique that assists the patient toward reality. *Validation therapy* is a technique that encourages the confused patient to explore his or her thoughts. Generally, reality orientation is used with patients who are temporarily or mildly confused, while validation therapy is more effective with patients who are severely confused or have advanced Alzheimer's disease. The patient's care plan will indicate which of these techniques is appropriate.

Reality Orientation

Reality orientation helps the confused patient with reality by frequent reminders of who he is, where he is, and what time it is. Always call the patient by name and identify yourself when you begin communication. Repeat the date, time, and place to the patient throughout the day. Give careful explanations of your intentions. Draw the patient's attention to clocks, calendars, and bulletin boards that may be posted. Reading material, radio, and television help keep the patient informed about current events. (See Figure 27–6.)

Reality orientation should not be used when patients become frustrated and angry. Being corrected may cause them to stop interacting with others. These reactions tend to increase instead of decrease confusion.

Validation Therapy

The word "validate" means to confirm or support. In validation therapy, you are supporting the patient's right to personal beliefs and feelings. It involves responding to what the patient is saying rather than trying to give correct information. You are looking for meaning in the patient's confused mind. Validation therapy helps make the patient feel less isolated. It is an attempt to restore the pa-

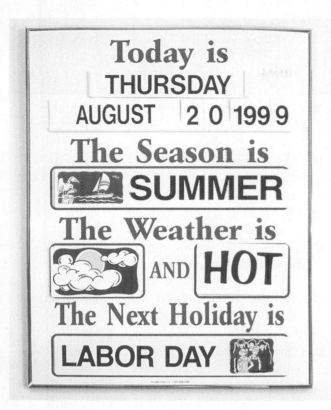

FIGURE 27–6
Calendars and bulletin boards inform patients of current events, and provide reality orientation.

tient's ability to interact with others and helps to validate the emotions that are being experienced.

When using validation therapy, you are not agreeing with the patient's false beliefs. You are simply encouraging the patient to explore and discuss them. Exploration of false thinking may lead to more normal thoughts based on reality. For example, the patient may say, "I have to go to the office now." An appropriate response might be, "What kind of work did you do at the office?" To remind the patient of the reality that he no longer goes to the office would only upset him.

Validation therapy can be useful with patients who are having delusions or hallucinations. It is important to remember that the patient really believes what he or she is saying. Hallucinations appear to the patient as though they actually exist. If you argue or correct the patient, he or she loses trust in you. Usually, the patient is frightened, so reassurance is necessary.

The Aggressive/Combative Patient

Even though aggression may seem to happen suddenly, it actually follows a progressive cycle.

The cycle usually involves four stages, which include certain behaviors:

- **Anxiety:** muscle tension, restlessness, pacing, and crying
- **Defensive behavior:** shouting, threatening, cursing, stubbornness, and lack of cooperation
- **Physical aggression:** hitting, kicking, scratching, and biting
- **Rage:** uncontrollable physical attacks on anyone or anything nearby

Whatever actions that you take need to occur before the patient becomes defensive. If you can find out what is upsetting the patient and relieve the anxiety and tension, there is a possibility of avoiding a combative episode. Once the patient starts acting out physically, your only solution is to protect the patient, other patients, and yourself from harm. It is difficult to work with patients who are so aggressive that they interfere with their own care.

Causes of Aggressive/Combative Behavior

Combative behavior usually occurs as a result of anger or fear. These feelings are frequently caused by misunderstanding. Other causes of aggressive/combative behavior include

- Hearing loss or vision loss—may not be able to understand due to sensory impairment.
- Mistaken identity—confusing a person for someone else with whom they are angry.
- Loss of control over one's life—someone making decisions for them.
- Physical discomfort, illness, and medications—may also cause aggressive behavior.
- Frustration—being rushed or unable to perform simple tasks.

Providing Care for the Aggressive/Combative Patient

Do not react defensively to the patient's anger. Try to discover the reason for the patient's angry words and actions. Respond calmly and use body language that is nonaggressive. Avoid using the "cowboy stance," facing the patient with your feet apart and your hands on your hips (see Figure 27–7A). What message does that send? It says that you are the boss and the patient must do as you say. A better position is standing at an angle to the patient with your hands at your side (see Figure 27–7B). This is less threatening to the patient and is also safer for you if you need to move quickly out of the way.

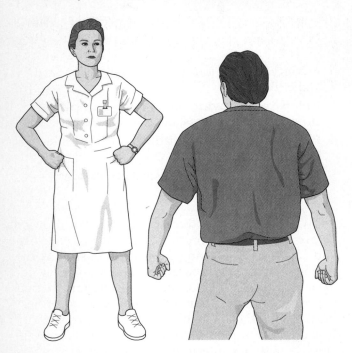

A. The "cowboy stance" may seem threatening to the patient.

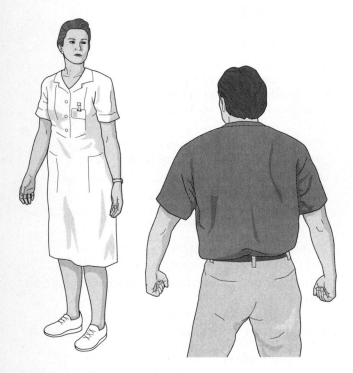

B. This stance is less threatening to the patient.

FIGURE 27–7
Use body language that is nonaggressive.

Guidelines for Care of the Aggressive/Combative Patient

- Get your own feelings under control first. It is alright to be angry but you must not respond in anger.
- Look for the cause of the behavior and fix it if you can. Check understanding.
- Leave and come back later, if possible.
- Return control to the patient. Allow choices when possible.
- Be aware of warning signs of anger, such as muscle tension, restlessness, pacing, crying, and loud speech.
- Offer distractions. Food or a change of activity may work.
- Use empathy and do not be judgmental.
- Communicate and reassure. Most combative behavior can be prevented by talking.
- Do not threaten the patient by your words or actions. Be aware of your nonverbal communication.
- Keep your voice tones smooth and supportive. Use simple, direct, clear language.
- Sit down, if possible. You will appear less threatening.
- Do not use touch without the patient's permission. It may be taken as a threat.
- Acknowledge the patient's feelings and offer reassurance. Patients have a right to be angry.
- Restraints should be used as a last resort. They only increase the patient's anger.

dren. Illness may cause depression if the ability to be independent and to run one's own life is threatened. Some elderly patients are depressed due to losses they have suffered. They may give up and lose the motivation to participate in any part of life.

The Depressed Patient

Depression is a type of reversible dementia that can be treated and frequently cured. It is a serious mental condition that can affect men, women, and chil-

Symptoms of Depression

Physical symptoms of depression include decreased energy, fatigue, poor hygiene and grooming, slow movement, sleep problems, constipation, and changes in appetite and weight. Severe depression can lead to confusion, chronic illness, and death. Psychosocial symptoms of depression include deep sadness, low self-esteem, feelings of worthlessness, lack of interest in activities, social withdrawal, negative reactions, and difficulty in decision making. Observing and reporting signs of depression are im-

Signs and Symptoms of Depression

Physical

Fatigue and lack of energy

Moves slowly

Poor appetite and picks at food

Refuses to eat or overeats

Weight loss or gain

Constipation

Sleep problems

Poor hygiene and grooming

Vague physical complaints, such as backache or headache

Psychological

Deep sadness

Frequent crying

Social withdrawal

Negative reactions

Lack of interest in activities

Difficulty making decisions

Rejection of family and friends

Talk of suicide

Verbal Responses

"I'm not good for anything."

"Nobody cares about me."

"I might as well be dead."

"I don't care."

"I might as well give up."

FIGURE 27–8 Signs and symptoms of depression.

portant in preventing its negative effects on the quality of the patient's life. Always report observations such as crying, withdrawal, refusal to eat, or any comments about suicide. (See Figure 27–8.)

Caring for the Depressed Patient

Supportive care provided by a sensitive and empathetic nursing assistant can help the patient cope with depression. Because the depressed patient feels unloved and unwanted, having someone who

Guidelines for Care of the Depressed Patient

- Encourage the patient to express feelings.
- Listen attentively. Do not be afraid of silence.
- Avoid comments such as "Don't cry" or "Everything will be all right."
- Use praise and encouragement frequently.
- Use empathy. Think about how you would feel in the patient's situation.
- Acknowledge each patient's special qualities and individual characteristics.
- Encourage and promote self-care and independence.
- Encourage activity and exercise, but do not force the depressed patient to participate.
- Take the patient outside in the fresh air, if possible.
- Check frequently to meet the patient's needs.
- Always report signs of depression to the nurse.

can be depended upon for social contact, acceptance, and support is valuable. (See Figure 27–9.) The guidelines above will help you care for depressed patients.

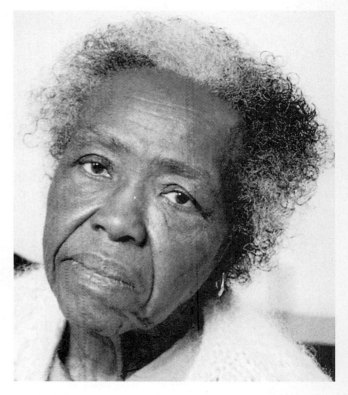

FIGURE 27–9
Observe and report any signs or symptoms of depression.

Review

Read each sentence and fill in the blank with the vocabulary term that best completes the sentence.

1. _____ is a general impairment of brain function that interferes with normal social and occupational activities.
2. False ideas or beliefs are called _____.
3. _____ is a technique that reminds patients of time, place, and person.
4. A technique used to encourage confused patients to explore their thoughts is called _____.
5. _____ are false perceptions related to reality; seeing or hearing things that do not exist.

Remember

1. Dementia is difficult for families and friends to understand, because their loved one may look healthy.
2. Multi-infarct dementia is usually caused by a series of small strokes.
3. As a result of confusion and wandering, the patient with Alzheimer's disease is at risk of accidents and injuries.
4. Provide a calm, quiet, safe environment for patients with Alzheimer's disease.
5. Reality orientation assists confused patients toward reality.
6. Validation therapy encourages the confused patient to explore false beliefs and feelings.
7. Aggression follows a progressive cycle, even though it seems to happen suddenly.
8. Combative behavior usually occurs as a result of anger or the feeling of losing control over one's life.
9. Depression is a type of dementia that can be treated and frequently cured.
10. Encourage depressed patients to express their feelings.

Reflect

Read the following case study and answer the questions.

Case Study

Doris Jones, a nursing assistant, is caring for Mrs. Santos, a patient who is in the middle stage of Alzheimer's disease. She is confused, aggressive, and eating poorly. She wanders into other patients' rooms and picks arguments with them. Her husband comes almost every day to help her with lunch and dinner. She gets hostile and angry with him, and he sometimes leaves in tears.

1. What are the symptoms associated with the middle stage of Alzheimer's disease?
2. How can Doris protect Mrs. Santos when she is wandering?
3. How can Doris handle Mrs. Santos's aggressive behavior?
4. What can Doris do to help Mr. Santos cope with his wife's hostility?

Respond

Choose the best answer for each question.

1. Which of the following statements about multi-infarct dementia is true?
   A. It is caused by a virus.
   B. It is reversible.
   C. It is the result of a series of small strokes.
   D. It is the result of a series of heart attacks.
2. Which of the following are symptoms of middle-stage Alzheimer's disease?
   A. Paranoia
   B. Hallucinations
   C. Delusions
   D. All of the above

3. Suspicious thinking that one is being treated wrongly, harassed, or persecuted is called
   A. Paranoia
   B. Hallucinations
   C. Delusions
   D. All of the above

4. An increase in confusion and agitation at the end of the day is called
   A. Evening syndrome
   B. Sundowner's syndrome
   C. Alzheimer's syndrome
   D. Confusion syndrome

5. What is the best way to care for a patient who wanders into another patient's room?
   A. Restrain him.
   B. Lock him in his room.
   C. Tell him to go to his own room.
   D. Take him for a walk.

6. An elderly Cuban patient reacts inappropriately to your question. What is your best response?
   A. "Are you crazy or something?"
   B. "Why can't you people speak English?"
   C. "Let me rephrase that question."
   D. "Poor thing. You just don't understand."

7. Which of the following is the best example of reality orientation?
   A. "Good morning, Mrs. Smith. I'm Jan, your nursing assistant for today."
   B. "Hi there. I'm going to help you with your bath."
   C. "Don't you know it's morning and bath time?"
   D. "Do you want to take a bath now, Granny?"

8. To confirm or support someone's beliefs is to
   A. Expectorate
   B. Validate
   C. Aerate
   D. Ventilate

9. The first stage in the cycle of aggressive/combative behavior is
   A. Rage
   B. Physical aggression
   C. Anxiety
   D. Defensive behavior

10. What is the best response to use when caring for a depressed patient?
    A. "Don't worry. Everything will be all right."
    B. "Would you like to talk about it?"
    C. "Cheer up and don't look so sad."
    D. "Let me tell you a funny story."

Chapter Twenty-Eight

The Patient *with* HIV (Human Immunodeficiency Virus) Infection

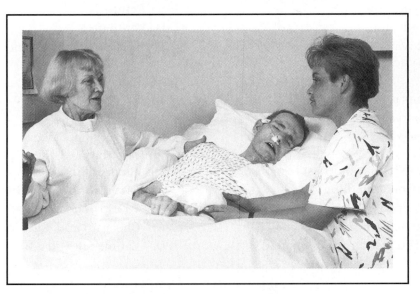

OBJECTIVES

After studying this chapter, you will be able to —

1. Identify four possible symptoms of HIV infection.

2. Identify four alternative therapies used to treat HIV infection.

3. Describe three cultural barriers that may interfere with effective HIV prevention and treatment.

4. Identify four measures to meet the physical needs of the HIV-infected patient.

5. List four measures to meet the psychosocial needs of the HIV-infected patient.

6. List three guidelines for care of children with HIV infection.

7. List four guidelines for assisting family and friends of HIV-infected patients.

emaciated   Excessively thin.

lesion   A wound or sore.

The focus of this chapter is on providing care to patients infected with HIV (human immunodeficiency virus). Even with recent medical advances in treatment, HIV infection remains a worldwide epidemic. As a nursing assistant, you may care for HIV-infected patients in hospitals, long-term care facilities, and home health. Many are in hospice programs. In order for you to become an effective caregiver, you will need to be knowledgeable about the effects of HIV infection and the special care that infected patients require. Although HIV infection was addressed in Chapter 5, a brief review of the disease is presented here.

HIV infection is a disease that destroys the immune system and leaves the body unable to fight infection. It is caused by a virus called human immunodeficiency virus that enters the bloodstream and takes over the body's defense cells (see Figure 28–1). The HIV-infected person can easily become ill with a serious infection or cancer. The most serious stage of disease is called AIDS (acquired immune deficiency syndrome).

HIV infection is diagnosed by a blood test for the antibody to the HIV virus. An antibody is a substance that is produced by the immune system when a foreign body such as a virus invades the human body.

HIV is transmitted by contact with infected blood or other infected body fluids. The majority of

HIV transmission involves sexual contact or sharing drug needles and syringes with an infected person. An infected mother may transmit the infection to her baby. In the past, some people acquired the disease through transfusion with HIV-infected blood. Because of changes in blood collecting and testing, transmission by blood transfusion is very unlikely today.

HIV infection does not easily occur, and every exposure does not result in infection. HIV is not spread by insects, sneezing and coughing, or touching an infected person. The risk of health care workers getting infected with HIV on the job is very slight if standard precautions are followed. Only a small number of health care workers have documented work-related HIV infection. Most of these individuals are nurses and laboratory technicians who were infected as a result of needle sticks and sharps injuries.

Standard Precautions

Part of providing care for HIV-infected patients is being familiar with infection control procedures. Although HIV is a fragile virus that is easily killed and not readily transmitted, you must protect yourself when coming into contact with body fluids. The Centers for Disease Control and Prevention (CDC) and Occupational Safety and Health Administration (OSHA) mandate the use of standard precautions, a method of infection control in which all human blood and other body fluids and substances are considered infectious. Standard precautions must be followed when you care for **any** patient. Early symptoms of HIV infection are similar to many other conditions, and many patients infected with HIV have no symptoms at all. HIV patients are not routinely placed in isolation. Once a person is infected with HIV, he or she can infect other people. That is one of the reasons why the use of standard precautions is so important.

Opportunistic Diseases

An opportunistic disease is a disease that invades the body when the immune system is weak or damaged. Pneumonia, cancer, thrush, tuberculosis, fungal infections, herpes, and shingles are examples of

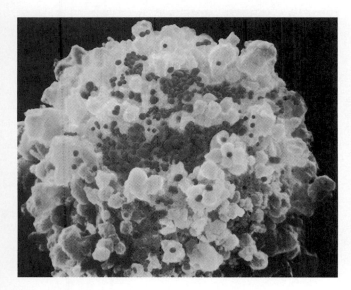

FIGURE 28–1
The AIDS virus.

opportunistic diseases that may occur in patients with HIV infection.

One of the deadliest of the opportunistic diseases is pneumocystis carinii pneumonia (PCP). This rare form of pneumonia infects approximately 75 percent of all AIDS patients at some point and is frequently the cause of death. Symptoms include dyspnea (difficulty breathing), cough, and fever. Some medications used to treat PCP have serious side effects, such as anemia and liver damage.

Much of the care and treatment of HIV-infected patients is directed toward treating the opportunistic diseases. For example, the HIV-infected patient with Kaposi's sarcoma (KS), a rare form of cancer, would receive cancer treatment as well as treatment for AIDS.

Signs and Symptoms of HIV Infection

People who are infected with HIV may be healthy for long periods of time before disease symptoms appear. The first noticeable symptoms are often those of an opportunistic disease. Patients may have white patches on the inside of the mouth (thrush), or they may have the dyspnea and cough of pneumonia.

Early symptoms of HIV infection may include fatigue, weight loss, dry cough, dyspnea, chills, fever, and night sweats. Glandular pain and swelling are common. Severe diarrhea, nausea, vomiting, and lack of appetite may occur. Rashes and *lesions* (sores) may appear on the skin or mucous membranes. Headache, weakness, numbness, dizziness, seizures, blindness, loss of memory, concentration, irritability, and mood swings indicate nervous system involvement. (See Figure 28–2.)

Care and Treatment of HIV-Infected Patients

Early care and management of HIV infections involves promoting a healthy lifestyle, educating patients, and providing counseling. HIV-infected patients are warned to avoid reexposure. Studies have shown that repeated exposures to HIV increase the risk of infected persons developing AIDS. Patients may question you about the disease. They may feel more comfortable talking to you than to a nurse or doctor. Answer honestly and correctly, and refer them to the nurse when appropriate.

Since there is still no cure for HIV infection, most of the treatment of infected patients involves relieving symptoms and treating opportunistic diseases. Care is also directed toward relieving symptoms caused by the treatment. The majority of medicines used to treat HIV infections have serious side effects, such as nausea, vomiting, and diarrhea. They may destroy healthy body cells and further weaken the immune system (see Figure 28–3).

It can be difficult for patients to follow complicated treatment plans. Most drug regimes consist of multiple drugs taken frequently, sometimes as often as 20 pills a day for the rest of the patient's life. There may be drug interactions between medicines given to treat HIV and medicines given for opportunistic diseases. They must also be concerned with drug interactions with food. Patients get discouraged because their treatment is making them feel worse. It is important to encourage compliance because current medications are allowing AIDS patients to live longer and more productive lives.

Symptoms of HIV Infection	
Fatigue	Dyspnea
Weakness	Dry cough
Loss of appetite	Chills
Weight loss	Fever
Nausea	Night sweats
Vomiting	Skin rashes and lesions
Diarrhea	Gland pain and swelling

FIGURE 28–2 Signs and symptoms of HIV infection.

HIV/AIDS Medications and Side Effects
AZT (Zidovudine)—anemia, nausea, vomiting, kidney problems, blood cell damage, fatigue
ddI (Didanosine)—nausea, diarrhea, pancreatitis, nerve damage
ddC (Zalcitabine)—pancreatitis, oral ulcers, nerve damage
ABC (Abacavir)—headache, nausea, vomiting, diarrhea, fatigue
Nevirapine—rash
Effavirenz—central nervous system effects
Saquinavir (protease inhibitor)—nausea, vomiting, diarrhea, rash, hair loss, hyperglycemia

FIGURE 28–3 Medications used to treat HIV infection have serious side effects.

Alternative and Holistic Treatment

Patients with HIV infection may turn to alternative therapies to promote healing and increase comfort. These therapies, combined with traditional drugs and treatment, may be used to enhance the patient's quality of life. Some alternative therapies include:

- Special diets aimed at slowing weight loss
- Exercise programs such as tai chi and yoga
- Herbal medicines and homeopathic medicines, including vitamins and minerals
- Massage therapy and relaxation techniques
- Stress management, meditation, hypnosis, and imagery

Alternative therapies must be carefully evaluated. If patients ask you about this type of treatment, encourage them to talk to their doctors.

Cultural Barriers

Cultural barriers may interfere with effective HIV prevention and treatment. Despite all the HIV/AIDS education in the United States, there remains a widespread belief that "only gays and drug addicts get AIDS." This leads to false beliefs that the disease is a punishment for doing something wrong. Foreign-born citizens and aliens may have a distrust for government agencies. They avoid seeking treatment because they fear being deported back to their birth country. Language barriers may interfere with understanding and compliance with a treatment regime. Working with these patients can be a challenge. Your reassurance and encouragement can improve their well-being and quality of life.

Physical Needs of the HIV-Infected Patient

HIV infection may affect every system of the body, creating multiple physical and psychosocial problems. Remember that physical needs are the most basic of all human needs and must be met before higher needs can be addressed.

Pain and Comfort

One of the first of the physical needs to be met is that of comfort. A patient who is not comfortable may not feel like eating, sleeping, exercising, or following the plan of care. Comfort can relate to any part of the body and frequently involves pain relief.

One of your responsibilities as a nursing assistant is to observe and report signs and symptoms of pain. Do not attempt to assess the intensity of the patient's pain. Some people are able to function with severe pain, while others are disabled by slight discomfort. Report all patient complaints of pain to the nurse immediately. Observe for nonverbal signs of pain, such as facial expressions and restlessness. Comfort measures such as repositioning and backrubs may help to relieve pain.

Respiratory Distress

Observe breathing regularity and depth while measuring respirations. Listen for coughing, wheezing, and other abnormal lung sounds. Observe skin color and nail beds for paleness or cyanosis (bluish color due to lack of oxygen). Assist a patient who is in respiratory distress to a sitting or upright position, if possible. Patients in respiratory distress may be upset, anxious, and frightened. Stay with the patient during episodes of severe dyspnea. Reassure patients by checking on them frequently.

Fluids and Nutrition

Loss of appetite, weight loss, nausea, vomiting, and diarrhea may occur. Observe for signs of dehydration and other fluid balance disorders. (See Figure 28–4.) Intake and output, calorie count, and body weight may need to be measured. Perform and record these procedures accurately and report any unusual observations. Provide mouth care frequently if the patient is nauseated or vomiting. The patient may be on a special diet of highly nutritional foods, and small feedings may be offered more frequently. Let the nurse know if the patient is not eating well.

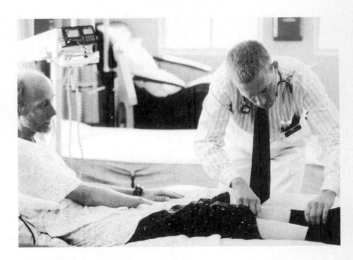

FIGURE 28–4
It is important to observe AIDS patients for dehydration and other signs of fluid imbalance.
David Weintraub, Photo Researchers, Inc.

Special Skin Care

Encourage mobility, exercise, and activity as tolerated. Assist the patient to change position frequently. Use pressure-relieving equipment, when ordered, to protect bony prominences. Change the incontinent patient immediately and do not allow urine or feces to remain on the skin. Report red spots or skin injuries to the nurse immediately.

Patients with Kaposi's sarcoma bruise easily, so gentle touch is necessary. Be careful when providing personal care or when moving patients. Provide soft-bristled toothbrushes or cotton swabs to avoid irritating the gums or mucous membranes of the mouth.

Weakness and Fatigue

Assist the patient with activities of daily living while still promoting independence. Encourage the use of canes and walkers to prevent falls. Observe for signs of fatigue and be ready to assist if the patient becomes tired. Provide a restful, quiet environment to promote relaxation.

Aching muscles and joints must be handled carefully to prevent further discomfort. Lift and turn the patient gently, using equipment such as a turn sheet or hydraulic lift when appropriate. Get help, if necessary, because two people make procedures easier and less painful for the patient. Provide passive range-of-motion exercises in which you do most of the work. Observe the patient's strength and report changes so that activity can be increased or decreased as necessary.

Reduced Resistance to Infection

AIDS patients are more susceptible to infection than are other patients. Wash your hands and remind patients and visitors to wash their hands. Let your employer know if you are not feeling well or have been exposed to an infectious disease. Remember, you are trying to protect the susceptible AIDS patient from infection.

AIDS Dementia Complex

AIDS dementia complex is the most common nervous system disorder that is seen in AIDS patients. Symptoms include forgetfulness, loss of recent memory, and a loss of concentration. Depression, lack of motivation, and social withdrawal are not uncommon. Blindness, tremors, loss of balance, dizziness, and seizures threaten the patient's safety. Patients may become irritable, angry, or combative. Confusion and disorientation may occur, and patients may not be able to recognize family members. Care of patients suffering from AIDS dementia complex is similar to that of patients who have other forms of dementia. A review of Chapter 27 will help you to understand more about the dementias. Follow the guidelines found in that chapter for care of the confused patient.

Psychosocial Needs of the HIV-Infected Patient

Patients with HIV infection face the same psychosocial problems that may occur with any other serious illness. They must deal with the fact that they have a progressive disease that may cause pain and disfigurement. Many of these patients are young and unprepared for death. They may experience a bewildering array of emotions, including frustration, anger, anxiety, and fear. If sexual activity or drug abuse is involved, the patient may feel guilt or shame. Some HIV-infected patients feel rejected by society and abandoned by their loved ones. Depression is common.

HIV-infected individuals also face problems that are unique to the disease. One of the most difficult issues is telling friends, family members, health care workers, or employers about their infection. The possibility of rejection or discrimination is very real. Even though discrimination against HIV-positive patients is illegal, it still occurs.

Financial problems can occur as the HIV-infected patient tries to maintain adequate income. Fatigue and weakness may interfere with job performance. Loss of employment may result in a loss of income and insurance benefits. The cost of treating HIV infection is very high, and financial resources can soon be exhausted.

Emotional support from family and friends, health care providers, and community groups is essential to the well-being of the HIV-infected patient. As a nursing assistant, you can do much to help the patient deal with the effects of this devastating disease. Creating an atmosphere of acceptance and reassurance may encourage the patient to express his or her feelings. Listen attentively and avoid making judgments. Remember that confidentiality is a major issue in caring for the HIV-infected patient. Keep information you have learned about the patient to yourself.

Counseling

Early counseling can be very helpful to the HIV-infected patient. The counselor will assess the emotional impact on the patient, identify previously used methods of stress management, and evaluate the quality of the patient's support system.

Information is offered regarding what to expect during the course of the disease, and questions are encouraged. The patient is informed that he or she is infected for life and can infect others. The patient's age, culture, and language are taken into consideration by the counselor.

Counselors also give patients information about available community services. The National AIDS Hotline, operated by the CDC, provides information concerning transmission, prevention, testing, and local referrals. This information is available in English, Spanish, and for the hearing impaired (see Figure 28–5). The hotline operates 24 hours a day, 7 days a week.

Let the nurse know if a patient requests advice. Some patients may want to talk to you about their concerns. Although it is important that you listen, be careful about answering questions and avoid giving advice.

Self-Image

Self-image is one's view of oneself. It is similar to self-esteem, except the focus is on body appearance. Symptoms of AIDS may negatively affect the patient's self-image and can result in withdrawal and social isolation. Rashes, lesions, and cancer tumors may be disfiguring, and treatments may cause hair loss. Weight loss may cause the patient to look sick and *emaciated* (very thin). (See Figure 28–6.)

Helping the patient to be clean and well-groomed can improve self-image. Make a point of touching the AIDS patient and not just during routine care. A pat on the hand or shoulder can be very reassuring. Your touch says more than words can and helps the patient to feel accepted.

Social Isolation

Social isolation may be caused by the patient's reaction to disease or by the attitude of society toward the AIDS patient. A poor self-image or guilt feelings may cause an infected person to withdraw from social interactions. Sometimes a patient is too weak or too sick to participate. Fear of catching AIDS

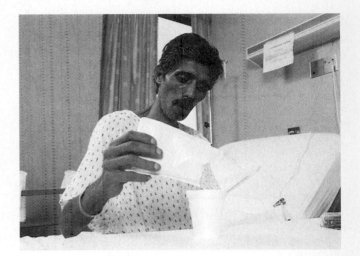

FIGURE 28–6
Weight loss may cause a patient to look sick and emaciated.

may cause people to avoid HIV-infected individuals. Lack of correct information about the disease may cause unnecessary fears and precautions.

Include the AIDS patient in activities and provide activities that take into consideration the patient's physical and emotional condition. Help them to dress, comb their hair, and look their best. Encourage family members and friends to visit.

Suicide

Studies have shown an increase in suicide rates in patients who are HIV positive. This is one of the reasons that counseling is so important. The counselor can assess the seriousness of the suicide danger. The patient's state of mind can range from occasional suicidal thoughts to an actual attempt at suicide. For many patients, the thought of pain and suffering may be more than they can bear. Patients with weak support systems or a previous history of psychological disorders are more at risk than others. Report any talk about suicide to the nurse immediately. All suicide threats should be taken seriously.

Nursing Attitude

In order to provide effective care for the HIV-infected patient, you will need to develop a caring, nonjudgmental attitude. This may involve considering your own beliefs about sexuality and morality. You may need to develop an understanding and acceptance of lifestyles that are different from your own. The HIV-infected patient needs an environment of acceptance and encouragement.

Tact, sensitivity, and empathy are necessary in caring for the patients. When you confront your fears, you will realize that most of those fears are

National AIDS Hotline
1–800–342–AIDS
1–800–344–SIDA (for Spanish speakers)
1–800–AIDS–889 (for the hearing-impaired)
The national AIDS hotline operates 24 hours a day, 7 days a week.

FIGURE 28–5   National AIDS hotline telephone numbers.

caused by lack of knowledge. Learning as much as you can about HIV infection will help you to properly care for HIV-infected patients. Remember that the patient with HIV infection is entitled to the same gentle loving care that you give to other patients.

Care of Children with HIV Infection

Caring for children with HIV infection can be a heartbreaking task. It is not easy to watch the suffering of helpless infants and children. Most of them are too young to understand what is happening and why they are so sick. Many are infants under the age of two.

The incidence of HIV infection in children is increasing, not only in the United States, but also worldwide. If this trend continues, AIDS will soon become one of the leading causes of death in children. The majority of HIV infection in infants and children is the result of mother-to-baby transmission. HIV infection may be transmitted from an infected mother to her child during pregnancy, at delivery, or through breast-feeding. (See Figure 28–7.)

Many times the mother of the infected baby is also sick. Pregnancy tends to speed up progression of the disease. This creates a situation in which a sick mother is trying to care for a sick infant. Many HIV-infected children are not being cared for by their natural mothers, because their mothers are either sick or dead. Separation from parents can cause the child to feel rejected or abandoned.

Older children may feel that somehow they are to blame for their illness. They may think they are

Guidelines for Care of Children with HIV Infection

- Children have special needs and cannot be treated like small adults.
- Each child is an individual with his or her own needs.
- Children should receive honest information at their level of understanding.
- Children should be taught handwashing and other infection-control measures when possible.
- Encourage independence while protecting the child's safety.
- Provide appropriate activities that do not cause the child to become overtired.
- Make mealtime pleasant and fun.
- Touching, hugging, and rocking the child can help to relieve anxiety and discomfort.
- Encourage family participation whenever possible.

being punished for bad behavior. It is important to explain that the disease is causing their pain and suffering and that it has nothing to do with their behavior. Teenagers may feel guilty if they have had unprotected sex or have used drugs. They are also concerned with the image that society has of AIDS patients.

Adults should be as honest as possible with children who are HIV infected. Children are far better at understanding and accepting the truth than we think they are. Telling a child an untruth may cause distrust and fear. The child's age must be taken into consideration, and information should be appropriate. Some parents prefer that a child not be told the truth, and you may disagree with their decision. Remember that parents have the right to decide what the child is to be told, so do not take it upon yourself to try to change the situation. The amount of information given to the child is included in the child's plan of care. Checking the care plan on a daily basis will help you to avoid saying the wrong thing.

The goal of caring for HIV-infected children is to try to keep their lives as normal as possible for as long as possible. In the early years of the AIDS epidemic, HIV-infected infants frequently lived out their lives in hospitals. Improvements in treatment now allow HIV-infected children to stay healthy longer and to lead more normal lives.

The picture of pediatric HIV infection is changing. In the early days of the epidemic, children were not diagnosed until they were already very ill. Death usually occurred in infancy or early childhood. There were also a number of older children who

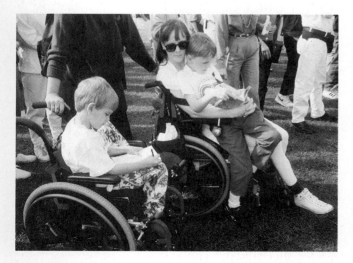

FIGURE 28–7
The incidence of HIV infection in children is increasing worldwide.
Vanessa Vick, Photo Researchers, Inc.

had been infected by blood transfusions. Many of them, like Ryan White, became public figures because of discrimination they experienced. Sadly, most of this group of young people have died.

Today, infants are being diagnosed at birth or even before birth. Women who are HIV positive are being treated during the pregnancy. With modern treatments, infected children are living longer. Some patients may spend their entire childhood living with HIV infection. Early diagnosis, specific treatments, and supportive care are vital to improve survival.

Family and Friends of HIV-Infected Patients

Family members of HIV-infected patients face many emotional issues. Disagreements about the patient's lifestyle choices may have damaged family relationships. There may be anger and frustration on both sides. It is very important that you do not "take sides" in these issues. You want to be a supportive listener to the patient and to the family. Avoid giving advice or being judgmental. Be aware that if you get involved in family disagreements, there is a good chance that you may become the target of their anger. Let the nurse know if family visits are upsetting to the patient.

Family members may want to talk to you about their problems. Since they see you caring for their loved one on a daily basis, they may develop trust in you and regard you as a friend. They may ask you questions that they are afraid to ask others. Sometimes they just want to be heard and are not looking for answers. If the family keeps asking you questions that you cannot answer, gently suggest that they talk to the nurse. (See Figure 28–8.)

The families of HIV-infected children may need special help. Since the majority of HIV-infected children were infected before birth, they usually come from families in which one or both parents are also infected. There may be a history of drug abuse or risky sexual practices. The parents are usually suffering from extreme guilt feelings. It will take all your skill to know how to respond to these individuals.

In many instances, you may not be dealing with the traditional family. HIV-infected children are often cared for by foster parents who, while not really related, may have formed extremely close bonds with the children. Grandparents or other family members may care for the HIV-infected children because the parents are ill or dead. Grandparents are dealing not only with the illness of their grandchild, but they are also grieving for their adult child.

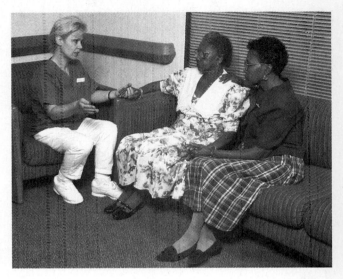

FIGURE 28–8
Encourage family members to express their feelings.

Family may consist of the partner and friends of the HIV-infected homosexual patient. Many homosexual couples live together for years, and their lifestyle may closely resemble that of married couples. The patient's companion should be treated with the same compassion and respect that traditional family members receive. If your own feelings and beliefs conflict with those of the patient, yours must be set aside and not interfere with the way that you treat others.

Guidelines for Assisting Family and Friends of HIV-Infected Patients

■ Respect the family's right to make decisions.
■ Support the family's priorities regarding needs, choices, and values.
■ Respect the family's culture and lifestyle choices.
■ Encourage family members to express their emotions.
■ Listen to family members and do not be judgmental.
■ Avoid getting involved in family disagreements.
■ Refer the family to the nurse with questions that you do not feel prepared to answer.
■ Help family members to follow infection-control practices.
■ Help family members secure correct information about HIV infection.

Caregiver Stress

Caregiver stress may involve family members and friends or health care workers. It is stressful caring for any patient who is dying, and especially so when the patient has AIDS. Concerns may include communicable disease, infection control, homosexuality, drug abuse, sexually transmitted disease, confidentiality, public opinion, and death. Caregivers may feel helpless and powerless against this terrible disease. There are times when nothing you do seems to help, and you feel that you have failed.

The fear of contracting HIV infection is always a factor. The caregiver of the homebound patient must also be concerned about protecting other members of the household. Many times people overreact and take more precautions than are necessary. This not only increases the fear, but it also is upsetting to the patient.

As a nursing assistant, you will need to consider your own feelings about caring for AIDS patients. You may be concerned about protecting your family as well as yourself. You should confront those feeling before you decide on a career in health care. Schedule a conference with your instructor if you have doubts about caring for AIDS patients. Generally, the more you learn about the disease, the more comfortable you will be in caring for HIV-infected patients. (See Figure 28–9.)

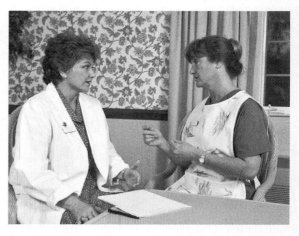

FIGURE 28–9
Talk to your instructor if you have concerns about caring for AIDS patients.

Review

Read each sentence and fill in the blank with the vocabulary term that best completes the sentence.

1. The medical term for very thin is _____.
2. A/an _____ is a wound or a sore.
3. The most serious stage of HIV infection is called _____.
4. _____ is a method of infection control in which all blood and other body fluids are considered infectious.
5. A substance produced by the immune system when a foreign body invades is called a/an _____.

Remember

1. The risk of getting HIV infection on the job is very slight if you follow standard precautions.
2. People who are infected with HIV may be healthy for long periods before disease symptoms appear.
3. Early care of HIV-infected patients emphasizes a healthy lifestyle, family support, education, and counseling.
4. It is important to encourage compliance because current medications are allowing AIDS patients to live longer and more productive lives.
5. Report all patient complaints or observations of pain to the nurse immediately.
6. Confidentiality is a major issue when you are caring for HIV-infected patients.
7. Providing an atmosphere of acceptance and reassurance will help the patient to express feelings.
8. The goal of caring for HIV-infected children is to keep their lives as normal as possible for as long as possible.
9. Your own feelings and beliefs must be set aside and not interfere with the way that you treat others.
10. Support the family's priorities regarding needs, choices, and values.
11. Generally, the more you learn about the disease, the more comfortable you will be in caring for HIV-infected patients.

Reflect

Read the following case study and answer the questions.

Case Study

Brad Barron is a 28-year-old hospital patient who has AIDS. Frequent episodes of nausea and vomiting have left him weak and emaciated. A water mattress is being used to protect his fragile skin. Greg, his companion, comes in daily to assist with his care and offer emotional support. When Brad's parents visit, their quarrels with Greg often leave everyone in tears. You feel sorry for Greg, who seems so devoted to Brad. You think the parents should stay away if they're going to cause so much trouble.

1. What measures can you take to protect Brad's skin from breakdown?
2. What can you do to relieve the discomfort of the nausea and vomiting?
3. What might be causing the quarrels between Brad's loved ones?
4. Should you take sides in this issue since you believe the parents are behaving badly? Explain your answer.

Respond

Choose the best answer for each question.

1. HIV infection is caused by
   A. A bacteria
   B. A virus
   C. A spore
   D. None of the above
2. The risk of health care workers getting HIV on the job is very high.
   A. True
   B. False
3. Which of the following statements about alternative treatments is FALSE?
   A. Alternative therapies have not been approved and do not work.
   B. Hypnosis and imagery may reduce stress.
   C. Massage therapy helps with relaxation.
   D. Alternative therapies may be combined with traditional treatments.
4. What is your best response to the comment that "Only gays and addicts get AIDS"?
   A. "You obviously don't know much about AIDS."
   B. "You're right. We just have to keep away from them."
   C. "Anyone can get AIDS."
   D. "AIDS is God's punishment."
5. How can you protect the skin of a patient who has Kaposi's sarcoma?
   A. Use gentle touch when turning him.
   B. Provide a soft-bristled toothbrush.
   C. Use pressure-relieving equipment.
   D. All of the above.

6. The most common nervous system disorder seen in HIV-infected patients is
   A. Multi-infarct dementia
   B. Alzheimer's disease
   C. Parkinson's disease
   D. AIDS dementia complex
7. Which of the following statements about children with HIV infection is TRUE?
   A. Children rarely get infected with HIV.
   B. AIDS will soon be one of the leading causes of death in children.
   C. Most children are infected as teenagers.
   D. Avoid telling children the truth about HIV.
8. A mother of a child dying of AIDS tells you that she feels guilty because she can't care for her child at home. What is your best response?
   A. "You're doing the best you can for your child."
   B. "Children are better off in the hospital."
   C. ""Why don't you take her home and try again."
   D. "Maybe you didn't try hard enough."
9. A visitor asks you how her niece became infected with HIV. What is your best response?
   A. "I don't know. I didn't ask."
   B. "She was injecting illegal drugs."
   C. "You'll have to talk to your niece about that."
   D. "It's none of your business."
10. A co-worker is upset and crying because one of her patients died of AIDS. What is your best response?
    A. "You're not acting very professional."
    B. "Maybe you should take the day off."
    C. "It's okay to cry."
    D. "Crying won't help."

Chapter Twenty-Nine

The Surgical Patient

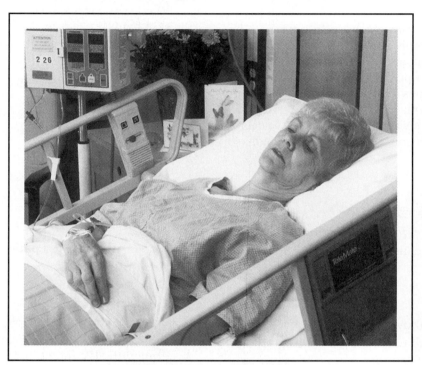

O B J E C T I V E S

After studying this chapter, you will be able to

1. List two recent trends in surgical care.

2. Explain the importance of psychological preparation for surgery.

3. List three physical preparations for surgery.

4. Identify four measures used to promote patient comfort.

5. List five postoperative observations that should be reported to the nurse immediately.

6. Perform the procedures described in this chapter.

anesthesia   The loss of sensation caused by a medication given before surgery.

anesthesiologist   A medical doctor specially trained to administer anesthesia and life support during a surgery.

embolus   A blood clot that breaks loose and travels through the bloodstream.

gurney   A type of stretcher or carrier used to transport patients.

postoperative (postop)   Refers to the period after a surgery.

preoperative (preop)   Refers to the period prior to a surgery.

thrombus   A stationary blood clot.

Changes in Surgical Care

In recent years many changes have taken place in surgical care. Surgery is being done today in less time and with less human suffering than ever before. There are changes in both preop and postop care. The term *peroperative (preop)* means "before surgery." The term *postoperative (postop)* means "after surgery." This chapter addresses these changes while focusing on basic nursing care of surgical patients.

One of the most important changes involves the development of new, improved surgical techniques, such as lasers. Laser surgery can be done safely, quickly, with a shorter recovery time, and fewer complications. Newer methods of *anesthesia* (the loss of sensation caused by a medication given before surgery) have also helped make surgery safer.

In the past, patients were admitted to the hospital at least a day before surgery for surgical preparations. Care plans were developed and staff members and patients began to get acquainted. Necessary laboratory tests and x-rays were taken during that period. The night before surgery certain preoperative procedures, such as skin preparations and bowel routines, if ordered, were done.

Today, patients may have their preop lab work done as an outpatient and usually come to the hospital early on the day of surgery. Preparation for surgery is done the morning of surgery or by the patient at home the night before. These patients do not come to the regular nursing unit until after surgery. This means that patients are not familiar with the area or the staff.

Changes in Preoperative Care

Most preop procedures are done in the surgical area just before surgery. Infection control studies have shown that there is less chance of infection if the patient receives preoperative medications and skin preparations (skin prep) in the surgical area rather than on a regular nursing unit. These procedures, once done by nurses and aides on the nursing unit, are now being done by surgical nurses and technicians.

Changes in Postoperative Care

Patients are getting up and moving about sooner than they used to, resulting in fewer complications. Patients are being discharged much faster, sometimes while they are still very sick. They may go to a subacute facility or be cared for at home by a home health agency or by family members. Early discharge has brought about rapid growth in these types of health care services.

Outpatient Surgery

There has also been an increase in the number of outpatient or same-day surgeries. Outpatient surgery is surgery that is done on the day of admission, with the expectation of going home the same day. This type of surgery may be done in the doctor's office, in an independent outpatient surgical facility, or in an outpatient surgery department within the hospital. Outpatient surgery is a time-saving, cost-saving measure that has proven, for the most part, to be safe and effective. Patients are carefully monitored after surgery and admitted to a hospital if complications occur. (See Figure 29–1.)

Types of Surgery

Surgery involves cutting into the patient's body. It may be done to repair an injury, remove a body part, diagnose disease, relieve symptoms, or improve appearance. There are basically two types of surgery: elective and emergency. Elective surgery is surgery that the patient elects, or chooses, to have done. It is planned and scheduled ahead of time. Emergency surgery is surgery that is done immediately to relieve an acute condition. It is unplanned and unscheduled.

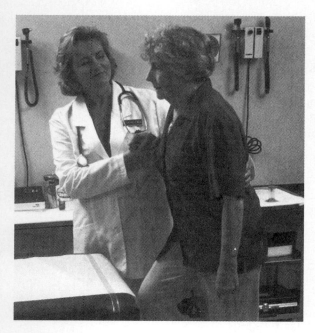

FIGURE 29–1
In some areas, nursing assistants are trained to work in outpatient surgery.

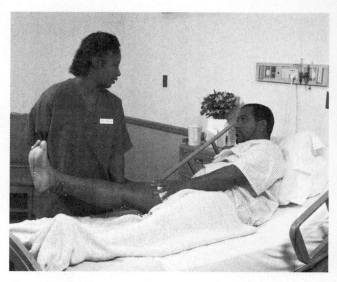

FIGURE 29–2
You may help the patient practice foot and leg exercises preoperatively.

Care of the surgical patient can be divided into three periods: preoperative (before surgery), operative (during surgery), and postoperative (after surgery). As a nursing assistant working in a hospital, you may be involved in the care of the patient before and after surgery. In a long-term care facility, a subacute unit, or home health setting, you may care for a patient who is recovering from surgery.

Psychological Preparation for Surgery

Regardless of modern advances and improvements, surgery remains a stressful event. Patients may be frightened because they do not know what to expect. They may be anxious about the outcome of the surgery and whether or not they will feel better afterwards. Most patients are concerned about pain, and they may be worried about anesthesia or dying. Psychological preparation helps to relieve anxiety and reduce stress.

Many people give information to the patient. The doctor reviews the surgical procedure and explains it in everyday language that the patient can understand. Nurses give preop instructions and teach exercises and breathing routines that the patient will need to follow after surgery. The *anesthesiologist* (a doctor who administers anesthesia) will discuss the type of anesthetic that will be used. Some hospitals have a special team that does preop teaching.

No matter how much information the patient has been given, you may still be asked many questions. It is important that you know the general surgical routine so that you can answer correctly. Refer technical questions to the nurse or physician. However, many questions are simple, such as "Will they take me to surgery on a stretcher?" Sometimes the patient knows the answer and is only seeking reassurance. Let the nurse know if the patient keeps asking questions or doesn't seem to understand. Remember to protect the patient's confidentiality by keeping information that you have learned private.

Preoperative Teaching

Nurses are responsible for preoperative teaching. Patients who are prepared and informed before surgery are usually more able to cooperate after surgery. As a nursing assistant, your responsibility is to reinforce what has been taught. You may be asked to help the patient with procedures such as breathing routines and foot and leg exercises. (See Figure 29–2.)

Preoperative Care

Preoperative care begins when the doctor tells the patient that surgery is needed. The preoperative period for elective surgery could be several days or weeks, while for an emergency surgery it might be only a few minutes.

Physical Preparations

Physical preparations that may be necessary before surgery include rest and sleep, food and fluid restrictions, bowel and bladder elimination, personal care, and skin preparations. These procedures may be done in the hospital, in an outpatient facility, or in the home.

Rest and Sleep

The patient needs a good night's rest and sleep the evening before surgery. Because of the psychological stress involved, sleep does not come easily to many people facing surgery. A medication may be ordered to help the patient sleep. You can help the patient relax by giving a backrub, repositioning, and straightening bed linen. Try to keep the environment quiet and peaceful. Usually, visitors are encouraged to leave early. Soothing music on the radio or television may be helpful, but avoid stimulation.

Food and Fluid Restrictions

The surgical patient will usually be NPO after midnight the night before surgery. This means the patient cannot take food, water, or any other fluid by mouth. An IV (needle into the vein) may be inserted to provide fluids.

Place an NPO sign over the bed and explain what it means to the patient and visitors. Empty the water pitcher and turn the glass upside down on the tray. Some facilities prefer to remove the pitcher and glass from the room to prevent mistakes. The patient who is NPO will need frequent oral care to prevent drying of the lips and mucous membranes of the mouth.

The patient will usually be NPO for a period after surgery. A postop nutritional routine may begin with a clear liquid diet, followed by a full liquid diet, and then a soft diet. Within a few days, most patients progress to their normal dietary pattern. A description of the different types of diets is given in Chapter 22.

Bowel and Bladder Elimination

An enema may be ordered the night before surgery or just prior to surgery, depending on the type of surgery planned. The purpose is to cleanse the bowel and to help prevent complications such as nausea, vomiting, and incontinence. In some facilities you will be allowed to administer the enema; in others you will assist the nurse. It is your responsibility to know what is expected of you and to follow facility policy.

An indwelling catheter may be inserted into the bladder to drain urine. The catheter may be removed after surgery or left in place for a few days. As a nursing assistant, you will be responsible for care of the catheter after it is inserted. You may be asked to empty and measure the urine in the drainage bag just before the patient goes to surgery.

Personal Care

You are responsible for assisting the surgical patient with personal care. A bath or shower the night before and the morning of surgery is no longer routine. However, most people want to take a bath or shower and a shampoo before surgery because it helps them to relax and feel better. The nurse will let you know what you are expected to do.

Assist the patient in changing into a hospital gown before the preop medication is given. You may need to remove nail polish from the patient's fingernails and toenails so that the surgical team can check the patient's circulation during surgery and the recovery period. Combs, clips, and pins should be removed from the hair.

Patients who wear dentures may need to remove them before surgery. Since many people are reluctant to be without their dentures, this task should be done as close as possible to the time of surgery. If the patient leaves dentures in the room, they should be stored in the bedside table, in a labeled, covered container filled with cool water.

Glasses, contact lenses, hearing aids, and jewelry are removed for safekeeping. A wedding ring or religious medal that the patient does not want to remove may be secured with gauze or tape. Items that are not removed should be noted on the chart. For your own protection, it is wise to let the nurse handle jewelry and money. These items should not be left at the bedside. Information is recorded in the chart as to the location of the patient's valuables.

Skin Preparations

The purpose of preoperative skin preparation is to have the patient's skin as clean and free from microorganisms as possible. The risk of infection is very great during surgery. A surgical opening through the skin invades the body's first line of defense against pathogens.

Skin preparations may include removal of hair by shaving. The skin area to be prepared includes the site of the surgical incision, plus a certain amount of the surrounding area (see Figure 29–3). The area to be prepared is determined by the surgeon's preference and facility policy. If you are doing the skin prep, be very careful not to nick or cut the patient. Check with the nurse to determine exactly what area to shave.

The Preoperative Checklist

In most facilities, a preoperative checklist is used to show that preparations for surgery have been completed (see Figure 29–5 on page 392). You may be asked to sign the list for tasks that you have done.

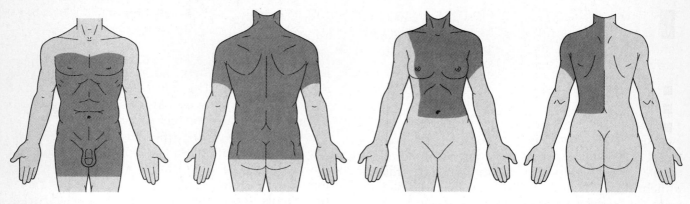

A. Abdominal prep for stomach
   or intestinal surgery.

B. Back prep.

C. Anterior and posterior prep for breast surgery.

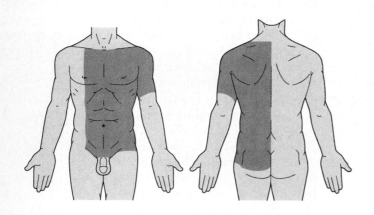

D. Chest prep for thoracic (heart or lung) surgery.

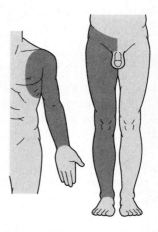

E. Prep for surgery of an extremity (arm or leg).

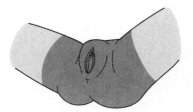

F. Vaginal prep for surgery of excretory
   organs and female reproductive organs.

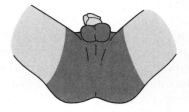

G. Scrotal prep for surgery of excretory
   organs and male reproductive organs.

FIGURE 29–3 Areas to be shaved in preparation for surgery.

You are not responsible for everything on the list, so only sign for what you actually do. The list must be completed before the patient goes to surgery.

The patient must sign a consent form before going to surgery. A signed consent form provides written documentation of the patient's permission for surgery. The doctor, nurse, or admissions clerk is responsible for getting the consent form signed. Nursing assistants do not obtain the consent for surgery.

Preoperative medication may either be given at the bedside or in the surgical area. The medication makes the patient feel drowsy and relaxed. Side

rails must be up, and the patient should not get out of bed after the medication has been given. If the patient needs to urinate, provide a bedpan or urinal. Observe medicated patients frequently. Some people, particularly children and the elderly, may become confused. During this period, the patient is dependent on staff to meet their safety needs.

The patient is usually transferred to surgery by nurses or technicians from the surgical unit. A stretcher will be used, so you will need to bring the patient's bed up to the height of the stretcher. You may be asked to help move the patient from the bed to the stretcher.

Procedure for Shaving the Operative Area (Skin or Surgical Prep)

Beginning Steps

- Identify the patient and explain the procedure.
- Collect necessary equipment and supplies.
- Wash your hands and use standard precautions.
- Protect the patient's privacy.
- Use correct body mechanics.

1. Raise the side rails, raise the bed to a comfortable working height, and lock the brakes.
2. Lower the rail on your working side.
3. Cover the patient with a bath blanket and fold the top linens to the foot of the bed. Place a disposable pad under the area to be shaved.
4. Place the prep kit on the overbed table and open the kit.
5. Position and drape the patient, using the disposable drape from the kit, and exposing only the area to be shaved.
6. Add warm water to the basin and put on gloves.
7. Moisten the soap-filled sponge in the basin of water and work up a lather over the area to be shaved.

8. Holding the skin taut with one hand, shave in the direction of hair growth (see Figure 29–4).
9. Rinse the razor frequently and keep the razor and the skin wet and soapy.
10. Rinse the skin thoroughly and pat dry. Ask the nurse to check the shave.
11. Check the skin carefully to see that no hair remains. Observe for cuts and nicks.
12. Remove the waterproof pad and drapes. Discard the razor in a puncture-proof sharps container.
13. Remove gloves and wash your hands. Discard gloves in the proper container.
14. Remove the bath blanket and straighten the top linens.

Ending Steps

- Check to see that the patient is comfortable.
- Lower the bed and raise the side rails, if appropriate.
- Place the call signal within the patient's reach.
- Wash your hands.
- Report and record your observations.

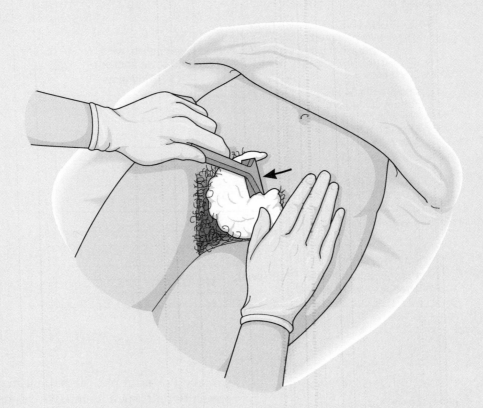

FIGURE 29–4
Holding the skin taut with one hand, shave in the direction of hair growth.

```
┌─────────────────────────────────────────────────────────────┐
│  IMMEDIATE PREOPERATIVE CHECKLIST                             │
│  Name                                    Date                 │
│  ═══════════════════════════════════════════════════════     │
│                                                               │
│  PATIENT IDENTIFICATION                                       │
│     ID on and accurate (name and numbers)   ☐ Yes    ☐ No     │
│     Comments _____        │
│                                                               │
│  PLANNED PROCEDURE                                            │
│     Patient's statement of: _____   │
│  ───────────────────────────────────────────────────         │
│  Patient verifies side:   ☐ Right    ☐ Left       ☐ N/A       │
│  ALLERGIES                                                    │
│     any known allergies:    ☐ Yes    ☐ No                     │
│     Specify if yes _____   │
│  ───────────────────────────────────────────────────         │
│  NPO STATUS                                                   │
│     NPO since midnight      ☐ Yes    ☐ No                     │
│  ───────────────────────────────────────────────────         │
│  PREGNANCY                                                    │
│     Patient   ☐ Denies   ☐ Confirms   ☐ Unsure   ☐ N/A        │
│     Comments _____                        │
│  PERSONAL POSSESSIONS                                         │
│     Dental appliance        ☐ Yes    ☐ No  _____   │
│     Prostheses/Implants     ☐ Yes    ☐ No  _____   │
│                                                               │
│     Valuables:       Item              Disposition            │
│     _____    _____│
│     _____    _____│
│     _____    _____│
│  ═══════════════════════════════════════════════════════     │
│  HEIGHT_____ WEIGHT_____ lb/kg   ☐ Actual   ☐ Est.        │
│                                                               │
│  VITAL SIGNS   B/P___   T___   P___   R ___   Time ___        │
│  PREOPERATIVE PREPARATION                                     │
│     Physically prepared:    ☐ Yes    ☐ No                     │
│        (personal clothes, glasses, contacts, nail polish, wigs,│
│        dentures, jewelry removed and hospital gown applied)   │
│                       Yes      No        Comments             │
│  Med. sheets to OR     ☐       ☐      _____        │
│  Patient voided preop  ☐       ☐      _____        │
│  Preop meds given      ☐       ☐      _____        │
│  Meds/supplies to OR   ☐       ☐      _____        │
│  Side rails up         ☐       ☐      _____        │
│  Patient instructed    ☐       ☐      _____        │
│  to stay in bed                                               │
│  Preoperative treatments _____    │
│  PATIENT IDENTIFIED IN OR DEPT. BY DR. _____      │
│  ═══════════════════════════════════════════════════════     │
│  COMMENTS: _____   │
│  _____ │
│                                                               │
│  READY FOR OR              Date _____       │
│     Preoperative unit RN/LPN (initials)  _____ │
│     Preoperative RN (initials)           _____ │
└─────────────────────────────────────────────────────────────┘
```

FIGURE 29–5   A sample preoperative checklist.

The Operative Period

Your responsibilities while the patient is in surgery will depend upon where the patient will go after surgery. For example, the patient may be going to a specialty unit, such as intensive care. If the patient is to return to the room, you will need to prepare the room for postoperative care. Sometimes this information is not known until after surgery. The nurse will let you know what you are supposed to do.

Family members and visitors should be directed to the proper waiting area. If the family is going to wait in the patient's room, you might suggest that they step out for a snack or a cup of coffee while you prepare the room. Questions about the progress of the surgery should be referred to the nurse.

If the patient is not coming back to the room, the patient's belongings must be taken to the new location. Make sure that you collect everything that belongs to the patient. Handle the patient's belongings with respect and pack them carefully. Remove equipment and discard disposables according to facility policy. Strip the bed and place the linen in the soiled linen hamper.

Preparing the Room

If the patient is coming back to the room, you will need to strip the bed and make a surgical bed. (See Figure 29–6.) This procedure is described in Chapter 16. Move chairs and other furniture out of the way to clear a path for the *gurney* (a type of stretcher used to transport patients). Clear the bedside stand and overbed table for the supplies the patient will need after surgery. The following list of supplies and equipment should be in the room:

- Blood pressure cuff and stethoscope
- Thermometer

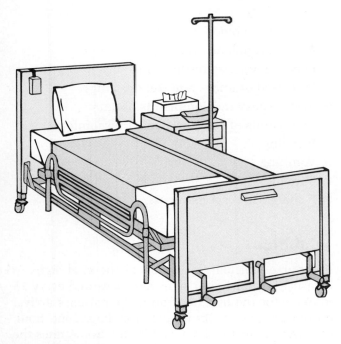

FIGURE 29–6
Prepare a surgical bed and provide supplies that will be needed.

- Emesis basin
- Box of tissues
- IV pole
- Vital signs flow sheet
- Intake and output form

The nurse will let you know if any other supplies or equipment are necessary.

Anesthesia

When patients arrive in the operating room, they are usually drowsy from the preoperative medication. The anesthesiologist administers an anesthetic, a medicine that causes a loss of sensation in one part or in all of the body and may cause unconsciousness. There are three basic types of anesthesia: general anesthesia, local anesthesia, and spinal anesthesia.

General anesthesia causes unconsciousness and a loss of sensation in the entire body. Patients are in a deep sleep and feel nothing. The postop effects of general anesthesia may include confusion, sleepiness, agitation, slowed respirations, slow blood flow, changes in blood pressure, slowed peristalsis, and weakness. Patients will be sleepy for several hours, sometimes for an entire day. However, they should awaken easily and be able to respond when called by name. They gradually become more awake until full consciousness returns. Nausea and vomiting may occur after this type of anesthesia. Patients are usually NPO for a period.

Local anesthesia causes a loss of sensation in the operative site only. Patients are awake during the surgery but feel no pain. A medication to relax the patient may be given with this type of anesthesia. The effects of local anesthesia generally wear off in a few hours. Patients are awake and usually able to eat and drink.

Spinal anesthesia involves the injection of medication directly into the spinal canal. It causes a loss of sensation in all parts of the body below the site of injection. This type of anesthesia does not produce unconsciousness, the patient is awake. A medication is usually given to relax the patient and reduce anxiety. After spinal anesthesia, the patient is unable to move and has no feeling in the lower part of the body for several hours. Patients are alert and usually able to eat and drink. Sometimes the doctor will order that the patient be kept flat for 12 hours.

Even though you are not involved in administering anesthesia, it is important that you know which type was used and what effects are expected. This information helps you to care for the surgical patient postoperatively.

Postoperative Care

Recovery Room

Immediately after surgery the patient goes to the recovery room. This unit may be called postanesthesia recovery (PAR) or postanesthesia care unit (PACU). Patients are cared for in this area while they are recovering from anesthesia. The patient will stay in recovery until his or her vital signs and other conditions are stable. The recovery room nurse will notify the nursing unit when the patient is ready to be transferred.

Care of the Patient from the Recovery Room

Recovery room nurses or technicians bring the patient to the room. The nurse who will be responsible accepts the patient to the nursing unit. You may be asked to help transfer the patient from the stretcher to the bed. Raise the side rails immediately to prevent the patient from falling. Have an extra blanket available because many postop patients complain of feeling cold.

The nurse will carefully examine the patient, noting tubes, IVs, catheters, and casts. Dressings will be observed for bleeding or other drainage. Vital signs will be taken and compared to the recovery room report. The nurse will call the patient's name to check the level of consciousness. When the examination is completed, side rails will be raised and the call signal placed within reach. Family members are usually waiting anxiously to see the patient.

The patient must be monitored carefully for the next few hours. A patient who has just returned from the recovery room is very vulnerable, and safety is a major issue. Keep the side rails raised when you are not caring for the patient and make sure the call signal is within the patient's reach. Nausea and vomiting are common postop problems. If the patient is not fully conscious, aspiration may occur. Aspiration (choking by inhaling food or fluid into the lungs) can cause pneumonia. Observe the postop patient frequently and, if vomitng occurs, turn the patient to the side and place an emesis basin under the chin (see Figure 29–7). Notify the nurse immediately, but do not leave the vomiting patient alone.

You may be asked to help with tasks such as measuring vital signs, reminding the patient to cough and breathe deeply, and assisting the patient with foot and leg exercises. Your responsibilities may also include helping the patient with turning

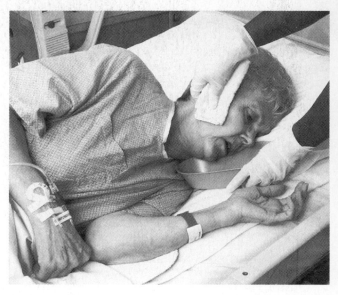

FIGURE 29–7
If vomiting occurs, turn the patient's head to the side to prevent aspiration.

and positioning, providing restorative skin care, and assisting with elimination. If the patient is on intake and output, all fluids that are taken in and all that are eliminated must be measured and recorded. If the patient does not have a catheter, you will need to measure and record the first voiding. Report this information to the nurse. Although you will not be responsible for changing dressings, you must observe the amount and type of drainage. As you care for the patient, it is important to observe changes in the patient's condition. Observations that should be reported to the nurse immediately include:

- A change in blood pressure
- A weak, rapid, or irregular pulse
- Labored or noisy respirations
- Increased drainage and wet dressings
- Restlessness and complaints of thirst
- Complaints of pain, nausea, or discomfort
- Bleeding
- Vomiting
- Choking
- A change in responsiveness

Vital Signs

The nurse will tell you which of the vital signs to measure. Usually vital signs are measured every 15 minutes for the first hour after the patient's arrival on the unit, every 30 minutes for the second hour, and every hour for the next 4 hours. Sometimes the patient is attached to machines that automatically measure vital signs.

If vital signs are back to normal at the end of that period, the preop routine ends and the regular routine will be followed. If vital signs are not stable or have not returned to normal levels, the postop routine will be followed for as long as necessary. The nurse will tell you if there are changes in the routine.

Vital signs are usually recorded on a postoperative flow sheet (see Figure 29–8). This document shows the flow of vital signs readings over a period of several hours. The flow sheet is usually left at the bedside until completed. Accurate measuring, recording, and reporting of vital signs are essential.

Comfort and Pain Control

Keeping the patient comfortable after surgery involves several nursing measures: positioning, mouth care, hygiene, warmth, and pain control.

Providing good personal care and hygiene is important. Straightening the linen and keeping the patient clean and dry promote comfort. Frequent mouth care may be necessary. The patient may be cold, and extra blankets might be helpful. But the most important comfort measure is pain control

Pain is a common postsurgical complaint. Proper pain assessment and control is essential to recovery because pain affects sleep, appetite, and healing. Self-reporting of pain is the most reliable assessment tool. Only the patient knows whether pain is present and to what degree. Since nursing assistants provide so much of the care, it may be you to whom the patient complains about pain. Be aware of nonverbal complaints of pain such as anxiety, restlessness, and grimacing. Remember that culture affects how people respond to pain. In some cultures, complaints of pain are considered cow-

POSTOPERATIVE VITAL SIGNS FLOW SHEET

Time	Blood Pressure	Temperature	Pulse	Respirations	Initials
11 AM	114/70	97.6	68	12	PG
11:15	119/70	97.6	70	14	MA
11:30	112/70	97.6	66	12	MA
11:45	114/68	97.8	68	14	MA
12:15	114/70	98	70	14	PG
12:45	116/70	98	72	14	MA
1:45	116/70	98.2	74	16	MA
2:45	116/72	98.4	76	16	MA
3:45	116/72	98.4	76	16	JS
4:45	116/72	98.6	76	16	JS

Initials	Signature	Initials	Signature
PG	Peggy Grubbs Rn		
MA	Mary Ash CNA		
JS	Joe Stevens CNA		

Fran K. Levy
Rm 212A

FIGURE 29–8   A sample postoperative flow sheet.

ardly. Observe and listen carefully, and report your observations to the nurse promptly.

A patient-controlled analgesia (PCA) pump may be used to relieve pain. In this system, as the name implies, the patient controls his or her pain medication. The pump is preset to control the amount of medication given and to prevent an overdose. Although you do not adjust the pump, you need to be aware of how it works. A needle is inserted into the tissue under the patient's skin. Tubing connects the needle with the PCA pump. (See Figure 29-9.) When caring for a patient with a PCA pump, be careful not to dislodge the needle. Do not pull on the tubing or allow it to twist or kink. Avoid getting the pump wet, and report any beeping sound to the nurse immediately.

Turning and Repositioning

Generally, surgical patients are turned and repositioned every 2 hours after surgery. Turning and repositioning help to prevent complications such as pneumonia, blood clots, and pressure sores. Activity increases circulation and helps to clear the respiratory tract of secretions. Remember to check the dressing each time you turn the patient and report new drainage to the nurse immediately.

In the immediate postoperative period, patients may need considerable help and encouragement in turning and repositioning. It may be painful to move, or the patient may be concerned about injuring the surgical site or pulling out stitches. Using a turn sheet makes repositioning the patient easier and less painful. Get help, if necessary, to make the procedure more comfortable.

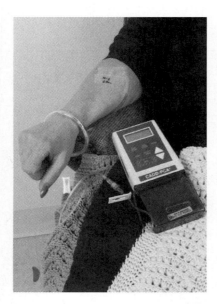

FIGURE 29-9
A patient-controlled analgesia (PCA) pump.

The nurse will tell you if there are any turning restrictions or special orders. For example, after some types of surgery, the patient must not be positioned on the operative side. It may be necessary to keep the bed flat, or an extremity may need to be elevated on a pillow. The patient should be positioned in correct body alignment; use pillows for support, if necessary.

Keep IV tubing, catheters, and other tubing clear while you are turning the patient. Check to see that the tubing is not kinked or twisted. Record the time, the position, and the patient's reaction each time the patient is turned. Let the nurse know if the patient refuses to turn or complains of pain during the procedure.

In most types of surgery, patients are encouraged to get up and walk within a few hours or the next day after surgery. Early ambulation has proven to be effective in preventing many postoperative complications and in assisting the patient to recover faster.

Deep Breathing and Coughing Exercises

Deep breathing and coughing exercises are necessary after surgery to prevent respiratory complications, such as pneumonia. Coughing helps clear mucus that has accumulated during the surgery. Mucus plugs can obstruct the airway, interfere with breathing, or cause infection. Deep breathing exercises help circulate air throughout the lungs and aid in the exchange of oxygen and carbon dioxide. The nurse will tell you how often the exercises are to be done and how many deep breaths and coughs are required. Preoperative teaching helps the patient to perform the exercises postoperatively. Immediately following postop is not a good time to try to teach the patient new procedures. The procedure for deep breathing and coughing exercises is located on the facing page.

Foot and Leg Exercises

Foot and leg exercise help to stimulate circulation and prevent blood clots. When circulation slows, blood tends to pool in one place and a *thrombus* (blood clot) may form. A blood clot that travels through the bloodstream is called an *embolus*. An embolus that lodges in one of the vessels of a vital organ, like the lungs or heart, can result in death. A doctor's order for foot and leg exercises will be necessary if the patient has had leg surgery; otherwise, they are a part of the postop routine.

These exercises were practiced by the patient before surgery, so teaching is not required postoperatively. At first, you may need to assist if the patient is very weak. However, patients should be encouraged to do the exercises independently whenever

Procedure for Deep Breathing and Coughing Exercises

Beginning Steps

- Identify the patient and explain the procedure.
- Collect necessary equipment and supplies.
- Wash your hands and use standard precautions.
- Protect the patient's privacy.
- Use correct body mechanics.

1. Raise the side rails, raise the bed to a comfortable working height, and lock the brakes.
2. Lower the rail on your working side.
3. Assist the patient to a semi-Fowler's or Fowler's position, if allowed.
4. Ask the patient who has had chest or abdominal surgery to place one hand on either side of the rib cage or over the operative site, or hold a pillow firmly over the operative site (see Figure 29–10).
5. Ask the patient to take a slow, deep breath, inhaling through the nose.
6. Ask the patient to hold the breath for 3 to 5 seconds, if possible.
7. Ask the patient to breathe out slowly through the mouth.

8. Ask the patient to repeat the steps three or four times.
9. Ask the patient to interlace the fingers over the pillow to splint the operative site.
10. Provide the patient with tissues and place the emesis basin within reach.
11. Put on gloves.
12. Ask the patient to take a deep breath and cough, with the mouth open, while breathing out. This step should be repeated three or four times, if possible.
13. Use the tissues to wipe the mouth and dispose of tissues in the emesis basin.
14. Empty and clean the emesis basin and return equipment to its proper place.

Ending Steps

- Check to see that the patient is comfortable.
- Lower the bed and raise the side rails, if appropriate.
- Place the call signal within the patient's reach.
- Wash your hands.
- Report and record your observations.

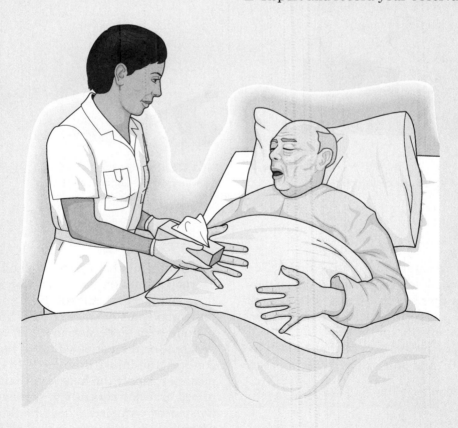

FIGURE 29–10
Hold a pillow firmly over the operative site to make deep breathing and coughing easier.

Procedure for Foot and Leg Exercises

Beginning Steps

■ Identify the patient and explain the procedure.
■ Collect necessary equipment and supplies.
■ Wash your hands and use standard precautions.
■ Protect the patient's privacy.
■ Use correct body mechanics.

1. Raise the side rails, raise the bed to a comfortable working height, and lock the brakes.
2. Lower the rail on your working side.
3. Assist the patient to a supine position.
4. Ask the patient to wiggle the toes and make circles with the toes three to five times.
5. Assist the patient to bend one foot upward and downward three to five times (see Figure 29–11). Repeat with the other foot.

6. Assist the patient to bend and straighten one knee three to five times. Repeat with the other knee.
7. Assist the patient to raise and lower one leg three to five times (see Figure 29–12). Repeat with the other leg.

Ending Steps

■ Check to see that the patient is comfortable.
■ Lower the bed and raise the side rails, if appropriate.
■ Place the call signal within the patient's reach.
■ Wash your hands.
■ Report and record your observations.

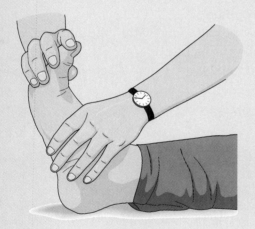

FIGURE 29–11
Assist the patient to bend the foot upward and downward.

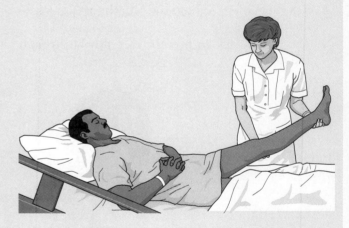

FIGURE 29–12
Assist the patient to raise and lower the leg.

possible. Try to coordinate foot and leg exercises with the turning schedule. Assist the patient to perform the exercises three to five times every 1 or 2 hours, when awake. Foot and leg exercise can be done while the patient sits on the edge of the bed, once the patient has progressed to that level. The procedure for foot and leg exercises is located above.

Elastic Support Hose

Elastic support hose may be ordered postoperatively for certain patients. They are used to improve circulation and help prevent blood clots. The elastic exerts pressure on the veins, which promotes blood flow to the heart. Elastic hose may also be called antiembolism stockings or TED hose. They come in various sizes, so be sure to use the size that has been ordered for the patient. Elastic hose can cause discomfort and injury if not applied correctly. It is important to apply the hose before the patient gets out of bed. Check frequently to see that the hose are not twisted or wrinkled. They should be removed and reapplied at least twice a day, or as ordered by the physician. Follow the guidelines in Chapter 24 for applying support hose.

Review

Read each sentence and fill in the blank with a vocabulary term that best completes the sentence.

1. _____ is the loss of sensation caused by a medication given before surgery.
2. The term _____ means "before surgery."
3. The term _____ means "after surgery."
4. The medical term for a blood clot that breaks loose and travels through the bloodstream is a/an _____.
5. A/An _____ is a type of stretcher used to transport patients.

Remember

1. Surgery is being performed today in less time and with less human suffering than ever before.
2. Patients who are prepared before surgery are more able to cooperate after surgery.
3. The purpose of a preoperative skin prep is to have the patient's skin as clean and free from microorganisms as possible.
4. A preoperative checklist is used to show that preparations for surgery have been completed.
5. Side rails should be raised after the patient has had preoperative medication.
6. A patient who has just returned from the recovery room is dependent on the staff for safety.
7. Let the nurse know immediately if the postop patient's blood pressure drops or the pulse is irregular.
8. Generally, postop patients are turned and repositioned every 2 hours to prevent complications.
9. If the patient is nauseated, the head should be turned to the side to prevent aspiration.
10. It is important to keep the patient comfortable and pain controlled after surgery.
11. Deep breathing and coughing exercises help clear mucus from the respiratory tract.
12. Foot and leg exercises help to stimulate circulation and prevent blood clots.

Reflect

Read the following case study and answer the questions.

Case Study

Mrs. Talltree is a 72-year-old Native American patient who had abdominal surgery yesterday. She has an IV in her left arm and a Foley catheter that was inserted before surgery. Mrs. Talltree seldom complains, although she appears to be in pain. Kevin has been assigned to assist her with coughing and deep breathing exercises, and with foot and leg exercises.

1. What effect might Mrs. Talltree's culture have on her comfort level?
2. What signs and symptoms will Kevin need to watch for to determine if Mrs. Talltree is having pain?
3. How can Kevin make it easier for Mrs. Talltree to do coughing and deep breathing exercises?
4. What is the purpose of foot and leg exercises?

Respond

Choose the best answer for each question.

1. Surgery that the patient chooses to have done and that is scheduled ahead of time is called
   A. Emergency surgery
   B. Elective surgery
   C. Postop surgery
   D. Psychological surgery
2. A doctor who administers medication that causes the patient to lose sensation during surgery is a/an
   A. Internist
   B. Urologist
   C. Anesthesiologist
   D. Psychiatrist

3. The medical abbreviation for "nothing by mouth" is
   A. IV
   B. NG
   C. NPO
   D. PRN

4. The patient refuses to remove her wedding ring before surgery. What is your best response?
   A. Secure the ring with tape or gauze.
   B. Tell her she must remove the ring. It is facility policy.
   C. Ignore the ring. It's not your responsibility.
   D. Ask the patient's husband to remove the ring.

5. Choking by inhaling food or fluid into the lungs is called
   A. Sterilization
   B. Aspiration
   C. Respiration
   D. Expectoration

6. The postop patient's blood pressure has dropped from 150/80 to 100/60. What should you do?
   A. Chart the blood pressure. It is within normal levels.
   B. Report the blood pressure to the nurse immediately.
   C. Shake the patient. Movement will cause the blood pressure to rise.
   D. None of the above.

7. Who can usually make the best assessment of the patient's pain after surgery?
   A. The nursing assistant
   B. The nurse
   C. The family
   D. The patient

8. A PCA pump is used for treating
   A. Pain
   B. Nausea
   C. Incontinence
   D. Diarrhea

9. The primary purpose of elastic support hose after surgery is
   A. To make the legs look slimmer
   B. To improve urination
   C. To prevent nausea
   D. To improve circulation

10. The postop patient is too sleepy to do foot and leg exercises. What is your best response?
    A. Wait until he is awake to do the exercises.
    B. Wake him up and make him do the exercises.
    C. Do the exercises for the patient.
    D. Remind the patient to do the exercise later.

Chapter Thirty

Maternal *and* Child Health

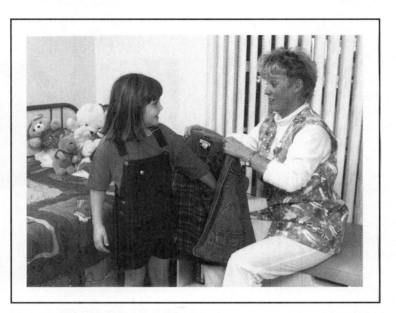

Glossary

circumcision   The surgical removal of the foreskin from the penis.

fetus   The developing unborn child, from the eighth week of pregnancy to birth.

maternity care   The health care of the pregnant woman before, during, and after childbirth.

pediatrics   The branch of medicine concerned with the care of infants and children.

postpartum   The period of time following the delivery of a baby.

umbilicus   The scar that marks the former attachment of the umbilical cord; the navel or belly button.

This chapter provides a broad overview of the care of new mothers, newborns, infants, and children. It briefly touches on *maternity care* (care of the pregnant woman before, during, and after childbirth). It addresses nursing care of the patient during the *postpartum* period (the period following delivery). However, information regarding pregnancy, labor, and delivery are not included. Keep in mind that the simple process of childbirth involves several branches of medicine that cannot be adequately covered in one chapter. This chapter also includes *pediatrics*, the branch of medicine that is concerned with the care of infants and children. As a nursing assistant, you may care for maternity patients, newborns, infants, and children of all ages. Special training is usually required to work in any of these areas.

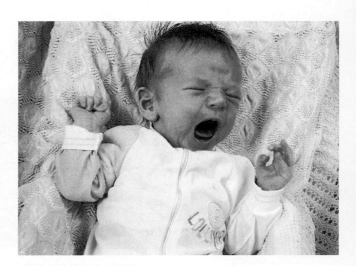

FIGURE 30–1
It is important to remember that newborns are individuals too.

Changes
in Maternity Care

In the early days of this country, babies were born at home. Later, maternity care switched to hospitals, where mothers and babies were separated from their families. Frequently, mothers and babies were also separated, with the baby being cared for in the nursery.

Realizing that the birth of a child affects the entire family, maternity care today is more family oriented. Family-centered care provides an excellent example of holistic nursing by recognizing the needs of the new mother, the newborn, and other family members, as well. The involvement of family members provides support and an opportunity for bonding (the development of a close, loving relationship) with the new baby. Birthing rooms, rooming-in, and alternative birthing centers have been developed to meet this need. The focus is on keeping mother and baby together in one room with relaxed visiting rules. Allowing other children in the family to visit helps relieve some of their anxiety on the arrival of a new sibling. Holistic care also includes an awareness of cultural diversity. Religious rites and customs are followed as closely as possible. Each patient is recognized as an individual with preferences and beliefs that are meaningful. It is important to remember that newborns are individuals as well (see Figure 30–1).

Childbirth is viewed as a normal, natural process and not as an illness. Fathers are encouraged to be with the mother during labor, delivery, and postpartum. In most areas, they are allowed to attend the delivery, even if the patient has a cesarean section, in which the *fetus* (unborn child) is delivered through a surgical incision into the abdominal wall and uterus. Mother and child are discharged on the second or third day after delivery, if there are no complications.

Postpartum Care

As a nursing assistant working in maternity, you will be assisting the nurse in caring for the patient during the postpartum period. As you provide care, observe carefully for signs of postpartum complications, such as hemorrhage (severe bleeding) or infection.

Observing for Hemorrhage

In the immediate postpartum period, the new mother must be closely observed for signs and symptoms of hemorrhage. Vital signs should be carefully measured and recorded. Report changes to the nurse immediately, particularly if there is a drop in blood pressure or a rise in pulse rate. Observe the color, texture, and warmth of the skin. Skin that is cold, pale, ashen, or cyanotic may indicate severe blood loss or shock. Check the perineal area and the pad for the amount and color of drainage. When changing the pad, check the rectal area to make sure that the patient is not lying in blood that may have leaked through the pad.

Observing the Uterus

Observe the size and firmness of the uterus. A soft, enlarged uterus may indicate excessive bleeding. The nurse will massage the top of the uterus to stimulate the muscles to contract and firm up the uterus. In some areas, nursing assistants are allowed to perform this procedure. If you are allowed, you will need special training to learn how to massage the uterus correctly. Never attempt this procedure if you have not had proper training.

Preventing Infection

Another postpartum concern is the prevention of infection. In the early 1900s, postpartum infection was one of the leading causes of death of new mothers. Keeping the patient in one area for labor, delivery, and postpartum helps to reduce the chance of infection. Report any changes in color or odor of drainage that might indicate infection. Also, report temperature elevations, no matter how slight. Use standard precautions and follow aseptic practices at all times.

Encouraging Urinary Elimination

The new mother may have trouble urinating. Tissue swelling, trauma during delivery, and the position of the uterus can affect the patient's ability to empty the bladder. If the patient is unable to urinate, turn on a faucet, place the patient's fingers in warm water, or pour warm water over the perineum to encourage urination. Measure the urinary output and report the amount to the nurse. Let the nurse know if the patient complains of discomfort or is unable to void.

Providing Perineal Care

The nurse will teach the new mother how to do her own perineal care (peri-care). The patient will be provided with a squeeze bottle filled with warm water and instructed to rinse the area each time she voids or has a bowel movement. She will be taught infection control techniques, such as washing her hands before and after peri-care, drying from front to back, and discarding soiled pads and tissues properly. Remind the mother to wash her hands before applying a clean pad and to avoid touching the inside of the pad. You will need to reinforce the teaching and assist her as necessary. If you need to provide peri-care for her, follow the procedure described in Chapter 20.

Assisting with Breast Care

The mother should wash her breasts at least once a day with soap and water and wear a well-fitted brassiere for support. If breast pads are used inside the brassiere to absorb milk leakage, they should be changed frequently. Report any complaints of breast pain, soreness, or other discomfort. If the mother is nursing, lotion may be used to keep the nipples soft. If the mother is not breastfeeding, the doctor may order medications to dry up her milk.

Care of the Newborn

For the first six weeks of life, the baby is called a neonate or newborn. During the neonatal period, the baby must adjust to living outside the uterus and adapt to changes that take place in its body systems. The neonatal period is a very vulnerable time. In fact, three fourths of infant deaths occur in the first six weeks of life. The neonate is totally dependent on others for survival.

As soon as the baby is born, a complete physical assessment is done by the nurse or physician. Heart rate, respiratory effort, muscle tone, reflexes, and skin color are evaluated. The neonate is weighed and measured, and vital signs are taken. (See Figure 30–2.) A bath may be given to clean the baby. The neonate must be kept warm because its temperature has not yet stabilized. For the first few hours after birth, the newborn is observed very carefully.

Infection Control

The newborn must be protected from infection. The immune system is not well-developed at birth, and the newborn is highly susceptible. Nursery workers usually wear clean scrub gowns, rather than their own uniforms. Follow standard precautions and use aseptic techniques, such as handwashing before and after each infant contact. The hands and the forearms must be scrubbed before entering the nursery. Do not come to work if you are ill, and let

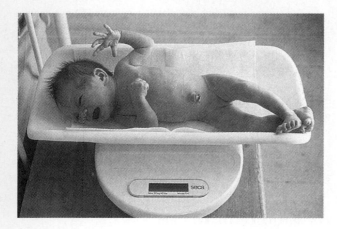

FIGURE 30–2
The neonate is weighed and measured soon after birth.

the nurse know if you have a cold, earache, or stomach upset.

Nursing Care of the Newborn

If you work in the newborn nursery, you will provide much of the baby's personal care, such as bathing, dressing, changing, and feeding. You will need to be skilled in performing procedures and in making observations. Changes in the newborn can occur rapidly and dramatically. Vital signs and weight must be measured accurately.

Nursing care should involve the whole family. How the parents, grandparents, and siblings react will affect the health and the future of the newborn. You can help in the bonding process by calling their attention to the baby's responses to their caregiving efforts. Encourage the parents to handle, examine, and dress their baby.

Discharge

Discharge planning for a neonate prepares the baby and the family for care at home. If necessary, the mother will be taught how to bathe, feed, dress, and care for her baby. Arrangements will be made for home health care services, if needed. Your responsibilities in the discharge process may include the following:

- Assist the mother to dress the newborn in its own clothing.
- Wrap the baby in a blanket.
- Collect the patient's personal belongings.
- Make sure that equipment and formula are ready.
- Check to see that the mother has received and understands the discharge instructions.
- Transport mother and baby by wheelchair to the discharge area.

Always check the baby's identification bracelet with that of the mother. Stay with the mother and baby in the discharge area until they leave.

Introduction to Pediatrics

It is essential that pediatric (infants and children) care be family oriented. Since most children do not care for themselves, the mother and other caregivers should be included in their care in the health care facility. When a child is sick, the whole family is affected, and their needs must be considered as well as those of the infant or child.

Children are not little adults. They lack the maturity and understanding of most adults. Small children may not understand what is happening to them or what is expected of them. They may not be able to follow directions or make wise decisions. They are not able to protect themselves and must rely on others for safety. Their helplessness may lead to fear and anxiety. When communicating with children, you must talk to them at their level and in language they can understand. Children are individuals, each with his or her own needs. Unlike adults, children continue to grow and mature while they are patients in the health care facility. Their needs keep changing as they move from one stage of development to another.

Meeting the needs of pediatric patients requires special knowledge and training. Procedures will need to be altered to accommodate the child's size and understanding. For example, to measure a child's vital signs, you will need a blood pressure cuff small enough to fit the child's arm. Be aware that the normal range of vital signs vary according to age. A pulse of 120 might be normal for a newborn but abnormal for an older child. Measuring pediatric vital signs is addressed in detail in Chapter 21.

Caring for infants and children can be challenging, frustrating, delightful, exhausting, and rewarding. Your reward for this kind of nursing may include smiles, pats, and hugs. At the end of a long, tiring shift, there is nothing more satisfying than to have a 3-year-old put her arms around you and whisper, "I love you."

Care of the Infant

The infant stage is from birth to two years of age. In the health care facility, we must help meet all their basic needs for food, water, sleep, elimination, temperature control, safety, and security. Routine care involves feeding, bathing, diapering, dressing, and measuring the infant's weight, height, and vital signs.

Guidelines for Infant Safety

- Keep crib side rails in the up position when you are not providing care.
- Keep one hand on the infant when a side rail is down.
- Do not leave the infant alone on an unprotected surface, such as a changing table or in a bathtub.
- Wash your hands and forearms before handling the infant.
- Use both hands to lift the infant.
- Support the infant's head and neck.
- Hold the infant securely, using one of the techniques shown in Figure 30–3.
- Protect the infant from drafts.
- Check the temperature of bottles and bath water to prevent burns.
- Secure safety straps in infant seats and high chairs.
- Keep small objects out of the infant's reach.
- Place the baby in a safe place while performing chores or answering the telephone.

The infant's psychosocial needs, such as love, caring, and social contact, must also be met.

Infants need love if they are to grow and thrive. Love is expressed through gentle handling of the infant while holding or providing care. Smiles, hugs, and soft voice tones show affection and help the infant to feel wanted. Infants cry when they have needs because they cannot tell us what they want. Meeting these needs helps to accomplish the major developmental task of infancy, which is learning to trust.

Safety

Safety is an important factor when you are caring for infants because they are unable to protect themselves. At home, parents and other family members assume that responsibility. In the health care facility, infants depend on you and other health care workers for safety and security.

Extra precautions are necessary when you are caring for an infant at home. Do not hold the baby while cooking, washing dishes, or doing other household chores. Do not talk on the telephone while holding the baby. If the telephone rings, ask the caller to call back later or ask them to hold while you return the infant to the crib and raise the side rails.

Feeding the Infant

The infant's nutritional needs can be met by breastfeeding, bottle-feeding, or a combination of the two. The parents make this decision based on various factors, such as cultural influences, the mother's occupational status, and finances. Support their decision and do not try to influence them one way or another.

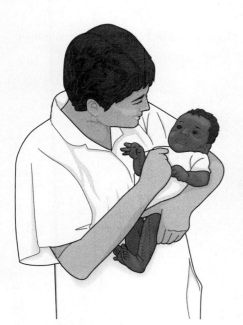

A. Hold the infant in the crook of your arm.

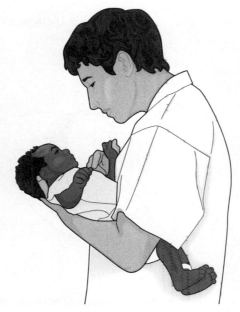

B. Hold the infant under one arm, with the hand of that arm supporting the head and neck.

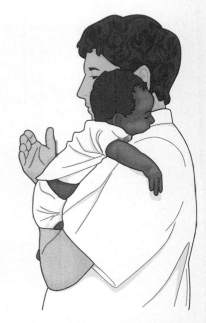

C. Hold the infant upright over your shoulder. Support the back, head, and neck with your hand.

FIGURE 30–3 Techniques for holding or carrying the infant.

Guidelines for Assisting with Breast-Feeding

■ Protect privacy by pulling the curtain, closing the door, and providing a baby blanket to cover the breast. A "Do Not Disturb" sign may be placed on the door.

■ Remind the mother to wash her hands before handling her breasts.

■ Assist the mother to wash her nipples, if necessary. Wash with a circular motion, from the nipple outward.

■ Assist the mother to a comfortable position.

■ Bring the infant to the mother.

■ Remind the mother to hold the infant close to her breast.

■ Have the mother stroke the infant's cheek with her nipple (see Figure 30–4A).

■ Remind the mother to keep breast tissue away from the infant's nose with her thumb or fingers (see Figure 30–4B).

■ To remove the breast from the infant's mouth, the mother will need to break the seal by inserting her little finger into the corner of the infant's mouth and gently pushing away the breast (see Figure 30–4C).

■ Help the mother to burp the infant (see Figure 30–6 on page 409).

■ Return the infant to the crib and change the diaper if necessary.

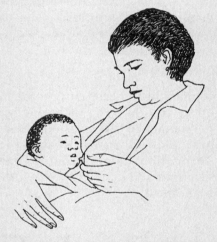

A. Have the mother stroke the infant's cheek with her nipple.

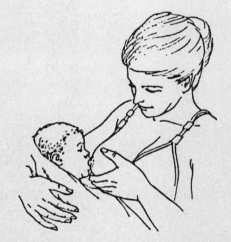

B. Use the thumb or fingers to keep breast tissue away from the infant's nose.

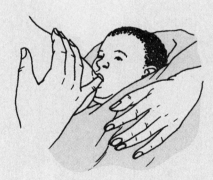

C. The mother can insert her little finger into the corner of the infant's mouth and gently push away her breast.

FIGURE 30–4 Breast-feeding the infant.

Assisting with Breast-Feeding

If the mother has chosen to breast-feed, the infant will be put to the breast within a few hours after delivery. Nurses teach breast-feeding techniques and are available to assist if necessary. Breast-feeding is a normal, natural act that mother and baby soon learn. You can help by encouraging the mother and reinforcing the teaching. You can assist the mother to get ready for breast-feeding by helping her with hygiene, assisting her to a comfortable position, and bringing the baby to her.

The breast-feeding routine and length of nursing vary. These decisions are made by the mother and reinforced by the baby. Call the nurse if either the mother or the baby has difficulty with breast-feeding.

Assisting with Bottle-Feeding

A bottle-fed infant is given formula that is prescribed by the doctor. The infant may receive all of his or her feedings from the bottle, or bottle-feeding may be used to supplement breast-feeding. The bottle may also be used in weaning the baby from the breast or in giving the baby water between breast-feeding. It is important to hold the infant securely during the entire procedure. Never leave the infant with a bottle propped in its mouth. The infant could vomit or aspirate (choke) while you are not watching. Feeding time should be a pleasant experience for both you and the baby. Provide a calm environment, talk softly to the baby, and do not hurry or force the baby to eat too much. The procedure for bottle-feeding the infant begins on page 408.

Diapering the Infant

The infant's diaper should be changed as often as needed. Check the diaper for dampness or soiling at regular intervals. The baby's skin is delicate and may become irritated very quickly by the wet diaper. Let the nurse know if the infant has diarrhea (frequent, watery stool). Diarrhea can cause dehydration very quickly in an infant, and if not treated promptly, death may result.

Diapers come in a variety of sizes and may be reusable or disposable. Reusable diapers are made of a soft, cotton cloth and must be washed, rinsed, and dried. Disposable diapers are used once and discarded in a special container. Never attempt to flush a disposable diaper down the toilet because it can clog the plumbing. Wear gloves while changing the baby or handling used diapers.

Diapering provides an excellent opportunity for communication. Talk softly to the baby during the procedure. Even though your words are not understood, the sound of your voice is comforting. Your nonverbal communication is even more important. Touch, smiles, and gentle handling all tell the infant that you care. The procedure for diapering the infant is located on page 410.

Care of the Umbilical Cord

The umbilical cord is a long, flexible organ that connects the mother to the fetus before birth. The cord is attached to the baby at the *umbilicus* (the navel or belly button). It carries blood, oxygen, water, and nutrients from the mother to the fetus and carries waste products from the fetus to the mother. Shortly after delivery, the doctor clamps and cuts the cord. Within 7 to 10 days, the stump of the baby's cord dries, shrinks, discolors, and falls off. When the cord comes off, there may be a slight oozing of blood, but it is not painful.

The cord forms a portal of entry for microorganisms until the stump completely heals. It is important to keep the cord stump clean and dry. Cord care is performed each time the diaper is changed and is continued for 1 or 2 days after the cord comes off. Guidelines for cord care are located on page 410.

Circumcision Care

Male newborns may be circumcised before they are discharged from the hospital. In *circumcision*, excess tissue called the foreskin is cut from around the end of the penis. This procedure is not routine and depends on the wishes of the parents. Check the circumcision each time the diaper is changed and apply the diaper loosely to avoid irritation. The area may look red and swollen, so you will need to observe carefully for signs of infection. Observe for adequate voiding. Report any odor, drainage, or bleeding to the nurse. Circumcisions usually heal quickly without complications. The mother is taught how to care for the circumcision at home.

Bathing the Infant

Bath time provides an opportunity to demonstrate the tender, loving care that is so important to infants and children. Take time while bathing the infant to touch, hold, and cuddle. Talk to the baby and smile. You might be lucky and get a smile in return from the baby.

Bath time is also an excellent time for observation. Carefully inspect areas where skin folds occur, such as the neck, axilla, and groin. Note the baby's movements during the bath and its response to the procedure. Never leave the baby unattended on the bath table or in the tub.

Procedure for Bottle-Feeding the Infant

Beginning Steps

■ Identify the patient and explain the procedure.
■ Collect necessary equipment and supplies.
■ Wash your hands and use standard precautions.
■ Protect the patient's privacy.
■ Use correct body mechanics.

1. Test the fluid for temperature if the bottle has been heated. Some facilities serve the formula at room temperature.
2. Pick up the infant and hold it in your arms during feeding. Sit in a comfortable chair.
3. Hold the infant in the crook of your arm, with the infant's head slightly raised (see Figure 30–5).
4. Place a diaper, washcloth, or bib under the infant's chin.
5. Tip the bottle upright until the nipple is filled with fluid.
6. Place the nipple in the infant's mouth. Usually if you stroke the infant's cheek, it will turn toward the nipple and open its mouth.
7. Hold the bottle so that the nipple is filled with fluid during the entire feeding.
8. Allow the infant to feed at its own speed.
9. At regular intervals, remove the nipple from the infant's mouth and burp the infant.
10. Place the infant in one of the following positions for burping. Use both hands for support.
    a. Lift the infant to your shoulder (see Figure 30–6A).
    b. Place the infant in a sitting position in your lap (see Figure 30–6B).
    c. Lay the infant across your lap (see Figure 30–6C).
11. Repeat the feeding and burping sequence until the feeding is completed or the infant is satisfied.

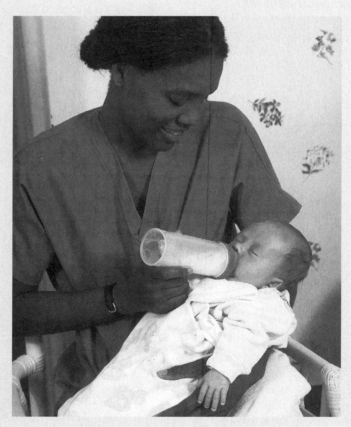

FIGURE 30–5
Hold the infant in the crook of your arm, with the infant's head slightly raised.

Procedure for Bottle-Feeding the Infant (cont.)

12. Clean excess milk from the infant's face and neck.
13. Place the infant in the crib on its back or side. Placing the infant on its abdomen is no longer recommended because the infant could smother.
14. Discard disposable bottles and nipples. In the home, bottles to be reused are washed with a bottle brush in warm, soapy water. Rinse the bottles well and air dry. Although sterilizing bottles is no longer routine, the home care plan will indicate if sterilization is necessary.

Ending Steps

■ Wash your hands.
■ Report and record your observations.

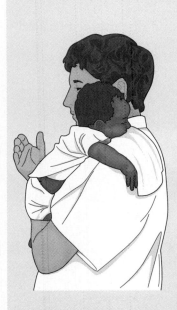
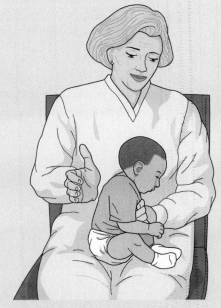
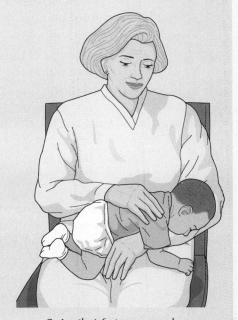

A. Lift the infant to your shoulder.   B. Place the infant in a sitting position in your lap.   C. Lay the infant across your lap.

FIGURE 30–6 Positions for burping the infant.

A sponge bath is usually given until the cord falls off and the circumcision heals. After that, a tub bath may be preferable.

Care of the Toddler

The toddler age includes children between two and three years of age. Some children are weaned and potty-trained before their second birthday, while others continue to take the bottle and wear diapers. Procedures for diapering, bottle-feeding, and bathing toddlers are similar to those of the infant. The major difference is that toddlers are able to get around without help and so are no longer totally dependent on others. However, toddlers who are sick at home or in a health care facility may revert back to infantile behavior. It is important not to scold or make fun of the child. Accept the behavior and continue to offer affection and reassurance.

The toddler needs a consistent, but not rigid, schedule. The child's need for independence often collides with the adult's need for control. Establishing a routine in which such things as mealtime and bedtime usually occur at the same time every day helps to discourage arguments, as does offering choices whenever possible. For example, allowing a 3-year-old to choose which juice he wants to drink with his lunch can work for both you and the toddler. You get him to drink something nutritious and he gets what he wants (see Figure 30–9 on page 412).

Two major issues of the toddler stage are weaning from the bottle and toilet-training. While the toddler is in the health care facility, it is important to continue whatever training has been started at home. This information should be included in the care plan. Remember that decisions on these issues are made by the parents, and you must support them whether you agree or not.

Procedure for Diapering the Infant

Beginning Steps

■ Identify the patient and explain the procedure.
■ Collect necessary equipment and supplies.
■ Wash your hands and use standard precautions.
■ Protect the patient's privacy.
■ Use correct body mechanics.

1. Lower the crib side rail on your working side.
2. Place the waterproof pad under the infant.
3. Put on gloves.
4. Unfasten the dirty diaper. If pins are used, close them and place them out of the infant's reach.
5. Fold the front part of the diaper down between the thighs.
6. Grasp the infant's ankles and lift the buttocks (see Figure 30–7).
7. If the infant has had a bowel movement, use a clean corner of the diaper to remove as much of the stool as possible.
8. Fold the diaper so that urine and feces are inside, and place it out of the infant's reach.
9. Clean the genital area from front to back with a wet washcloth or disposable wipes. Use a mild soap if facility policy permits. Rinse and gently pat dry.
10. Apply cream or lotion, if ordered.
11. Grasp the infant's ankles and lift the buttocks. Place a clean diaper under the buttocks.
12. Bring the loose part of the diaper up between the thighs and over the front. Adjust it for a snug fit.
13. Secure the diaper in place. Disposable diapers have adhesive strips; pins are used for cloth diapers. If you are using pins, place the fingers of one hand under the diaper to prevent sticking the infant with the point of the pin.

14. Remove equipment and supplies from the crib and raise the side rails.
15. Return equipment to its proper place and put soiled linens in the soiled linen hamper.
16. Discard the disposable diaper in the container. Stool should be rinsed from the cloth diaper before placing it in the container. Use standard precautions to avoid contamination of yourself with splashes.
17. Remove your gloves and discard them according to facility policy.

Ending Steps

■ Wash your hands.
■ Report and record your observations.

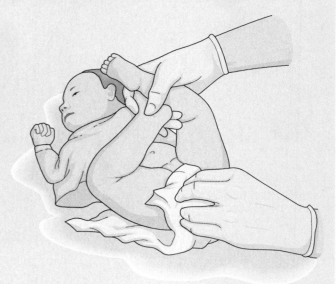

FIGURE 32–7
Grasp the ankles and lift the buttocks to remove or place a diaper under the infant.

Guidelines for Cord Care

■ Keep the cord stump clean and dry.
■ Place the diaper below the cord stump.
■ If alcohol is ordered to promote drying, apply the alcohol with a cotton ball to the base of the stump.
■ Avoid pulling on the stump. It will fall off by itself.
■ Report redness, bleeding, drainage, or odor to the nurse.
■ Give the infant sponge baths until after the cord falls off.

Hospitalization and separation from parents and family is very difficult for toddlers. They may fear that their parents have abandoned them and will never return. Most facilities encourage parents to stay with their child during hospitalization. Family visits and participation in the toddler's care helps to relieve anxiety. You can help by holding and rocking the children. Offer your love and affection and reassure them that their family will be back soon.

Procedure for Giving an Infant a Sponge Bath

Beginning Steps

- Identify the patient and explain the procedure.
- Collect necessary equipment and supplies.
- Wash your hands and use standard precautions.
- Protect the patient's privacy.
- Use correct body mechanics.

1. Fill the bath basin with warm water, between 100° F and 105° F. Check the temperature with a bath thermometer or the inside of your wrist.

2. Put on gloves (and a gown if required).

3. Moisten a cotton ball or gauze in the warm water and clean one of the baby's eyes, wiping from the inner aspect (next to the nose) to the outer aspect. Discard that cotton ball. Repeat this step for the other eye, using a clean cotton ball (see Figure 30-8).

4. Moisten a cotton ball and clean the outer nostril. Discard the cotton ball. Repeat this step for the other side of the nose, using a clean cotton ball.

5. Wet the washcloth and wash the infant's face with warm water. Do not use soap.

6. Pat the face dry with the towel.

7. Wash the scalp by making a soapy lather with your hands.

8. Pick up the infant and hold it over the bath basin. Use one arm and hand to support the infant.

9. Rinse the soap off the scalp with a wet washcloth and dry gently with a towel.

10. Wash the neck and ears, paying special attention to skin folds on the neck and behind the ears.

11. Rinse thoroughly to remove all the soap and pat dry.

12. Lay the infant back on the bath table. Remove the diaper and other clothing and cover the infant with a towel.

13. Moisten a cotton ball and cleanse the diaper area. Wash from front to back using a separate cotton ball for each stroke.

14. Using a wet soapy washcloth, wash the entire front of the infant's body, or you may apply soap to your hands and wash the infant with your hands. Pay special attention to skin creases and folds, and do not get the cord wet.

15. Rinse and dry thoroughly.

16. Turn the infant over and wash the entire back of the body.

17. Rinse and dry thoroughly.

18. Give cord care and clean the circumcision according to facility policy.

19. Apply lotion or oil if ordered.

20. Diaper the infant. Remove and discard your gloves.

21. Dress the infant, comb the hair, and wrap it in a small blanket.

22. Place the infant in the crib and raise the side rails.

Ending Steps

- Wash your hands.
- Report and record your observations.

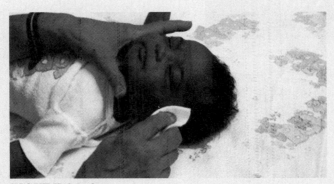

FIGURE 30–8
Clean away from the inner aspect of the baby's eye.

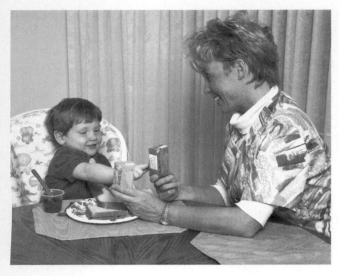

FIGURE 30–9
Allowing the toddler to make decisions helps build independence.

Safety Concerns

One of your major responsibilities when you are caring for toddlers is to protect their safety. Accidents are one of the leading causes of death among small children. Because they are mobile, toddlers are able to get into many unsafe situations. Their desire to touch, taste, and smell everything can create problems. Keep in mind the curiosity of toddlers, and be aware of hazards that may exist. This danger is especially true at home where electrical cords, kitchen stoves, and swimming pools beckon them. Toddlers can move quickly, so watch them carefully at all times. It is also important that you know how to respond if an emergency occurs, such as choking or bleeding. It will be helpful to review the emergency procedures that are explained in Chapter 7.

Guidelines for Care of the Toddler

- Protect the child's safety.
- Allow choices and promote independence.
- Offer love, affection, and reassurance.
- Observe, record, and report physical and psychosocial changes.
- Measure, record, and report weight, height, and vital signs.
- Assist with routine care, such as feeding, bathing, and dressing.
- Assist with examinations and treatments.
- Assist with weaning and toilet training.

Developmental Task of Toddlers

The developmental task for toddlers is to gain independence, and care must be given with that thought in mind. Encourage them to do as much as possible for themselves. Select clothing that is easy to put on and remove. Pants and shorts with an elastic waist are better than those with zippers, buttons, or suspenders. Finger foods and special utensils make it easier for toddlers to learn to feed themselves.

Communication

Use simple words and short sentences when communicating with toddlers. Their attention span is short, and if your message is lengthy, they may lose interest before you finish. However, do not hesitate to explain what you are doing and what you expect from the child. Make eye contact with the toddler, just as you would with an adult. This may involve getting down to the child's level or bringing the child up to your level. Keep your voice tones warm, soft, and friendly. Make sure your verbal and nonverbal communications agree. If they do not, the child will be more likely to believe the nonverbal message.

Nutrition

Toddlers need fewer calories than infants because growth has slowed. However, the toddler should be eating more solid food in order to get all the necessary nutrients. Appetite may vary from day to day, and most toddlers are learning to feed themselves. Special equipment such as scoop plates and two-handled cups make it easier for them to eat independently. Food may need to be chopped or cut in small pieces for easier chewing and swallowing. Small portions of food, attractively served, are less likely to overwhelm toddlers. Dishes should be of plastic or some other unbreakable material, because toddlers may drop or even throw dishes on the floor. Never leave a child unattended in a high chair or while eating.

*C*are of the Preschool-Age Child

The preschool age includes children between the ages of 3 and 6. Normal, healthy 6-year-olds can run, jump, and climb with ease. They can carry on conversations and express their needs verbally.

Safety

During the preschool years children begin assuming some responsibility for their own safety. However, they still need supervision to protect them from danger. Because preschool children spend more time away from home, they must be made aware of the risks they might encounter. It is important that they learn about traffic and crossing streets safely. Preschoolers should know their own name, address, and telephone number. They should be taught not to talk to strangers and what to do in an emergency.

Developmental Tasks

Because the major developmental task of preschool children is to develop initiative, preschool children need to be allowed to do as much as possible for themselves. Sometimes in our sympathy for sick children, we want to do everything for them. You can remind or assist them without taking over. Praise and encouragement for their efforts help build confidence, which leads to initiative.

Provide opportunities for play because play allows the preschool child to practice new skills, strengthen coordination, and expend energy. Children tend to act out their feelings during play. You may learn how the preschool patient feels about illness by observing him or her at play. (See Figure 30–10.)

Communication

Communication skills dramatically increase during the preschool years. Preschoolers learn by questioning, watching, and imitating others. Questions should be answered simply and honestly. Lengthy explanations may cause confusion and are usually not necessary.

The preschool children's response to illness includes many fears. They usually fear pain and mutilation (destroying or crippling part of the body) rather than death. Children of this age may be frightened of you and other health care workers who are in uniform. They may believe that you are a bad person who has come to hurt them. It is important to explain procedures to them in language they can understand. Be honest and do not tell them something will not hurt unless that is true. If the children lose trust in you, the fear may only become worse.

Personal Care

The preschool child does not require the amount of physical care of the infant or the toddler. The 3-year-old will need assistance with bathing, oral care, and grooming. However, by the age of 6 most children are able to do much of their own personal care. Personal care routines are similar to those of adults and include a daily bath and weekly shampoo. Often the first trip to the dentist is made during these years, and the child is taught to brush the teeth on a regular basis. Your responsibilities focus on supervising and assisting, rather than doing everything for the child.

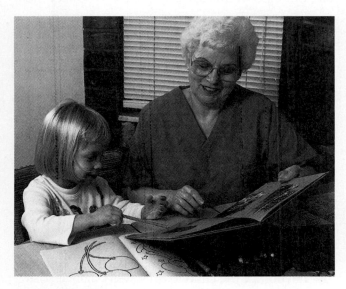

FIGURE 30–10
Provide opportunities for the preschool child to play.

Guidelines for Care of the Preschool Child

- Protect the child's safety.
- Allow the child to do as much as possible for himself or herself.
- Offer praise and encouragement to build confidence.
- Provide opportunities for play.
- Answer questions honestly and simply.
- Explain procedures before you begin.
- Supervise and assist the child in personal care activities.
- Encourage family visits and participation.
- Provide a well-balanced diet, which includes foods the child prefers.
- Provide warmth and affection.
- Observe, record, and report your observations promptly.

Nutrition

Preschool children need to eat a well-balanced diet. By this age, most children can feed themselves and have developed definite likes and dislikes. Adjusting to hospital food may be very difficult, especially if a restricted diet is ordered. The hospital diet should include as many of the child's favorite foods as possible. The preschool child's appetite varies under normal circumstances, and illness may make it worse. Mealtime should be pleasant and enjoyable, so avoid scolding and coaxing. Building rapport (a trusting relationship) may help because children of this age are usually anxious to please people they like. Let the nurse know if the child does not seem to like the food or is not eating well.

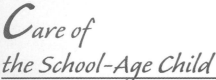

Care of the School-Age Child

The school-age group includes children between the ages of 6 and 12. Because of the six-year age range, a lot of variation occurs. School-age children have a better understanding of illness and are more able to cooperate in their treatment. These children need love and affection as much as younger children, so continue to offer it. They may be missing their parents and other family members, so encourage family visits and participation.

Safety

This age group continues to be at risk for accidents. In their efforts to please friends and classmates, they may place themselves in dangerous situations. Because American children are maturing earlier, it is important to begin sex education during these years. School-age children need to be informed of the danger of using alcohol or drugs. Although parents are responsible for teaching their children about these subjects, be prepared to answer questions as honestly as possible.

Developmental Tasks

The major developmental task of school-age children is to gain competency by learning to perform tasks correctly. Illness can interfere with the school-age child's ability to develop competency. If physical, emotional, and social limitations are present, the child must learn to adapt to those limitations. As a nursing assistant, you can help the child to function as normally as possible. (See Figure 30–11.)

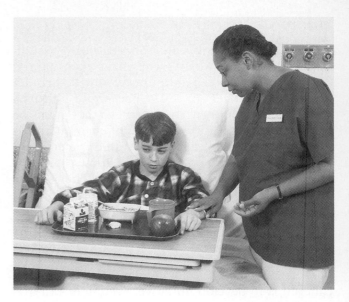

FIGURE 30–11
Help the school-age child to function as normally as possible.

Part of the care plan will involve the continuation of educational studies at home or in the health care facility. The local school will usually provide the necessary materials, equipment, and personnel. Provide play opportunities that are appropriate to the child's needs. Vary activities so that some activities are with other children and others require individual effort.

Activities of Daily Living

Healthy school-age children are usually able to do their own personal care and other activities of daily living. However, the child who is sick will need your assistance. Encourage self-care as much as possible. Children of this age group tend to be very mod-

Guidelines for Care of the School-Age Child

- Protect the child's safety.
- Provide play activities appropriate to the child's age.
- Offer love, affection, and reassurance.
- Assist with homebound educational needs.
- Encourage self-care as much as possible.
- Protect the child's modesty.
- Assist with activities of daily living when necessary.
- Encourage family visits and participation.
- Encourage the child to eat a well-balanced diet.
- Observe, record, and report your observations.

est, so protect privacy at all times. A well-balanced diet is necessary for health and development. Vary the diet because school-age children are usually more willing to try new foods.

Care of the Teenager

The teenage group includes children between the ages of 13 and 18. This time period is also called adolescence. The many physical and psychosocial changes that take place during these years make it difficult for the teenager to adjust. Both girls and boys reach full sexual maturity during this time.

Teenagers are concerned about body image and personal appearance. Their chief concern about an injury or illness may be its effect on the way they look. They may avoid their friends and family because they are embarrassed about wounds, scars, injuries, and tubes. Privacy of body, belongings, and information must be maintained and protected.

Developmental Tasks

The major developmental task of adolescence is to gain self-identity. Teenagers fear the loss of independence when they are patients in a health care facility and may resist treatment. They may also have a problem with authority figures and dislike being told what to do. One way to handle their resistance is to include them in the development of the care plan and encourage them in the decision-making process. This involvement helps to give them back the control that they feel they are losing. Separation from friends may cause anxiety and uncertainty. The availability of a telephone is important, because it allows the patient to keep in touch with peers. (See Figure 30–12.)

Basic Needs

Healthy teenagers are usually able to meet their own personal needs, but when they are sick, your assistance may be needed. Encourage independence and assist only as necessary. Frequent praise and encouragement help to relieve some of the uncertainty that teenagers frequently experience.

Teenagers need to eat a well-balanced diet that is high in calories to meet the tremendous growth during these years. They are often concerned about the effects of food on their body image. Girls may worry about their weight and go on fad diets. Both boys and girls may develop poor eating habits by skipping meals and munching on snacks. Exercise is as important as diet because it helps to build muscle tone and firm the body.

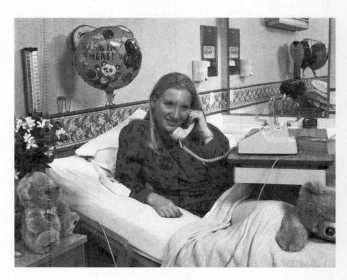

FIGURE 30–12
The hospitalized teenager can keep in touch with friends by telephone.

Many teenagers meet the need for exercise through athletic activities.

Drug and Alcohol Abuse

In the health care facility, you may care for children who have drug or alcohol problems. One of your responsibilities is to observe and report signs and symptoms of substance abuse. Encourage patients to express their feelings and concerns. Listen objectively and try to be supportive and nonjudgmental. Let the nurse know if the teenager wants to discuss the problem or seek help. Signs and symptoms of drug or alcohol abuse are included in the following list. Notify the nurse if you observe any of these signs and symptoms:

- A change in personality
- Watery eyes or a change in pupil size
- Needle marks on the skin, especially on the inner arm
- Drowsiness and a short attention span
- Loss of interest in school and surroundings
- Slurred speech
- Staggering gait
- Restless, combative, or violent behavior
- Poor appetite, nausea, and stomach pain
- Confusion, hallucinations, and paranoia
- Dizziness or loss of consciousness

Teenagers are difficult patients, but despite their prickly personalities, they can be loving and appreciative. Teenagers respect honesty even when it hurts, so do not hesitate to give them the facts. Remember, however, that you can supply the information, but they are the ones who must make decisions that can affect their futures dramatically.

Review

Read each question and fill in the blank with the vocabulary term that best completes the sentence.

1. Care of the pregnant woman before, during, and after childbirth is called _____.
2. _____ is the period following delivery of the baby.
3. The correct medical term for the navel or belly button is the _____.
4. The _____ is the developing unborn child, from the eighth week of pregnancy to birth.
5. The surgical removal of the foreskin from the penis is called _____.

Remember

1. Today, childbirth is viewed as a normal, natural process, not as an illness.
2. During postpartum, the new mother must be closely observed for signs and symptoms of hemorrhage or infection.
3. The neonate is totally dependent on others for survival.
4. Always check the infant's identification bracelet with that of the mother.
5. When a child is sick, the whole family is affected.
6. Talk to children at their level and in a language they can understand.
7. Never leave an infant with a bottle propped in its mouth.
8. The infant's diaper should be changed frequently to avoid irritation of delicate skin.
9. Never leave the infant unattended on the bath table or in the tub.
10. Toddlers need reassurance that their parents will return and have not abandoned them.
11. Play helps the preschool child practice new skills and strengthen coordination.
12. You may need to assist the school-age patient with educational studies.
13. Include the teenage patient in care planning and decision making.
14. One of your responsibilities is to observe and report signs and symptoms of substance abuse.

Reflect

Read the following case study and answer the questions.

Case Study

Molly Price gave birth to her first child, a son named Lester, two days ago. Molly, who is 17, lives on a small farm with her 19-year-old husband. They have no family nearby. Molly entered the health care system when the birth of her child was imminent. She had no prenatal care and knew nothing about caring for babies. Lester is a normal, healthy baby and Molly is nursing him. Although she has plenty of breast milk, Lester is not nursing well. Molly is anxious about caring for his umbilical cord and his circumcision. As a home health aide you are part of a team assigned to the Price family.

1. How can you assist Molly with the breast-feeding routine?
2. List four guidelines for cord care.
3. What observations should you remind Molly to make when caring for the baby's circumcision?
4. How can you help Molly bond with her new baby?

Respond

Choose the best answer for each question.

1. The branch of medicine that is concerned with the care of infants and children is
   A. Psychiatry
   B. Pediatrics
   C. Gynecology
   D. Geriatrics

2. The development of a close, loving relationship between a mother and baby is called
   A. Mentoring
   B. Maturing
   C. Bonding
   D. Immobilizing

' 3. Which of the following are signs of hemorrhage?
   A. A drop in blood pressure
   B. A rise in pulse rate
   C. Pale, cold skin
   D. All of the above

4. Which of the following is NOT a measure used to encourage urination?
   A. Pour cold water over the perineum.
   B. Turn on a faucet.
   C. Place the patient's fingers in warm water.
   D. Give the patient a glass of water to drink.

5. The medical term for a newborn in the first six weeks of life is
   A. Fetus
   B. Umbilicus
   C. Neonate
   D. Toddler

6. Which of the following is NOT a guideline for infant safety?
   A. Raise the crib rails when you leave the baby in the bed.
   B. Support the baby's neck and head when carrying it.
   C. Use both hands to lift the baby.
   D. Shift the baby to the other arm while talking on the telephone.

7. What is the major developmental task of toddlers?
   A. Gain independence
   B. Develop initiative
   C. Develop trust
   D. Gain self-identity

8. Which of the following statements about play is TRUE?
   A. Play serves no useful purpose.
   B. Preschoolers are too young to learn by playing.
   C. Play strengthens coordination.
   D. All of the above.

9. A 10-year-old patient is concerned that her illness will cause her to fail in school. What is your best response?
   A. "School is the least of your worries right now."
   B. "Oh, I'm sure you'll do fine."
   C. "Failing school isn't the end of the world."
   D. "Your school will help you keep up."

10. A teenage patient tells you that he has been using marijuana after school. What should you do?
   A. Call the police. Marijuana is illegal.
   B. Report the information to the nurse.
   C. Keep still. It's none of your business.
   D. Report the information to his parents.

Chapter Thirty-One

Subacute Care

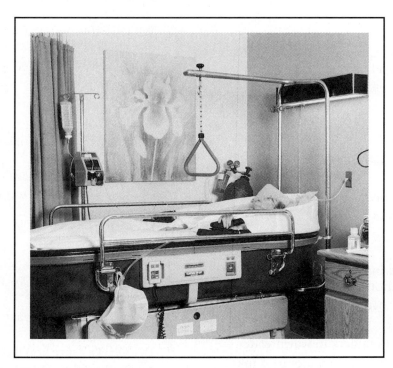

Nellcor Puritan Bennett

OBJECTIVES

After studying this chapter, you will be able to

1. Describe the four types of subacute care units.

2. List six guidelines for care of the ventilator patient.

3. Identify three guidelines for care of the patient with a tracheostomy.

4. List four guidelines for care of the patient with an infusion therapy pump.

5. Identify four guidelines for care of the patient with an enteral nutrition pump.

6. List three guidelines for care of the patient with a gastrointestinal suction pump.

7. List four guidelines for care of the dialysis patient.

dialysis Artificial filtration of waste products from the blood.

intubation The insertion of a tube into the trachea to provide a pathway for air to enter the lungs.

mechanical ventilator A machine that provides artificial respiration of the lungs.

shunt A connection created between two blood vessels.

tracheostomy A surgical opening into the windpipe to promote unobstructed breathing.

Subacute care is medical and nursing care provided to patients who require a lower level of care than that provided in acute care hospitals. These patients often have complex, long-term problems. Many require rehabilitation or special equipment such as ventilators and pumps.

This chapter identifies the types of patients who may be cared for in a subacute care unit and the qualities necessary to work in this area. It describes the care of the patient with specific, complex, physical needs.

The Development of Subacute Care

Subacute care was developed as a result of efforts to reduce the high cost of medical care. Until recently, patients who required long periods of hospitalization remained in acute care hospitals. For example, some ventilator patients were cared for indefinitely in expensive hospital rooms. Now these patients are moved from acute care hospitals into more cost-effective subacute facilities.

A subacute care unit may be located in a long-term care facility, a hospital, or an independent facility.

There are basically four types of subacute care units:

- **Traditional subacute:** Provides respiratory care, rehabilitation, and nutritional assistance 24 hours a day
- **General medical–surgical subacute:** Provides care for patients who require medical care at least once a week, and who also need rehabilitation and nursing services
- **Chronic subacute:** Provides care for patients who are chronically ill and have little hope of recovery
- **Long-term transitional subacute:** Provides care for patients who are ventilator patients or have long-term complex medical problems

In subacute care, patients may need a variety of complicated machines and equipment. Many times the patient's life is dependent on the correct operation of a machine such as a ventilator. One of the most common complaints of patients in these situations is that caregivers are more interested in the machinery than they are in the patient. It is important that you do not become so machine oriented that you lose sight of the patient.

Personal Qualities Necessary for Subacute Care

Staff members in subacute care units must have excellent technical skills. They must be able to perform procedures correctly and quickly. People skills—the ability to communicate, build rapport, and empathize—are equally important. If you work in subacute care, you will need all these skills plus those of observing, reporting, and recording.

There is an important role for nursing assistants in subacute care. These patients will need assistance with personal care, moving and transferring, and other activities of daily living (ADLs). Subacute care provides an opportunity for you to learn about complex technical skills.

Care of the Patient on a Mechanical Ventilator

A *mechanical ventilator* is a machine that provides the patient with artificial respirations. It assists in the circulation and exchange of gases in the lungs. In the alveoli of the lungs, oxygen is exchanged for carbon dioxide, a gas that is the waste product of respiration (see Figure 31–1). In order to remain healthy, a person must move enough gasses into and out of the alveoli to maintain metabolism. When this movement does not occur naturally, mechanical ventilation is necessary. It will be helpful to review the respiratory system as explained in Chapter 10.

Ventilators come in various sizes, shapes, and designs and do not all operate in the same way. Most are equipped with many controls, dials, measurements, and alarms that allow for adjustment to meet individual patient needs. An example of a ventilator is shown in Figure 31–2.

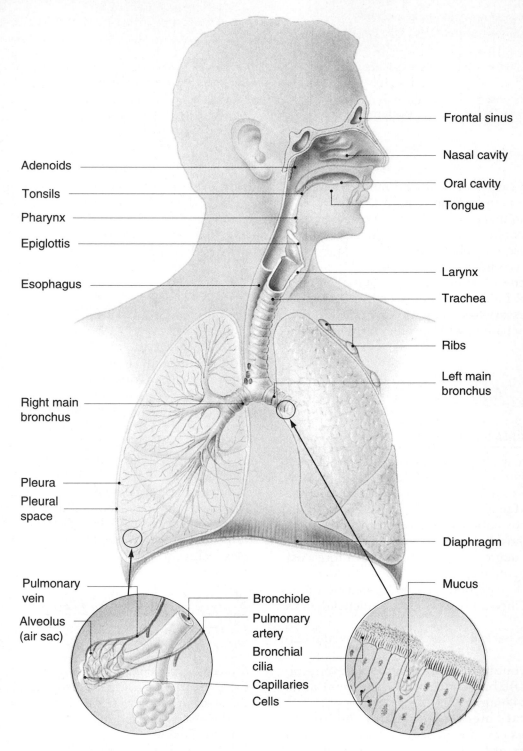

FIGURE 31–1
Oxygen and carbon dioxide are exchanged in the alveoli of the lungs.

Intubation

Mechanical ventilation requires *intubation* (the insertion of a tube into the trachea). The tube may be inserted through the nose or mouth into the trachea or directly into the trachea through an incision in the neck called a *tracheostomy* (a surgical opening into the windpipe). The intubation tube is called an endotracheal tube, or in the case of a tracheostomy, a tracheostomy tube.

Meeting the Patients' Needs

Most patients who are on mechanical ventilation are totally dependent on others to meet their needs. Movement is restricted because the tubes

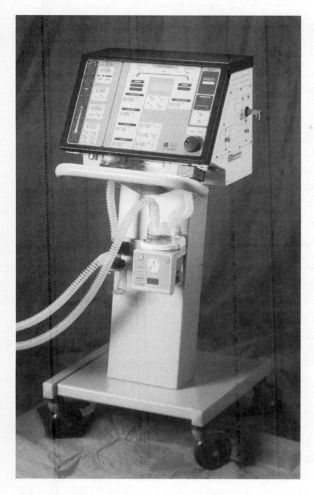

FIGURE 31–2 The 740 ventilator system.
Nellcor Puritan Bennett

attaching the patient to the ventilator can become twisted or disconnected. Ventilator patients cannot speak while attached to the ventilator and must depend on nonverbal communication unless they are able to write. Some ventilator patients are comatose. Personnel who work with ventilator patients need special training in order to monitor the complex, sophisticated equipment and to provide safe care.

Psychological Needs

Ventilator patients who are conscious are usually anxious and frightened. Their very existence depends on a slim tube connected to an electrical machine. Their total dependency on others can create feelings of hopelessness and despair or frustration and anger. Their difficulty in trying to communicate can be overwhelming.

Psychological support is necessary in any disease, but in respiratory care it is even more essential. Emotional stress has a direct effect on the respiratory and cardiovascular systems. One of

your most important responsibilities will be to help the ventilator patient meet psychological needs.

Provide an environment that is as calm and quiet as possible. This is not easy because the equipment itself may be noisy and the activity around the patient may be confusing. Move quietly yourself and avoid unnecessary noise. Discussions with other members of the health care team should take place away from the patient's bedside. Even comatose patients seem to react to a noisy atmosphere.

Reassurance is important to ventilator patients. You cannot promise that patients will get better, but you can assure them that someone will be available to help meet their needs. You can assist the patient to communicate. If the patient is able to write, keep a pencil and notepad within reach. A communication board, in which the patient signals yes or no to a picture on the board may be helpful. One of the best ways to reassure patients is by performing your duties confidently and competently. (See Figure 31–3.)

The ventilator panel should be turned away from the patient, if possible. The alert patient will watch the dials and measurements and may become unnecessarily alarmed. Never make statements in front of the patient that might indicate something is wrong. A simple statement, such as "I don't think this machine is working right," could cause the patient or the family to panic.

Place the call signal within reach, even if the patient is comatose. Fasten it in place, if necessary, to keep it from being mislaid. Answer call signals im-

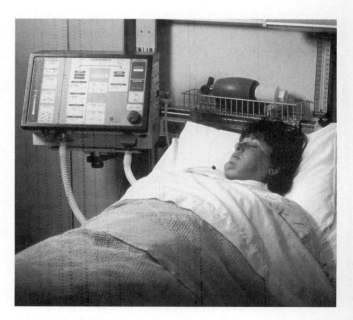

FIGURE 31–3
Ventilator patients need support and reassurance.
Nellcor Puritan Bennett

mediately, no matter how often they are used. Patients who are constantly using the call signal for no apparent reason are usually afraid. The quicker you respond to the signal, the sooner they will feel safer and more secure. Your prompt answer to their calls for help is a form of reassurance.

Physical Needs

Most of the time you will work with a nurse when you are providing physical care for the ventilator patient. Even routine tasks such as bathing or bedmaking become complex when the patient is on a ventilator. Two people are needed for procedures that require moving the patient. One person does the actual moving, while the other person protects tubes and wires and monitors the equipment. Nursing assistants are not allowed to adjust the ventilator dials or controls.

Procedures should be planned and coordinated as much as possible to allow the patient to have periods of uninterrupted rest. Bathing, bedmaking, turning, physical therapy, medication, and other treatments should be done within specific blocks of time; otherwise, the patient will soon be exhausted.

Physical care not only increases patient comfort, but it also provides psychological support. Gentle handling and touching of the patient shows affection and caring. A refreshing bath and clean bed linen help produce relaxation and relieve stress.

Turning and Positioning

Turn and reposition the patient at least every two hours to prevent complications. Care must be taken not to pull, twist, or disconnect tubing. Make sure the tubes are functioning and that the patient is not lying on them. If the ventilator must be moved in order to reach the patient, be careful that tubing and other attachments do not become kinked, damaged, or disconnected. Closely observe the pressure gauge on the ventilator. A sudden drop in pressure indicates a leak or a disconnected tube. Notify the nurse immediately if this should occur.

Vital Signs

The vital signs of ventilator patients are measured on a regular basis, and you may be asked to perform this task. However, most patients are connected to a machine that measures the vital signs and prints the readings on a screen. This machine provides measurements quickly and accurately without disturbing the patient.

Operating and Monitoring the Ventilator

Monitoring and adjusting the mechanical ventilator is not a nursing assistant responsibility. However, after you have worked with a particular machine for a while, you may have a fairly clear idea of how it works. Pay attention to dials and gauges, and observe them for changes as you provide care. Notify the nurse immediately if an alarm sounds or if you think something is wrong. Do not attempt to adjust the machine yourself.

Weaning the Patient

Some patients are able to be removed from the ventilator permanently or for a time. This removal is not done suddenly but is a gradual process. "Weaning" the patient usually begins with removing the patient from the ventilator for 5 to 10 minutes every hour. If that period is tolerated, the patient is removed for longer periods until he or she is "weaned" and is no longer dependent on the ventilator.

As a nursing assistant, you must **never** remove a patient from a ventilator. However, you may be asked to sit with patients while they are off the machine. This is a difficult time for patients, and they will need your support and reassurance. You may be asked to measure patients' vital signs during this period. Reassure patients that they will be returned to the ventilator immediately if they request it.

Care of the Patient with a Tracheostomy

A tracheostomy is performed to establish an artificial airway when the natural airway is damaged or is not adequate. A surgical incision is made through the neck into the trachea and a tube is inserted. The patient breathes through the tube rather than through the nose or mouth. The tracheostomy may be temporary or permanent. (See Figure 31–4.)

As you have already learned, intubation is necessary when the patient is on a ventilator. Intubation through the mouth or nose is very uncomfortable. The patient cannot eat, drink, or talk and may feel smothered. This type of intubation is done in an emergency situation and for short-term conditions, such as during surgery. If the patient is going to require long-term ventilator care, a tracheostomy may be the better choice.

When used with a ventilator, the outer end of the tube is fitted with an adaptor for attachment to the ventilator tubing. The end of the tube closest to

Guidelines for Care of the Ventilator Patient

- Remember that you are caring for a patient, not a machine.
- Offer your support and reassurance.
- Assist the patient with communication needs.
- Place the call signal within the patient's reach and answer it promptly.
- Get help before moving the patient.
- Ask the nurse to check the patient after you have completed a task.
- Coordinate procedures to allow the patient periods of uninterrupted rest.
- Handle the patient gently.
- Turn and reposition the patient at least every two hours.
- Provide frequent oral care.
- Take care not to pull, twist, or disconnect tubing.
- Move the ventilator machine carefully and observe the gauge for changes.
- Measure, record, and report vital signs accurately.
- Notify the nurse immediately if an alarm sounds, the pressure gauge drops, or you observe anything unusual.

the patient's neck usually has an inflatable cuff. The cuff is inflated inside the trachea to prevent oxygen from leaking out around the tube and into the mouth or nose. An inflated cuff assures that gases, forced by the machine, are delivered to the lungs.

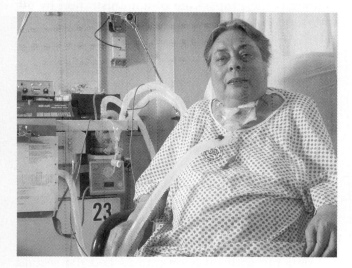

FIGURE 31–4
A tracheostomy provides an artificial airway.

The tube fits into the tracheostomy stoma and is secured by tapes, ties, or Velcro fasteners. The outer edge or flange of the tube has a hole on each side where a tie or tape may be inserted. The ends of the ties are secured at the back of the neck. A tracheostomy that is not attached to a ventilator does not usually have an internal cuff.

Tracheostomy patients whose cuffs are not inflated may be able to speak by covering the outer opening of the tube with a finger. Speech therapists work with patients who have permanent tracheostomies to teach them how to talk with the tube open. This process requires dedication and practice, and patients will usually welcome your support and encouragement.

In most areas, nursing assistants are not allowed to perform tracheostomy care. It involves sterile technique, which is not routinely included in nursing assistant training. However, you may be providing care for tracheostomy patients, so it is helpful to have some idea of what is involved. The tracheostomy stoma (mouth of the surgical opening) may be covered by a loose, nonstick dressing. A "Y" split is cut in the dressing so that it can be slipped under the edge of the tube. The new tracheostomy wound and the skin around it are cleaned and the dressing is changed several times a day, as needed. The tape or ties may also need to be changed if they become wet or soiled. Avoid wetting the dressing while assisting the patient with bathing and personal care. Never cover the opening or allow water to enter the tracheostomy or the patient may suffocate.

If the tube has an inner cannula (a tube inside a tube), it must be removed and cleaned once each shift or more frequently if needed. This procedure is done by a nurse or respiratory therapist, because it requires disconnecting the patient from the ventilator. A spare tracheostomy tube is kept at the bedside in case the tube needs to be replaced suddenly.

Suctioning the Airway

Artificial airways interfere with the patient's ability to cough and clear the airway of mucus. Secretions accumulate and can interfere with ventilation. Mechanical suction may be necessary to remove secretions and clear the airway. There are also situations in which the natural airway will need to be suctioned.

When the nurse suctions a patient on a ventilator, a small-diameter catheter is inserted into the tracheostomy tube, using sterile technique. (To suction patients who are not intubated, a catheter is inserted through the nose.) The catheter is attached to tubing that is connected to a collection

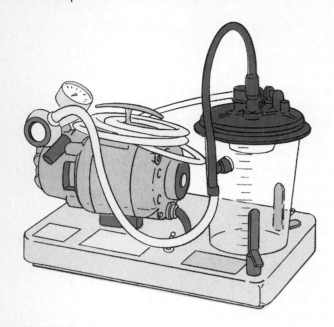

FIGURE 31–5
Mechanical suction may be necessary to remove secretions and clear the airway.

bottle. Tubing from the collection bottle is connected to a portable suction pump or to a wall suction outlet (see Figure 31–5). It may be your responsibility to empty, measure, and record the contents of the collection bottle. Wear gloves and follow standard precautions when performing this procedure.

In most areas, nursing assistants are not allowed to suction patients. However, you are re-

Guidelines for Care of the Patient with a Tracheostomy

- Support and encourage the patient who is learning to speak with a tracheostomy.
- Make sure that the tracheostomy tapes or ties are securely fastened.
- Avoid wetting the tracheostomy dressing while providing care.
- Check to see that a spare tracheostomy tube is available.
- Report unusual observations to the nurse promptly.
- Notify the nurse if the patient appears to need suctioning.
- Reassure the patient and family members.
- Follow standard precautions and wear gloves and mask when assisting with tracheostomy care or suctioning.

sponsible for observing the patient and the equipment and letting the nurse know if a problem occurs. Indications that suctioning may be required include bubbling or rattling respirations, shortness of breath, or any other form of dyspnea (difficult breathing).

Always wear gloves when assisting the nurse with tracheostomy care or suctioning. Sometimes more protective clothing, such as a gown, mask, or goggles, will be necessary. Dispose of contaminated materials according to facility policy. Follow standard precautions and wash your hands before and after the procedure.

Care of the Patient with a Pump

A patient may be connected to a pump for infusion therapy (injection or infusion of fluids or medications directly into a vein), for enteral nutrition (delivery of nutrients directly into the digestive system), or for gastrointestinal suctioning.

Infusion or Intravenous Therapy

Infusion or intravenous (IV) therapy may be necessary to replace body fluids, to administer medications, or to deliver nutrition directly into the bloodstream. A needle or special catheter is inserted into a peripheral (surface) vein or into a central vein closer to the heart. Tubing connects the needle or catheter to a container of fluid. When a pump is used, the tubing between the needle or catheter and the container is threaded through the pump. The pump is an electronic device that regulates and maintains the proper rate of administration by exerting pressure on the fluid or on the tubing. The rate of administration is calculated and the pump preset by the nurse.

The pump is usually lightweight and hangs on an IV pole (see Figure 31–6). It is equipped with an alarm that sounds when something is wrong. Most pumps have back-up batteries in case of power failure. There are also portable battery-operated pumps that are small enough to fit in the palm of the hand. This type of pump is used for patients who require minimal care. It allows for maximum mobility and is often used in home care. You will often care for a patient who has an IV. Two sets of guidelines are included here to assist you. The first concerns providing nursing care for patients with infusion pumps and the second focuses on how to change the clothes of a patient with an IV.

Guidelines for Care of the Patient with an Infusion Therapy Pump

- Follow universal precautions and wear gloves if contact with body fluids is likely.
- Protect the site of infusion and keep the dressing dry.
- Observe for complications.
- Handle IV tubing carefully without putting pressure on it.
- Keep the solution container above the site of insertion.
- Handle the pump carefully and avoid dropping or jarring it.
- Call the nurse if the dressing at the insertion site becomes wet.
- If an alarm sounds, check the tubing to see that it is not kinked or under the patient's body. If the alarm continues to sound, call the nurse.

Guidelines for Changing the Clothes of a Patient with an IV

- Remove clothing first from the unaffected arm (the arm without the IV).
- Carefully slide the sleeve down over the arm, over the site of the IV, and then off the arm.
- Remove the IV bag or bottle from the pole and slide it down the sleeve.
- Do not lower the bag below the IV site.
- Return the bag to the pole.
- Place clothing first on the affected arm (the arm with the IV).
- Remove the bag from the pole and slip it through the sleeve as if it were part of the patient's hand.
- Slide the sleeve over the tubing, hand, arm, and IV site, and onto the shoulder.
- Ask the nurse to check the IV as soon as you have finished dressing the patient.

The nurse is responsible for starting and stopping the IV, for hanging IV fluids, for changing the IV site dressing, and for setting, operating, and adjusting the pump. Nursing assistants do not do any of these procedures. Never disconnect the solution from the pump or turn off the pump alarm.

Enteral Nutrition

Patients may receive enteral nutrition because they have difficulty swallowing, are unable to eat, or cannot meet nutritional needs orally. Either a nasogastric (NG) tube is inserted through the patient's nose into the stomach, or a gastrostomy (G) tube is inserted through a surgical incision in the abdominal wall into the stomach. NG tubes are generally used for short-term therapy, and G tubes are used when the patient is to be tube-fed for a long time. (See Figure 31–7.)

The feeding tube is connected to a container of commercially prepared formula that is ordered by the doctor. The tubing is threaded through the pump, which is set to deliver a certain amount of feeding over a specific period of time. Unlike the infusion therapy pump, which runs continuously, some feeding pumps are turned off and the patient is disconnected from the pump when the feeding is complete. Others feed the patient small amounts continuously. The pump has an alarm that sounds if the feeding tube becomes plugged. Check the tubing for kinks if the alarm sounds, and notify the nurse if the alarm continues. The administration of the feeding and operation of the pump is usually the responsibility of the nurse. The following guidelines will help you to carry out your responsibilities.

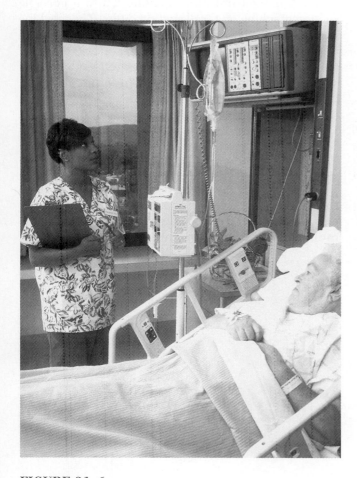

FIGURE 31–6
The infusion pump maintains the rate of administration by exerting pressure on the fluid or the tubing.

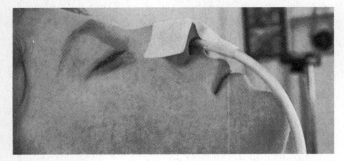

A. A nasogastric tube may be attached to a feeding pump for enteral nutrition.

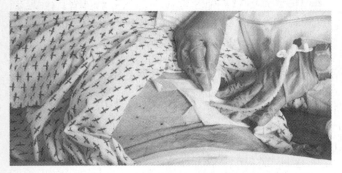

B. A G tube may be attached to a feeding pump for enteral nutrition.

FIGURE 31–7 Enteral nutrition pumps.

In home health you may have additional duties. You may be asked to shop for the feeding, store it, and prepare it for the patient's use. In some areas you may also be allowed to hang the feedings. It is your responsibility to know the policy where you work. Care of the patient receiving tube feedings is also discussed in Chapter 22.

Guidelines for Care of the Patient with an Enteral Nutrition Pump

- Position the patient in a Fowler's or semi-Fowler's position during the feeding and for at least 30 minutes after the feeding.
- Change the tape and give skin care daily if the NG tube is taped to the nose.
- Check the nose for irritation and report any redness, rash, or bleeding to the nurse.
- Provide frequent oral and nasal care.
- Keep the skin around the G tube site clean and dry.
- Report redness, leakage, or drainage around the G tube.
- Report to the nurse if the patient complains of nausea or fullness.
- Report episodes of diarrhea, including the time, amount, and consistency of stool.
- If the feeding pump alarm sounds, check the tube for kinks, straighten the tubing, and if it continues to sound, notify the nurse.

Guidelines for Care of a Patient with a Gastrointestinal Suction Pump

- Check for leaks in the tubing or the system.
- Keep collection containers below the level of the bed, unless instructed otherwise by the nurse.
- Empty drainage containers only when instructed by the nurse.
- Measure, describe, and record contents of the drainage container.
- Check to see that tubing does not become disconnected.
- Let the nurse know if the amount of drainage in the container increases rapidly or if drainage stops.

Gastrointestinal (Stomach) Suctioning

Suctioning may be necessary to remove fluid, blood, or wastes from the patient's stomach. (See Figure 31–8.) A nasogastric tube is connected to a portable suction machine or a wall suction outlet. The machine may be set to suction constantly at low-level or intermittently (not continuously), coming on and going off at intervals. This type of suctioning frequently follows surgery and is not often used in subacute care. However, if you are caring for a patient with this type of pump, the following guidelines will be helpful.

Dialysis

Dialysis is artificial filtration of waste products from the blood. It is used when the kidneys fail to function. Without dialysis, waste products would accumulate in the blood and result in death. Usually,

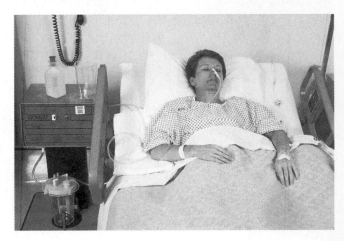

FIGURE 31–8
Portable suction is used to remove fluids from the body.

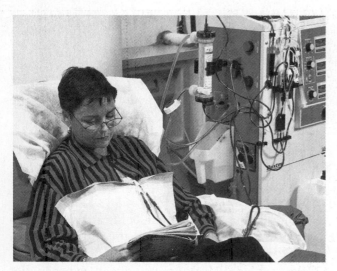

FIGURE 31–9
In hemodialysis the blood is circulated outside the body through an artificial kidney machine.

dialysis is a temporary procedure used until the kidneys start functioning again or a kidney transplant is performed. The two types of dialysis are hemodialysis and peritoneal dialysis.

Hemodialysis

In hemodialysis the blood is circulated outside the body through an artificial kidney machine. The machine removes the waste products from the blood, and returns the cleansed blood to the body. (See Figure 31–9). A *shunt* (a connection between two blood vessels) is created between an artery and a vein to remove and return the blood. Dialysis may be necessary several times a week and the process takes about four hours to complete.

Peritoneal Dialysis

In peritoneal dialysis, solution is introduced through a catheter into the peritoneal (abdominal) cavity. The waste products are drawn into the dialysis solution and drained by another catheter out of the body. Peritoneal dialysis is a sterile procedure performed by the nurse.

Nursing Care of the Dialysis Patient

Patients receiving dialysis are usually on a special diet with fluid restrictions. Accurate, daily weight measurement is necessary to evaluate fluid balance. During dialysis treatment, patients' vital signs are measured at regular intervals. If the patient is not on a vital signs monitor, you will need to measure and record them carefully.

Guidelines for Caring for a Patient on Dialysis

- Measure vital signs accurately.
- Avoid taking the blood pressure in the arm used for dialysis.
- Measure and record all intake and output.
- Weigh the patient at the same time each day with the same clothing.
- Encourage the patient to follow diet and fluid restrictions.
- Observe the patient for weakness after a dialysis treatment.

Observations to Report to the Nurse
- Changes in weight, vital signs, or intake and output (I&O)
- Patient complains of abdominal pain or pain at the shunt site
- Swelling of hands, feet, or face
- Shortness of breath
- Leaks or kinks in the dialysis tubing

Review

Read each sentence and fill in the blank with the vocabulary term that best completes the sentence.

1. A _____ is a machine that provides a patient with artificial respirations.
2. The insertion of a tube into the trachea is called _____.
3. A _____ is a surgical opening into the windpipe.
4. Artificial filtration of waste products from the blood, used when the kidneys aren't functioning is called _____.
5. A _____ is a connection created between two blood vessels.

Remember

1. Subacute care provides care to patients who need a lower level of care than is provided by acute care hospitals.

2. Mechanical ventilation is necessary when a patient does not move enough gases into and out of the alveoli to maintain metabolism.

3. One of the best ways to reassure patients is by performing your duties competently.

4. As a nursing assistant, you must never remove a patient from a ventilator.

5. Remember that you are caring for a patient, not a machine.

6. A tracheostomy is performed to establish an artificial airway when the natural airway is inadequate.

7. Handle the infusion pump carefully and avoid dropping or jarring it.

8. When dressing a patient with an IV, place clothing first on the affected arm (the arm with the IV).

9. If the feeding pump sounds, check the tube for kinks and notify the nurse if it continues to sound.

10. Empty drainage for gastrointestinal suctioning only when you are instructed to do so by the nurse.

11. Dialysis is used to artificially filtrate waste products from the blood when the kidneys fail to function.

12. Patients on dialysis are usually on a special diet with fluid restrictions.

13. When caring for a dialysis patient, report changes in weight, vital signs, or I&O promptly.

Reflect

Read the following case study and answer the questions.

Case Study
Bethel is a nursing assistant who works in a subacute unit of a long-term care facility. Her assignment for the day includes Mr. Fielder, a patient with a tracheostomy; Mrs. Oberon, with an IV in her left hand; 9-year-old Janet, receiving a hemodialysis treatment; and Mrs. Dooley who is in rehabilitation following a stroke that left her temporarily paralyzed.

1. List four guidelines for caring for Mr. Fielder's tracheostomy.

2. Describe how you would change Mrs. Oberon's hospital gown. It does not have snaps on the shoulder.

3. When caring for Janet, name three observations you would need to report to the nurse.

4. Describe some of the rehabilitation therapy you might assist Mrs. Dooley in performing.

Respond

Choose the best answer for each question.

1. Which of the following patients would be most likely to receive care in a subacute unit?
   A. A pregnant patient, ready to deliver
   B. A patient needing emergency care
   C. A patient with severe chest pain
   D. A patient on a mechanical ventilator

2. The chronic subacute unit cares for patients who
   A. Are chronically ill and have little hope of recovery
   B. Are on a mechanical ventilator
   C. Are recovering from acute heart attacks
   D. All of the above

3. Which skills are necessary for staff members working in subacute care?
   A. Technical skills
   B. Ability to communicate
   C. Good observational skills
   D. All of the above

4. Oxygen and carbon dioxide are exchanged in the
   A. Kidney
   B. Alveoli
   C. Heart
   D. Pancreas

5. Which of the following statements about care of the ventilator patient is FALSE?
   A. Keep the environment calm and quiet.
   B. Reassure the patient frequently.
   C. Turn the ventilator control panel toward the patient.
   D. Two people are needed when moving the ventilator patient.
6. Which of the following statements about tracheostomy patients is TRUE?
   A. Untie the tracheostomy tapes when bathing the patient.
   B. Gloves are not necessary when assisting with tracheostomy care.
   C. Keep water out of the tracheostomy tube.
   D. All of the above.
7. Keep the IV solution bag or bottle above the site of insertion.
   A. True
   B. False

8. A nasogastric tube is inserted
   A. Directly into the stomach
   B. Through the nose into the stomach
   C. Directly into the peritoneal cavity
   D. Through the abdominal wall into the bladder
9. Blood is circulated outside the body through an artificial kidney machine during
   A. Hemodialysis
   B. Peritoneal dialysis
   C. Gastric suctioning
   D. Tracheostomy care
10. Which of the following is NOT a guideline for caring for a patient on dialysis?
    A. Measure all the intake and output.
    B. Encourage the patient to follow the diet.
    C. Encourage the patient to drink a lot of fluid.
    D. Report changes in weight to the nurse.

Chapter Thirty-Two

The Home Health Aide

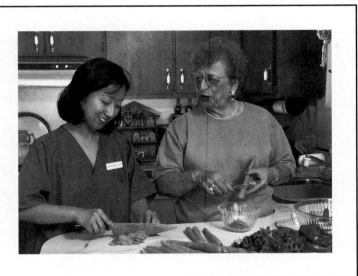

OBJECTIVES

After studying this chapter, you will be able to

1. Describe two differences between home health and hospital nursing.

2. List four services provided by home health agencies.

3. Identify four responsibilities of the home health aide.

4. Identify three tasks that the home health aide is not allowed to perform.

5. List six guidelines for assisting the patient with medication.

6. Describe three personal and professional qualities of the home health aide.

7. Identify four patient's rights in home health.

8. Explain the responsibilities of the home health aide regarding abuse and domestic violence

9. Describe two ways that cultural diversity affects the duties of the home health aide.

Glossary

integrated care team   The group of people directly involved in the care of the home health patient.

Modern developments in technology and increased acuity levels (a measurement scale defining how sick a patient is and the amount of care needed) has changed the practice of home health dramatically. There is now equipment available to provide advanced, in-home medical services such as ventilators, dialysis, and infusion therapy. In an effort to cut costs, patients are being discharged from acute care hospitals while they are still sick and in need of medical and nursing care. The least expensive place to care for these patients is in their own homes. These changes have led to an explosion of growth in the home health industry.

Because of this growth, there is a national shortage of qualified, well-trained home health care workers. Home health aides are in particularly short supply. Special home health training programs have been developed all across the country to meet the need. Many experienced health care workers are leaving hospitals and nursing homes to move into the home health care field. This chapter addresses the role of the home health aide, how it differs from other types of nursing, and the requirements for employment in this area. In some parts of the country, home health patients are called clients. However, use of the term is not universal, and this text will use the more familiar term "patient."

How Home Health Differs

There are many differences between home health and other types of health care. The major difference is in the setting. Home health care is delivered in the patient's home rather than a health care facility. You are a guest of the patient and the patient's family.

It is their territory, and they are in charge. For example, a health care facility can enforce a "no smoking" rule, whereas in the home, that decision is up to the patient and the family.

There are other important differences to consider. While a wealth of positive opportunities awaits you in the home health field, there are some negatives as well. The following lists of advantages and disadvantages to working in home health care may help you decide whether home health is for you.

Advantages of Working in Home Health

- You will usually care for only one patient at a time.
- There are more opportunities to practice holistic and humanistic care.
- There is time to build rapport with patients and families.
- You will have more control over the amount of time you work.
- You can choose when and where you want to work.
- There are more opportunities for independence and autonomy (control of one's own life).
- The hourly pay scale is often higher than for similar jobs in other health care settings.
- There is freedom from constant supervision.

Disadvantages of Working in Home Health

- You will need dependable transportation, and the mileage, wear and tear on your own vehicle adds up.
- There is a lack of in-home supplies—you will need to carry anticipated supplies with you (see Figure 32–1).
- You will need to be flexible and able to adapt skills and procedures to the home setting.
- It is more difficult to follow safety and infection precautions in the home.

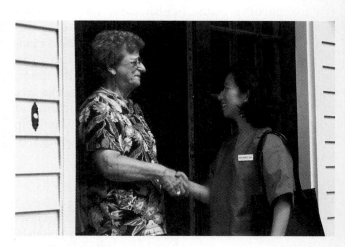

FIGURE 32–1
In home health, you may need to carry supplies with you.

- You must be motivated and self-directed. There is no one to remind you what to do next.
- You will have to work around pets, children, and family members.
- There is no job security. You choose when to work, but the employer chooses when to call you to work.
- There is no on-site supervisor. You must make careful observations and decide when to call the nurse.
- There are no co-workers to call on when you need help.

A lot depends on your personality and work habits. The very thing that attracts one person to home health will repel others. For example, you might like the autonomy and self-direction that home health provides while another person would feel more comfortable with nurses and other supervisors in the building. You might find it challenging to work when you want to, and in a different place every day, while someone else would prefer a routine job with a steady paycheck. Thankfully, the health care field is wide enough to accommodate the needs of many different workers. As you can see, there are both advantages and disadvantages to working as a home health aide. Before making a decision, you need to consider what works best for you.

Home Health Agencies

Some home health agencies are privately owned, some are owned by hospitals, and others are governmental agencies. However, the majority are owned and operated by large national corporations. They are licensed and regulated by local, state, and federal governments.

Laws have been passed and regulations put in place regarding home health care. The Omnibus Budget Reconciliation Act (OBRA) not only addressed quality patient care but also included standards of training, continuing education, and conditions of employment for home health aides. Careful screening and background checks are mandatory, and many states require certification of home health aides. These laws and regulations help to protect the patient and improve the quality of home health care.

Managed Care

In managed care systems, the case manager reviews patient needs, costs, and quality of care and coordinates the many services that patients may receive from a variety of providers. The emphasis in managed care is to use hospitals only as acute care settings. Because the number of hospital days is reduced, patients are discharged earlier. Patients are frequently referred to a home health agency where care can be delivered at less cost. The home health aide plays an important role in managed care. Your observations and prompt reporting help the patient to recover more quickly. Your accurate and timely charting helps the case manager to evaluate the patient's progress.

Home Health Services

Home health agencies provide health care services to patients in the patient's own home. These services may include:

- Skilled and nonskilled nursing care
- Rehabilitation
- Social services and counseling
- Nutritional education and planning
- Patient and family education
- Housekeeping and household management
- Respite care (providing relief for the caregiver)

Integrated Care Team

Home health care is delivered by a group of well-trained, dedicated health care workers who work together as a team. The *integrated care team* is composed of all the people who are directly involved in the care of the patient. The team may include doctors, nurses, aides, homemakers, social workers, rehabilitation therapists, a dietitian, chaplain, and other specialists. The patient and the family are truly at the center of the team. Because family members may serve as caregivers, they must be aware of the patient's plan of care.

The team meets on a regular basis to develop, evaluate, and revise the patient's plan of care. The purpose of the team is to provide expert advice and participation from every team member. The home health aide is an important member of the integrated team. Although you may be working by yourself in the patient's home, you are never really alone. The nurse supervisor and other team members are standing behind you, ready to assist as necessary.

Responsibilities of the Home Health Aide

The home health aide works as a member of the integrated care team under the supervision of the nurse. Your role will depend on the assignment you receive and on the individual patients for whom you care. Your assignment may vary widely from day to day. For example, you might be assigned six patients who need personal care services. Usually, one hour is planned for each patient. You will go to the first patient's home and assist with bathing, dressing, grooming, or whatever is included in the plan of care. Before you leave, you must carefully and accurately document what you have done. Then you go to the next patient's home and meet the individual needs of that patient. This process is repeated until you have completed your assignments. Obviously, you will need to be efficient and organized in order to keep this kind of schedule. You will need to plan your day carefully to spend more time with patients and less time driving.

You might also be assigned to go to a patient's home for 3 or 4 hours, 2 or 3 times a week. While there you may help the patient with personal care, do the laundry, take the patient grocery shopping, or whatever is called for in the plan of care. Some patients need assistance 24 hours a day. In that situation, you might work an 8-hour shift in the same patient's home for several weeks or months. The reason for this variety is that home health services are provided on an "as needed" basis, and all patients do not have the same needs.

Although the role varies, the most common responsibilities of the home health aide involve assisting with personal care and housekeeping. When you are hired, the agency will give you a copy of your job description or an outline of your duties. It also includes the limits of your responsibility. You are a home health aide, and while you may do some cooking and cleaning, you are not the primary cook or housekeeper. Responsibilities of the home health aide may include the following:

■ Assisting with personal care such as bathing, dressing, and grooming.
■ Assisting with other ADLs, such as ambulation, toileting, and feeding.
■ Assisting with devices that aid mobility, such as canes, walkers, and wheelchairs.
■ Assisting with range-of-motion exercises (see Figure 32–2).
■ Measuring intake and output.
■ Measuring vital signs.
■ Assisting with medications.
■ Observing, recording, and reporting.
■ Maintaining a clean, safe environment.
■ Following standard precautions and aseptic practices.
■ Providing household management and light housekeeping.
■ Planning meals.

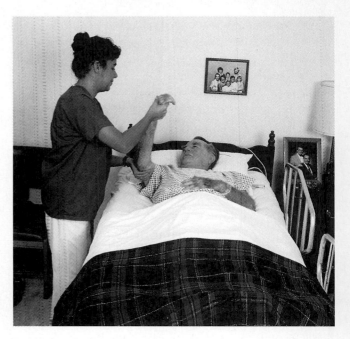

FIGURE 32–2
The home health aide assists the patient with range-of-motion exercises.

■ Purchasing groceries and preparing meals.
■ Assisting the patient to eat.

There are some tasks that the home health aide is not allowed to do. These tasks may not be the same in all sections of the country. In most areas, the home health aide is **not** allowed to:

■ Perform sterile procedures
■ Irrigate body cavities (including procedures such as enemas and colostomy irrigations)
■ Insert urinary catheters
■ Administer medication
■ Apply heat (such as heating pads and hot water bottles)
■ Perform any procedure that has not been taught

Holistic Health Care

Holistic health care focuses on the psychological and social aspects of the patient's recovery, as well as on medical progress. As a home health aide, you should treat each patient as an individual and acknowledge that each person has unique needs. Home health lends itself well to this type of care and is more able to meet the needs of the whole person.

Home health provides many opportunities for restorative care. For some patients, regaining or maintaining independence is essential to remaining in their own homes. They will need praise and encouragement to continue rehabilitation pro-

Guidelines for Assisting the Homebound Patient with Medication

- Check the patient's medication list.
- Check the prescription label.
- Make sure you have the right patient, the right medication, the right time, the right amount, and the right route.
- Place the medication within the patient's reach.
- Loosen container lids.
- Tell the patient the name of each medication.
- Support the patient's hand as he or she pours the medication into a medicine cup or the hand.
- Give the patient a glass of water. (See Figure 32–3.)
- Check to be sure the patient swallows.
- Return medications to the proper place.
- Document the medication taken and the time. Also document and report any effects of the medication that you observe or any patient complaints.
- Remember that a patient has a right to choose whether or not to take any medication or treatment.
- Document and report if the patient doesn't take a medication or is taking over-the-counter drugs such as aspirin or cough medicine.

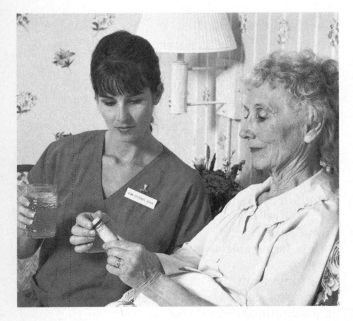

FIGURE 32–3
Give the patient a glass of water to take her medicines with.

grams that began in hospitals and nursing homes. Reinforce the instructions given in the use of adaptive equipment. Be alert for environmental barriers such as throw rugs or a step-down from one room to another. You may also need to help family members assume the role of caregivers. Be cheerful and positive. Your attitude can influence the success or failure of rehabilitation.

Assisting with Medication

In some areas of the country, home health aides are allowed to assist the patients with medication. Because home health aides are **not** allowed to administer medication, it is important that you know the difference between administering and assisting with medication. Administering medication means to pour the medication from the bottle into a medicine cup and give that medication to the patient. Assisting with medication means observing and supervising patients while they take their own medication. You are not allowed to pour medication into a medicine cup or actually place the medication in the patient's mouth.

Personal and Professional Qualities of the Home Health Aide

In order to be a successful home health aide, you will need to develop the personal and professional qualities described in Chapter 2. Although it is important to be caring, sensitive, empathetic, and considerate, certain qualities are emphasized in home health.

Flexibility

Flexibility is the ability to adjust to change. This quality is necessary because your assignment varies so often. You will have to adapt the skills and procedures you have learned to meet the conditions in the home without sacrificing safety principles. You will also need to learn how to develop rapport with a variety of patients and family members. Every day you may work with new people with different personalities and expectations.

Dependability

Dependability is an important asset in any job, but it is essential in home health. You will probably be the only person scheduled at a patient's home at a certain time. If you are late or do not come to work, the agency will have to try to find someone to work in your place, or the patient will have to do without assistance for that day. If you are not where you are supposed to be when you are supposed to be there, many people will be inconvenienced.

Honesty

You must be absolutely honest. Patients may have money, jewelry, or valuables around their home. Misuse of patients' belongings is a violation of patients' rights (a form of material abuse) and is illegal. You must also be honest about your work activities. You must document when you arrive, when you leave, and what you have done. Your employer and the patient will depend on you to be totally honest, sincere, and truthful.

Legal and Ethical Issues

Home health aides should follow the legal and ethical guidelines presented in Chapter 3. In addition, there are some areas of special concern in home health.

Confidentiality

Confidentiality is especially important in home health. Because you are in the patient's home, you may see and hear things that the family considers private. You may pick up personal mail and read it to the patient. (See Figure 32–4.) You may notice objects and notes as you clean the house. You might also witness a serious argument between your patient and a family member. Although you would need to report that information to your supervisor, it is not the business of the patient's friends and neighbors. Do not discuss the patient's affairs with anyone other than your supervisor.

Privacy

Maintain privacy of the patient's body, of his or her belongings, and of information. Protect privacy

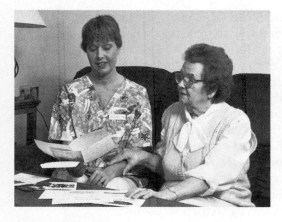

FIGURE 32–4
Protect the confidentiality of the patient.

while performing procedures or assisting with personal care. Do not disturb the patient's belongings unnecessarily. Find out from the patient or the family where things are located that you will need, and avoid searching through drawers and cupboards. Do not borrow anything from the patient, even if you have permission.

Limitations

Work within the limits of the care plan. Your assignment will clearly define your role, and a copy of the plan will be placed in the home. Do not perform tasks that are not included on your assignment. If a patient or family member asks you to do something that is not a part of your assignment, tell that person that you will have to check with the supervisor first. Call the supervisor immediately for directions. The care plan should identify the family member who is in charge. If another family member or friend asks you to do differently, refer that person back to the designated family member or to your supervisor.

Boundaries

It is easy to develop a relationship with patients or family members in the home. Sometimes this relationship can go beyond professional boundaries. Be friendly and helpful, while avoiding overinvolvement. Do not reveal more of your personal life than is appropriate or pry into the patient's private life. Avoid getting personally involved in the patient's problems. Let the nurse know if the problem is having an impact on the patient's health. The nurse will contact the appropriate person or agency.

Gifts

Patients or family members may want to give you a gift to show their appreciation. Tactfully explain that a gift is not necessary and that you are not allowed to accept it. Never ask for money, and if the patient tries to give you money, respectfully refuse. Sometimes gifts are offered with the expectation of getting extra services. Report all offers of gifts to your supervisor.

The Patient's Bill of Rights

Patients in all health care organizations have certain rights, and home health is no exception. Although some rights, such as privacy, are basic and are included in the hospital or long-term care bill of rights, others are specific to home health. For example, home health patients have the right to request preferred caregivers. The patient may request a certain home health aide because he or she "fits into the family," or "is strong and able to lift." Figure 32–5 includes a list of patient's rights in home health.

Abuse and Domestic Violence

Treat your patients kindly and gently and do not do anything that might appear to be abusive. Be careful what you say. A comment such as, "If you don't eat your dinner now, I won't fix you anything later," sounds threatening. While you may only be joking or trying to get the patient to eat, the comment could be considered assault (a threat to do harm).

You must also be aware of abuse in the home. Be sure to notify the supervisor if you suspect that abuse is taking place. Abuse can take many forms. In health care we automatically think about patient abuse, and our concern is protecting the patient. Patient abuse might be caused by a health care worker, a family member, or a friend. However, sometimes the patient is the abuser. This does not usually happen in the health care facility, because the individual who is being abused simply stays away from the facility. At home it is a different situation. Remember that the person who is being abused may not report the abuse and, in fact, may deny it. That does not relieve you of your responsibility to report the abuse.

You may witness domestic violence in the home. It may involve a spouse, a child, or another

Signs and Symptoms of Abuse in the Home
Fear and anxiety
A change in personality
Withdrawal and quietness
Unusual behavior
Frequent injuries
Old and new bruises
Unclean living conditions
Unnecessary restraints
Depression
Patient complaints of items missing from the home
Physical neglect, such as poor hygiene
Frequent crying spells
Hostile, aggressive behavior
Secretiveness and refusal to talk
Suicide threats
Mood swings

FIGURE 32–6 Observing for signs and symptoms of abuse.

family member. Again, it is your legal responsibility to report the abuse, even if it does not involve your patient. Health care workers are in a unique position to observe abuse and can do much to prevent it from continuing. A review of Chapter 3 will help you recognize signs of abuse and the proper action to take. Signs and symptoms of abuse are listed in Figure 32–6.

Family Interactions

A family consists of a group of people who live together under the same roof. The traditional example of a husband, wife, and two children as the typical family is no longer true. Families today might include an unmarried man and woman (with or without children), two people of the same sex, several unrelated people, or a single parent. The intergenerational family in which several generations share a home still exists, particularly in certain cultures. One of the most common family groups consists of two parents, each with minor children of their own, who marry or live together. This is sometimes called a "blended family." Whomever the patient considers family should be treated as family.

When you work in home health, you are providing care in the family home. The first time you

The Patient's Bill of Rights in Home Health
1. The right to be treated with consideration and respect
2. The right to privacy and confidentiality
3. The right to participate in developing the care plan and the discharge plan
4. The right to be informed of the charges for services, regardless of payment
5. The right to informed consent before service
6. The right to continuity of care
7. The right to know the name, classification, and responsibilities of assigned personnel
8. The right to request preferred caregivers
9. The right to be free from abuse
10. The right to refuse care, treatment, and medication and to be informed of the consequences of such actions
11. The right to be informed of the procedure for reporting complaints to the agency
12. The right to be informed of these rights, in writing

FIGURE 32–5 The home health care Patient's Bill of Rights.

come to the home, you are a stranger, and the family members may feel uncomfortable having you there. They may feel guilty, as though somehow they have failed. These kinds of feelings could cause them to resent you and even to react in anger. Do not take it personally, because it is generally not meant that way. Once the family members see that you are taking good care of the patient, they will usually be appreciative and welcome you into their home. Let the supervisor know if bad feelings continue to persist.

In home health, you will care for people of all ages and levels of need. Some live in beautiful, luxurious homes, while others live in poverty. Lifestyles, habits, values, and behaviors may differ from yours. Do not criticize or ridicule the way a family lives. While you always want to encourage cleanliness and good personal hygiene, you cannot change people's lifestyles. Regardless of where and how they live, or how they behave, family members have a right to be treated with respect and consideration.

Family relationships affect the atmosphere and attitude in the home. Some families are warm, kind, and supportive of their members, providing a happy home that is a pleasure in which to work. Other families seem filled with anger and conflict. Problems such as drug abuse, alcoholism, and unemployment may exist. As a home health aide, you must be able to function in any setting. You cannot become personally involved in the patient's family matters. Be empathetic, understanding, and nonjudgmental. Never take sides in family conflicts but remain neutral and be available to listen to both sides.

Families differ in their reaction to illness in the home. Family members need all the support and encouragement that you can give them. When possible, include them in the patient's activities (see Figure 32–7). Part of the patient's adjustment to illness depends on the strength of their support system. This system includes extended family members (relatives who are involved in the family, but do not live in the same home). Grandparents, aunts, uncles, nieces, nephews, and cousins may be a part of the extended family. Friends, coworkers, church members, and club members may also be included in the patient's support system.

The extended family and other members of the support system can sometimes make your job more difficult. In their efforts to be helpful they may create problems rather than solve them. For example, grandmother has a home remedy that she is certain would do the patient more good than the present medications, and a well-meaning uncle reminds you that it wasn't done that way when he was young. Usually these people are not familiar with the pa-

tient's care plan or your responsibilities in the home. You have to handle them with tact and diplomacy to avoid hurting their feelings. Listen to them, acknowledge their concerns, but continue to follow the patient's care plan.

Working around children can be a real challenge. Whether it's the baby crying, the toddler underfoot, or the schoolchild asking questions, you must be able to adapt. Safety of the children in the home is of utmost importance. You must respond to an unsafe situation or an emergency, even when the child is not your patient. However, do not assume responsibility of a child unless it is part of the care plan.

Many households include pets that are treated like family members. Dogs, cats, and other animals may be in the house, on the furniture, and in the patient's bed. Remember, this is the patient's home, not yours. Accept the fact that you will need to vacuum dog hairs off the sofa, disinfect countertops where the cat walked, and change the patient's bed linen more frequently. It can be a real challenge to perform your duties and protect your patient with a pet underfoot. Do not ask the patient to put the pet outside or in a special area while you are in the home. If you are allergic to or afraid of cats, dogs, or birds, let the supervisor know, and you will not be sent to a home where those pets are kept.

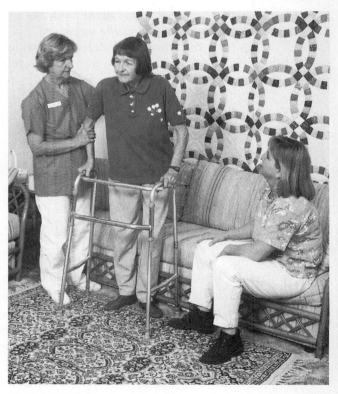

FIGURE 32–7
When possible, include family members in the patient's activities.

Cultural Diversity

As a home health aide, you will work in homes with patients from all cultures. You will need to be familiar with their customs and practices in order to provide quality patient care. Cultural diversity directly affects your duties as a home health aide, particularly if you are responsible for planning, cooking, and serving meals. Culture and religion often determine the types of food the patient eats and the manner in which it is prepared. Bathing, personal care routines, and clothing are also influenced by culture. If you are not sure what to do, check the care plan, which includes the patient's cultural needs and instructions for meeting those needs.

In some households, you elderly patient may be raising grandchildren. He or she may have many roles to fill—parent, grandparent, head of household, and patient. The children may act out because of their worry over the patient. Be supportive and allow them as much private time together as you can (see Figure 32–8). You can provide comfort and reassurance by taking good care of their loved one.

It will be helpful to review and follow the guidelines listed in Chapter 13, where cultural diversity was described in detail. The key is to respect and try to understand the culture of the patient with whom you are working.

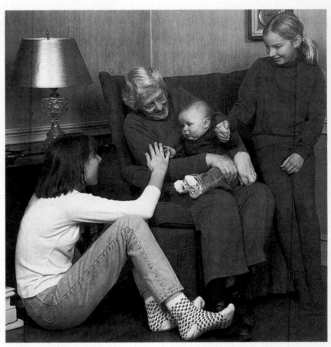

FIGURE 32–8
Allow the patient and the children private time together.

 ## *Review*

Read each sentence and fill in the blank with the vocabulary term that best completes the sentence.

1. _____ is a measurement scale that defines how sick a patient is and the amount of care that will be needed.
2. Control of one's life is called _____.
3. _____ is providing relief for the caregiver.
4. The group of people directly involved in the care of the home health patient is called a/an _____.
5. _____ is the ability to adjust to change.

 ## *Remember*

1. There is a national shortage of qualified, well-trained home health aides.
2. Home health allows you to work with more autonomy and independence.
3. Government regulations help to protect the patient and improve the quality of home health care.
4. The home health aide works as a member of the integrated team, under the supervision of a nurse.
5. The most common responsibilities of the home health aide involve assisting with personal care and housekeeping.
6. Home health aides are not allowed to administer medications.
7. Dependability is an essential quality of a home health aide.
8. Confidentiality is a major issue in home health.
9. Never accept gifts from patients or their family members.
10. It is your responsibility to report abuse in the home.
11. Tact and diplomacy may be necessary in dealing with the patient's friends and family.
12. Remember that it is the patient's home, not yours.
13. Respect and try to understand the culture of the patient with whom you are working.

Reflect

Read the following case study and answer the questions.

Case Study

Glenda is a home health aide whose assignment today includes Mrs. Benson, a 62-year-old patient with emphysema. Mrs. Benson has oxygen ordered PRN, by concentrator through a nasal cannula. She uses the oxygen frequently. She fatigues easily and can walk only a short distance with help. Her 25-year-old daughter and 2-year-old granddaughter live with her. The care plan calls for you to assist Mrs. Benson with a shower, shampoo, and personal care. You are also supposed to change the bed. You are scheduled to be there approximately one hour. The daughter asks you to look after the 2-year-old while she runs some errands.

1. What should you tell the patient's daughter about caring for the toddler?
2. Make a priority list showing how you would organize your tasks in the Benson home.
3. Identify safety rules you will need to observe because oxygen is being used.
4. How can you protect your back while making the bed? It is not a hospital-type bed.

Respond

Choose the best answer for each question.

1. Which of the following is an advantage of working in home health?
   A. It causes wear and tear on your car.
   B. You may work around children and pets.
   C. You care for only one patient at a time.
   D. There are no co-workers to ask for help.
2. OBRA regulations do not apply to home health.
   A. True
   B. False
3. Which of the following are members of the integrated care team?
   A. Home health aide
   B. Nurse supervisor
   C. Patient
   D. All of the above
4. Which of the following are responsibilities of the home health aide?
   A. Measuring intake and output
   B. Administering medications
   C. Ordering the diet
   D. All of the above
5. The patient asks you to help her with her medications. What should you do?
   A. Nothing. You are not allowed to help with medications.
   B. Pour the medication into a medicine cup.
   C. Remove the cap from the medicine bottle.
   D. Place the medication in the patient's mouth.
6. The patient asks you to wash the windows in her house. What is your best response?
   A. "I don't do windows."
   B. "I'll do the windows some other time."

C. "I'm sorry, but that's not in the care plan."
   D. "Your windows aren't that dirty."
7. The patient's husband wants to give you $50.00 for being so good to his wife. What should you do?
   A. Take it—$50.00 is a lot of money.
   B. Tell him to send the money to the office.
   C. Take it, but don't tell anyone.
   D. Tell him you're not allowed to accept money or gifts.
8. You observe the patient's son-in-law hit his wife. What should you do?
   A. Get out of there before he hits you.
   B. Report his actions to the nurse immediately.
   C. Ignore it. It's none of your business.
   D. Tell him you're going to call the police.
9. The patient has a small dog that stays in the house and you are allergic to dogs. What should you do?
   A. Ask her to put the dog outside while you're there.
   B. Lock the dog up in a spare bedroom.
   C. Ask the nurse to assign someone else to the patient.
   D. Stay as far away from the dog as possible.
10. Your patient is a young Hispanic woman. She is refusing to take her medication because her mother-in-law told her it was poison. What is your best response?
    A. Report the problem to your supervisor immediately.
    B. Tell the patient that she has to take the medication.
    C. Tell the mother-in-law that she is wrong.
    D. Place the medication in the patient's food.

Chapter Thirty-Three

Homemaking Skills

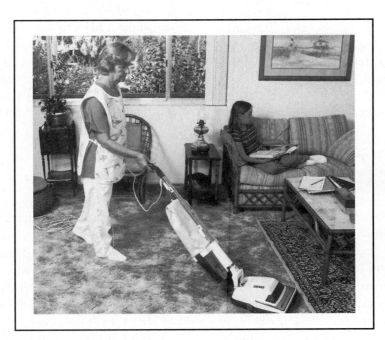

OBJECTIVES

After studying this chapter, you will be able to

1. List six guidelines for safety in the home.

2. List six guidelines for infection control measures in the home.

3. Describe two methods for organizing your work.

4. Identify four tasks that are included in light housekeeping and two that are not.

5. List four guidelines for using cleaning products.

6. Describe four guidelines for laundry and care of clothing.

7. List six guidelines for grocery shopping.

8. Identify six guidelines for preparing food.

Glossary

homemaker   A person who performs household duties.

In order to become a successful home health aide, you will need to be both a competent nursing assistant and a skilled *homemaker* (a person who performs household duties). Although your assignment in home health varies, it will frequently include light housekeeping duties. You will need to be able to create a pleasant environment in a home that belongs to someone else and over which you have little control. That is not an easy task. Your duties will involve keeping the patient's home clean and safe.

Safety and Infection Control in the Home

Safety is always a major concern in nursing. Check the patient's home for safety hazards each time you come to work. Help the family correct problems such as throw rugs that might cause the patient to slip and fall. Let the nurse know about hazards you cannot correct. Remember, however, that you are not there to rearrange the patient's home; your goal is to make it as clean and safe as possible. Safety and infection control hazards to observe for in the home include:

- Throw rugs or loose carpeting
- Slippery floors
- Inadequate lighting
- Damaged equipment, such as walkers and wheelchairs
- Medications stored improperly
- Cleaning solutions not put away
- Overloaded electrical circuits
- Frayed electrical cords
- Careless smoking habits
- Unsafe heating devices
- Nonworking smoke detectors
- Unwashed dishes
- Open garbage containers
- Signs of insects or rodents

Safety in the Home

The family home can be hazardous to the patient's health and to yours. Most homes are designed primarily for comfort and attractiveness, rather than

Guidelines for Safety in the Home

- Use the guidelines for body mechanics and other safety measures that are found in Chapter 6.
- Report safety hazards promptly.
- Clean up spills immediately.
- Remove throw rugs or secure them to the floor.
- See that the patient wears proper footwear.
- Lock brakes on all wheeled equipment.
- Provide a bath mat or towel beside the bathtub or shower.
- Pick up toys and other objects that clutter floors and stairways.
- Read labels and directions before using supplies and equipment.
- Keep poisons out of the reach of children or confused adults and in a locked cabinet, if possible.
- Keep medications in their proper place and out of the reach of children or confused adults.
- Store sharp knives with the blades covered.
- Keep electrical equipment away from water.
- Empty ashtrays only after the ashes are completely cool.
- Stay with confused or weak patients while they smoke.
- Handle hot liquids and food carefully.
- Fill the bathtub and adjust the water temperature in the shower before the patient enters.

for safety. Safety features that are routine in a health care facility, such as hand rails in the hallways and grab bars in the bathroom, are not usually found in the home. More accidents occur at home than in almost any other setting, and the most common accident site is the bathroom.

Home Emergencies

It is important that you know what to do if an accident, a fire, or other emergency occurs while you are in the patient's home. Your supervisor will help you and the family make a plan to follow in case of fire. It will include identifying an escape route and in-

---

EMERGENCY TELEPHONE NUMBERS

Fire _____   Police _____

Ambulance _____   Poison Control _____

Physician _____   Family Member _____

Agency Supervisor _____

Patient _____

Address _____

Nearest Cross Street _____

Telephone _____

FIGURE 33–1
Keep a list of emergency telephone numbers at each telephone.

structions for getting the patient out of the home. Keep a list of emergency telephone numbers at each telephone. You will need to include telephone numbers for the fire department, police department, ambulance service, poison control, your supervisor, the patient's doctor, and the responsible family member. Also include the name of the patient, the home telephone number, and the address. In an emergency situation, you may not be able to remember this vital information. (See Figure 33–1.) If your area has 911 services, you will not have to use some of the individual telephone numbers. The procedure for calling 911 or activating EMS includes the following:

- Identify the type of emergency.
- Give the location, including the nearest cross street.
- Give the number of persons needing help.
- Identify the first aid that is being given.
- Do not hang up the telephone until you are told to.

It will be helpful to review Chapter 7 for detailed first aid and emergency information.

Workplace Violence

Workplace violence can be more dangerous in the home setting because you are there alone. Sometimes patients become violent and may try to hurt you or themselves. Family members or friends may argue or fight. It may suddenly become necessary to protect not only your patient but yourself as well. Do not argue or take sides and notify your supervisor immediately.

You will also need to protect yourself as you come and go from the patient's home. If you drive to work, try to park near the home in a visible area. Always lock your car when you leave it and immediately upon entering it. When you leave the house to go home, get your car keys out while you are still in the house, and carry them in your hand. Go directly to your car, get in, and lock the doors. Always be aware of your surroundings. If you ride public transportation, wait in a well-lit area and be observant for danger. Carry a flashlight at night and some sort of warning device. Even a child's whistle may make enough noise to scare off an attacker or summon help. If you are working in an unsafe section of town, try to arrange for someone to either pick you up at work or escort you to your car. If you see or hear anything suspicious, return to the patient's home and call for help. Workplace violence is discussed in more detail in Chapter 6. Dealing with aggressive/combative patients is addressed in Chapter 27.

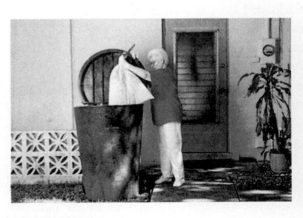

FIGURE 33–2
Place trash in a covered container.

Guidelines for Infection Control in the Home

■ Use aseptic technique and follow standard precautions.
■ Wash your hands frequently.
■ Wear gloves when appropriate.
■ Maintain a clean environment.
■ Wash soiled dishes and utensils promptly.
■ Wash fruits and vegetables before serving.
■ Store food at the correct temperature.
■ Disinfect kitchen surfaces daily.
■ Dispose of garbage properly.
■ Dispose of contaminated supplies correctly.
■ Clean bathrooms daily.
■ Handle soiled linen as little as possible.

Infection Control in the Home

Although the patient is at less risk of infection in the home than in a health care facility, maintaining infection control can be a challenge. The equipment and supplies that you take for granted in the health care facility may not be available in the home. Even washing your hands can be a problem if the washbasin is at the other end of the house from where you are working. A review of Chapter 4 will be helpful at this time. (See Figure 33–2.)

Guidelines for Disposing of Regulated Medical Waste

■ Flush human waste products down the toilet immediately.
■ Clean up blood and bloody fluids immediately and flush them down the toilet if possible.
■ Wash contaminated clothes in hot water, separately from other clothes.
■ Double bag contaminated dressings and cleaning rags in plastic and discard in a special container.
■ Double bag contaminated disposable medical equipment in plastic and discard in a special container.
■ Discard used needles and contaminated sharps immediately into a puncture-proof container.
■ Check with your supervisor regarding the disposition of the special medical waste containers.

Regulated Medical Waste

Regulated medical waste includes blood, blood products, sharp medical objects such as needles, and items contaminated with blood or body fluids. Government regulations determine the disposal of medical waste. The purpose of the regulations is to protect the patient, health care workers, environmental workers, and the general public from bloodborne pathogens and other infectious agents. In hospitals and other facilities, the environmental services department is responsible for medical waste, but in the home the patient and members of the health care team must take care of the problem. Special containers are usually placed in the home to contain the various waste products. Disposing of the contents of the special containers depends on local regulations. The following guidelines will help you to properly deal with regulated medical waste.

Bloodborne Pathogens

The most common bloodborne diseases are HIV (human immunodeficiency virus) infection and HBV (hepatitis B virus) infection. You may care for patients with either of these diseases in home health. Detailed information on bloodborne diseases is given in Chapter 5.

As explained in earlier chapters, the best way to prevent the spread of bloodborne pathogens in the workplace is by following standard precautions. Wear gloves whenever there is a possibility of contact with body fluids such as blood, semen, vaginal secretions, saliva, urine, feces, vomitus, or wound drainage. Wash your hands before and after providing care for the patient.

At the present time, there is no cure for HIV infection and no vaccine to prevent its occurrence. However, there is a vaccine available that will prevent hepatitis B, the most common type of hepatitis that occurs in health care settings. The vaccine provides immunity to hepatitis B and has few side effects or reactions.

Hospitals and long-term care facilities are required to provide the vaccine, at no cost, to all employees who may come in contact with body fluids and who choose to receive it. The requirements for home health agencies are not as clear-cut, and practices vary. It is important to find out what the agency's policy is before you go to work, because the hepatitis vaccine is expensive.

Organizing Your Work

The organizational skills that you have learned as a nursing assistant will be very useful to you in home

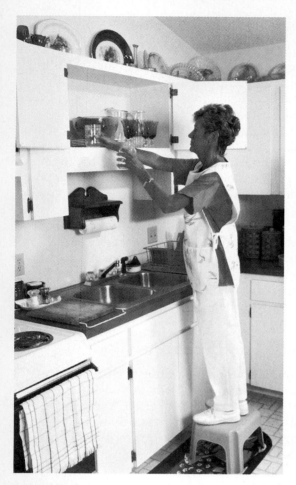

FIGURE 33-3
Use your spare time for chores such as straightening the kitchen cabinets.

health. Planning your schedule and making a list will help you to avoid wasting time. Begin your shift by checking your assignment sheet. Even if you are going to the same house every day, your daily schedule will vary. Some tasks are done on a daily basis, while others are done less frequently. Make a list of your duties and establish priorities. Setting priorities involves rating each task in its order of importance.

The first time that you go to a patient's home, ask a family member to show you where the patient's personal care items, linen, and cleaning supplies are kept. If you will be cooking for the patient, you will also need to locate the food, dishes, and utensils that will be required. Get instructions for operating household appliances such as the washer, the dryer, and the dishwasher.

Group tasks together whenever possible. For example, if you need to grocery shop for the patient, check your list for other tasks that can be done at the same time. You might be able to do the grocery shopping, leave clothes at the dry cleaner, and pick up the patient's medication from the drugstore in

one trip. While the patient is resting, you can wash the dishes and clean the kitchen. Start the laundry early in your shift. Clothes can be washing, rinsing, and drying as you care for the patient and do other household tasks.

Collect your equipment before you begin a task. Put cleaning supplies in a basket or box and carry them with you. That way, whatever you need will be handy. The most efficient way to work is to perform one task throughout the house before you begin another task. For example, you might sweep all the floors or dust all the furniture at one time. If this is not possible, the next best way is to clean one room at a time.

If you finish your daily chores early, check your assignment for tasks that are done less frequently. You might use this time to clean the refrigerator or straighten kitchen cabinets. Do not use work time for personal telephone calls or other personal activities. Not only is that a waste of time, it is also dishonest. While you are in the home, your time belongs to the patient, so use the time wisely and efficiently. (See Figure 33-3.)

Basic House Cleaning

As a home health aide, your responsibilities may include light housekeeping duties. These tasks include sweeping, dusting, doing the patient's laundry, picking up clutter, cleaning the bathroom, and cleaning the kitchen. Light housekeeping does **not** include such tasks as washing windows, cleaning carpets, moving furniture, or mowing lawns.

Your assignment sheet will include a general idea of your housekeeping duties. Whatever tasks that you do must be documented completely and accurately. Your agency may provide a flow sheet on which you simply check off the household tasks that you have completed.

Sometimes the patient or family member may ask you to do a household chore that is not on your assignment sheet. Never argue with the patient, a family member, or a friend of the patient. If you are not sure if a request is appropriate, your best response would be "I'll need to check with my supervisor first." Let your supervisor know if this kind of situation occurs frequently.

Cleaning Equipment and Supplies

Cleaning equipment in the home may include a vacuum cleaner, broom, mop, dustpan, toilet brush, and feather duster. Cleaning supplies include cleaning cloths, paper towels, garbage bags, garbage cans, and cleaning products. Check to see what equipment and supplies are already in the

Guidelines for Using Cleaning Products

- Store cleaning products in their original containers, out of the reach of children or confused adults.
- Read the label before using any product.
- Follow the directions on the label.
- Scrub surfaces carefully to avoid scratches or other damage.
- Wear rubber gloves to protect your skin when you are using cleansers.
- Call for help if accidental poisoning occurs. Poison Control will need the name of the product and a list of the ingredients, so keep the container at hand when you make the call.

home and make a list of needed items. Go over the list with the patient and the family to determine if they have preferences regarding the type of product you are to use.

Some homes will have all kinds of equipment, gadgets, and supplies, while others may not even have the bare necessities. Keep the household budget in mind. Do not ask the family to buy expensive equipment or supplies just to make your job easier. Learn to make do with whatever is in the home. Diluted household bleach will effectively clean and disinfect counters, sinks, tubs, and toilets. A mixture of vinegar and water will clean glass and mirrors as well as commercial cleaners.

Use cleaning products carefully and read the labels on the containers. Rubber gloves may be necessary to protect your hands (see Figure 33–4). Many

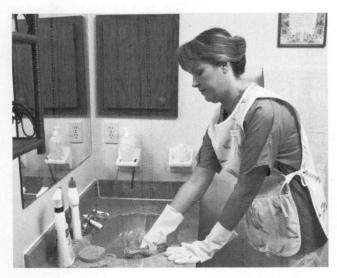

FIGURE 33–4
Wear rubber gloves when using commercial cleansers.

of these products are toxic (poisonous) and irritating to the skin. Never mix cleaning products together because the combination can cause a dangerous chemical reaction. For example, bleach or ammonia used individually are excellent cleaning agents. Mixed together they produce a toxic gas that can cause severe injury or death. The following guidelines will help you to use cleaning products effectively and safely.

The Patient's Bedroom and Living Room

The patient's bed may be set up in his or her own bedroom or in another part of the house. It may even be located in a section of the living room. Wherever the bed is located is considered the patient's unit and should be treated as such. The bed and other equipment may belong to the patient, or it may be rented from an equipment company. Hospital beds, special mattresses, overbed tables, wheelchairs, mechanical lifts, and other types of medical equipment are available for home health patients.

Keep the patient's room as neat and tidy as possible. Do not, however, remove personal items such as photographs and mementoes. Allowing the patient to surround herself with things that have special meaning is important to the healing process. The patient spends a lot of time in this room, and it may be the only part of the house that the bedbound patient sees. Avoid clutter on table and dresser tops, as well as on the floor. Try to create an atmosphere that is pleasant and peaceful. Provide privacy whenever necessary by closing the door and the window drapes. If the patient's bed is in the living area, use screens or curtains. Privacy is just as important at home as it is in the health care facility.

In home care, daily changing of bed linens is not usually necessary. Once or twice a week may be sufficient, unless the patient is in bed most of the time. Of course, a wet or soiled bed is changed immediately. It may be necessary to adapt the bedmaking procedure if the patient does not have a hospital bed. Remember that only the steps change, not the principles. For example, even if you cannot raise the bed to a correct working height, you can still follow the rules of body mechanics. Stand with your feet apart, your knees bent, and keep your back as straight as possible. Make as much of the bed as you can from one side before going around to the other side. When the procedure has been completed, the bed linen should be clean, neat, and unwrinkled.

Furniture is dry-dusted daily and polished weekly. Floors should be swept or vacuumed daily, and mopped once a week, unless something is spilled on the floor. All spills should be cleaned up immediately. If the patient eats in the room, disinfect table surfaces before each meal. Line wastebaskets with plastic bags and empty them daily. Lamps and light fixtures should be kept clean and free from dust or smudges. Weekly chores also include vacuuming upholstered furniture, polishing wood surfaces, and cleaning mirrors and the glass on framed pictures. Your goal is not just to keep the room clean, but also to remove dust particles before they can cause problems.

Collectibles and other ornaments should be hand-washed or cleaned once a month. Handle delicate items carefully to avoid damaging them. If you are not sure how to clean an item, wipe it gently with a soft, dry cloth. Books and book shelves should be cleaned at regular intervals. Remove the books from the shelves for cleaning and put them back in the same order that you found them. Do not rearrange furniture or other items without permission from the patient or the family.

The Bathroom

The bathroom provides an ideal environment for the growth of microorganisms. Think about the areas that are warm, dark, and damp, such as behind the toilet and under the washbasin. Daily cleaning is necessary to prevent the spread of microorganisms and to eliminate odors. Surfaces to be cleaned and disinfected in the bathroom include the following:

- Washbasin and faucets
- Bathtubs, showers, faucets, and shower curtains or doors
- Toilet bowls, seats, and outside surfaces
- Countertops and mirrors
- Toothbrush, glass, and soap containers
- Towel bars and toilet tissue holders
- Window sills
- Floors

Empty the wastebasket daily and wash the basket once a week. Put soiled towels and washcloths in the laundry and replace them with clean ones. Replace toilet tissue, facial tissue, and soap, as necessary. A deodorizer in the bathroom helps to keep down odors. When weather permits, open the bathroom window while you are cleaning the area.

Check the bathroom frequently to see that the toilet has been flushed and that spills have been cleaned up. Wipe off the washbasin after you or the patient uses it. Dry surfaces in the tub or shower after each use to help prevent mildew. A bleach solution will remove mildew from wall surfaces, shower curtains, and shower doors.

The Kitchen

The kitchen also has many areas that encourage the growth of microorganisms, such as under the sink, stove, and refrigerator. Regular cleaning helps to keep these areas clean and controls the spread of microorganisms. Daily housekeeping chores in the kitchen include the following:

- Clean the sink and countertops after each use.
- Clean the outside surfaces of the stove, refrigerator, and other appliances. (See Figure 33–5.)
- Clean up spills immediately.
- Wash the dishes after each meal.
- Store leftovers in covered containers in the refrigerator.
- Empty the garbage.
- Sweep the floor and mop, if necessary.

The floor should be mopped at least once a week. Cabinet and drawer fronts are also cleaned weekly. Straighten the cupboards and drawers whenever it seems necessary. If you put things back where they belong when you are through using them, these areas will stay neat and orderly. Clean the interior of the refrigerator, the oven, and the microwave at regular intervals.

Garbage may need to be separated before discarding. There may be special containers for paper, metal, and wet garbage. Be aware of and follow recycling procedures in the area. If the home has a garbage disposal, follow instructions as to what goes into the disposal and what does not. The same is true of a trash compactor. Dispose of medical waste properly.

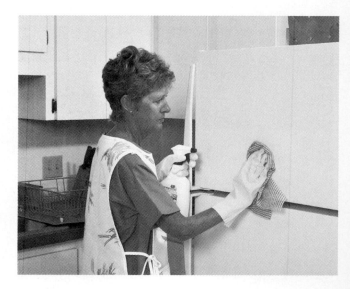

FIGURE 33–5
Clean the outside surfaces of the refrigerator daily.

Washing Dishes

When washing dishes by hand, rinse the sink and fill it with hot, soapy water. Wash glasses and cups first, then silverware, plates, and bowls. Pots, pans, and skillets should be washed last. Rinse the dishes under hot water and place them in a drainer to dry. If a dishwasher is used, the dishes are usually rinsed first. Arrange the dishes and add detergent according to the manufacturer's instructions. Only dishwasher-safe dishes and utensils should be placed in the dishwasher. It is better to handwash an item if you are not sure. Remove the dry dishes from the drainer or the dishwasher and put them away before you leave for the day.

Laundry and Care of Clothing

As a home health aide, you will frequently be asked to do the patient's laundry. Clean clothing and linens may help the patient feel better and improve self-esteem. Think about how you feel when you put on clean clothing or lie down on fresh, clean sheets. On the other hand, an accumulation of dirty clothes may create an odor and make the house look untidy. It also provides a reservoir for microorganisms.

Check clothing labels for washing instructions and to determine if the garment is to be hand-washed, machine-washed, or dry cleaned. Find out from the patient or a family member what their preferences are regarding washing procedures and products. Make sure that you have all the necessary supplies before you begin.

Sort the clothes according to color, fabric, and degree of soiling, and wash them separately. For example, it is best to wash all white clothes together, particularly if you are going to add bleach. They are usually washed in hot water for a longer period than are colored clothes. Delicate fabrics, however, require gentle washing in warm or cold water for a shorter period. Use your common sense. What would happen if you washed a dark blue sweatshirt with a new white towel? You would probably end up with a dingy blue towel and a dark shirt covered with white fuzz.

While sorting the clothes, you should also check for spots and stains. There are commercial products available that will remove many types of stains. If you do not have one of those products, try soaking the item in cold water and scrubbing it with a small amount of detergent applied directly to the spot. Whenever possible, stains should be treated as soon as they occur. Check the pockets of clothing for loose change, pens, and other items. A tube of lipstick left in a sweater pocket can cause a disaster in the dryer. Even a facial tissue can make a mess in the washer or dryer.

Make sure that you know how to operate the washing machine and the dryer correctly. Many washers have simple instructions printed on a label inside the lid. Distribute the clothes evenly in the washer and do not overload it. Follow directions for adding detergent, bleach, and fabric softener. Set the washer for the proper temperature, time, and water level.

Remove clothes from the washer as soon as the load is finished. Wet clothes may mildew or sour, and they provide an ideal environment for the growth of microorganisms. Either hang the clothes on a clothesline or place them in the dryer. Set the dryer for the correct time and temperature. Some fabrics should not be placed in the dryer. They need to be put on hangers and hung on a rod or line to dry. Follow the directions on the clothing label for drying the garment.

Place clothes in a clean basket when you remove them from the dryer or the clothesline and avoid unnecessary wrinkling. Clothes made from wash-and-wear fabrics should be removed immediately and hung to dry. Clothes to be ironed should be folded and placed in a separate basket. Involve the patient in folding the clothes, if possible. Take the basket of dry clothes to the couch or the bed and encourage the patient to help in folding the laundry. This can give the patient a feeling of usefulness and help in maintaining independence. Return clothing and linen to their proper places after they are folded. (See Figure 33–6.)

Guidelines for Laundry and Care of Clothing

- Check clothing labels for washing and drying instructions.
- Collect your supplies before you begin.
- Sort clothes as to color, fabric, and degree of soiling.
- Treat for spots and stains before washing.
- Check the pockets of clothing for loose change and other items.
- Be sure that you know how to operate the washer and dryer.
- Distribute clothes evenly in the washer and avoid overloading.
- Remove clothes from the washer as soon as they are done.
- Fold clothes as soon as you take them from the dryer.

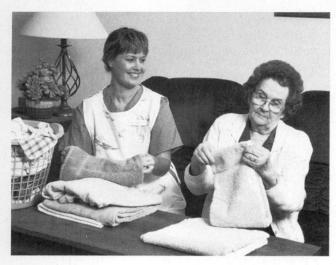

FIGURE 33–6
Helping to fold clothes may give the patient a feeling of usefulness.

Food Planning and Preparation

In some homes you may be responsible for planning and preparing food. Your duties may include planning menus, grocery shopping, cooking, and serving meals to the patient. You may already have gained experience in these tasks in your own home. However, there are some skills that will make grocery shopping, cooking, and mealtime easier and more enjoyable.

Food Planning

Food planning begins with a nutritional assessment of the patient by the nurse and the development of a nutritional care plan. The patient and the family are involved in the planning process. The care plan describes the patient's physical and psychological limitations and the ability for self-care. It identifies the type of diet that is ordered and foods that are restricted. The patient's normal eating habits are determined, and cultural, religious, financial, and personal preferences are considered. Check the nutritional care plan before you begin planning meals.

Plan the menus for a full week to avoid frequent trips to the store. All meals, snacks, and between-meal nourishments must be considered. The menus should provide the patient with a well-balanced diet that is both pleasing and nutritious. Involve the patient in planning the menus, if possible. Appetite often improves when the patient has had a choice in selecting the food. The daily diet should contain a variety of foods that include the following:

- 6 to 11 servings of bread, cereal, rice, and pasta
- 3 to 5 servings of vegetables
- 2 to 4 servings of fruits
- 2 to 3 servings of milk, yogurt, and cheese
- 2 to 3 servings of meat, poultry, fish, dry beans, eggs, and nuts

Fats, oils, and sweets should be used sparingly. These guidelines are included in the Food Guide Pyramid, developed by the U.S. Department of Agriculture. Refer to Chapter 22 for detailed information regarding nutrition and fluids.

Make a shopping list after you have planned the menus. Go over the menus to determine which ingredients are on hand and which ones you will have to buy. Check the supply of staples such as flour, sugar, and spices. Include cleaning supplies, paper goods, and any other items that are needed in the home. Ask the patient to go over the list and make suggestions, if needed.

Shopping

Check with the patient or family member to see if there is a certain grocery store that he or she wants you to use. If not, select one that is close to the patient's home and that has competitive prices. It is usually best to do as much of your shopping as you can at one store. When you go from store to store hunting specials and bargains, you will usually spend more money. You will also need to consider the expense of the car and your time.

Involve the patient in grocery shopping, if possible. Grocery store aisles are wide enough for wheelchairs, and some stores provide motorized carts for the convenience of their shoppers. Shopping provides an opportunity for exercise and socialization. It also helps the patient to feel needed and useful.

Let the supervisor know when you will be out of the home and the approximate amount of time that you will be gone. If the patient does not go with you, make arrangements for someone to stay with the patient until you get back. This would be a good time for a visit from a friend or neighbor.

Storing Groceries

Put the groceries away in the proper place as soon as possible after you return to the patient's home. Meats, poultry, fish, and frozen foods should be placed in the freezer, unless you are going to use them immediately. Dairy products and most fresh vegetables and fruits are placed in the refrigerator. Dried, canned, bottled, and packaged food should be placed in the cupboards. Rotate foods by placing the items that you have just purchased behind items that are already in

Guidelines for Grocery Shopping

■ Check newspaper ads for specials and coupons.

■ Check items off your shopping list as you put them into the cart.

■ Start at one side of the store and go up and down the aisles to the other side.

■ Read the content label on the package. The ingredient that is listed first is present in the greatest amount. The label may also include a list of calories and nutrients per serving (see Figure 33–7).

■ Compare the cost of different sizes and brands by reading the unit price, which lets you know which brand or size costs less.

■ Plain or store brands are usually cheaper than name brands.

■ Check package labels for sodium, sugar, and fat if your patient is on a special diet.

■ Buy the size item that is best for your patient. A large package is not a bargain if most of it is wasted.

■ Buy less expensive cuts of meat for use in stews and casseroles.

■ Buy fruits and vegetables that are in season.

■ Select nourishing snacks.

■ Pick up perishable foods, such as milk and frozen foods, last.

■ Purchase some convenience foods that the patient may fix when you are not there.

■ Save grocery shopping receipts for the patient or family member.

Nutrition Facts

Serving Size 1 cup (49g)
Servings Per Container about 10

Amount Per Serving	Cereal	Cereal with 1/2 cup Skim Milk
Calories	170	210
Calories from Fat	5	5
	% Daily Value**	
Total Fat 0.5g*	1%	1%
Saturated Fat 0g	0%	0%
Polyunsaturated Fat 0g		
Monounsaturated Fat 0g		
Cholesterol 0mg	0%	0%
Sodium 0mg	0%	3%
Potassium 200mg	6%	11%
Total Carbohydrate 41g	14%	16%
Dietary Fiber 5g	21%	21%
Insoluble Fiber 5g		
Sugars 0g		
Other Carbohydrate 36g		
Protein 5g		
Vitamin A	0%	4%
Vitamin C	0%	2%
Calcium	2%	15%
Iron	8%	8%
Thiamin	8%	10%
Riboflavin	2%	10%
Niacin	15%	15%

FIGURE 33–7
Check the content label for ingredients, calories, and nutrients.

the cupboard. This procedure helps ensure that the food will be fresh and avoids spoilage and waste. Canned foods should be stored away from any heat source, such as the stove or hot water heater.

Cleaning supplies and paper goods should be stored as close as possible to the area where they will be used. Store dishwashing detergent and paper towels under the sink, toilet tissue and bathroom cleanser in the bathroom, and laundry detergent in the laundry area.

Preparing Food

The ability to prepare food that is appetizing and nutritious is an important skill that will be useful on the job and in your personal life. If you are already an accomplished cook, remember that you are cooking for the patient, not for yourself. The patient's diet may determine how the food is prepared as well as which foods are selected. Consider any

problems the patient may have with chewing, swallowing, and digestion. Limit the amount of salt that you use and be careful with seasonings. Avoid frying foods, even if your patient is not on a special diet.

It will be helpful to prepare a sink or dishpan of hot, soapy water to clean up dishes and utensils as you cook. Wash your hands before beginning to prepare food and after you have handled meat, poultry, and fish. Wash knives and cutting boards between items. Put away ingredients such as flour and sugar as soon as you are through using them. Clean the outside of oil and syrup bottles before you put them back in the cupboard.

Do whatever you can to make the food look appetizing. Avoid overcooking, which destroys vita-

Guidelines for Preparing Food

- Wash your hands before preparing food.
- Bake or broil foods rather than fry them.
- Be creative with leftovers.
- Avoid keeping hot or cold food at room temperature for any length of time.
- Divide leftovers into serving size portions and freeze for later use.
- Trim meat before cooking to avoid excess fat.
- Use the oven for more than one food at a time.
- Select the right size pan for the burner.
- Turn the handles of pans toward the center of the stove.
- Never leave pans unattended on the stove.
- Turn off the stove as soon as you are through using it.
- Clean up as you go.

Guidelines for Using a Microwave Oven

- Follow the instructions in the owner's manual.
- Use only microwave-safe containers in the oven. Wood or fine china can be damaged.
- Avoid using aluminum foil, metal, or metal-trimmed dinnerware in the oven.
- Do not attempt to operate the oven empty or with the door open.
- Use the correct time and power settings and avoid overcooking food.
- Know what foods cannot be cooked in the oven. For example, whole eggs may explode.
- Cover food to help prevent drying out or splashing.
- Use a temperature probe to be sure that microwaved meat is done all the way through.
- Wipe up spills immediately and clean the oven after each use.

mins as well as changes the appearance of the food. Think about how the food will look on the plate when you serve it, and provide a variety of colors and textures. A meal consisting of foods that are all the same color would not look very inviting nor would it produce a well-balanced meal. A variety of color is not only attractive, it is nutritious (see Figure 33–8).

Microwave Cooking

Many people today use a microwave oven to cook or reheat food. It can be a clean, fast, efficient method of cooking when done properly. Check with the patient or family before using the microwave, and read the owner's manual if it is available. The following guidelines will help you to use the microwave oven safely and efficiently.

Serving the Food

Encourage your patient to eat in the dining room whenever possible. Occasionally, the patient may want to eat in the living room or on the porch when the weather is nice. If the patient must eat in bed, he or she should sit up as straight as possible. Elevate the bed so the patient is in a high Fowler's position. If the bed is not adjustable, pillows may be used to prop the patient up straight.

The traditional three meals a day, served at set times, may not suit the patient. Encourage the patient to set a schedule that he or she prefers. Some patients may prefer several small meals during the day. The patient with a poor appetite may eat better when not faced with a lot of food at one time.

Meals are more enjoyable in a relaxed and attractive setting. Make sure the area is neat and clean when the patient is ready to eat. Use a tablecloth or placemat, if available, and place some flowers on the table. Even a single blossom or a piece of greenery in a vase or bottle can help the room look more cheerful. Some people enjoy music while they are eating. Encourage visitors to stay so the patient will not have to eat alone (see Figure 33–9).

The patient may need help getting ready for mealtime. Offer toileting and assist as necessary

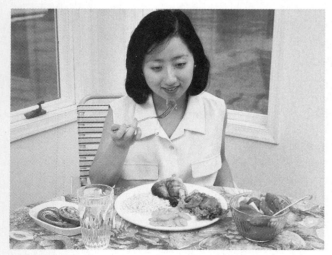

FIGURE 33–8
A variety of colors and textures makes a meal more attractive as well as nutritious.

with oral care and handwashing. Make sure that the patient's clothes are clean and neat and the hair is combed. Most people feel more like eating when they are clean and well groomed. Remind patients who need them to wear their glasses or hearing aid.

Encourage the patient to eat as independently as possible. Fill cups and glasses about three-fourths full for easier handling. Check to see if the patient uses any adaptive equipment, such as a scoop plate or special utensils. If the patient has trouble grasping a fork or spoon, you can make a built-up utensil by wrapping tape or gauze around the handle. Detailed information regarding assisting the patient with dining is found in Chapter 22.

Snacks and Between-Meal Nourishment

Provide nourishing snacks for the patient to eat between meals. Many people like a light snack before retiring for the night. Fresh fruit, cheese and crackers, graham crackers, and peanut butter are examples of nutritious and attractive snack foods. Avoid snack foods that are high in fats and sugar, such as doughnuts and pie. A glass of milk or juice is better than a carbonated beverage, and the patient should avoid caffeine late in the evening.

Some patients may drink liquid supplements for between-meal nourishment. The doctor may order this type of feeding for patients who are not eating well. Find out if the patient likes the supplement chilled or at room temperature. Ice cream or fruit may be added if allowed on the patient's diet.

Cleaning Up After Meals

After the patient has completed the meal, you will need to clean up the kitchen and meal site. Discard leftovers or put them into the refrigerator in covered containers. Wash the dishes and put them away when they are dry. Clean the stove, sink, and countertops in the kitchen. Wipe up spills and crumbs from the table and sweep the floor, if necessary. When you are through, the kitchen and dining room should be ready for the next meal.

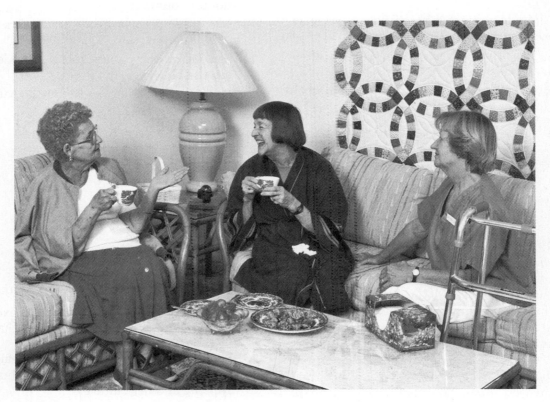

FIGURE 33–9
Encourage visitors to stay so that the patient will not have to eat alone.

Review

Read each sentence and fill in the blank with the vocabulary term that best completes the sentence.

1. A _____ is a person who performs household duties.
2. Disease-causing microorganisms transmitted by contact with blood or blood products are called _____.
3. _____ are waste materials contaminated by blood or body fluids. Disposal of these wastes are regulated by the government.
4. Setting _____ is rating each task in order of its importance.
5. The medical term for poisonous is _____.

Remember

1. More accidents occur at home than in any other setting.
2. Use aseptic technique and follow standard precautions to prevent the spread of microorganisms in the home.
3. It is important to know what to do if an emergency occurs in the patient's home.
4. Government regulations determine the disposal of medical waste such as blood and contaminated items.
5. Know how to protect yourself from workplace violence.
6. Make a list of your duties in the home and establish priorities.
7. Whatever tasks that you do in the patient's home must be documented.
8. Use cleaning products carefully and read the labels on containers.
9. Clothing and household linen must be handled carefully and correctly.
10. Involve the patient in planning menus whenever possible.
11. Read the content label on the food package before you buy it.
12. Remember that you are cooking for the patient, not for yourself.
13. Use only microwave-safe containers in the microwave oven.
14. Encourage the patient to eat as independently as possible.
15. Provide nourishing snacks for the patient to eat between meals.

Reflect

Read the following case study and answer the questions.

Case Study

You are a home health aide who has been assigned to care for Mrs. Lopez in her home from 8 a.m. until 12 noon three times a week. Mrs. Lopez, who is Hispanic, has terminal cancer. She eats poorly, has lost a lot of weight, and is very weak. Her daughter and two small grandchildren live with her. Your assignment includes assisting Mrs. Lopez with her bath and personal hygiene, changing the bed, and washing the bed linen. You also have to prepare breakfast when you arrive and lunch before you leave. The daughter asks you to change the children's beds and do their laundry when you do her mother's.

1. List the order in which you will do the tasks for Mrs. Lopez.
2. How will you handle the daughter's request to do the children's beds and laundry?
3. Plan a daily menu for the two meals you will prepare, taking into account Mrs. Lopez's poor appetite and her culture.
4. What restorative measures can you use to promote Mrs. Lopez's independence?

Respond

Choose the best answer for each question.

1. Which of the following are safety hazards to observe for in the home?
   A. Safety bars in the bathroom
   B. Throw rugs on the floor
   C. Smoke detectors in the home
   D. Closed garbage containers in the kitchen

2. The most common accident site in the home is the
   A. Bedroom
   B. Living room
   C. Hallway
   D. Bathroom

3. What is the proper way to dispose of contaminated surgical dressings in the home?
   A. Flush them down the toilet.
   B. Discard them in the bathroom trash can.
   C. Double bag and place them in a special container.
   D. Wash them in hot water and then discard them.

4. Which of the following tasks would be highest on your priority list?
   A. Change the bed.
   B. Clean the bathroom.
   C. Feed the patient.
   D. Do the laundry.

5. Which of the following are NOT light housekeeping duties?
   A. Doing the patient's laundry
   B. Cleaning the patient's room
   C. Cleaning the kitchen
   D. Washing the windows

6. You are providing the patient's husband with a list of cleaning supplies that are needed. Which is the best response?
   A. "A bottle of bleach will take care of a lot of cleaning."
   B. "Try to find that cleaning solution that was advertised on television."
   C. "I'll need separate cleaning solutions for the kitchen and the bathroom."
   D. "I know what I like, so let me pick up the cleaning supplies."

7. It is safer to wear rubber gloves when using cleaning solutions.
   A. True
   B. False

8. Which of the following is a daily housekeeping chore in the home?
   A. Emptying the garbage
   B. Doing the laundry
   C. Straightening the kitchen cabinets
   D. Polishing the living room floor

9. Which of the following is a guideline for grocery shopping?
   A. Shop for specials in all the local stores.
   B. Buy the most expensive brands.
   C. Read the contents label on the package.
   D. Pick up perishable foods first.

10. The patient is weak and has limited use of his arms. Which of the following is the most restorative?
    A. Feed the patient yourself.
    B. Make the patient feed himself.
    C. Assist the patient as necessary with feeding.
    D. Ask a family member to feed the patient.

Chapter Thirty-Four

Employability Skills

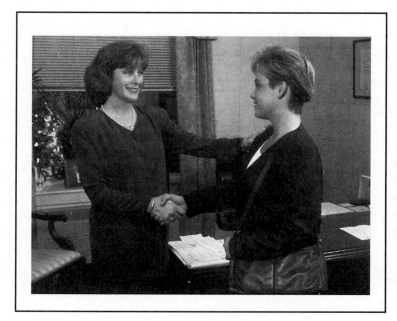

OBJECTIVES

After studying this chapter, you will be able to

1. Make an action plan for successful employment.

2. Prepare a resume or personal information sheet.

3. List four guidelines for conducting a job search.

4. Fill out a job application form correctly.

5. Identify four guidelines for a successful job interview.

6. List six guidelines for surviving the probationary period of employment.

7. List four guidelines for resigning from a job.

mentor A trusted, experienced person who influences, guides, and directs another person.
networking Communicating and interacting with people who have similar interests and goals.

resume A brief, written summary of an individual's work experience and qualifications.

Even with a nationwide shortage of nursing assistants, certain employability skills are necessary to get a job and keep it. Employability skills include making an action plan, preparing a resume, conducting a job search, filling out an application, participating in an interview, and performing satisfactorily on the job. This chapter presents information to help you attain those skills. It would also be helpful to review the material in Chapter 2 concerning job qualifications and performance.

Making an Action Plan

Good career decisions do not just happen—they are carefully planned and developed. A career action plan consists of:

- Setting goals
- Preparing a *resume* (a brief, written summary of an individual's work experience and qualifications)
- Conducting a job search
- Getting hired for a job
- Retaining the job
- Receiving good evaluations

Setting Goals

Deciding where you want to go and what you want to achieve in your career allows you to focus your energies in that direction. First, set a long-range goal and then set short-range goals to help you get there. For example, if your ultimate goal is to be a pediatric nurse, becoming a nursing assistant is a great beginning. Completing a licensed nursing program and taking a pediatric study course are also steps toward your long-range goal.

Be realistic and set goals that you feel you can meet. Becoming a pediatric RN next year is not a realistic goal. It takes several years of hard study to become a registered nurse. But do not sell yourself short. Develop a positive attitude, believe that you

will succeed, and keep working toward your long-range goal. It is amazing what you can accomplish one step at a time. Be honest and make sure the goals are your own. The fact that your grandmother and your mother are nurses does not mean that you have to be a nurse. Don't get involved in someone else's dream.

Let others know what your goals are. Your family, friends, instructor, or employer may be able to help you. Family members and friends can provide support and encouragement that will help you meet your goals. Most employers are glad to see that an employee wants to continue his or her education. The employer may be willing to provide financial assistance with scholarships or loans. Your instructor can help you select the appropriate programs to enter when you complete the nursing assistant course.

Preparing a Resume

A resume or personal information sheet contains most of the information you will need when applying for a job (see Figure 34-1). Type or print the information clearly, using correct grammar and spelling. Try to keep it brief enough to fit on one or two pages. Have someone check it over when you are finished. A neatly prepared resume helps you appear professional, even if a resume is not required. Plus, you will have at your fingertips all the information needed for the job application form. Update your resume periodically to keep it current and reflect your accomplishments. A resume includes:

- **Personal data.** List your name, address, and telephone numbers.
- **Education and training.** Start at the last school you attended and work backward.
- **Work history.** Work backward from your present job. Include job title, dates you worked there, your supervisor's name, and the name, address, and telephone number of each employer.
- **Special abilities and strengths.** Identify your strengths such as being organized, dependable, or flexible. Typing or computer skills are helpful.

PAULA SMITH
555 Knox Street
Collegeville, PA 10001
717-555-5555 Home
717-555-0000 Office

OBJECTIVE	Seeking an entry level position as a nursing assistant.
STRENGTHS	Results oriented; Adaptable to challenges; Establishment of excellent patient relations.
EXPERIENCE	
Nursing Assistant	Nursing Assistant for 32 bed dementia unit, Lansdale Convalescent Home, Lansdale, PA 20002; 20xx–20xx.
Intern	One Year ICU Unit Intern, Sacred Heart Hospital, 103 Main Street, Norristown, PA 30003; 20xx–20xx.
EDUCATION	
Nursing Assistant Certification	North Montco Technical Career Center, Lansdale, PA 20002
ORGANIZATIONS	National Honor Society; Health Occupations Students of America; Vocational Student Organization.
CONFERENCES	Vocational Student Organization Conference 20xx.
AWARDS AND ACHIEVEMENTS	First Place Award in State Competition for Nursing Assistants; Leadership Certificate for demonstration of skills.
SPECIAL COMPETENCIES	Fluent in Spanish.
REFERENCES	Furnished upon request.

FIGURE 34–1
A sample resume.

- **Interests and hobbies.** Include community activities and special things that you are interested in or like to do.
- **Honors and awards.** List and be able to provide copies if necessary.
- **References.** Include names, addresses, and telephone numbers of three or four people who know you well. It is helpful to have professional people such as your pastor or your instructor for your references. Get their permission first and do not include relatives.

Conducting a Job Search

Unlike many other occupations, conducting a search for a health care job is fairly easy. There are job openings available in almost all parts of the country. Your nursing assistant certificate indicates that you have been properly trained and are competent to do the job. That makes you a valuable potential employee. Sometimes the hardest part is deciding which job you want to accept.

Guidelines for Conducting a Job Search

- Talk with friends and family who may know of job openings. Discuss your goals with your instructor, other students, and medical people you already know or have met during your training. This is called *networking* (communicating with people who have similar interests and goals).
- Check newspaper advertisements. Look in the "Want Ad" section under "Help Wanted—Medical." You will see ads for nurses, nursing assistants, and other health care workers. Be aware that some facilities that are chronically short of help may run an ad whether they have immediate openings or not.
- Contact employment offices. Counselors there will be able to help you. Some government agencies offer free services, while most private agencies charge a fee. Discuss financial costs before you sign up with the agency.
- Check out work sites. Visit hospitals, nursing homes, and other health care facilities where you are interested in working. Find out the name of the person who does the hiring, and call for an appointment.
- Contact the person who does the hiring in the facility in which you did your clinical training. These people know the quality of training you received, and they have had a chance to observe you. Your instructor may be able to help you set up an appointment with the proper person.

You may have several job offers to consider. Your decision will have an impact on your life and on your goals. Think about the distance from your home and the availability of transportation. Sometimes facilities that are located in a rural area or those that are not on a bus line will pay a slightly higher salary to attract employees. Remember that the extra cost of transportation and time may cancel out the salary differential.

Salary is often not the most important consideration. Most health care facility salaries are competitive. That means the pay is about the same at all of them when other factors are considered. Pay attention to the benefits offered. Health care plans, life insurance, vacation and sick leave, and scholarship opportunities are all important.

Observe how employees interact with one another and how they treat patients. Is the atmosphere pleasant and happy? Observe safety and infection control practices. Is this a safe place to work? Remember, if you take the job, you will be spending a third of your day in this building with these people.

Obtaining a Job

The first real step in obtaining a job is to pick up an application form. Come alone and dress professionally. Remember that you will be making a first impression on someone, even if it is only the receptionist. Be prepared to fill out the application and participate in an interview the same day. This sometimes happens when there is a severe shortage of help. It is best to fill out the application the same day you pick it up. This saves time and demonstrates your efficiency.

Filling Out a Job Application

Gather everything you will need ahead of time and place it in a folder or briefcase. Documents you will need include your Social Security card, driver's license or other photo identification, your nursing assistant certificate, and any other training certificates. Bring your resume and any written references you may have. Include pens and pencils. If you need glasses to read, be sure and bring them with you.

When filling out the application form, use a typewriter or print clearly with a pen. Use correct spelling and grammar. Read the questions carefully and follow directions. Be honest. Lying on an application form is cause for dismissal. Fill in all the blanks because an incomplete application form may be discarded. Your resume or personal information sheet will contain most of the information necessary to fill out the form. (See Figure 34–2.)

Interviewing for a Job

An interview is a meeting between a job applicant and a prospective employer that provides an opportunity for an exchange of information. The interview is the most important part of the hiring process. It does not matter how great your qualifications are—if you do not do well on the interview, you probably will not be hired. Your civil rights should be protected during the interview. Civil rights laws in this country make it illegal to discriminate based on age, sex, religion, race, ethnic origin, or physical handicap. It is illegal for the employer to discriminate in hiring or any other part of the employment process.

You will need to collect some information before the interview. Find out what kind of patients are cared for in the facility. Are they a mix of all ages, or are most patients elderly? Does the facility

EMPLOYMENT APPLICATION
(Please print plainly)

Personal Information

Date:_____

1. Name_____
           (Last)   (First)   (Middle)

2. Soc. Sec. No.:_____

3. Present Address:_____
             (No.)   (Street)   (Apt. No.)

   _____
       (City)   (State)   (Zip)

4. Number of years at the above address:_____

5. Phone Number:_____
       (Area Code)   (Number)

Educational Background

Type of School	Name and Address	How Many Years Attended	Graduated	Course or Major
Grammar or Grade			__Yes __No	
High School			__Yes __No	
College			__Yes __No	

Work History (List in order, last or present employer first)

Dates From To	Name, Address and Telephone Number of Employer	Rate of Pay Start Finish	Supervisor's Name	Reason for Leaving

Describe in detail the
work you did:

Dates From To	Name, Address and Telephone Number of Employer	Rate of Pay Start Finish	Supervisor's Name	Reason for Leaving

Describe in detail the
work you did:

May we contact the employers listed above? _____ If not, indicate below which one(s) you do not wish us to contact and why. _____

Personal References

List three people who can give you personal references. (You may exclude former employees, relatives, members of the clergy, or persons whose titles or business addresses might indicate your race, color, religion, sex, age, national origin, ancestry, or disability.)

Name and Occupation   Address   Telephone Number

1._____
   (Name)   (Occupation)

2._____
   (Name)   (Occupation)

3._____
   (Name)   (Occupation)

FIGURE 34–2
A sample job application form.

specialize in one type of illness? In a hospice, for example, all the patients are terminally ill. Are you ready for that at this stage of your career? Having that kind of information allows you to ask intelligent questions and make relevant comments during the interview. Know how to get to the facility and where to park. Learn the numbers of the buses if using public transportation. Find out how long it will take you to get there from where you live. A trial run beforehand will help to answer these questions and make you feel more confident.

During the interview, you may be asked questions about your interests and goals. The interviewer will be evaluating your answers and your communication skills. He or she will be looking for responses that indicate compassion and empathy. Avoid negative answers. Examples of the kinds of questions you may be asked include "Why do you want to work here?" and "Why did you go into nursing?". Think carefully before you respond. Be prepared to ask questions yourself, about insurance and other benefits. Find out if there is a credit union available. When discussing salary, ask about promotions and raises and where there is a shift differential.

Keep an open mind about the hours you will work and what you will do. Many facilities start all new employees on the evening or night shift because these shifts are hardest to fill. If you have a shift preference, make that clear during the interview so that your name can go on the waiting list. If you are flexible about when and where you are willing to work, you are more likely to be hired. This is especially true if you have limited experience. The following guidelines will help you have a successful interview.

Guidelines for Interviewing for a Job

- Dress conservatively in business attire.
- Follow good personal hygiene and grooming practices.
- Be on time or a few minutes early.
- Introduce yourself and greet the interviewer by name.
- Listen attentively to the interviewer and do not interrupt.
- Think before you respond and answer all questions truthfully.
- Be prepared to ask pertinent questions.
- Be aware of cultural diversity.
- Thank the interviewer as you leave.

Retaining the Job

Good job performance and positive evaluations will help you retain your job and receive promotions. Job performance includes your work habits, your communication and interpersonal skills, and your competency (the knowledge and skill required to perform tasks correctly). Chapter 2 offers guidelines for personal hygiene and appearances, managing stress, and developing professionalism. A review of that material would be helpful.

Orientation

Orientation is mandatory for all new employees and may last for one day or several weeks. The purpose is to familiarize you with the work environment. Orientation is usually held during the day, regardless of the shift that you will be working. Part of the time will be spent in the classroom learning the facility's policies and procedures. You will be informed of safety and infection control practices. Fire and other emergency management procedures will be explained. You will be given a copy of your job description and an employee handbook. Then you will receive clinical orientation to the nursing unit, where you will learn the routine and the location of equipment and supplies. You may be assigned to a mentor (a trusted, experienced person who influences, guides, and directs another person). Or you may work with another employee on the "buddy system" for a period of time. This is the time to ask questions and learn your role and responsibilities.

The Probationary Period

The first three to six months of employment are known as the probationary period. During that time, the employer is evaluating your skills and competence. You can be let go at any time if your performance is not satisfactory. The decision for permanent employment is not made until the end of the probationary period. The following guidelines will help you to survive the probationary period.

Employment Evaluations

Nurses are evaluating your performance all the time, especially when you are a new employee. Evaluations are based on the quality of your work and your professionalism. Organizational abilities, communication skills, and interactions with others are observed. Special attention is given to your ability to think and problem solve. Attending available in-service training programs and continuing your education will help your evaluation. Promotions

Guidelines for Surviving the Probationary Period

- Be at work on time, as scheduled.
- Carry out your responsibilities to the best of your ability.
- Be cooperative and get along with your co-workers.
- Express a willingness to learn.
- Be flexible and willing to adapt to change.
- Follow facility policies.
- Accept criticism positively.
- Improve your performance skills.
- Earn high evaluations.

and pay raises are based on evaluations, although seniority is also involved. The nursing supervisor will do your first formal evaluation when you complete the probationary period (see Figure 34–3) and at regular intervals during your employment.

Submitting a Resignation

Eventually, you may wish to change jobs and move on in your career. Never leave without giving notice. Generally, a two-week notice or the length of one pay period is sufficient. Your resignation will be noted in your employee files, so do it properly. A resignation should always be in writing to the person in charge of hiring, although you may want to personally inform your supervisor. (See Figure 34–4.)

Guidelines for Resigning from a Job

- Give two weeks' written notice, when possible.
- If you have a positive reason for leaving, say so. However, it is not necessary to give a reason.
- Leave with good feelings, if possible. Avoid expressing anger or criticism.
- State the last day of your employment.
- Avoid calling in sick during the resignation period.
- Thank the employer for the opportunity to have worked there.

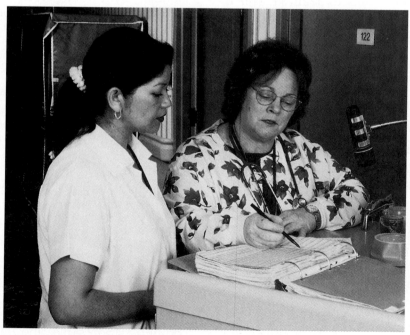

FIGURE 34–3
Nurses will be evaluating your performance all the time.

102 Center Street
Smalltown, FL 33555

March 6, 2002

Geneva L. Johnson
Director of Nurses
City Hospital
224 Main Street
Tampa, FL 33610

Dear Ms. Johnson:

This letter is to notify you that I am resigning my job as a nursing assistant at City Hospital. My last day of work will be March 20, 2002.

I have enrolled in the nursing program at Sarasota Community College and will be moving there to be near the school. It will be too far away for me to commute to City Hospital.

I have enjoyed working with the patients and staff at City Hospital. Thank you for giving me the opportunity to work there.

Sincerely,

Margaret Brown, CNA

FIGURE 34–4
A sample resignation.

Review

Read each sentence and fill in the blank with the vocabulary term that best completes the sentence.

1. A _____ is a brief, written summary of an individual's work experience and qualifications.
2. Communicating with people who have similar interests and goals is called _____.
3. An _____ is a meeting between a job applicant and a prospective employer to exchange information.
4. The knowledge and skill required to perform tasks correctly is called _____.
5. A _____ is a trusted, experienced person who influences, guides, and directs another person.

Remember

1. Good career decisions need to be carefully planned and developed.
2. When planning your career, set long-range goals and then set short-range goals to help you achieve them.
3. A resume contains most of the information you will need when applying for a job.
4. Networking will help you find a job in health care.
5. The interview is the most important part of the hiring process.
6. Dress conservatively and be on time for the job interview.
7. Good job performance and positive evaluations will help you retain your job and receive promotions.
8. Orientation is given to new employees to familiarize them with the work environment.
9. During the probationary period, the employer is constantly evaluating your skills and competence.
10. When resigning from a job, give a two weeks written notice, if possible.

Reflect

Read the following case study and answer the questions.

Case Study

Dan Truman has successfully completed a nursing assistant training program and passed the competency tests required in his state. Dan's mother is a registered nurse, as is his best friend. His long-range goal is to be a surgical or recovery room nurse. His instructor has helped arrange an interview at the facility where he received his clinical training. However, Dan has heard that a nursing home far out in the suburbs is offering a higher salary. Dan is not sure where he wants to work.

1. What short-range goals will help Dan reach his long-range goal?
2. What networking can Dan do to help him find a job?
3. How can Dan make a good impression in the job interview?
4. What factors must Dan consider when deciding where he wants to apply for a job?

Respond

Choose the best answer for each question.

1. Employability skills include
   A. Preparing a resume
   B. Filling out an application
   C. Participating in an interview
   D. All of the above
2. Which of the following is the best example of a long-range goal in health care?
   A. Passing the anatomy/physiology test
   B. Taking a course in geriatrics
   C. Becoming a pediatric nurse
   D. Demonstrating competency in a procedure
3. Which of the following would NOT be included in your resume?
   A. Your name and address
   B. Your children's names
   C. Your educational background
   D. Your work history
4. What documents will you need when applying for a job?
   A. Social Security card, photo identification, and nursing assistant certificate
   B. Social Security card, insurance card, and birth certificate
   C. Birth certificate, credit card, and nursing assistant certificate
   D. Social Security card, birth certificate, and photo identification
5. An employer can refuse to hire you if you are over 65 years of age.
   A. True
   B. False

6. During a job interview at a nursing home, you are asked why you want to work there. What is your best response?
   A. "You pay more than anyone else."
   B. "I like working with elderly people."
   C. "I live right down the street."
   D. "I don't like caring for children."

7. During your orientation, your "buddy," another nursing assistant, asks you to do something that you've never done alone. What is your best response?
   A. "Okay, I'll try to do it."
   B. "I can't do that by myself."
   C. "I've never done that alone. Would you help me."
   D. "Why do you ask? You know I've never done that."

8. Which of the following is NOT a guideline for surviving the probationary period on a new job?
   A. Express a willingness to learn.
   B. Accept criticism positively.
   C. Follow facility policies.
   D. Work only in areas that you like.

9. Promotions are based on your performance, skill, and seniority.
   A. True
   B. False

10. Which of the following is appropriate when submitting a resignation?
    A. Let the supervisor know that she is the reason you are quitting.
    B. Give a two-week written resignation.
    C. Give your notice at the last minute to avoid unpleasantness.
    D. Call in sick the last three days of the resignation period.

Chapter Thirty-Five

Surveys and Accreditation

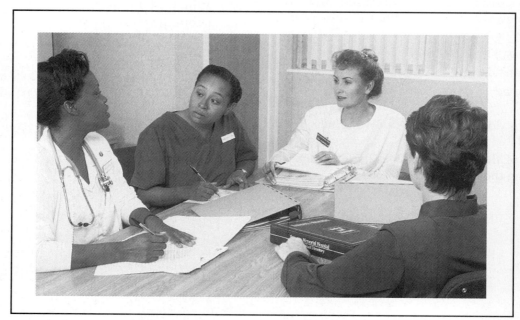

O B J E C T I V E S

After studying this chapter, you will be able to

1. List six guidelines for following standards of care.

2. Explain the purpose of quality assurance.

3. Briefly describe the survey process in health care facilities.

4. Identify three regulatory agencies that may survey health care facilities.

5. Describe your responsibilities regarding mandatory in-services.

6. List six guidelines for participating in a successful survey.

accreditation A process in which a regulatory agency recognizes that a facility has met accepted standards.

quality assurance A program in which health care facilities evaluate the services they provide by comparing them to accepted standards.

The goal of the medical community is to provide quality health care to all patients regardless of age, sex, race, ethnic origin, or the ability to pay. This care requires that health care workers use techniques and procedures that result in the best possible outcome for patients. In addition, the patient must be satisfied with the care. Medical and nursing ethics exist throughout the system, beginning with the Hippocratic oath to "do no harm." Thus, the foundation for quality health care was laid down centuries ago.

The problem has always been how to ensure that quality care is being delivered in all health care settings. The establishment of standards of care or standards of practice provide a basis for measurement and evaluation. Government agencies conduct periodic surveys to determine if the standards are being met. This chapter explains the purpose of standards of care and quality assurance. It describes the survey and accreditation process and includes guidelines for nursing assistants to follow.

Standards of Care

Standards of care have been established to ensure that patients receive quality health care from all practitioners. This means that a specific health care worker must provide the same knowledge, care, and skill that a similarly trained person would provide under the same circumstances in the same locality. The law requires reasonable, ordinary care that does not expose patients to undue risk. The standards depend on your training, skill, education, and the responsibility given you. If you act outside your area of competence and as a result the patient is injured, you may be guilty of negligence. As a nursing assistant, you should never take on a task or duty for which you have not been trained. Many procedures you perform could result in harm to the patient if not done properly (see Figure 35–1).

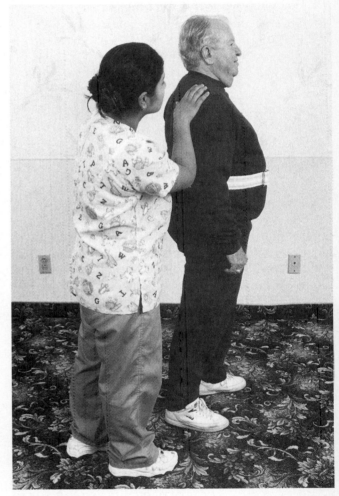

FIGURE 35–1
Many procedures you perform could result in harm to the patient if not done properly.

Guidelines for Following Standards of Care

- Be aware of and protect patient's rights.
- Perform procedures correctly and do not perform procedures that you have not been trained to do.
- Follow facility policies and procedures.
- Follow the care plan for each patient.
- Protect the patient's safety at all times.
- Use aseptic practices and standard precautions with all patients.
- Be aware of cultural diversity.
- Treat all patients with courtesy and respect.
- Document your care accurately.
- Observe and report changes in the patient's condition.
- Perform your duties in an ethical and legal manner.

Quality Assurance

Quality assurance is a program by which health care facilities evaluate the services they provide by comparing them to accepted standards. The program includes methods to identify and correct problems. Patient care is assessed on a continuous basis, and changes are made, as necessary, to improve the quality of care. Medical records such as nursing notes and progress reports are reviewed. Quality assurance programs are required by law in order to achieve and maintain *accreditation* (a process in which a regulatory agency recognizes that a facility has met established standards).

A quality assurance committee, composed of various members of the health care team, is established by the facility. As a nursing assistant, you may be a member of the committee. The role of the committee is to identify issues to be reviewed, perform the assessment and review, and to maintain accurate records. The goal of quality assurance is to improve patient care so that there is no difference between the quality of care desired and the quality of care delivered.

All health care employees play a role in quality assurance. As a nursing assistant, you have a responsibility to report issues that you believe may be harmful to patients. You have a duty to bring patient complaints to the attention of your supervisor. You are also responsible for keeping careful and accurate medical records of the care you provide.

The Survey Process

Health care facilities are regulated by federal and state governmental agencies. These agencies set standards of care for each level of health care. Facilities are licensed by the state in which they operate. Additional certification is necessary if a facility cares for Medicare and Medicaid patients. Legislation provides the basis for many facility policies and procedures that are designed to assure quality care for all patients.

Many different government and private agencies conduct surveys of health care facilities. A survey is a review and evaluation to ensure that standards of care are being met, that patients' rights are being protected, and that quality of life for patients is being enhanced. Each facility is evaluated and given a rating by the survey team. Surveyors review every department of the facility (see Figure 35–2). They evaluate nursing care, safety and infection control, patients' rights, dietary procedures, housekeeping, record keeping, staff to patient ratios, and employee education. The survey team identifies problems and deficiencies and recommends penalties when necessary. The facility is responsible for correcting the problems and deficiencies. Penalties may include fines, license revocation, withdrawal of reimbursement, and closure. The survey team will make follow-up visits to determine if deficiencies have been corrected.

Regulatory Agencies

One of the agencies that regulate health care facilities is the Joint Commission on Accreditation of

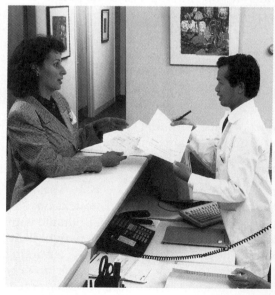

FIGURE 35–2
Surveyors review every department of the facility.

Health Care Organizations (JCAHO). Hospitals must be accredited by this agency in order to receive federal funds, such as Medicare. See Figure 35–3 for the functions evaluated by JCAHO surveyors.

The Health Care Financing Administration (HCFA) is another organization that conducts surveys. This agency has regulatory powers over any health care facility that receives federal funds. The Occupational Safety and Health Administration (OSHA) also does surveys. OSHA has the power to enforce regulations concerning the health and safety of employees. The use of standard precautions is an example of OSHA regulations. The role of OSHA has been addressed in earlier chapters of this textbook.

The survey team will divide into small groups that go to different areas of the facility. They will observe the care, go over the records, interview patients, and talk to staff members. You may be observed while you are providing patient care. Do not be nervous. Surveyors will be looking for the same things your instructor did during your training period. They will observe safety and infection control practices, your communication skills, and

your competency in performing procedures. Attention will be given to how well you protect patient's rights. The surveyor may ask you questions. Answer truthfully and completely, while being mindful of patient confidentiality.

Staff Education and Training

One of the areas that surveyors concentrate on is employee education and training. There are standards relating to orientation, continuing education, and competency. JCAHO, OSHA, and other regulatory agencies require periodic updates on certain topics such as safety, infection control, and patients' rights. These mandatory programs must be presented to all employees on a regular basis. The facility is responsible for maintaining accurate records of attendance.

Program content must meet the curriculum standards set up by the agency. It must be adapted as necessary to meet the needs of a culturally diverse workforce. Staff development nurses who are responsible for the training programs must be sure that information is accurate and current. Skills competencies are evaluated at regular intervals. For example, nursing assistants may be required to demonstrate the ability to correctly measure vital signs.

You are responsible for attending the in-services and training programs offered in your facility. There must be documented records that you have attended all the mandatory programs. Be aware of the in-service calendar and make plans to attend. Pay attention during the program so that you will be an informed, competent employee (see Figure 35–4).

Functions Surveyed for JCAHO Accreditation

Patient-Focused Functions

- Patients' rights
- Organization ethics
- Assessment of patients
- Care of patients
- Education of patients and significant others
- Continuum of care

Organizational Functions

- Improving organizational performance
- Leadership: planning, directing, and integrating services
- Management of the environment of care
- Management of human resources: orientation, training, competence assessment, and staff rights
- Management of information
- Surveillance, prevention, and control of infection
- Governance of the facility
- Management
- Credentialing of medical and nursing staff

FIGURE 35–3 Functions surveyed for JCAHO accreditation.

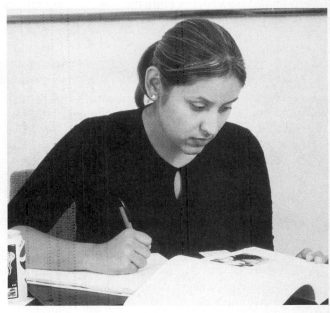

FIGURE 35–4
Pay attention during the in-service programs.

Preparing for a Survey

A health care facility cannot really prepare for a survey because there are so many agencies involved. Sometimes the facility will know the date of an intended survey, but most of the time they will not know. A survey team will suddenly appear, ready to inspect the facility on a normal day. The best way to prepare for a successful survey is to always provide the type of care that meets the standards.

Guidelines for Participating in a Successful Survey

- Follow the guidelines for standards of care given earlier in this chapter.
- Communicate with patients while providing care.
- Maintain a professional appearance.
- Treat each patient as an individual.
- Encourage patient independence.
- Maintain patient privacy and confidentiality.
- Keep patient comfort uppermost in your mind.
- Listen respectfully to patients and report complaints to the nurse immediately.
- Answer call signals promptly and politely.
- Provide empathy and emotional support as necessary.
- Keep your work area neat and clean.
- Be aware of the facility's emergency plan.
- Attend in-services and other training programs.
- Cooperate with other members of the health care team.
- Cooperate with members of the survey team.
- Answer the surveyors' questions completely and truthfully.

Review

Read each sentence and fill in the blank with the vocabulary term that best completes the sentence.

1. _____ have been established to ensure that all similarly trained persons provide quality health care.
2. _____ is a program in which health care facilities evaluate the services they provide by comparing them to accepted standards.
3. A process in which a regulatory agency recognizes that a facility has met established standards is called _____.
4. A/an _____ is a review and evaluation conducted by a regulatory agency in a health care facility to ensure that standards are met.
5. The agency that has the power to enforce regulations concerning the health and safety of employees is called _____.

Remember

1. The goal of the medical community is to provide quality health care to all patients.
2. Standards of care have been established to ensure that patients receive quality health care from all practitioners.
3. The standards depend on your training, skill, education, and the responsibilities given to you.
4. Always perform procedures correctly and do not perform procedures that you have not been trained to do.
5. The goal of the quality assurance committee is to improve patient care so that it meets accepted standards.
6. Federal and state agencies conduct surveys to ensure that standards of care are being met.
7. JCAHO is an agency that accredits health care facilities, which receive federal funds.
8. OSHA is an agency that is concerned with the health and safety of employees.
9. Members of the survey team may observe you while you are providing patient care.
10. There are standards that relate to the orientation, education, and competency of employees.
11. The best way to prepare for a survey is to always provide the type of care that meets the standards.
12. Cooperate with members of the survey team and answer their questions completely and truthfully.

Reflect

Read the following case study and answer the questions.

Case Study

When Angela arrives at work, she learns that the state survey team is in the building. Because she was running late, Angela's appearance is untidy. This makes her feel uncomfortable and nervous. She has trouble concentrating on her work and as the day progresses she falls behind in her duties. One of her patients, Mr. Deal, is in a restorative feeding program. Knowing how slowly he feeds himself, she decides to feed him his lunch. A survey team member, who has been observing her, asks her if Mr. Deal isn't supposed to be feeding himself.

Angela tells the surveyor that Mr. Deal refused to feed himself, although that is not true.

1. How could Angela have avoided getting so nervous and upset at the beginning of her shift?
2. What should Angela have done about Mr. Deal's lunch?
3. Was Angela's response to the surveyor appropriate? Explain your answer.
4. List four guidelines Angela could have followed during the survey?

Respond

Choose the best answer for each question.

1. Quality health care does NOT require that patients be satisfied with their care.
   A. True
   B. False
2. The standards of care that apply to a nursing assistant in Florida are the same as those of
   A. A registered nurse in Florida
   B. A physician in Florida
   C. Another nursing assistant in Florida
   D. All of the above
3. If you act outside your area of competence, and as a result a patient is injured, you could be guilty of
   A. Assault and battery
   B. Invasion of privacy
   C. Negligence
   D. Slander
4. Which of the following is NOT a guideline for following standards of care?
   A. Tell your best friend what a patient did.
   B. Use standard precautions.
   C. Be courteous and respectful.
   D. Document the care you gave.
5. The quality assurance committee is composed of
   A. Doctors
   B. Nurses
   C. Nursing assistants
   D. All of the above

6. What agency is responsible for accrediting hospitals that care for Medicare patients?
   A. JCAHO
   B. OBRA
   C. OSHA
   D. CDC
7. A surveyor hears you say to a patient, "Come on, honey, and let's get you bathed." What did you do wrong?
   A. Nothing. You were trying to be kind.
   B. You violated the patient's right to respect.
   C. You are guilty of negligence.
   D. You violated the patient's right to privacy.
8. You must attend all mandatory in-services.
   A. True
   B. False
9. The best way to prepare for a successful survey is to
   A. Have more employees on duty during the survey
   B. Plan a nice dinner for the survey team
   C. Provide the type of care that meets the standards
   D. Plan special patient activities during the survey
10. Which of the following is a guideline for participating in a successful survey?
    A. Encourage patient independence.
    B. Answer call signals promptly.
    C. Protect patients' rights.
    D. All of the above.

Glossary

A

abandonment   Being left without care or support.

abbreviation   A shortened form for writing a word or phrase.

acceptance stage   The last stage of grief, during which the grieving person is calm and peaceful.

accountability   To accept responsibility for your own actions.

accreditation   A process in which a regulatory agency recognizes that a facility has met accepted standards.

activities of daily living (ADLs)   Personal care activities that individuals usually perform every day.

acute illness   An illness that begins suddenly and continues for a short period of time.

adolescence   The period of life from puberty to adulthood.

advance directive   A document giving instructions regarding a person's desires about health care treatment in the event that he or she is no longer able to voice such desires.

ambulate   To walk.

amputation   Surgical removal of all or part of an extremity.

anatomy   The study of body structure.

anesthesia   The loss of sensation caused by a medication given before surgery.

anesthesiologist   A medical doctor specially trained to administer anesthesia and life support during a surgery.

anger stage   The second stage of grief, during which the grieving person becomes hostile.

aphasia   A loss of speech.

apical pulse   The number of heart beats per minute as heard over the apex of the heart.

asepsis   A condition free from pathogens.

aspiration   Choking due to inhaling food or fluid into the airway.

assault   Any threat to do bodily harm.

assess   To examine or evaluate.

atrophy   A wasting and decrease in size of muscle tissue.

autonomy   The ability to be in control of one's own life.

axilla   The armpit.

B

bargaining stage   The third stage of grief, during which the grieving person attempts to gain more time.

battery   The act of touching another person's body without permission.

biohazardous waste   Material that has been contaminated with blood or body fluids.

blood pressure   A measurement of the amount of force the blood exerts against the artery walls.

bloodborne pathogens   Disease-causing microorganisms that are found in blood, human blood components, any body fluid that contains blood cells, and products made from human blood tissue.

body alignment   Positioning the body in correct anatomical position.

body mechanics   The process of using the body safely and efficiently.

body temperature   A measurement of the amount of heat in the body.

C

calorie   A unit of heat produced as the body oxidizes food.

cardiac arrest   Condition in which the heart stops beating.

cardiopulmonary resuscitation (CPR)   Emergency procedure used to restore heart and lung function.

care plan   A written document outlining the care of an individual patient.

cell   The unit of structure of all animals and plants; the smallest unit of the body that performs all vital life functions. The basic building block of the body.

central processing unit (CPU)   The "brain" or controlling part of a computer.

chain of command   The order of authority within a facility.

chromosomes   Structures found in the nucleus of a cell that contain information that controls heredity.

chronic illness   An illness that progresses slowly, or gradually, over a long period of time.

circumcision   The surgical removal of the foreskin from the penis.

closed bed   A method for making a bed in which the blanket and bedspread cover the sheets.

colostomy   A surgically created opening through the abdominal wall into the colon.

comatose   A condition in which a person is unconscious.

communicable disease   A disease that spreads easily from one person to another.

communication   The exchange of thoughts, information, and ideas.

communication block   Anything that interferes with communication.

communication impairment   A disability that interferes with communication.

competency   The knowledge and skill required to perform tasks correctly.

confidentiality   The act of keeping information about patients private and disclosing it only to appropriate health care team members.

constipation   Infrequent, difficult defecation of hard, dry stool.

contagious   Condition of being easily transmitted.

contamination   The condition of items or areas that have been exposed to disease-causing microorganisms.

contracture   Shortening and wasting of muscle tissue due to lack of use.

convalescence   The period of recovery after an illness or injury.

cross-training   An approach to health care education that involves training a staff member to perform basic skills that have traditionally been considered the responsibility of another member of the health care team.

cyanosis   A bluish discoloration of the skin due to lack of oxygen.

D

dangling   Sitting on the side of the bed with the feet hanging down.

defecation   The process of eliminating solid waste from the body through the anus.

dehydration   Lack of adequate fluid in the body.

delusions   False ideas or beliefs.

dementia   A general impairment of brain function that interferes with normal social and occupational activities.

denial stage   The first stage of grief, during which the grieving person refuses to believe what is happening.

dentures   A partial or complete set of artificial teeth.

depression stage   The fourth stage of grief, during which the grieving person becomes saddened and quiet.

dialysis   Artificial filtration of waste products from the blood.

diastole   The stage of the cardiac cycle during which the heart is relaxing and filling with blood.

diastolic pressure   A measurement of blood pressure against the artery wall when the heart is relaxing between beats (diastole).

digestion   The process of physical and chemical breakdown of food so that it can be used by the body.

disinfection   The process of destroying pathogens on objects and surfaces.

disoriented   Confused as to time, place, and/or person.

dysphagia   Difficulty chewing and swallowing.

dyspnea   Labored or difficult breathing.

dysuria   Painful urination or difficulty urinating.

E

edema   Swelling of a body part due to fluid in the tissues.

emaciated   Excessively thin.

embolus   A blood clot that breaks loose and travels through the bloodstream.

emesis   Vomitus.

emesis basin   A small, kidney-shaped pan used for oral care, spitting, or vomiting.

empathy   The ability to share another person's point of view and understand his or her feelings.

empowerment   To give power to a person; to enable a person to make decisions independently.

enema   Procedure to introduce fluid into the lower colon and rectum for the purpose of removing feces.

environment   The surroundings, conditions, and influences that affect an organism.

epidemic   The incidence of an infectious disease affecting a large number of people in a certain area.

ethics   Guidelines for right and wrong behavior.

F

false imprisonment   The act of restricting or restraining a person's movements without proper consent.

fecal impaction   A large amount of hard, dry, stool overloading the bowel.

feces   The solid waste products that remain after the body has absorbed all nutrients and water from ingested food.

fetus   The developing unborn child, from the eighth week of pregnancy to birth.

fever   A body temperature that is above normal.

first aid   The immediate care given for injury or sudden illness.

flaccid   A condition of having little or no muscle tone; limp or flabby.

flatus   Air or gas expelled from the digestive tract.

flexibility   The ability to adjust to change.

Fowler's position   A sitting or semi-sitting position.

fracture   A break in a bone.

G

gatch handle   Crank handle located at the foot of a hospital bed, used for changing bed positions.

geriatric   Refers to the aging person.

gerontology   The branch of science that studies aging.

glossary   A collection of specialized terms with the meaning of each term.

graduate   A calibrated container for measuring fluids.

gurney   A type of stretcher or carrier used to transport patients.

H

hallucinations   False perception unrelated to reality; may be seeing, hearing, or smelling nonexistent things.

hardware   The physical equipment used by a computer to process data.

Heimlich Maneuver   Procedure performed to dislodge a foreign body from the airway.

hemiplegia   The condition of paralysis of one side of the body.

hemorrhage   Severe bleeding.

heredity   Characteristics passed down from one's ancestors.

HIV (human immunodeficiency virus) infection   A disease that destroys the immune system and leaves the body unable to fight infection.

holistic health care   An approach to health care in which the whole person is treated, both physically and emotionally. It involves treatment of both the physical illness and the person's emotional response to the illness.

homemaker   A person who performs household duties.

hormones   Chemicals secreted by the endocrine glands directly into the bloodstream. These chemicals regulate and control the functions of other organs and glands.

hospice   A type of health care agency that treats patients who are terminally ill and offers support services to their families.

humanistic health care   An approach to health care in which each person is treated as an individual. A person's culture and beliefs are considered as well as their illness or disease.

hydration   The amount of fluid in the body.

hygiene   The observance of rules for health and cleanliness.

hyperglycemia   A condition of abnormally high glucose levels in the blood; high blood sugar.

hypertension   A condition of consistently elevated blood pressure above 140/90; high blood pressure.

hypoglycemia   A condition of abnormally low glucose levels in the blood; low blood sugar.

hypotension   An abnormally low blood pressure reading.

I

immobilize   To position a limb or body part to prevent movement.

immunization   A procedure to make a person more resistant to a specific disease.

incident report   A specific form used for recording the details surrounding an accident or error.

incontinence   The inability to control urine or feces.

infection The invasion and growth of disease-causing microorganisms in the body.

infectious Capable of spreading infection.

inflammation The body's response to injury or disease, evident by the presence of redness, swelling, heat, and pain.

initiative The power or right to take independent action in a situation.

intake and output (I & O) A record of all fluids taken into the body and all fluids eliminated from the body.

integrated care team The group of people directly involved in the care of the home health patient.

integrity The state of being whole or complete.

integument The anatomical name for the skin.

intimacy A personal relationship involving love or affection.

intravenous (I.V.) A needle or special catheter placed within a vein.

intubation The insertion of a tube into the trachea to provide a pathway for air to enter the lungs.

invasion of privacy Failure to protect a person's body from exposure or failure to keep personal information confidential.

isolation The practice of separating the infected patient from others to prevent the spread of infection.

J

job description A list of tasks and responsibilities to be performed in a certain job.

L

lateral position Lying on either side.

lesion A wound or sore.

licensed practical nurse (LPN) Health care team member who is educated and licensed to assist the registered nurse in planning and providing nursing care.

M

maternity care The health care of the pregnant woman before, during, and after childbirth.

mechanical ventilator A machine that provides artificial respiration of the lungs.

Medicaid State-funded program designed to help meet the medical needs of low-income families.

Medicare Federal program that helps provide medical and hospital care to persons who are 65 years or older or are permanently disabled.

menarche A female's first menstrual period.

menopause The period of life when menstrual periods cease.

menstruation The periodic discharge of the lining of the uterus when fertilization of the egg does not occur.

mentor A trusted, experienced person who influences, guides, and directs another person.

metabolism The processes of physical and chemical change within the cell that produces energy for growth and repair.

microorganism General term for any small plant or animal that cannot be seen without the aid of a microscope.

mobility One's ability to move about.

motivation The internal feeling or external stimulus causing one to take action.

N

N.P.O. Abbreviation for the Latin phrase, "non per os," which means "nothing by mouth."

negligence Failure to give proper care, which results in harm to the patient or the patient's property.

neonate An infant in the first six weeks of life.

networking Communicating and interacting with people who have common interests and goals.

nocturia Excessive urination during the night.

nonpathogens Microorganisms that are not harmful and do not cause infection.

nonverbal communication The exchange of information without using words.

normal flora Microorganisms that live and grow in certain locations of the body.

nursing assistant (N.A.) Health care team member who provides care for the patients under the supervision of a nurse.

nutrients Substances contained in foods that are necessary for metabolism.

nutrition The intake and metabolism of food by the body.

O

obese Condition of excess fat resulting in the individual being more than 20% to 30% over ideal body weight.

objective observations Information that can be observed by seeing, hearing, smelling, or touching.

observation The process of noticing facts and events.

occupied bed A method of bedmaking in which the linens are changed while the patient remains in the bed.

Omnibus Budget Reconciliation Act (OBRA) Federal act whose purpose is to improve the quality of health care. This act addresses the safety, happiness, and well-being of patients.

open bed A method of bedmaking in which the top linens are turned down for a patient who will be returning to the bed soon.

oral hygiene Cleaning and care of the mouth, teeth, and gums.

organ A group of similar tissues that work together to perform a particular function.

organize To arrange information, tasks, or things in an orderly manner.

ostomy A surgical procedure to form an artificial opening from an organ to an exit site.

oxygen A colorless, odorless, gas, that is essential to life.

P

P.O. Abbreviation for the Latin phrase "per os," which means "by mouth."

paralysis The inability to move a body part.

paranoia Suspicious thinking that one is being treated wrongly, harassed, or persecuted.

paraplegia The condition of paralysis of the lower half of the body.

pathogens Harmful microorganisms that can cause infection upon entering a person's body.

patient's bill of rights A list of the basic rights to which all patients are entitled. Such lists exist for different health care settings.

pediatrics   The branch of medicine concerned with the care of infants and children.

peers   Those who have equal standing in age or rank.

perineal care (peri-care)   Cleansing the genital and anal areas.

peristalsis   The wavelike muscular contractions of the digestive system that propel food through the digestive tract.

physiology   The study of body function.

pollution   Contamination of the environment.

postmortem care   Care of the body after death.

postoperative (post-op)   Refers to a period after a surgery.

postpartum   The period of time following the delivery of a baby.

prefix   The element of a medical term found at the beginning of the word.

prejudice   A dislike or hatred of a particular culture, race, or group of people.

preoperative (pre-op)   Refers to the period prior to a surgery.

pressure ulcer   A breakdown of skin tissue caused by the interruption of blood flow to the area.

priority, prioritize   To arrange information or tasks in their order of importance.

prone position   Lying on the abdomen with the face downward or to the side.

prosthesis   A device that replaces or assists the function of a body part.

psychosocial   Related to emotional, mental, spiritual, sexual, and social factors.

puberty   The developmental period of life in which secondary sex characteristics appear and reproduction can occur.

pulse   Heartbeat felt as blood pushes through arteries.

Q

quadriplegia   The condition of paralysis of both arms and legs.

quality assurance   A program in which health care facilities evaluate the services they provide by comparing them to accepted standards.

R

range-of-motion exercises   Movements of joints through the normal area of movement.

rapport   Mutual trust.

reality orientation   A technique used with confused patients involving repeated verbal and nonverbal information to remind them of time, place, and person.

recording   Writing information on the correct form; also called charting or documenting.

registered nurse (RN)   Health care team member who is educated and licensed to assess, plan, provide, coordinate, and evaluate nursing care.

rehabilitation   The process of restoring the patient to as nearly normal function as possible.

reporting   The act of communicating information to the proper person.

respiration   Breathing; the process of inspiration and expiration.

respiratory arrest   A condition in which breathing stops.

respite care   A program to provide relief for the caregiver.

restorative care   A type of nursing care that assists patients in meeting their needs as independently as possible.

restraint   Any device that restricts movement or normal access to one's body.

resume   A brief, written summary of an individual's work experiences and qualifications.

root   The element of a medical term that represents the foundation of the word.

S

seizure   The sudden contraction of muscles caused by abnormal brain activity, also called a convulsion.

self-actualization   To prove oneself as real or worthy; self-fulfillment.

sexually transmitted disease (STD)   A disease in which the major route of transmission is through sexual contact.

shunt   A connection between two blood vessels.

slander   To injure the name and reputation of another person by making a false statement.

software   The programs or sets of instruction that make a computer work.

specimen   A sample of fluid or tissue from a person's body.

sphygmomanometer   An instrument for measuring blood pressure.

spirituality   The relationship with one's self, nature, and a supreme being.

sputum   Mucus from the lungs.

standard precautions   Procedures to be used with all patients to protect the health care worker against exposure to blood, body fluids, and body substances.

sterile   The condition of being free from all microorganisms.

stethoscope   An instrument that amplifies body sounds.

stoma   The artificially created opening of an ostomy on the outside of the body.

stress   Mental and physical tension or strain.

subjective observations   Information that cannot be observed but must be communicated and described by the person experiencing it.

suffix   The element of a medical term found at the end of the word.

suffocation   A condition in which breathing stops due to lack of oxygen.

sundowner's syndrome   A condition in which confusion and agitation increase as the evening progresses.

supine position   Lying on the back with the face up.

suppository   A cone-shaped, semi-solid substance inserted in the rectum where it dissolves.

surgical bed   A method of bedmaking in which the top linens are folded to the side of the bed to accommodate the patient's return from surgery.

susceptible   One who is likely to develop an infection or disease when exposed to pathogens.

system   A group of organs that work together to perform one or more functions.

systole   The stage of the cardiac cycle during which the heart is contracting and pumping blood out through the blood vessels.

systolic pressure   A measurement of blood pressure against the artery wall when the heart is contracting (systole).

T

terminal illness An illness in which recovery is not expected.

thrombus A stationary blood clot.

tissue A group of similar cells that work together to perform a specific function.

toxic Capable of causing poisonous reactions.

tracheostomy A surgical opening into the windpipe to promote unobstructed breathing.

transmission-based precautions Procedures used when a patient is known to be infected or suspected of being infected with certain contagious diseases or conditions.

tympanic membrane Thin layer of tissue separating the outer ear from the middle ear; eardrum.

U

umbilicus The scar that marks the former attachment of the umbilical cord; the navel or belly button.

unlicensed assistive personnel (UAP) Unlicensed health care workers who assist nurses in providing patient care.

urinal A container into which male patients urinate.

V

validation therapy A technique used to encourage confused patients to explore their thoughts.

ventilate To supply the lungs with air.

verbal communication The exchange of thoughts, ideas, and information, using words.

vital signs Measurements of temperature, pulse, respiration, and blood pressure.

void To expel urine.

Anatomy *and* Physiology

ILLUSTRATIONS

PLATE 1:

MUSCULOSKELETAL SYSTEM

Skeleton

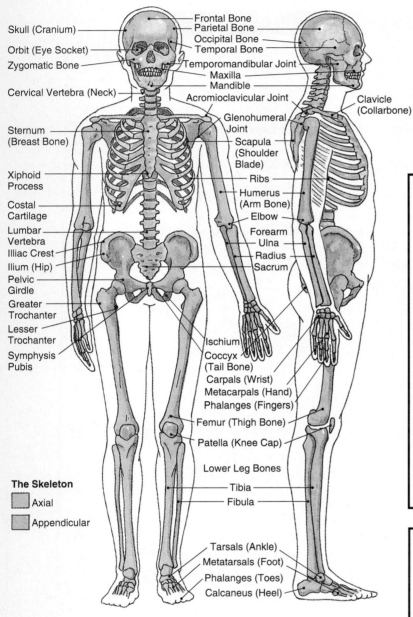

Skull (Cranium)
Orbit (Eye Socket)
Zygomatic Bone
Cervical Vertebra (Neck)
Sternum (Breast Bone)
Xiphoid Process
Costal Cartilage
Lumbar Vertebra
Illiac Crest
Ilium (Hip)
Pelvic Girdle
Greater Trochanter
Lesser Trochanter
Symphysis Pubis

Frontal Bone
Parietal Bone
Occipital Bone
Temporal Bone
Temporomandibular Joint
Maxilla
Mandible
Acromioclavicular Joint
Glenohumeral Joint
Scapula (Shoulder Blade)
Ribs
Humerus (Arm Bone)
Elbow
Forearm
Ulna
Radius
Sacrum

Clavicle (Collarbone)

Ischium
Coccyx (Tail Bone)
Carpals (Wrist)
Metacarpals (Hand)
Phalanges (Fingers)
Femur (Thigh Bone)
Patella (Knee Cap)
Lower Leg Bones
Tibia
Fibula

The Skeleton
☐ Axial
☐ Appendicular

Tarsals (Ankle)
Metatarsals (Foot)
Phalanges (Toes)
Calcaneus (Heel)

The skeleton is a living framework made by the joining of bones. It serves to provide support, body movement powered by muscular contractions, protection for the vital organs and other soft structures, blood cell production, and storage for essential minerals. There are 206 bones in the adult body, forming the two divisions of the skeletal system. The axial skeleton is comprised of skull, vertebrae, rib cage, and sternum. The upper and lower extremeties and the shoulder and pelvic girdles form the appendicular skeleton.

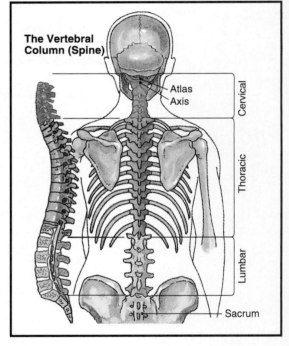

The Vertebral Column (Spine)

Atlas
Axis

Cervical
Thoracic
Lumbar

Sacrum

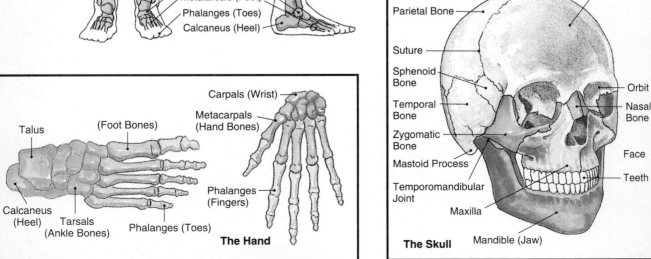

Talus
(Foot Bones)
Calcaneus (Heel)
Tarsals (Ankle Bones)
Phalanges (Toes)

Carpals (Wrist)
Metacarpals (Hand Bones)
Phalanges (Fingers)
The Hand

Cranium
Parietal Bone
Suture
Sphenoid Bone
Temporal Bone
Zygomatic Bone
Mastoid Process
Temporomandibular Joint
Maxilla
Mandible (Jaw)

Frontal Bone
Orbit
Nasal Bone
Face
Teeth

The Skull

PLATE 2:

MUSCULOSKELETAL SYSTEM

Muscles

The tissues of the muscular system comprise 40% to 50% of the body's weight. The skeletal muscles of the body are voluntary muscles, subject to conscious control. They exhibit the properties of excitability; that is, they will react to nerve stimulus. Once stimulated, skeletal muscles are quick to contract and can relax and very quickly be ready for another contraction. There are 501 separate skeletal muscles that provide contractions for movement, coordinated support for posture, and heat production. Muscles connect to bones by way of tendons.

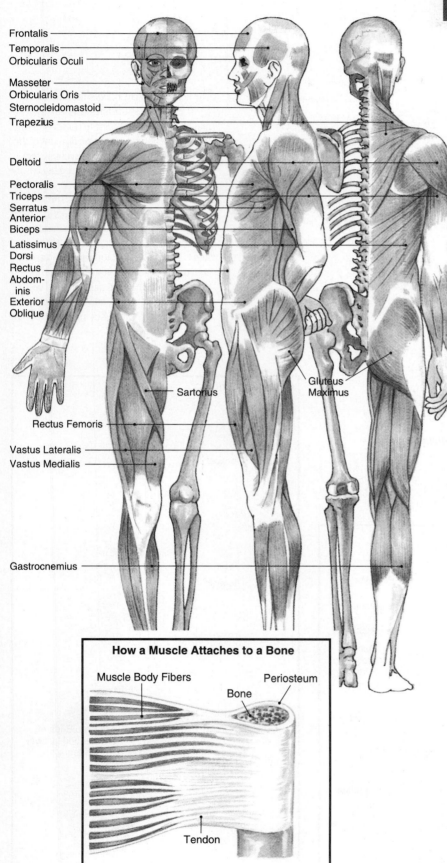

Frontalis
Temporalis
Orbicularis Oculi

Masseter
Orbicularis Oris
Sternocleidomastoid
Trapezius

Deltoid

Pectoralis
Triceps
Serratus Anterior
Biceps

Latissimus Dorsi
Rectus Abdominis
Exterior Oblique

Sartorius

Gluteus Maximus

Rectus Femoris

Vastus Lateralis
Vastus Medialis

Gastrocnemius

How a Muscle Attaches to a Bone

Muscle Body Fibers

Periosteum

Bone

Tendon

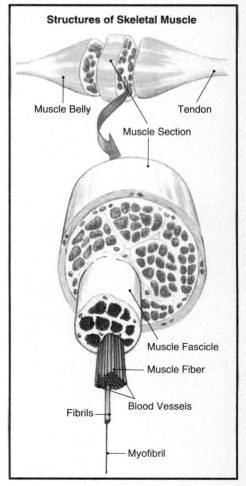

Structures of Skeletal Muscle

Muscle Belly

Tendon

Muscle Section

Muscle Fascicle

Muscle Fiber

Blood Vessels

Fibrils

Myofibril

PLATE 3:

NERVOUS SYSTEM

Brain and Spine

The Brain

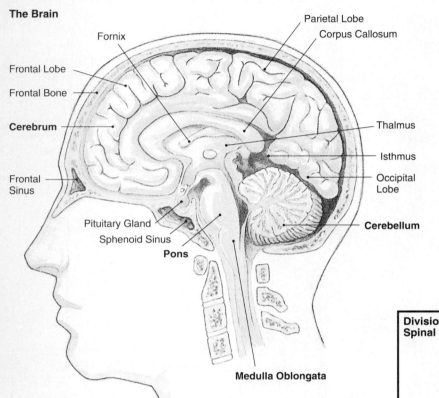

The nervous system includes the brain, spinal cord, and nerves. Structures within the system may be classified according to divisions: central, peripheral, and autonomic divisions of the nervous system. The central nervous system includes the brain and spinal cord. The sensory (incoming) and motor (outgoing) nerves make up the peripheral nervous system. The autonomic nervous system has structures that parallel the spinal cord and then share the same pathways as the peripheral nerves. This division is involved with motor impulses (outgoing commands) that travel from the central nervous system to the heart muscle, blood vessels, secreting cells of glands, and the smooth muscles of organs. The impulses will stimulate or inhibit certain activities.

The Spinal Cord

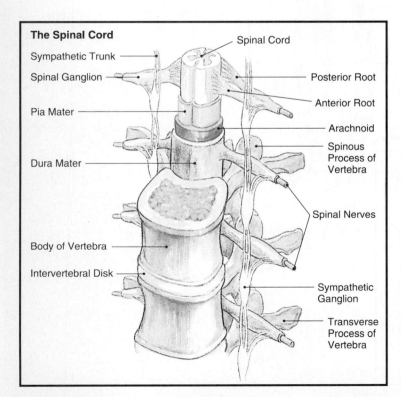

Divisions of the Spinal Cord

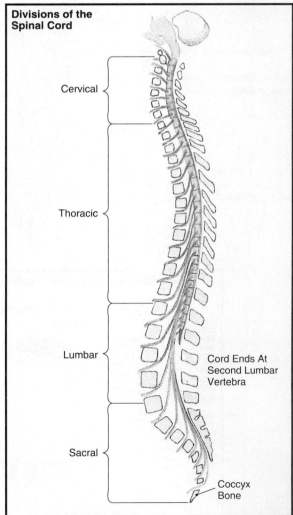

PLATE 4:

NERVOUS SYSTEM

Nerves

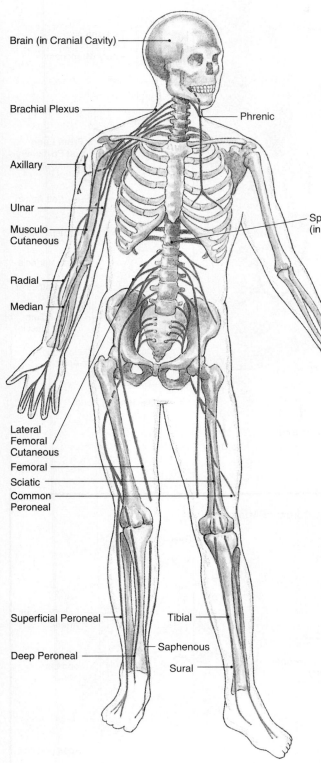

Brain (in Cranial Cavity)

Brachial Plexus

Phrenic

Axillary

Ulnar

Musculo Cutaneous

Spinal Cord (in Spinal Cavity)

Radial

Median

Lateral Femoral Cutaneous

Femoral

Sciatic

Common Peroneal

Superficial Peroneal

Tibial

Deep Peroneal

Saphenous

Sural

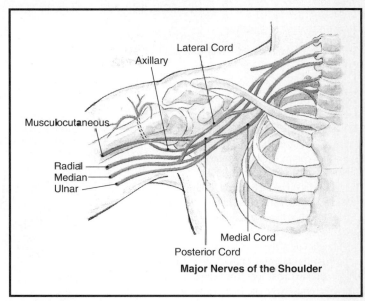

Lateral Cord

Axillary

Musculocutaneous

Radial
Median
Ulnar

Medial Cord

Posterior Cord

Major Nerves of the Shoulder

AUTONOMIC NERVOUS SYSTEM

The autonomic nervous system affects the heart, blood vessels, digestive tract, salivary and digestive glands, pancreas, liver, spleen, anal sphincter, kidneys, urinary bladder, urinary sphincter, adrenal glands, thyroid gland, gonads, genitalia, nasal lining, larynx, bronchi, lungs, iris and ciliary muscles of the eyes, tear glands, and hair muscles. Impulses can increase or slow heart rate, stimulate dilation or constriction of blood vessels, cause glands to secrete or decrease secretion, initiate or inhibit contractions in the bladder, stimulate or decrease a wave of muscle contraction along the digestive tract, and many other essential body activities.

Sympathetic (partial representation)   **Parasympathetic**

Dilates

Constricts

Brain Stem

Spinal Cord

Cillary Ganglion

Dilates Bronchi

Constricts Bronchi

Accelerates

Celiac Ganglion

Slows Rate

Decreases Gastric Juices

Increases Gastric Juices

Sympathetic Trunk

PLATE 5:

CARDIOVASCULAR SYSTEM

Heart

The heart is a hollow, muscular organ that pumps 450 million pints of blood in the average lifetime. Its superior chambers, the atria, receive blood. Both atria fill and then contract at the same time. The inferior chambers are the ventricles. They pump blood out of the heart. Both ventricles fill and then contract at the same time. When the atria are relaxing, the ventricles are contracting.

The right side of the heart receives blood from the body and sends it to the lungs (pulmonic circulation). The heart's left side receives oxygenated blood from the lungs and sends it out to the body (systemic circulation).

The heartbeat originates at the sinoatrial node (pacemaker) and spreads across the atria to stimulate contraction. After a slight delay, the impulse is sent from the atrioventricular node, down the bundles of His, and out across the ventricles. This stimulates the ventricles to contract while the atria are relaxing.

The heart muscle (myocardium) receives its blood supply by way of the right and left coronary arteries. These vessels are the first branches of the aorta.

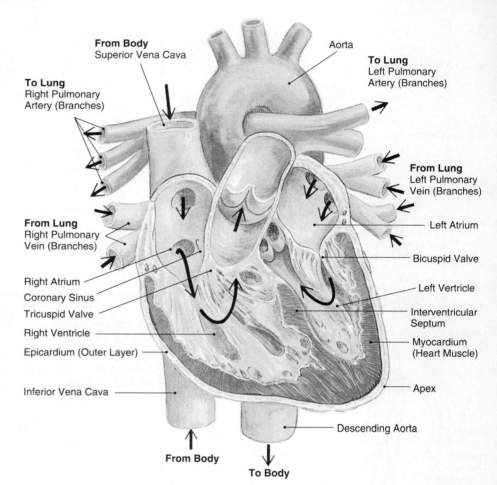

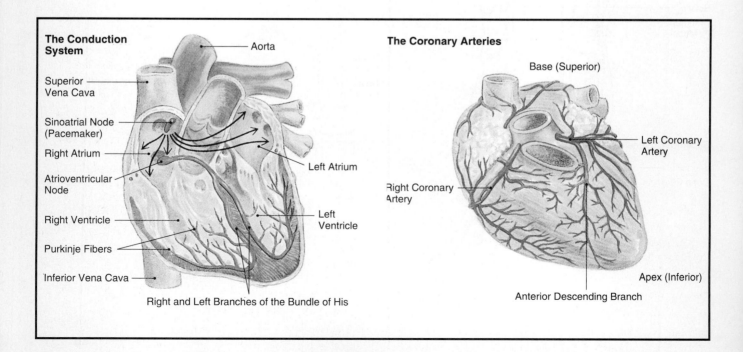

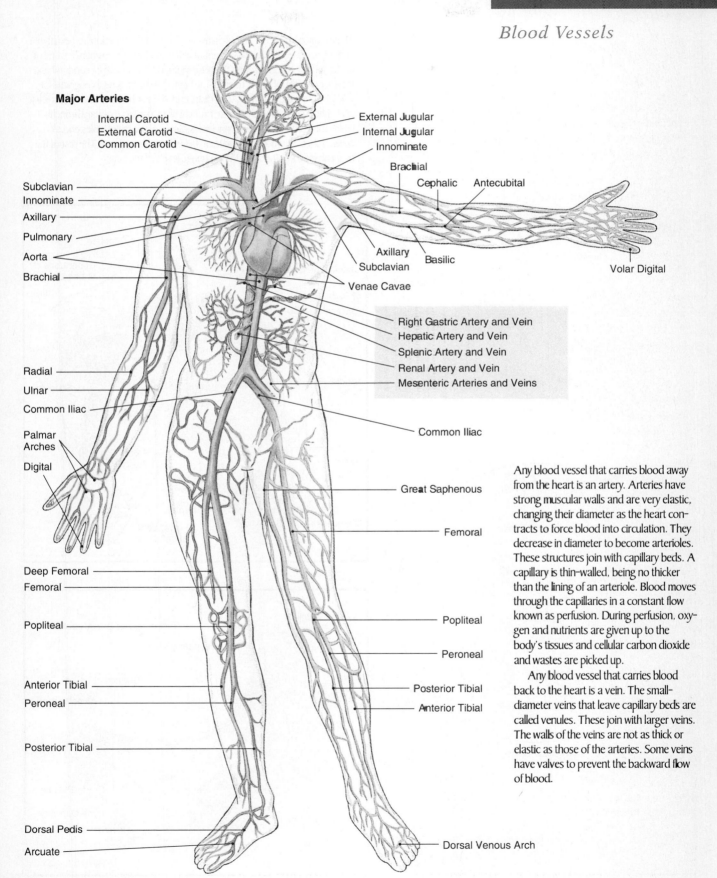

Major Arteries

Internal Carotid
External Carotid
Common Carotid

External Jugular
Internal Jugular
Innominate
Brachial
Cephalic   Antecubital

Subclavian
Innominate
Axillary
Pulmonary
Aorta
Brachial

Axillary
Subclavian   Basilic
Venae Cavae

Volar Digital

Right Gastric Artery and Vein
Hepatic Artery and Vein
Splenic Artery and Vein
Renal Artery and Vein
Mesenteric Arteries and Veins

Radial
Ulnar
Common Iliac

Palmar
Arches
Digital

Common Iliac

Great Saphenous

Femoral

Deep Femoral
Femoral

Popliteal

Popliteal

Peroneal

Anterior Tibial
Peroneal

Posterior Tibial
Anterior Tibial

Posterior Tibial

Dorsal Pedis

Arcuate

Dorsal Venous Arch

Any blood vessel that carries blood away from the heart is an artery. Arteries have strong muscular walls and are very elastic, changing their diameter as the heart contracts to force blood into circulation. They decrease in diameter to become arterioles. These structures join with capillary beds. A capillary is thin-walled, being no thicker than the lining of an arteriole. Blood moves through the capillaries in a constant flow known as perfusion. During perfusion, oxygen and nutrients are given up to the body's tissues and cellular carbon dioxide and wastes are picked up.

Any blood vessel that carries blood back to the heart is a vein. The small-diameter veins that leave capillary beds are called venules. These join with larger veins. The walls of the veins are not as thick or elastic as those of the arteries. Some veins have valves to prevent the backward flow of blood.

PLATE 7:

RESPIRATORY SYSTEM

The airway consists of structures involved with the conduction and exchange of air. Conduction is the movement of air to and from the exchange levels of the lungs. Air enters through the nose (primary) and mouth (secondary) and travels down the pharynx to enter the larynx. After passing through the larynx, air enters the trachea. At its distal end, the trachea branches into the left and right primary bronchi. These bronchi branch into secondary bronchi, which then branch into the bronchioles. Some of the bronchioles end as closed tubes. Air movement in them helps the lungs expand. The rest of the bronchioles carry the air to the exchange levels of the lungs.

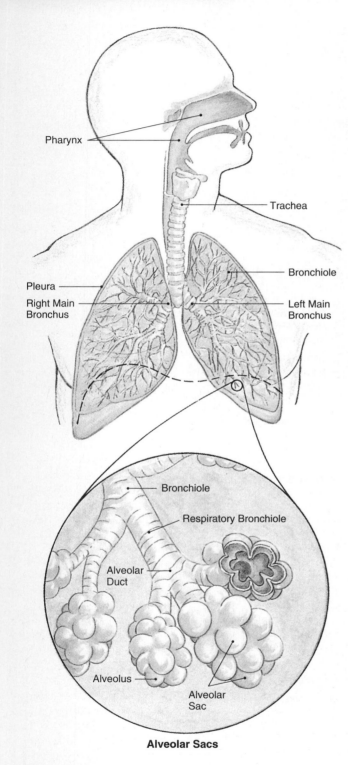

Pharynx

Trachea

Pleura

Bronchiole

Right Main Bronchus

Left Main Bronchus

Bronchiole

Respiratory Bronchiole

Alveolar Duct

Alveolus

Alveolar Sac

Alveolar Sacs

The respiratory bronchioles turn into alveolar ducts. These form alveolar sacs that are made up of the alveoli. Gas exchange takes place between the alveoli and the capillaries in the lungs.

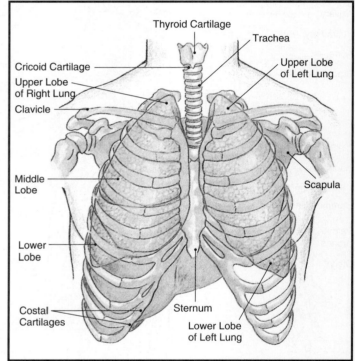

Thyroid Cartilage

Trachea

Cricoid Cartilage

Upper Lobe of Left Lung

Upper Lobe of Right Lung

Clavicle

Middle Lobe

Scapula

Lower Lobe

Costal Cartilages

Sternum

Lower Lobe of Left Lung

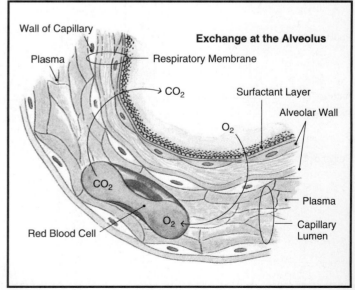

Wall of Capillary

Exchange at the Alveolus

Plasma

Respiratory Membrane

CO_2

Surfactant Layer

O_2

Alveolar Wall

CO_2

O_2

Plasma

Red Blood Cell

Capillary Lumen

DIGESTIVE SYSTEM

The digestive system includes the digestive tract and various supportive structures and accessory glands. The tract begins at the oral cavity with the teeth and tongue. The salivary glands release saliva into the mouth to moisten food for swallowing. The tract continues down the throat to the esophagus, through the cardiac sphincter, and into the stomach. Acid and digestive enzymes are added to the food to produce chyme. The chyme passes through the pyloric sphincter to enter the small intestine. Digestive enzymes from the pancreas and bile from the liver are added to the chyme. The processes of digestion and absorption are completed in the small intestine. Wastes are carried through the ileocecal valve into the large intestine. The wastes are moved to the rectum, from where they can be expelled through the anus.

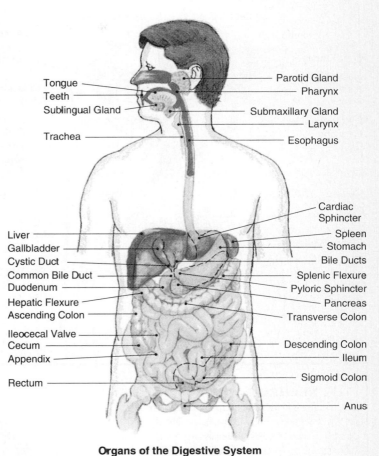

Organs of the Digestive System

Liver, Stomach, and Pancreas

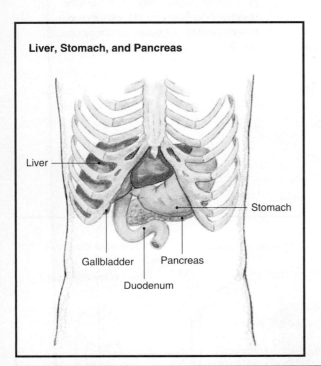

Small Intestine

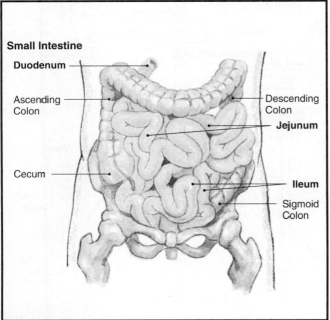

Large Intestine

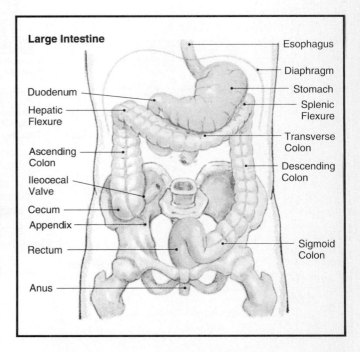

PLATE 9:

Urinary System

Organs of the Urinary System

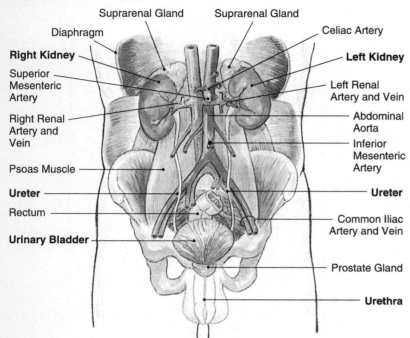

- Diaphragm
- Suprarenal Gland
- Suprarenal Gland
- Celiac Artery
- **Right Kidney**
- **Left Kidney**
- Superior Mesenteric Artery
- Left Renal Artery and Vein
- Right Renal Artery and Vein
- Abdominal Aorta
- Inferior Mesenteric Artery
- Psoas Muscle
- **Ureter**
- **Ureter**
- Rectum
- Common Iliac Artery and Vein
- **Urinary Bladder**
- Prostate Gland
- **Urethra**

The urinary system is part of the body's excretory structures (urinary system, lungs, sweat glands, and intestine). The kidneys remove the wastes of chemical activities (metabolism) in the body. These wastes are removed from the blood to produce urine. At the same time, the kidneys remove certain excess compounds, regulate the blood pH (acid−base balance), and the concentration of sodium, potassium, chlorine, glucose, and other important chemicals.

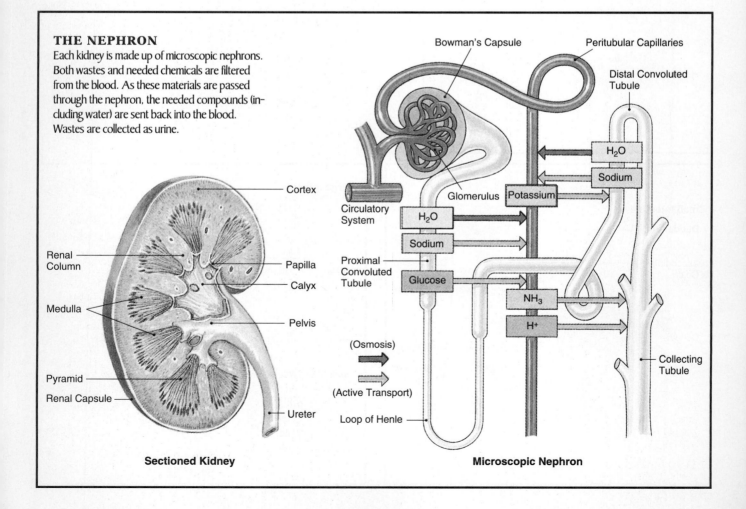

THE NEPHRON
Each kidney is made up of microscopic nephrons. Both wastes and needed chemicals are filtered from the blood. As these materials are passed through the nephron, the needed compounds (including water) are sent back into the blood. Wastes are collected as urine.

- Bowman's Capsule
- Peritubular Capillaries
- Distal Convoluted Tubule
- H_2O
- Sodium
- Glomerulus
- Potassium
- Circulatory System
- H_2O
- Sodium
- Cortex
- Renal Column
- Papilla
- Calyx
- Proximal Convoluted Tubule
- Glucose
- NH_3
- Medulla
- H^+
- Pelvis
- (Osmosis)
- (Active Transport)
- Pyramid
- Renal Capsule
- Collecting Tubule
- Ureter
- Loop of Henle

Sectioned Kidney

Microscopic Nephron

The reproductive system consists of the organs, glands, and supportive structures that are involved with human sexuality and procreation. In the male, spermatozoa and the hormone testosterone are produced in the testes. The female produces ova (eggs) and the hormones estrogen and progesterone in her ovaries. The union of ovum and sperm produce a single cell called a zygote. Through growth, cell division, and cellular differentiation (the formulation of specialized cells) the new individual develops and matures.

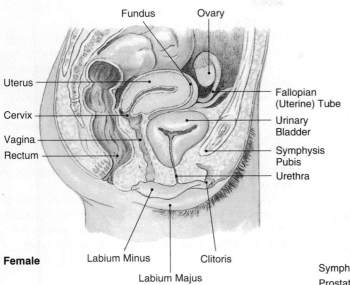

Female

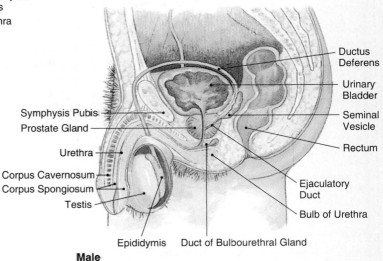

Male

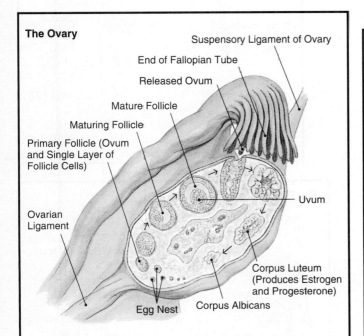

The Ovary

The developing ovum and its supportive cells are called a follicle. Each month, follicle–stimulating hormone (FSH) from the pituitary gland starts the growth of several follicles. Usually, only one will mature and release an ovum (ovulation). During its growth, the follicle produces estrogen. After ovulation, the remaining cells of the follicle form a specialized structure that produces both estrogen and progesterone.

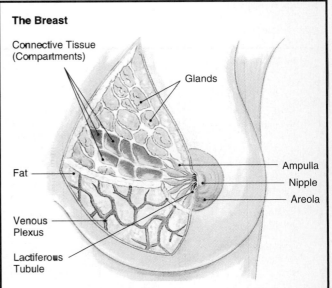

The Breast

The breasts contain the mammary glands that produce milk (lactation). A mammary gland is a highly modified form of sweat gland. Estrogen stimulates the growth of the ducts, while progesterone stimulates the development of the secreting (milk-producing) cells. Lactic hormone from the pituitary stimulates milk production. Another pituitary hormone, oxytocin, stimulates the milk-producing cells to eject their milk into the ducts.

PLATE II:

INTEGUMENTARY SYSTEM

The Skin

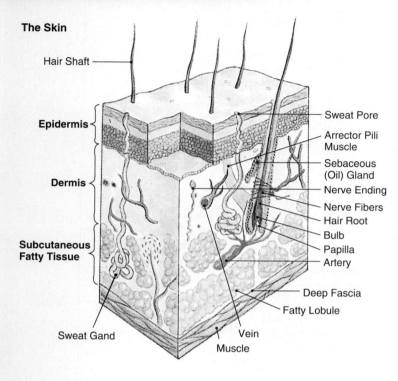

- Hair Shaft
- Epidermis
- Dermis
- Subcutaneous Fatty Tissue
- Sweat Gand
- Sweat Pore
- Arrector Pili Muscle
- Sebaceous (Oil) Gland
- Nerve Ending
- Nerve Fibers
- Hair Root
- Bulb
- Papilla
- Artery
- Deep Fascia
- Fatty Lobule
- Vein
- Muscle

SKIN

The skin is the largest organ of the body. In the adult the skin covers about 3000 square inches (1.75 square meters) and weighs about 6 pounds. It is involved with protection, insulation, thermal regulation, excretion, and the production of vitamin D.

The Peritoneum

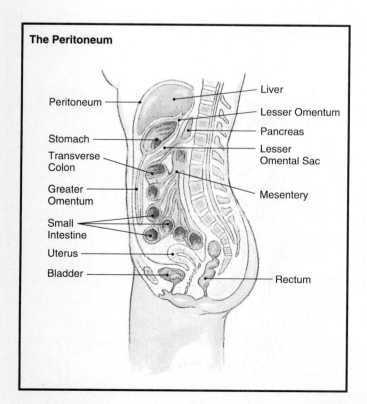

- Peritoneum
- Stomach
- Transverse Colon
- Greater Omentum
- Small Intestine
- Uterus
- Bladder
- Liver
- Lesser Omentum
- Pancreas
- Lesser Omental Sac
- Mesentery
- Rectum

MEMBRANES

Membranes cover or line body structures to provide protection from injury and infection. There are four major classes of membranes. Mucous membranes line those structures that open to the outside world (for example, the mouth, the airway, digestive tract, urinary tract, and vagina). Serous membranes line the closed body cavities and cover the outsides of organs. The cutaneous membrane is the skin. Synovial membranes line joints to reduce friction during movement.

A serous membrane that covers an organ is called a visceral layer. The term parietal layer is used for the part of the serous membrane that lines a cavity. The serous membrane in the thoracic cavity is called pleura (for example, the parietal pleura lines the chest cavity). In the abdominal cavity, it is called peritoneum (for example, the parietal peritoneum). A double layer of peritoneum is called mesentery. The membrane that lines the sac surrounding the heart is pericardium.

Synovial Joint

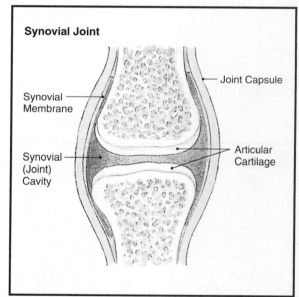

- Synovial Membrane
- Synovial (Joint) Cavity
- Joint Capsule
- Articular Cartilage

The Pleura

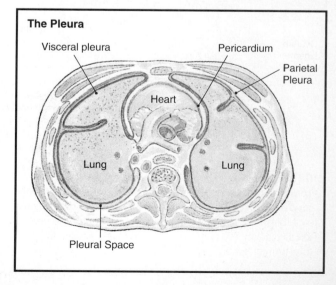

- Visceral pleura
- Pericardium
- Parietal Pleura
- Heart
- Lung
- Lung
- Pleural Space

The Eye

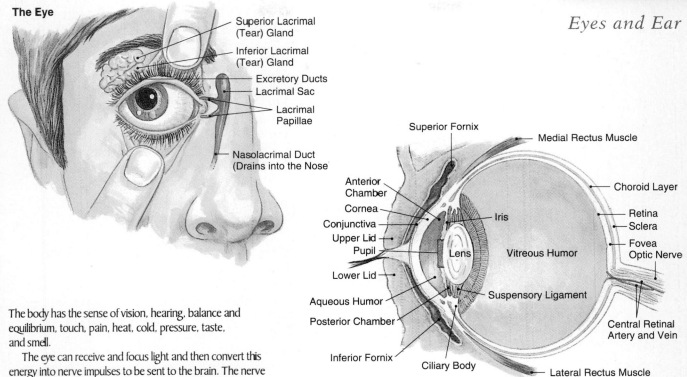

Superior Lacrimal (Tear) Gland

Inferior Lacrimal (Tear) Gland

Excretory Ducts
Lacrimal Sac

Lacrimal Papillae

Nasolacrimal Duct (Drains into the Nose)

Superior Fornix

Medial Rectus Muscle

Choroid Layer

Anterior Chamber

Retina
Sclera

Cornea

Iris

Conjunctiva

Upper Lid

Fovea
Optic Nerve

Pupil

Lens

Vitreous Humor

Lower Lid

Aqueous Humor

Suspensory Ligament

Posterior Chamber

Central Retinal Artery and Vein

Inferior Fornix

Ciliary Body

Lateral Rectus Muscle

The body has the sense of vision, hearing, balance and equilibrium, touch, pain, heat, cold, pressure, taste, and smell.

The eye can receive and focus light and then convert this energy into nerve impulses to be sent to the brain. The nerve impulses originate from the retina. Visual receptors in the retina called rods can work in low intensity light. They have no color function. The visual receptors called cones operate in high-intensity light and do receive colors.

The ear's functions include hearing, static equilibrium (balance while standing still), and dynamic equilibrium (balance when moving). The outer and middle ear are responsible for sound gathering and its transmission. The inner ear has the nerve endings for hearing and equilibrium.

The Ear

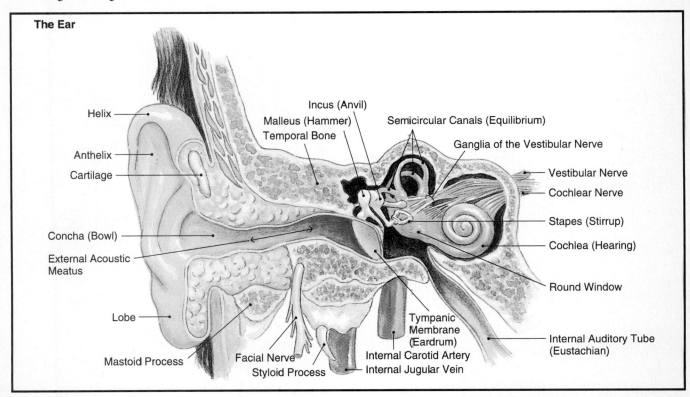

Helix

Incus (Anvil)

Malleus (Hammer)
Temporal Bone

Semicircular Canals (Equilibrium)

Ganglia of the Vestibular Nerve

Anthelix

Cartilage

Vestibular Nerve
Cochlear Nerve

Stapes (Stirrup)

Concha (Bowl)

Cochlea (Hearing)

External Acoustic Meatus

Round Window

Lobe

Internal Auditory Tube (Eustachian)

Mastoid Process

Facial Nerve
Styloid Process

Tympanic Membrane (Eardrum)

Internal Carotid Artery
Internal Jugular Vein

Index